To *Ganesha*
God of Beginnings,
Remover of Obstacles.
By His grace
All is done.

To my parents and extended family for
developing and strengthening the foundations of my internal lodestone
and awakening my intellectual curiosity.
Also to my wife, Manashi, for her generous kindness,
extraordinary patience and loving support.

Arun Shanbhag

To Brad, for your strength of character, maturity and humor.
Best wishes for success, personal and collegiate;
Steven, for your intellect, integrity and endless potential,
may you leverage these resources in life;
and Kristin, for your insight, determination and courage
as you have endured recent personal challenges.
As always, along with my wife, Kimberly,
they are the beginning, middle and continuation of my joy.

Harry E. Rubash

To my son Ross, whose inquisitiveness and passion are a source of motivation.
To my son Max, whose spirit and joie de vivre are a source of inspiration.
To my daughter Eve,
whose grace and poise are a source of pride;
and To my wife Faye,
whose support and love make it all worthwhile.

Joshua J. Jacobs

Joint Replacement and Bone Resorption

Joint Replacement and Bone Resorption

Pathology, Biomaterials, and Clinical Practice

Edited by

Arun Shanbhag

*Massachusetts General Hospital
Harvard Medical School
Boston, Massachusetts, U.S.A.*

Harry E. Rubash

*Massachusetts General Hospital
Harvard Medical School
Boston, Massachusetts, U.S.A.*

Joshua J. Jacobs

*Rush University Medical Center
Chicago, Illinois, U.S.A.*

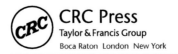

CRC Press
Taylor & Francis Group
Boca Raton London New York

CRC Press is an imprint of the
Taylor & Francis Group, an **informa** business

CRC Press
Taylor & Francis Group
6000 Broken Sound Parkway NW, Suite 300
Boca Raton, FL 33487-2742

First issued in paperback 2019

© 2006 by Taylor & Francis Group, LLC
CRC Press is an imprint of Taylor & Francis Group, an Informa business

No claim to original U.S. Government works

ISBN-13: 978-0-8247-2954-7 (hbk)
ISBN-13: 978-0-367-39180-5 (pbk)

Library of Congress Cataloging-in-Publication Data

Catalog record is available from the Library of Congress

**Visit the Taylor & Francis Web site at
http://www.taylorandfrancis.com**

**and the CRC Press Web site at
http://www.crcpress.com**

Foreword

Total joint replacement is an extraordinary success story. Over the last four decades, millions of patients have been able to return to active lifestyles with lasting relief of pain and persisting superior functional results. As a result of the efforts of numerous talented investigators, many of the issues responsible for failure have been addressed and resolved. However, osteolysis secondary to the periprosthetic tissue response to the presence of particulate wear debris has been one of the main causes of long-term failure and is a problem that persists to the present.

This book represents a timely contribution to literature on the subject. It represents an exhaustive review of the different facets of this condition written by those who have made important contributions. The clinical presentation, basic science issues, the pathobiology, the solutions and treatments, and the future perspectives are discussed in different chapters.

The recent introduction of wear-resistant surfaces is bound to change the clinical picture of osteolysis with the promise of a dramatic reduction in its incidence and consequently an improvement in the long-term survivorship of joint replacements. A drastic reduction in the wear rate should result in a corresponding reduction in the rate of occurrence of osteolysis. However, it is important not to be complacent about this subject and to take a realistic view of potential future events.

As recently reported, the revision burden for total hip arthroplasty in the United States is around 18% with a yearly incidence, in 2002, of about 12%. These rates are not decreasing with time. It is interesting to postulate about the reason for differences in failure incidence in the population at large and reports from individual centers where the failure incidence is typically substantially less than 10%. Surgical experience, surgical skills, and patient selection criteria are some of the variables that may play a role. Osteolysis must represent a substantial fraction of those failures. It is a late appearing phenomenon; in our experience the mean time of presentation was over 10 years following implantation. Furthermore, the rate of osteolysis increases as a function of time. The corollary is that there is a substantial population at risk, probably in the millions. Given that the widespread introduction of wear-resistant surfaces is only recent, those numbers at risk are bound to remain unchanged for quite a number of years. In addition, the use of wear-resistant surfaces has its own limitations and potential sources of failure. For example, acetabular orientation is a variable capable of changing the wear-resistant properties of the articular couple in a dramatic manner. This is true for hard-on-hard bearings and for highly cross-linked polyethylene as well. While acetabular orientation is a simple issue in the hands of the experienced surgeon, it can become a source of problems in the hands of the surgeon who performs limited numbers of surgeries (a frequent event in the United States), or with the use of minimally invasive techniques.

While polyethylene wear particles generated at the joint surface represent the bulk of the debris responsible for the cases of osteolysis seen today, there are other sources of particulate debris capable of producing a similar phenomenon. Corrosion products and particles generated due to impingement have all been implicated in the past. New prosthetic designs are being introduced with increasing degrees of modularity and the potential occurrence of long-term problems at these modular junctions cannot be totally ruled out. Thus, although the future looks promising with the potential for a drastic reduction in the occurrence of osteolysis, we are bound to see persisting problems of this nature in the foreseeable future.

The information assembled in this book will be invaluable for the orthopaedic surgeon and for the basic scientist and will continue to be a reference source for many years to come.

Jorge O. Galante, MD
Chicago, IL

Foreword

Peri-implant bone loss, variously termed "cement disease," "small particle disease," or osteolysis, represents one of the greatest solved puzzles of 20th century medicine. First observed by Sir John Charnley nearly 50 years ago, characterized pathologically by Prof. Hans Willert in the 1970s and increasingly understood on a cellular and molecular level (beginning with the landmark 1980s studies of Dr. Steven Goldring and colleagues) osteolysis—the inability of healthy bone to harmoniously co-exist with biomaterials particulates and degradation products—is now well on the way to becoming a rare clinical observation. From a 100% incidence in Charnley's otherwise successful first several hundred cases of total hip replacement (THR) arthroplasty, osteolysis—as a primary cause of surgical revision—has declined to a general prevalence of not more than 1 per year in every 300 contemporary total joint replacements, with reliable published reports of large clinical series well exceeding 10 years' minimum follow-up with no osteolytic failure of one or both major components of particular designs.

This has not been an easy victory. The splendid group of editors and authors of this work well represent the major contributors and their students who have been involved in this long campaign. The studies discussed here show the current level of understanding of the etiology, the biology, and the necessary clinical responses to osteolysis as well as summarizing earlier views and evidence. While some of the modern innovators in total joint replacement arthroplasty are no longer with us, those remaining must take great satisfaction in seeing this primary barrier to overcome their clinical aspirations.

In 1995, I undertook a study to estimate the incidence and prevalence of revision of THR arthroplasty in the United States. Despite the problem of obtaining reliable clinical data in a setting with no national databases, I reached several conclusions.[a] Although revision surgery represented about 18% of the clinical burden of THR arthroplasty, such procedures were probably <1.6% per year of the implanted total and that percentage had been declining steadily for the past five years. Furthermore, sometime in the early '90s, the number of patients reaching life's end each year with successfully functioning devices began to exceed the annual number of revisions and the curves were continuing to diverge. Only about 60% of those revisions could be ascribed primarily to osteolysis and its resulting clinical symptoms of pain and instability. Comparison with European databases suggested an even better experience for THRs and significantly lower incidences for total knee replacement.

Since then, all indications are that the situation has further improved. Various US national estimates now report that annual revision rates for all causes of <0.25% per year were achieved in the past decade in individual series and 0.5–1% per year in global, "all comers" populations. One need only to consider the improvements in fabrication and processing of polyethylene and the reintroduction of ceramic/ceramic bearing systems to conclude that contemporary THR recipients will experience both significantly lower annual and total doses of small particles than these patients, let alone the pioneers of 30–50 years ago.

Although it has been said that history cannot be written until all involved have been dead for 50 years, this work may prove to be a happy exception. Research continues and further elucidation will be gained, but I believe that this effort represents a mere tidying up and filling in of small blanks. This book may well become the definitive record of a "disease" caused and then essentially eliminated by the progress of medicine.

However, we should not become complacent. Engineering guidelines, both for optimal production, sterilization and storage of biomaterials, and for the design of joint replacement components made from them, are now definable and should be adhered to. Clinical insights pointing out the need for initial component stability, limitation in joint laxity, and exclusion of particles from fixation interfaces, should become more generally appreciated. On a more fundamental level, a focus on individual phenotypic and physiologic differences among patients is needed to further reduce atypical responses. Finally, the largely neglected subject of treatment of osteolysis in situ, by pharmacological and surgical interventions short of revision, should be emphasized.

---

[a] While I presented these results in several settings, they were, unfortunately, not published.

I believe that there are reasons for optimism. If our colleagues and their students can remember the past, we shall not be doomed, as George Santayana reflected, to repeat it. The editors and contributors to this work are to be commended for providing a sturdy and illuminating record to guide us in the times ahead.

Jonathan Black
King of Prussia, PA

Preface

Over the last four decades, investigators around the globe have toiled in clinics, in laboratories, and in operating rooms trying to understand the causes of bone resorption around joint replacements. What is the impact on patients? What is the role of the engineering materials used for joint reconstruction? What are the potential solutions? How do we implement them? What does the future hold for joint replacements? Their findings have been tucked away in tens of thousands of research articles within hundreds of journals. In this volume, an interdisciplinary team of thought leaders from around the world have synthesized the knowledge and compiled it into concise and authoritative chapters.

Periprosthetic bone resorption, or osteolysis, remains an important and common clinical problem and will continue to be so for the foreseeable future. Improvements in implant design and bearing materials have the potential to reduce the prevalence of this phenomenon in modern implant systems introduced since the mid-1990s. Long-term clinical outcomes with newer materials are not yet know. There are also large numbers of patients who have functioning devices that were implanted prior to that era. Furthermore, indications for arthroplasty have expanded and patient demographics have altered dramatically, resulting in recipients placing increasing demands on their artificial joints—they tend to be younger at the time of their surgery, are more active and live longer. These considerations curtail any sense of complacency with regard to the elimination of this pathological bone resorptive process.

This book is separated into five sections. In Section I—Clinical Picture—we have compiled the historical perspective of joint replacement surgery, as well as the early investigations that have shed light on the host tissue reaction to the implanted materials and factors that have been associated with osteolysis, clinical failure, and clinical success. In Section II—Basic Science—we have taken the opportunity to re-acquaint ourselves—the perennial students—with the fundamentals of material science, wear, and the immune response, so that we may better understand the cellular, molecular, and engineering underpinnings of joint replacements and the host response. This should permit us to critically evaluate the progress we have made and the challenges that stand before us. In Section III—Mechanisms of Peri-implant Bone Loss—we have brought together the strongest proponents of various hypotheses for implant loosening and permitted them to make their case. This provides the reader with the opportunity to hear it from "the horse's mouth" without the editorializing of critics and skeptics.

In Section IV—Solutions and Treatments—we asked leading clinicians, engineers, and scientists to summarize the latest developments in biomaterials science and surgical techniques. This section demonstrates the wide range of innovations that have taken root and aims to improve the quality of life of the patients we serve by extending the durability of joint replacements. The trajectory of these innovations gives us hope that joint replacement surgery may mature to the point when reconstruction will routinely last for the lifetime of the patient. In Section V—Future Directions—the contributors take a peek into the future of joint replacements and project how newer technologies could aid our understanding of the pathological processes of cartilage destruction, alter the course of arthritis and related diseases, offer opportunities for medical management and enhance surgical solutions.

This volume is intended as a ready reference to current knowledge in the field, with comprehensive treatment of each topic, written by those at the forefront of laboratory investigations and patient care. This book was written for the orthopaedic surgery resident and fellow, the biomedical engineering graduate student, and the orthopaedic researcher. Practicing clinicians will find a concise summary of the vast field of joint replacement. For those new to this information, this volume will provide a quick "entry" into a dynamic field.

Arun Shanbhag
Harry E. Rubash
Joshua J. Jacobs

Acknowledgments

The editors wish to express their gratitude to many authors and contributors who took time away from their laboratory, clinics, and families to contribute to this book. It is through their efforts that we have been able to compile this authoritative volume. We are also grateful to our students, fellows, and colleagues, whose energy, enthusiasm, and curiosity inspires us to seek and learn the truth. We acknowledge our many teachers and mentors who have guided us in our intellectual and personal pursuits, in particular Jonathan Black, William Harris, and Jorge Galante. We thank the diligent folks at Marcel Dekker, and now Taylor & Francis for agreeing to bring this to a wider audience and publishing it. Finally, we acknowledge the love and support of our families who have made this effort possible and meaningful.

Contents

SECTION II: BASIC SCIENCE

SECTION III: MECHANISMS OF PERI-IMPLANT BONE LOSS

Contributors

Sanjeev Agarwal Department of Orthopaedic Surgery, Massachusetts General Hospital, Harvard Medical School, Boston, Massachusetts, U.S.A.

James M. Anderson Institute of Pathology and Departments of Macromolecular Science and Biomedical Engineering, Case Western Reserve University, Cleveland, Ohio, U.S.A.

Thomas P. Andriacchi Department of Mechanical Engineering, Biomechanical Engineering, Stanford University, Palo Alto, California, U.S.A.

Per Aspenberg Department of Neuroscience and Locomotion, Section for Orthopaedics, Faculty of Health Science, Linköping University, Linköping, Sweden

Anuj Bellare Department of Orthopaedic Surgery, Brigham & Women's Hospital, Harvard Medical School, Boston, Massachusetts, U.S.A.

Richard A. Berger Department of Orthopaedic Surgery, Rush University Medical Center, Chicago, Illinois, U.S.A.

Cheryl R. Blanchard Corporate Research and Clinical Affairs, Zimmer, Inc., Warsaw, Indiana, U.S.A.

J. D. Bobyn Division of Orthopaedics, Montreal General Hospital, McGill University, Montreal, Canada

Stephen Burnett Central Dupage Hospital, Winfield, and Department of Orthopaedic Surgery, Rush University Medical Center, Chicago, Illinois, U.S.A.

David R. Cho New England Baptist Bone and Joint Institute, Rheumatology and Metabolic Bone Division, Beth Israel Deaconess Medical Center, Harvard Medical School, Boston, Massachusetts, U.S.A.

Robert F. Closkey Jr. Department of Biomedical Mechanics and Materials, Hospital for Special Surgery, New York, New York, and Department
of Orthopaedic Surgery, Community Medical Center, Toms River, New Jersey, U.S.A.

Tania N. Crotti New England Baptist Bone and Joint Institute, Beth Israel Deaconess Medical Center, Harvard Medical School, Boston, Massachusetts, U.S.A.

Craig J. Della Valle Department of Orthopaedic Surgery, Rush University Medical Center, Chicago, Illinois, U.S.A.

Daniel M. Estok, II Department of Orthopaedic Surgery, Brigham and Women's Hospital, Harvard Medical School, Boston, Massachusetts, U.S.A.

John Fisher Medical and Biological Engineering, School of Mechanical Engineering, University of Leeds, Leeds, U.K.

Victor Fornasier Department of Pathology, St. Michael's Hospital, University of Toronto, Toronto, Ontario, Canada

Elizabeth A. Fritz Department of Immunology/Microbiology, Rush University Medical Center, Chicago, Illinois, U.S.A.

Jonathan P. Garino Department of Orthopaedic Surgery, Hospital of the University of Pennsylvania, Philadelphia, Pennsylvania, U.S.A.

Grant E. Garrigues Department of Orthopaedic Surgery, Massachusetts General Hospital, Harvard Medical School, Boston, Massachusetts, U.S.A.

Tibor T. Giant Departments of Biochemistry and Orthopaedic Surgery, Rush University Medical Center, Chicago, Illinois, U.S.A.

Jeremy L. Gilbert Department of Bioengineering and Neuroscience, Syracuse University, Syracuse, New York, U.S.A.

A. H. Glassman The Ohio State University College of Medicine, The Halley Orthopaedic Clinic, Columbus, Ohio, U.S.A.

Steven R. Goldring   New England Baptist Bone and Joint Institute, Rheumatology and Metabolic Bone Division, Beth Israel Deaconess Medical Center, Harvard Medical School, Boston, Massachusetts, U.S.A.

Stuart B. Goodman   Department of Orthopaedic Surgery, Stanford University Medical Center, Stanford, California, U.S.A.

Nadim James Hallab   Department of Orthopaedic Surgery, Rush University Medical Center, Chicago, Illinois, U.S.A.

William H. Harris   Department of Orthopaedic Surgery, Orthopaedic Biomechanics and Biomaterials Laboratory, Massachusetts General Hospital, Harvard Medical School, Boston, Massachusetts, U.S.A.

Justin P. Hawes   Department of Orthopaedic Surgery, Hospital of the University of Pennsylvania, Philadelphia, Pennsylvania, U.S.A.

David R. Haynes   Department of Pathology, Adelaide University, South Australia, Australia

Kevin E. Healy   Departments of Bioengineering and Materials Science and Engineering, University of California at Berkeley, Berkeley, California, U.S.A.

Joshua J. Jacobs   Department of Orthopaedic Surgery, Rush University Medical Center, Chicago, Illinois, U.S.A.

Adam M. Kaufman   Department of Orthopaedic Surgery, Massachusetts General Hospital, Harvard Medical School, Boston, Massachusetts, U.S.A.

B. Kinner   Department of Orthopaedic Surgery, Brigham and Women's Hospital, Harvard Medical School, Boston, Massachusetts, U.S.A. and Department of Trauma Surgery, University of Regensburg, Regensburg, Germany

Georg Köster   University of Göttingen, Göttingen, Germany

Robert M. Leven   Department of Anatomy and Cell Biology, Rush University Medical Center, Chicago, Illinois, U.S.A.

John Lyon   Rush University Medical Center, Chicago, Illinois, U.S.A.

Eric L. Martin   Central Dupage Hospital, Winfield, and Department of Orthopaedic Surgery, Rush University Medical Center, Chicago, Illinois, U.S.A.

Dana J. Medlin   Corporate Research and Clinical Affairs, Zimmer, Inc., Warsaw, Indiana, U.S.A.

Calin S. Moucha   Department of Orthopaedic Surgery, Rush University Medical Center, Chicago, Illinois, U.S.A.

Orhun K. Muratoglu   Department of Orthopaedic Surgery, Orthopaedic Biomechanics and Biomaterials Laboratory, Massachusetts General Hospital, Harvard Medical School, Boston, Massachusetts, U.S.A.

Mark J. Neavyn   Department of Orthopaedic Surgery, Massachusetts General Hospital, Harvard Medical School, Boston, Massachusetts, U.S.A.

Wayne Paprosky   Central Dupage Hospital, Winfield, and Department of Orthopaedic Surgery, Rush University Medical Center, Chicago, Illinois, U.S.A.

Lisa A. Pruitt   Department of Mechanical Engineering, University of California at Berkeley, Berkeley, California, U.S.A.

Brian L. Puskas   Department of Orthopaedic Surgery, Massachusetts General Hospital, Harvard Medical School, Boston, Massachusetts, U.S.A.

Kenneth A. Roebuck   Department of Immunology/Microbiology, Rush University Medical Center, Chicago, Illinois, U.S.A.

Aaron Rosenberg   Rush University Medical Center, Chicago, Illinois, U.S.A.

Harry E. Rubash   Department of Orthopaedic Surgery, Massachusetts General Hospital, Harvard Medical School, Boston, Massachusetts, U.S.A.

Thomas P. Schmalzried   Joint Replacement Institute at Orthopaedic Hospital, Los Angeles, California, and Harbor-UCLA Medical Center, Torrance, California, U.S.A.

Rajiv K. Sethi   Department of Orthopaedic Surgery, Massachusetts General Hospital, Harvard Medical School, Boston, Massachusetts, U.S.A.

Arun Shanbhag   Department of Orthopaedic Surgery, Massachusetts General Hospital, Harvard Medical School, Boston, Massachusetts, U.S.A.

Ravi Shetty   Corporate Research and Clinical Affairs, Zimmer, Inc., Warsaw, Indiana, U.S.A.

Mauricio Silva Joint Replacement Institute at Orthopaedic Hospital, Los Angeles, California, and Harbor-UCLA Medical Center, Torrance, California, U.S.A.

M. Spector Department of Orthopaedic Surgery, Brigham and Women's Hospital, Harvard Medical School, VA Boston Healthcare System, Boston, Massachusetts, U.S.A.

Dale R. Sumner Department of Anatomy and Cell Biology, Rush University Medical Center, Chicago, Illinois, U.S.A.

M. Tanzer Division of Orthopaedics, Montreal General Hospital, McGill University, Montreal, Canada

Thomas M. Turner Department of Orthopaedic Surgery, Rush University Medical Center, Chicago, Illinois, U.S.A.

Robert M. Urban Department of Orthopaedic Surgery, Rush University Medical Center, Chicago, Illinois, U.S.A.

Amarjit S. Virdi Department of Anatomy and Cell Biology, Rush University Medical Center, Chicago, Illinois, U.S.A.

Fabian von Knoch Department of Orthopaedic Surgery, Massachusetts General Hospital, Harvard Medical School, Boston, Massachusetts, U.S.A.

Jeffrey Wiley Concord Orthopaedics, Concord, New Hampshire, U.S.A.

Hans Georg Willert University of Göttingen, Göttingen, Germany

Markus A. Wimmer Department of Orthopaedic Surgery, Rush University Medical Center, Chicago, Illinois, U.S.A.

Paul H. Wooley Department of Orthopaedic Surgery, Immunology, and Biomedical Engineering, Wayne State University, Detroit, Michigan, U.S.A.

Timothy M. Wright Department of Biomedical Mechanics and Materials, Hospital for Special Surgery, and Department of Orthopaedics, Weill Medical College of Cornell University, New York, New York, U.S.A.

1

Periprosthetic Osteolysis Around Total Hips and Total Knees

William H. Harris

Department of Orthopaedic Surgery, Orthopaedic Biomechanics and Biomaterials Laboratory, Massachusetts General Hospital, Harvard Medical School, Boston, Massachusetts, U.S.A.

The unraveling of the phenomenon of periprosthetic osteolysis is one of the most remarkable medical detective stories of the last 40 years. Special features of the development of understanding this unprecedented condition with its worldwide importance stem from the fact that it is an entirely new disease. No such disease has been recorded previously in the annals of medicine. It is, moreover, a man-made disease. It is a disease only of the second-half of the 20th century and beyond.

To unravel the identification, understand the mechanism, and develop innovative approaches that have a high probability of eliminating an entire worldwide unique disease constitutes an exciting chapter in the annals of contemporary medicine. Just as the history of the development of total hip replacement in its modern form was biphasic, so too, periprosthetic osteolysis paralleled those changes and showed its human manifestations in a biphasic pattern.

When Charnley (1) made his commitment to the development of an artificial joint, he based the selection of the polymer material for this plastic on metal articulation on the basis of his dominating assumption that he needed an articulation with an extremely low coefficient of friction. He chose polytetrafluorethylene (PTFE). Indeed, its coefficient of friction is exceedingly low. Note also that his initial concept was to develop a mechanical replacement of the arthritic hip joint by using an artificial socket surrounding a metal ball of 41.5 mm in diameter (2). Indeed, his first total hip replacements were of this size.

However, the wear of the PTFE led him to progressively reduce the diameter of the femoral head and increase the thickness of the plastic in an effort to both reduce the amount of wear and increase the duration over which the joint could function despite that wear. It was wear that led him ultimately to select a 22.25 mm femoral head in the development of the low friction arthroplasty (3).

Thus, from the start of total hip replacement surgery using plastic on metal articulations, the central disadvantage was the wear of those plastics available at that time.

From the experience of his first 300 or so consecutive cases of PTFE/ stainless steel total hip replacement operations, two extraordinary observations were made. The first was the exhilarating success of this remarkable and innovative concept of surgically treating arthritis of the hip in terms of the uniformly high level of functional capacity and pain relief that could be created, at least over the short term (4).

The second outstanding observation was the rapid wear of the plastic material and in many cases the appearance of a curious form of granulomatous reaction around the joints, which was often associated with rather pronounced resorption of bone adjacent to the total hip replacement implants (4). This was the first manifestation of this new disease, which we now call periprosthetic osteolysis, a bizarre condition not recognized at that time for what it really was. In his customary thoroughness, diligence, dedication, and creativeness, Charnley identified the granulomatous material and characterized its cellular contents. The tissue was largely fibrous and composed of macrophages (5). Active bone resorption was taking place. But the exact mechanism of this process remained unknown. In fact, Charnley published on cases of periprosthetic osteolysis, but because his early experience contained such a high incidence of deep infection, he felt that some of these cases of periprosthetic bone resorption must be examples of deep infection, even though in these cases he was unable to identify any bacterial organisms (6).

Because of the high incidence of rapid wear of the PTFE, and the high incidence of severe localized bone loss, Charnley abandoned PTFE and searched for a new material.

His extensive in vitro studies of many different polymers led to the introduction of ultra high molecular weight polyethylene (UHMWPE) in November of 1962 (7) and thus, the second phase of metal on plastic total hip replacement surgery was initiated.

Because the in vitro wear resistance of UHMWPE and subsequently the in vivo wear resistance was substantially better than that of PTFE, the issue of wear with its concomitant periprosthetic osteolysis disappeared, at least for a time. The wear rates of UHMWPE were substantially lower and the penetration of the femoral head into the plastic was dramatically retarded compared to the PTFE experience (8).

However, a few worrisome radiographic signs remained unexplained. One of these was the presence of a radiolucent line, perhaps a half-millimeter or a millimeter in thickness, that developed at the interface between the acetabular bone cement and the adjacent bone. While it was clear that this had to represent bone resorption, a multiplicity of theories abounded to explain it, including resorption secondary to stress shielding, excessive stress, toxicity from the methacrylate, low grade infection, osteocyte death secondary to the heat of polymerization of the methacrylate, and other unknown mechanisms. Still, the clinical success of the operation remained so striking that this type of radiographic change, without associated symptoms, did not receive much attention.

About 14 years after the introduction of UHMWPE, new disturbing observations were made, again reflecting rather extensive periprosthetic osteolysis. Willert et al. (9) in 1976 postulated the concept of particulate debris being released from the joint and migrating through the adjacent areas, including behind the acetabular component and into the femur. The same year, without fully understanding the nature of the disease, we published four alarming cases of patients with periprosthetic osteolysis (10). The radiographic appearance of periprosthetic osteolysis looked remarkably similar to a malignant disease form of resorption, either from metastatic malignancy, multiple myeloma, or other primary malignant diseases. Surprisingly, however, the histology of these tissues was not that of a malignant transformation, but rather that of massive amounts of macrophages, some fibrous tissue, some intense osteoclastic activity, and birefringent particles which could be demonstrated under polarized light (10).

In retrospect, there were substantial similarities between the periprosthetic osteolysis generated by the PTFE experience and these cases using the UHMWPE. The differences were that 14 years had passed and the rate of wear of the polyethylene was substantially less than PTFE. The similarity that was most striking, however, was that the mechanism by which this aggressive resorption was taking place remained unexplained.

The next important step in unraveling this condition was identification from our laboratory of the true nature of the so-called "fibrous membrane" associated with the periprosthetic osteolysis (11). Key observations at that time (1983) were that this membrane elaborated prostaglandin E2 (PGE2) and collagenase. We also showed that the membrane had the capacity to resorb bone when placed on the rat calvaria, and this resorptive activity could be partially inhibited by nonsteroidal anti-inflammatory agents.

These pivotal observations initiated detailed study of the biology of this process, leading to dramatic progress in unveiling the complex interactions which caused the increased osteoclastic activity (12). It is now clearly understood that central to this resorptive process is the elaboration of enzymes and cytokines, primarily from the macrophage but also from other cells after ingesting the micron and submicron particulate debris. Ultimately, this inflammatory response to the ingested particle leads to the activation of the osteoclasts, and thus the periprosthetic osteolysis. Because they had not yet been identified, IL-1, IL-6, and tumor necrosis factor alpha and TGF beta and other important factors in this cascade were not identified in our initial report on the PGE2 and collagenase.

Subsequently, extensive work identified the requirement that the particulate debris be, in general, less than 10 μm in size in order to be ingested by the macrophage, and that the bulk of the particulate debris generated in polyethylene on metal total hip replacement operations was micron and submicron particles of UHMWPE.

Thus, the first two central steps in the elaboration of the concept of this unique disease were the identification of the presence of the periprosthetic osteolysis as being a benign, noninfective process and secondly, the establishment of the relationship between the particulate debris, macrophage ingestion of the particles, and the cascade of cellular responses which lead to the activation of the osteoclast (12).

The next important step was an expanded understanding of the magnitude of the problem. Three recent reports provide some prospective on this issue. These are the reports by Clohisy and Harris (13) on the Harris-Galante porous (HGP) femoral stem at 10 years, the report from Capello (14) on the omnifit total replacement prosthesis at 10 years, and that by Engh (15) on the anatomic modullary locking (AML) prosthesis at 10 years. These findings are fortified by the report by Dorr on the anatomic porous replacement (APR) prosthesis at six years (16). These reports all show a striking incidence of periprosthetic osteolysis between 39% and 62%, 10 years after a total hip replacement. While these figures are selected representatives of the high end of incidence for this condition, all types of total hip implants show some level of periprosthetic osteolysis over time.

An additional demonstration from our laboratory on the nature of the radiolucent zone that developed behind the acetabular cement filled in another important aspect of periprosthetic osteolysis. Studies of autopsy-retrieved specimens showed that the thin, slowly progressing radiolucent line behind the cement of cemented acetabular components was, in fact, the same biologic process recognized in the more florid, so-called "balloon" manifestations of massive localized bone loss in the femur or pelvis from periprosthetic osteolysis (17). In other words, the radiolucent line at the cement–bone interface behind the acetabular component results from the progressive ingress of micron and submicron particles of UHMWPE from the articular surface, working their way behind the acetabular component. As they do, they are then ingested by macrophages and the resorptive process is initiated. When the osseous interface between the bone cement and the adjacent pelvis is completely or largely destroyed by this process, the acetabular component generally becomes loose. Thus, in many instances, the loosening of the acetabular component is a reflection also of periprosthetic osteolysis. To give an example of the magnitude of this aspect of periprosthetic osteolysis, consider the report by Schulte et al. (18) of the Charnley implants in the group of patients over 50. At 22 years, the acetabular loosening rate was 37% because of this linear form of periprosthetic osteolysis. Even more striking is the incidence of loose acetabular components in the report by Ballard et al. (19) at 16–22 years following Charnley total hip replacement in patients aged 50 years and younger. Fifty percent of the acetabular components were loose, again largely secondary to this slow linear form of periprosthetic osteolysis.

Similar findings have subsequently been reported for the role of periprosthetic osteolysis in producing femoral component loosening (20).

Consequently, periprosthetic osteolysis is now recognized as a disease of major importance in total hip replacement surgery with plastic on metal bearings. In fact, it is unquestionably the number one long-term complication of this type of surgery (21,22).

Periprosthetic osteolysis has certain particularly important characteristics. Among them are the facts that it increases progressively with time (13,23), is substantially worse around the acetabular component in younger patients (19), substantially worse in the younger than in the older age group (19,20), is accelerated if the component is loose, and can be made substantially worse under circumstances of those conditions that lead to a more rapid rate of wear. Rapid wear, for example, occurs more in males than in females (24), more in the young than the old, more with third body wear than without, and more with ethylene oxide sterilized than in gamma radiated UHMWPE (25). It also occurs more rapidly when conventional UHMWPE is used in conjunction with larger diameters of the femoral head such as surface replacements or 32 mm heads rather than with 22 mm heads (26,27).

It is important to recognize that the relationship of this disease to total knee replacement is substantially different than that in total hip replacement (28). One important reason for this is that in total knee replacement surgery, the oxidative imbrittlement and delamination of the polyethylene is a more common form of failure than is adhesive and abrasive wear. And yet, it is the adhesive and abrasive wear that has the characteristics of being able to generate the submicron particles. The big flakes, which are generally associated with delamination, do not incite the same macrophage response.

Nevertheless, there have been striking examples of periprosthetic osteolysis around total knee replacements, generally associated with implants which had either inferior polyethylene or inferior design such that the adhesive–abrasive wear of the polyethylene was accelerated (29,30). Thus, around total knee replacements, even over longer periods of time, periprosthetic osteolysis is less of a problem than it is around total hip replacements.

However, that does not mean that it is not a substantial factor in the list of long-term complications of total knee replacement as well. Similarly, although relatively small in numbers at this time because the total number of patients involved is small, it is now clear that a similar form of periprosthetic osteolysis occurs around total elbow replacements and total shoulder replacements if they survive long enough to allow this slowly developing biologic response to occur.

The next major advance in unraveling the conundrum of periprosthetic osteolysis was the question of why the particular wear characteristics UHMWPE led to the generation of the massive numbers of such tiny particles. The resolution of this came from the studies which identified the nature of the surface changes associated with gait in total hip replacement patients. The crucial observation was that the surface of the polyethylene becomes deformed in a process called large plastic strain deformation (31–34). The polyethylene surface becomes oriented in the direction of the principal motion, namely flexion and extension. While this process increases the wear resistance in the direction of flexion and extension, the reorientation of the fibers makes the polyethylene surface vulnerable to shear stresses, so that crossing patterns of motion create the particular wear circumstances that leads to the elaboration of the micron and submicron particles. In fact, we studied this phenomenon in the Boston hip simulator with experiments in which simply flexion–extension was introduced, rather than the complex motion associated with flexion and extension, internal and external rotation, and abduction and adduction. Under the flexion–extension motions no measurable wear of conventional polyethylene occurred over seven million gait cycles. However, repeating that very same study, but simply adding crossing motions by adding physiological rotations and abduction–adduction to the path of the femoral head led to wear of 30 mg per million cycles using a 32-mm head, all other conditions being kept identical to the pure flexion–extension experiment (32).

It was this observation that also led to the rejection of all previous unidirectional pin-on-disk data. The amount of wear that occurred under the traditional pin-on-disk testing, which was unidirectional (either reciprocating unidirectional or rotary unidirectional) (35), is substantially less than occurs in vivo in the hip. A more physiologic wear rate is produced by having crossing patterns in the pin-on-disk tester, which we then built into a bidirectional pin-on-disk simulator for screen testing of new materials (36). This type of device both reproduced a rate that was analogous to the wear rate in the hip in vivo and simultaneously confirmed the importance of crossing patterns in the specific wear mechanism of UHMWPE.

The reason that these observations on the mechanism of the surface deformation of polyethylene and their relationship to the generation of the submicron particles are important in the history of periprosthetic osteolysis is that the essential ingredient for overcoming periprosthetic osteolysis is to reduce or eliminate the micron and submicron particles. The specific suggestion that the wear mechanism involved large-scale strain at the surface (31) underlays the concept that cross-linking the polyethylene might be a fruitful approach to reducing particle generation.

In conjunction with Professor Ed Merrill at MIT, we created UHMWPEs that had been heavily cross-linked with electron beam radiation to 9.5 or 10 mrad to reduce wear (37). This material was then melted to eliminate the residual free radicals left behind from the irradiation. We demonstrated in the hip simulator that by doing so we had created an extra-ordinary reduction in particulate debris elaboration and that this dramatic reduction in wear occurred in a material which did not oxidize over time. Similar studies have been carried out using gamma irradiation with subse-quent melt annealing to reduce the incidence of free radicals (38).

Thus, in terms of plastic on metal total hip replacement surgery, a very important feature of the last decade of the 20th century was the elaboration of new forms of UHMWPE with improved wear resistance and improved oxidation resistance (37,38). These materials have the high probability of eliminating or substantially reducing periprosthetic osteolysis.

Concomitantly, other alternative bearing surfaces have been extensively studied that have substantially less wear. Contemporary metal on metal articu-lations substantially reduce the volume of particulate debris generated com-pared to the traditional UHMWPE (39–41). In hip simulator tests, they produce femoral head penetration rates comparable to the highly cross-linked, melted UHMWPE. The particles generated by the metal on metal articulation are an order of magnitude smaller and thus the number of particles produced is large. The long-range importance of this observation remains unknown.

Similarly, ceramic on polyethylene and ceramic on ceramic articula-tions have been followed for two decades (42). In the ceramic on ceramic experience, the volumetric generation of submicron particles is also substan-tially reduced compared to traditional polyethylene, but in simulator tests is comparable to the highly cross-linked polyethylenes. The data also suggests that the ceramic particles that are generated incite less of a macrophage response. A few examples of periprosthetic osteolysis surrounding total hip replacements in which ceramic on ceramic joints have been published (43–45).

Another very exciting aspect of this condition which grew out of the unraveling of the molecular biology of periprosthetic osteolysis is the phar-macological approach to its control. Beginning with the demonstration in dogs that alendronate can inhibit the lytic aspect of the macrophage response to particle debris even though the other cellular responses continue (46), further important possibilities for disrupting the biology of peripros-thetic osteolysis have been postulated including other bisphosphonates, TNFα inhibitors, and the possibility of blocking NFκB. Thus, dual avenues exist to reduce or prevent this disease, first by using better articulating surfaces to markedly decrease or essentially eliminate the particle generation, and secondly, to use the rapidly expanding understanding of molecular biologic pathways to inhibit key point or points in the progress of the cascade and thus reduce or prevent the bone lysis.

Thus, the story of periprosthetic osteolysis is unique at multiple levels. In the first place, this disease has never occurred before in the history of mankind. It is a unique disease precisely because it requires the continuous generation of submicron particles of nonresorbable materials within the body. This requisite debris generation occurs in total hip and total knee implants. Since they were invented in the second half of the 20th century, it follows that it is a disease not known prior to the past 43 years.

It is an extremely important disease because, over time, its incidence can be very high, its consequences can be severe, including loosening of the components, clinical failure because of pain and loss of function, the need for revision operation, and the need for extremely complex techniques to deal with the massive areas of bone loss secondary to the periprosthetic osteolysis.

It is unique also in the sense that the ultimate outcome of this unrestrained ingestion of the submicron particles of the polyethylene by macrophages is the elaboration of an extremely complex cascade of cytokines and enzymes. It is also unique in that the ultimate event generating the osseous pathology is the activation of a single cell type—the osteoclast.

Equally remarkable, perhaps, is the fact that within just over one generation, roughly from the initiation of the expanded understanding of this disease (about 1976 through to the present), the following sequence has occurred. This new disease has become recognized, the cellular mechanism of its occurrence has become identified, the mechanism of the submicron particulate elaboration has been defined, and improvements have been made in available materials for the articulations that have a high probability of either dramatically reducing or completely curing this worldwide disease. In the course of slightly over one generation, a unique, man-made, human disease has been created, identified, understood, and perhaps cured.

REFERENCES

1. Charnley J. Arthroplasty of the hip. A new operation. Lancet 1961; 1: 1129–1132.
2. Charnley J. Surgery for the hip joint. Present and future considerations. Br Med J 1960; 5176:821–826.
3. Charnley J, Kamangar A, Longfield MD. The optimum size of prosthetic heads in relation to the wear of plastic sockets in total replacement of the hip. Med Biol Engng 1969; 7:31–39.
4. Charnley J. Low Friction Arthroplasty of the Hip: Theory and Practice. New York: Springer, 1979:6.
5. Charnley J. Low Friction Arthroplasty of the Hip: Theory and Practice. New York: Springer, 1979:32ff.

6. Charnley J, Follacci F, Hammond B. The long-term reaction of bone to self-curing acrylic cement. J Bone Joint Surg 1968; 50B:822–829.
7. Charnley J. Low Friction Arthroplasty of the Hip: Theory and Practice. New York: Springer, 1979:7.
8. Charnley J, Halley D. Rate of wear in total hip replacement. Clin Orthop 1975; 112:170–179.
9. Willert H. Tissue reactions to plastic and metallic wear products of joint endoprostheses. In: Gschwend N, Debrunner H, eds. Total Hip Prosthesis. Huber: Bern, 1976.
10. Harris WEA. Extensive localized bone resorption in the femur following total hip replacement. J Bone Joint Surg Am 1976; 58:612–618.
11. Goldring S, et al. The synovial-like membrane at the bone–cement interface in loose total hip replacements and its proposed role in bone lysis. J Bone Joint Surg 1983; 65A:575–584.
12. Archibeck MJ, et al. The basic science of periprosthetic osteolysis. AAOS Instructional Course Lectures. San Francisco, 2001; 50:185–195.
13. Clohisy JC, Harris WH. The Harris-Galante uncemented femoral component in primary total hip replacement at 10 years. J Arthroplasty 1999; 14(8): 915–917.
14. Hellman EJ, Capello WN, Feinberg JR. Omnifit cementless total hip arthroplasty. A 10-year average followup. Clin Orthop Relat Res 1999; 364:164–174.
15. Zicat B, Engh C, Gokcen E. Pattern of osteolysis around total hip components inserted with and without cement. J Bone Joint Surg 1995; 77A:432–439.
16. Dorr LD, et al. Failure mechanisms of anatomic porous replacement I cementless total hip replacement. Clin Orthop Relat Res 1997; 334:157–167.
17. Schmalzried TP, et al. The mechanism of loosening of cemented acetabular components in total hip arthroplasty. Analysis of specimens retrieved at autopsy. Clin Orthop Relat Res 1992; 274:60–78.
18. Schulte K, et al. The outcome of Charnley total hip arthroplasty with cement after a minimum twenty-year follow-up. The results of one surgeon [see comments] [published erratum appears in J Bone Joint Surg Am 1993; 75(9): 1418]. J Bone Joint Surg 1993; 75A:961–975.
19. Ballard W, Callaghan J, Sullivan P. Total hip arthroplasty in patients under 50 using contemporary cement techniques. J Bone Joint Surg 1995; 77A: 585–589.
20. Smith SE, Estok DM II, Harris WH. 20-year experience with cemented primary and conversion total hip arthroplasty using so-called second-generation cementing techniques in patients aged 50 years or younger. J Arthroplasty 2000; 15(3):263–273.
21. Harris WH. Wear and periprosthetic osteolysis: the problem. Clin Orthop Rela Res 2001; 393:66–70.
22. Harris W. Osteolysis and particle disease in hip replacement. A review. Acta Orthop Scand 1994; 65:113–123.
23. Huddleston H. Femoral lysis after cemented hip arthroplasty. J Arthroplasty 1988; 3:285–297.
24. Schmalzried T, et al. Quantitative assessment of walking activity after total hip or knee replacement. J Bone Joint Surg Am 1998; 80:54–59.

25. Dowd JE, et al. Characterization of long-term femoral-head-penetration rates. Association with and prediction of osteolysis. J Bone Joint Surg Am 2000; 82-A(8):1102–1107.

26. Kabo JM. In vivo wear of polyethylene acetabular components. J Bone Joint Surg Br 1993; 75(2):254–258.

27. Livermore J. Effect of femoral head size on wear of the polyethylene acetabular component. J Bone Joint Surg 1990; 72(4):518–528.

28. Schmalzried T, et al. Polyethylene wear debris and tissue reactions in knee as compare to hip replacement prostheses. J Appl Biomater 1994; 5:185–190.

29. Engh GA, Parks NL, Ammeen DJ. Tibial osteolysis in cementless total knee arthroplasty. Clin Orthop Relat Res 1994; 309:33–43.

30. Cadambi A, et al. Osteolysis of the distal femur after total knee arthroplasty. J Arthroplasty 1994; 9(6):579–594.

31. Jasty M, et al. Wear of polyethylene acetabular components in total hip arthroplasty: an analysis of 128 components retrieved at autopsy or revision operation. J Bone Joint Surg Am 1997; 79:349–358.

32. Bragdon CR, et al. The importance of multidirectional motion on the wear of polyethylene. Proc Instn Mech Engrs 1995; 210:157–165.

33. Wang A, Polineni VK, Essner A. The significance of nonlinear motion in the wear screening of orthopaedic implant materials. J Test Eval 1997; 25:239.

34. Edidin AA, et al. Plasticity-induced damage layer is a precursor to wear in radiation-cross-linked UHMWPE acetabular components for total hip replacements. J Arthroplasty 1999; 14(5):616–627.

35. Rostoker W, Galante J. Some new studies of the wear behavior of ultrahigh molecular weight polyethylene. J Biomed Mater Res 1976; 10:303–310.

36. Bragdon CR, et al. A new pin-on-disk wear testing method for simulating wear of polyethylene on cobalt-chrome alloy in total hip arthroplasty. J Arthroplasty 2001; 16(5):658–665.

37. Muratoglu OK, et al. A novel method of crosslinking UHMWPE to improve wear, reduce oxidation and retain mechanical properties. J Arthroplasty 2001; 16(2):149–160.

38. McKellop H, et al. Development of an extremely wear-resistant ultra high molecular weight polyethylene for total hip replacements. J Orthop Res 1999; 17(2):157–167.

39. Schmidt M, Weber H, Schon R. Cobalt chromium molybdenum metal combination for modular hipprostheses. Clin Orthop Relat Res 1996; 329S:S35–S47.

40. Dorr LD, et al. Total hip arthroplasty with use of the Metasul metal-on-metal articulation. Four to seven-year results. J Bone Joint Surg Am Vol 2000; 82(6):789–798.

41. Schmalzried T, et al. Long-duration metal-on-metal total hip arthroplasties with low wear of the articulating surfaces. J Arthroplasty 1996; 11:322–331.

42. Hamadouche M, et al. Alumina-on-alumina total hip arthroplasty. J Bone Joint Surg Am 2002; 84A(1):69–77.

43. Shih C, et al. Localized femoral osteolysis in cementless ceramic total hip arthroplasty. Orthop Rev 1994; 23:325–328.

44. Wirganowicz P, Thomas B. Massive osteolysis after ceramic on ceramic total hip arthroplasty. A case report. Clin Orthop 1997; 338:100–104.

45. Yoon T, et al. Osteolysis in association with a total hip arthroplasty with ceramic bearing surfaces. J Bone Joint Surgery Am 1998; 80:1459–1468.
46. Shanbhag AS, Hasselman CT, Rubash HE. The John Charnley Award. Inhibition of wear debris mediated osteolysis in a canine total hip arthroplasty model. Clin Orthop Relat Res 1997; 344:33–43.

2

Fixation of Implants

Calin S. Moucha, Robert M. Urban, Thomas M. Turner, and Joshua J. Jacobs

Department of Orthopaedic Surgery, Rush University Medical Center, Chicago, Illinois, U.S.A.

Dale R. Sumner

Department of Anatomy and Cell Biology, Rush University Medical Center, Chicago, Illinois, U.S.A.

INTRODUCTION

Most clinicians and researchers in the field of implant fixation would probably agree that long-term success of an arthroplasty depends upon firm fixation of the implant to the host skeleton. Although no precise definition of "firm fixation"exists, conceptually, one may identify two critical phases: establishment and maintenance of fixation. The importance of each of these two phases may vary considerably depending upon whether implant stabilization is achieved mechanically or biologically.

Mechanical fixation of prosthetic implants is most commonly achieved using bone cement. Since the first uses of bone cement for this purpose (51,96), the properties of cements, implants, and techniques have improved dramatically (12,34,173,188). Modern cementation of endoprostheses is considered in detail elsewhere in the present volume. Here we describe the basic biology of cementless fixation.

DEFINITIONS

Biological fixation of implants occurs through osseointegration and bone ingrowth. Originally used to describe the phenomenon of vital bone tissue in contact with a metallic implant, the term osseointegration was later refined to mean a "direct structural and functional connection between ordered, living bone and the surface of a load-carrying implant" (30–32). Osseointegrated implants often have a soft-tissue layer at the implant-bone interface (1,61,64), and bone, bonded either physically and/or chemically to the surface, may or may not grow into the implant. Bone ingrowth, on the other hand, refers to new bone formation (known as osteogenesis) directly into the porous structure of an implant (227). The main focus of this chapter will be on bone ingrowth.

BONE INGROWTH AND FRACTURE HEALING

Bone ingrowth resembles fracture healing as both are well-orchestrated biological sequences involving the coordinated participation of several cell types (227). Similar to fracture healing, during which the local mechanical environment has a great impact on the type of ossification that leads to bone regeneration (49,241), a particular implant's initial stability is critical to its ultimate clinical outcome. An implant placed in a mechanically stable environment achieves final bone ingrowth through the same three phases that occur in fracture healing: inflammatory, reparative, and remodeling (88). After the initial inflammatory response, reparative woven bone is seen histologically at one to two weeks after implantation, followed by remodeling of lamellar bone by four weeks (Fig. 1). Under stable conditions, bone found in well-ingrown prostheses is intramembranous and not endochondral in origin. As evidenced by the lack type II and type X collagen synthesis, no cartilaginous anlage is ever present (35).

SURGICALLY INDUCED INJURY AND THE BIOLOGICAL RESPONSE

Much of the focus in cementless joint replacements has been on establishing the initial mechanical connection between the host bone and the implant. This is very different from cemented arthroplasties, where the main concern is often with intermediate-term and long-term failure (i.e., maintenance), especially of the acetabular component (89,126,208,216,264). Whereas in most instances of fracture healing an external callus first stabilizes the fracture site (165), this is not the case during prosthetic bone ingrowth in which early biologic stability occurs through a medullary "callus" (227). Assuming intact metaphyseal arteries and a stable surgically created mechanical environment (120), this medullary "callus" stabilizes the implant while intramembranous ossification occurs.

(A)

(B)

(C)

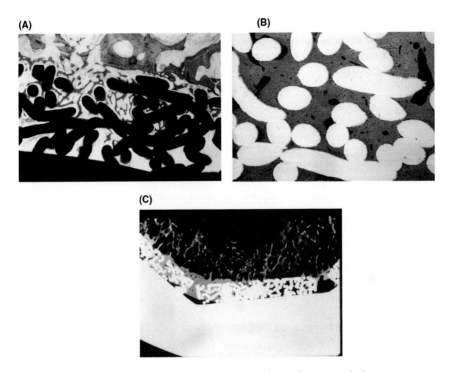

Figure 1 Images of bone ingrowth. (**A**) A section of an acetabular component retrieved postmortem after one month shows slender trabeculae of woven bone at the interface with the host bone and within the porous coating (undecalcified, ground section stained with basic fuschsin and toluidine blue). (**B**) A section from a well-fixed femoral hip stem revised after 26 months for distal endosteal osteolysis demonstrates dense haversian bone within the porous coating (backscattered-electron scanning electron micrograph). (**C**) A sagittal section of a total knee replacement femoral component revised after 37 months for failure of the patellar component reveals dense condensation of bone within the porous coating and at the interface between the porous coating and cancellous host bone of the femoral condyle (high-resolution contact radiograph of undecalcified section).

The initial surgical insult, in fact, stimulates mesenchymal stem cells residing within the marrow or along the endosteal surface of the bone to differentiate into osteoblasts. Even after reaming of the medullary cavity, the adult skeleton has considerable capacity to repair via an internal callus (193–195). The molecular biology of intramembranous bone formation in response to skeletal injury has been studied in several animal models (213,234,238). Following ablation of the rat tibial diaphysis, for example, there is a rapid increase in osteoblast cell density, and expression of the alkaline phosphatase, procollagen $\alpha 1$ (I) and osteopontin genes. Slightly later, osteocalcin and collagenase gene expression peaks. Consistent with previous

histologic observations that bone formation in this context is intramembranous, the type II collagen gene is never expressed (35). Woven bone is
present within a few days in rats and within one week in canines and
humans. This local microenvironment appears to be controlled by several
growth factors acting in an autocrine manner, including members of the
TGF-β superfamily and their receptors, as well as numerous other growth
factors and cytokines discussed in more detail elsewhere in this book.

Several investigators have also studied the organized interaction of cells
with various biomaterials (87,95,172,209,259). Frosch et al. (87) described the
growth, mineralization, and bone formation patterns of osteoblast-like cells in
titanium pore channels. Using porous titanium implants inserted into human
osteoblast-like cell cultures, they characterized three distinct cellular migration
and reorganization stages. During stage I, osteoblast precursor cells adhered to
the wall of the pores and migrated three-dimensionally into these channels by
forming foot-like protoplasmic processes. Stage II was notable for osteoblast-
like cell anchorage on the substrate wall by matrix proteins and the build-up
of a dense network of matrix proteins in the pores. Stage III consisted of
mineralization, during which the network of extracellular matrix proteins
and osteoblast-like cells began to form an osteon-like structure.

The differential responses of osteoblastic cells to titanium Ti–6A1–4V,
cobalt–chrome–molybdenum, hydroxyapatite ceramic, and ultra-high-
molecular-weight polyethylene have been described by several research
groups. Using a human bone marrow cell culture system, Wilke et al. (259)
showed differences in cell proliferation, cell differentiation, and production
of extracellular matrix when various substrates were compared. Hydroxyapatite, for instance, led to the highest level of cell proliferation. While titanium
samples exhibited the most B-cell and granulocyte proliferation, there did not
appear to be differences between the various materials with regard to T-cell
and monocyte proliferation. Shah et al. (209) more recently performed a
detailed morphometric analysis of human osteoblastic cell adhesion to the
titanium alloy Ti6A14V and cobalt–chrome–molybdenum. The kinetic profile
of adhesion was consistent with enhanced cell attachment upon rough titanium surfaces relative to rough cobalt–chrome–molybdenum. Focal adhesion
contacts, as indicated by vinculin immunostaining, were distributed throughout the cells adhering to titanium, but were relatively sparse and localized to
cellular processes on cobalt–chrome–molybdenum. Three-dimensional laser
scanning microscopy reconstruction analysis indicated the presence of vinculin at all membrane-to-surface contact points on both titanium and cobalt–
chrome. On titanium, these contact points closely followed the surface
contour, whereas, on cobalt–chrome, they were restricted to relative topographic peaks only. Actin cytoskeletal reorganization was prominent in cells
cultured on titanium, with stress fibers arranged throughout the cell body;
cobalt–chrome specimens, on the other hand, exhibited actin filaments that
were sparse and localized primarily to cellular extensions.

It is well accepted that osteoblasts (and osteocytes) interact with extracellular matrix proteins such as collagen types I and II, collagen fibers, osteopontin, osteonectin, fibronectin, fibrinogen, thrombospondin, and laminin (1). Both integrin and nonintegrin adhesion receptors mediate these interactions (201) via specific cell-binding domains (184,266). The connection between the bone matrix and the cytoskeleton appears to be a critical modality by which extracellular signals get transduced into intracellular messages (90). Differences between various biomaterials clearly exist with regard to the distribution of matrix proteins. Differential responses of osteoblasts to various substrates have also been demonstrated. As functional implications are the end-result of such pathways, further research in this arena using standardized models needs to be performed.

IMPLANT STABILITY AND MICROMOTION

Advancements in implant design (8), surgical technique (99) and patient selection have focused in part on providing adequate initial physical support for biologic fixation to occur. It is well accepted that relative motion between the implant and host bone influences the type of tissue that develops within a porous surface. This relationship, however, is poorly understood. Pilliar et al. (186) showed that relative displacement of less than 28 μm leads to bone ingrowth and that motion greater than 150 μm results in fixation provided solely by mature connective tissue (186). Micromotion has been studied extensively in several knee arthroplasty animal and human retrieval investigations (33,211,221,229,247). An animal study by Turner et al. (247) in particular confirmed that regions with relatively minimal micromotion (within a 1- to 3-mm radius around a tibial implant's peg) showed consistent bone ingrowth whereas other areas had a highly variable amount of ingrowth (Fig. 2). Subsequent human retrieval analyses confirmed these findings (229).

Results from roentgenstereometric (RSA) in vivo studies do raise some concern over the relatively high degree of micromotion that may be present in a variety of implants (121,122,176). As RSA techniques of measuring micromotion are being perfected (177), these types of studies, in conjunction with retrieval data, are expected to contribute greatly to our current knowledge on this important topic.

The role of initial stability on bone ingrowth also cannot be ignored when contemplating postoperative rehabilitation protocols. Heck et al. (102), using a canine model, studied the effect of overloading and underloading on tissue ingrowth into a porous-coated titanium segmental femoral prosthesis. The study concluded that reduced loading immediately following surgery improved the interfacial shear strength of the implants. Although studies in this arena are lacking, a recent human investigation concluded that when solid initial fixation is obtained intraoperatively using a fully

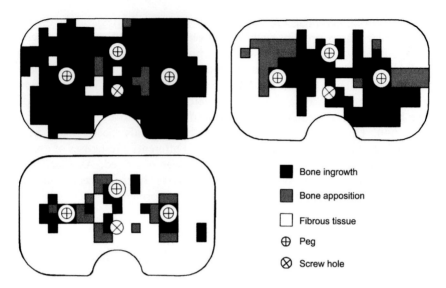

Figure 2 Distribution of bone ingrowth in a canine model. In the tibial component of cementless porous coated knee replacements, areas with relatively minimal micromotion (within a 1- to 3-mm radius around the tibial implant pegs) consistently achieve bone ingrowth, whereas other areas have highly variable amounts of bone ingrowth. Topographic distribution of bone in experimental canine tibial components (*clockwise from upper left*): 81.1% bone ingrowth and 3.7% appositional bone, 31.5% bone ingrowth and 10.8% appositional bone, and 12.0% bone ingrowth and 7.5% appositional bone. *Source*: From Ref. 247.

porous-coated femoral component and postoperative radiographs confirm appropriate canal fit, biological fixation occurs whether or not a partial or full weight-bearing postoperative protocol is followed (263). The type of loading, however, may be as critical as the amount (38). Novel methods of studying the effect of loading on micromotion have recently been proposed (94).

PORE SIZE

Several investigators have studied the relationship between pore size and bone ingrowth. For pore sizes less than 100 μm, increasing pore size has been shown to increase the strength of fixation (197,257). For pore sizes between 150 μm and 400 μm, pore size does not appear to affect the strength of fixation (26,62,144). Within this range of pore sizes, only one study has concluded that increasing pore size was associated with decreasing bone ingrowth and strength of fixation (54). Pore sizes greater than 400 μm have been shown to have lower strength of fixation than implants with pores in the 50–400 μm range (26). Within the generally accepted "optimal pore size range" of 100–400 μm, quantitative studies of bone ingrowth have shown differences between femoral and acetabular components. Turner et al. (245), using a canine model, compared bone ingrowth in fiber metal-coated (mean pore size 247 μm) and bead-coated (mean pore size 297 μm) femoral components, and reported more ingrowth in the fiber group than in the bead group (37.3% vs. 25.2%). Jasty et al. (119), reporting on porous coated canine acetabular components, found more bone ingrowth, as measured by backscattered scanning electron microscopy, within implants with 450 μm and 200 μm pores than in implants with 140 μm pores. These differences may be attributed in part to variability in the type of bone that an acetabular component is placed adjacent to (vascular, subchondral cancellous bone) as compared to a femoral component (relatively avascular, cortical bone). Methodological differences by which bone ingrowth was measured in these studies also accounts for some of the discrepancies. A more recent study challenges the traditional belief that the amount of new bone is even dependent on pore size (112). Possibly substantiating this more recent report, a material relatively new to the field of joint arthroplasty, tantalum, has also been shown to have bone ingrowth relatively independent of pore size (28). More investigations on the optimal pore size for bone ingrowth are warranted both for time-tested materials as well as for newer ones.

INTERFACE GAPS

Although initial bone apposition of a porous-surfaced implant is desirable, it is not always achieved surgically. Bone ingrowth is diminished when more than a critical distance is present between a porous surface and the host bone. Several investigators have studied this distance, often referred to as the interface gap. Both non-weight-bearing and weight-bearing models with a controlled gap and a stable implant have confirmed the inhibitory effect of an interface gap on bone ingrowth (27,45,65,98,202,205).

Sandborn et al. (205), using an adult dog model, surgically placed implants in the intramedullary canals of adult dogs producing uniform gap spaces 0.0–2.0 mm wide. After 3, 6, and 12 weeks in situ, histologic and microradiographic evaluations were performed. The results demonstrated that the initial apposition of a porous implant to the surrounding bone surface is not necessary for fixation by bone ingrowth. New bone grew up to and within the porous structure of an implant even when there was a gap as large as 2.0 mm. The rate and degree of maturity and mineralization, however, was enhanced when the gap width was 0.5 mm or less. A more recent study (65) also used skeletally mature adult mongrel dogs to examine interface gaps of 0.0, 0.5, 1.0, and 2.0 mm in implants treated or untreated with hydroxyapatite. Histological sections were prepared, and the amount of bone within the porous structure and the amount of the original gap that was filled with new bone were quantified with a computerized video image-analysis system. Both mechanical attachment strength as well as bone ingrowth were found to increase with the time after implantation and with a decrease in the size of the gap. Placement of the implant in proximal (cancellous) compared with distal (cortical) locations had no significant effect on the strength of attachment, bone ingrowth, or the filling of gaps. Implants with a large initial gap (1.0 or 2.0 mm), however, demonstrated greater attachment strength in cancellous bone than in cortical bone. With a few exceptions, hydroxyapatite-coated implants with an initial gap of 1.0 mm or less demonstrated significantly increased mechanical attachment strength and bone ingrowth at all time periods. Interface attachment strengths were positively correlated with bone ingrowth, the time after implantation, the use of a hydroxyapatite coating, and decreasing initial gap size.

The conclusion drawn from these investigations is that initial implant-bone apposition is a prerequisite for good biological fixation. Based mostly on animal models that mimic an optimal situation, it appears that bone ingrowth does not occur across a nongrafted 2 mm gap with regularity. Implant design, instrumentation, operative technique, and host bone status may individually or collectively result in an increased interface distance and a suboptimal environment for ingrowth.

Numerous reports of using various grafting materials to improve bone ingrowth can be found in the literature (65,67,107,116,130,143,146,147, 164,202,207,212,248). Most of these are either osteoconductive and/or osteogenic. Allogeneic bone and porous ceramics such as hydroxyapatite and tricalcium phosphate, serving as a "scaffold" for bone ingrowth, are considered osteoconductive. Autologous bone, on the other hand, is both osteoconductive and osteogenic (bone producing). Whereas bone ingrowth into porous structures leads to the formation of a microinterlock, host bone interaction with these grafts results in a chemical bond (115–117). In the presence of a mechanically stable implant compromised by interface gaps, these grafts act as effective facilitators of bone ingrowth into the porous structure of various prostheses. Because of the limited availability of allograft bone and the significant morbidity associated with harvesting autologous bone (138,267), however, much attention has recently been given to bone graft substitutes. Some of these substances promote mitogenesis of undifferentiated mesenchymal cells, leading to formation of osteoprogenitor cells that have osteogenic capacity, a process known as osteoinduction (250). Enhancing bone ingrowth using bone graft substitutes is discussed in a later section of this volume.

FACTORS KNOWN TO INHIBIT CEMENTLESS FIXATION

Increased gap interfaces, certain pore size ranges, and "excessive" motion have already been discussed as having potential detrimental effects on cementless fixation. Other local and systemic factors have also been reported to lead to inhibition on bone ingrowth. Irradiation starting above the

500–1000 rad range has been shown by several animal and human investigations to correlate with poor bone ingrowth potential (53,114,231,262). Recommendations for radiation dosing used for heterotopic ossification prophylaxis should be based in part on these studies. Additionally, as the number of patients surviving pelvic cancers treated with irradiation is increasing, so do the number of joint replacements done on these patients. In planning for the type of reconstruction to be performed, therefore, it is critical for the clinician to obtain a detailed history of the type and dose of radiation administered. If faced with an avascular acetabular bone bed, one must be prepared to implant a prosthesis that relies on mechanical rather than biological fixation.

Other factors that have been reported to inhibit ingrowth are medications that patients receiving joint arthroplasties may be taking perioperatively, including disodium (1-hydroxythylidene) diphosphonate (135), warfarin (42), warfarin sodium (coumadin) (149), cisplatin (149), and methotrexate (149). Cook et al. (58) have shown that perioperative administration of indomethacin does not significantly affect attachment strength or bone ingrowth into porous-coated implants except at early periods, in which cases a transient decrease in attachment strength occurs. Other authors also found this inhibitory effect of indomethacin, and also reported on similar effects of ibuprofen, and high-dose aspirin (243). In a more recent study, Goodman et al. (92), using a rabbit model, showed that Rofecoxib, a specific cyclooxygenase–2 inhibitor, decreased the area of osteoblasts per section area ($p = 0.014$) compared to controls.

In conclusion, any factor that inhibits fracture healing should be assumed to have a similar detrimental effect on bone ingrowth during cementless fixation. Aside from the factors discussed above, systemic statuses of the patient such as nutritional status (73), anemia (200), diabetes mellitus (151,163), and certain hormone deficiencies (254) have all been shown to have an inhibitory effect on fracture healing, and therefore may have similar effects on bone ingrowth.

CLINICAL BEHAVIOR OF CEMENTLESS FIXATION

It is beyond the scope of this text to provide a comprehensive review of the mammoth volume of literature on the clinical results of cementless joint arthroplasty. It is important, however, to give an overview of some clinical studies that have provided input into the basic science of bone ingrowth.

Primary Cementless Hip Arthroplasty

Cementless primary joint arthroplasty has been performed for almost 20 years, with encouraging clinical data available for several designs. Cylindrical stems, such as the fully porous-coated anatomic medullary locking (AML) femoral prosthesis (DePuy, Warsaw, Indiana), have demonstrated excellent long-term results (131,132,137,160). Other cylindrical designs, such as the Harris–Galante (Zimmer, Warsaw, Indiana) and anatomic porous replacement (APR)-1 (Intermedics Orthopaedics, Austin, Texas), have not possessed the same clinical success due to relatively high loosening and osteolysis (56,66,72,155). Anatomic stems, such as the porous-coated anatomic (PCA) stem (Howmedica, Rutherford, New Jersey), have demonstrated varying degrees of success, with some reports showing an increased loosening rate and a higher incidence of thigh pain compared with the cylindrical AML stems (46,97,157). Tapered stems, such as the Taperloc (Biomet, Warsaw, Indiana), Tri-Lock (DePuy, Warsaw, Indiana), and Zweymuller (Allopro, Bern, Switzerland) appear to demonstrate excellent clinical results as well. A variety of studies have shown that tapered stems can achieve predictable ingrowth with a relatively low incidence of thigh pain (40,69,110,111, 166,167,204). Clinical results (74) have confirmed autopsy study observations (249) that a proximal circumferential ingrowth capability on an implant is important for prevention of polyethylene debris entry into the medullary canal that can result in distal osteolysis. Engh et al. (79) reported a stem survival of 97% in patients with the circumferentially coated AML prosthesis at a mean follow-up of 11 years. As previously discussed, initial stability is thought to be critical to bony ingrowth (186). Early subsidence with a tapered prosthesis, however, has not necessarily been correlated with poor results (110,265). Interestingly, a canine study (52) investigating the effect of collarless versus collared prostheses showed no differences in subsidence, although the collarless prostheses had significantly greater bone ingrowth proximally ($p = 0.003$), lower cortical porosity ($p = 0.006$), and less proximal-medial radiolucency ($p = 0.03$). Overall clinical experience with newer implant designs of uncemented femoral stems continues to improve. A recent study (8) of second-generation cementless femoral components designed to provide more reliable ingrowth and to limit distal osteolysis by incorporating circumferential proximal ingrowth surfaces showed a 5% incidence of osteolysis proximal to the lesser trochanter and no evidence of osteolysis distal to it. The mean preoperative Harris hip score of 51 points improved to 94 points at the time of final follow-up and the overall survival of the femoral component at 10 years was 100%.

Although early and intermediate results of cemented all-polyethylene acetabular components have been excellent (191), long-term follow-up of this type of acetabular fixation has been more disappointing (124,152,208, 214,216,219,264). Cementation of metal-backed shells has proven to result in even worse short- (196) and long-term results (216). Although some of these poor results may be due to variability in interpreting radiographic signs suggestive of loosening (103,216), based on trends seen in the aforementioned studies, the rates of revision for cemented acetabular components certainly appears to be increasing. By using implants that rely on biological fixation, numerous attempts have been made at improving the results of cemented sockets. Nonporous coated threaded acetabular implants that relied on mechanical interlocking between the acetabular bone and the threads led to extremely high-failure rates (36,47,76,136,168,242). This was due, in part, to little surface area in contact with host bone and suboptimal ingrowth surface area. Porous coating or grit-blasting these types of shells helped improve performance somewhat (2,48,190). A recent study reported excellent early success of a hydroxyapatite-coated threaded component (84); interestingly, hydroxyapatite-coated smooth shells have resulted in quite poor results (48,84,156). While porous cups treated with hydroxylapatite and tricalcium phosphate led to early clinical results comparable to the non-coated porous cups (240), radiostereometric analysis of these cups revealed less tilting and diminishing radiolucencies in the treated group as compared to the controls. Porous-coated cementless acetabular components have fared well at mean follow-ups of 5–12 years, with revision rates generally being under 15% (8,55,78,101,131,133,134,153,178,206,215). Differences in success are quite obvious between these implants. The Harris-Galante-1 (Zimmer, Warsaw, Indiana) and the Acetabular Reconstruction Component (Howmedica, Rutherford, New Jersey) shells have been shown to have revision rates below 5%, while the PCA (Howmedica, Rutherford, New Jersey) components have led to revision rates approaching 15%. The AML system (DePuy, Warsaw, Indiana) has been reported to have a revision rate for loosening as low as 0.4% and as high as 15% (78,132). Differences between these components are related to many variables, including such things as the routine use of 32-mm heads and thin acetabular liners with some of the AML and PCA designs. Early- and intermediate-term revision rates appear to be comparable to those of cemented all polyethylene components. At 9–12 years, however, matched-pair analysis of cemented and cementless acetabular reconstructions in primary total hip arthroplasty showed that cementless cups had significantly lower rates of radiographic loosening (0% versus 30%) and osteolysis (7% versus 20%) as compared to cemented cups (57). Clinically, both types of fixation led to excellent results.

Primary Cementless Knee Arthroplasty

Cementless fixation of total knee replacements is much less commonplace than cemented fixation. Part of the lack of enthusiasm by many surgeons to perform such procedures may be related to the historically poor results of cementless metal-backed patellas (6,10,11,150,187,198,222). Due in part to improved instrumentation, component design, and a better understanding of knee joint biomechanics, several surgeons have reported more encouraging results of cementless total knee arthroplasty. Whiteside (258) reported on the 9 to 11 year follow-up of 163 knees (61% follow-up) implanted with cementless femoral and tibial components. Survival rate at 10 years using loosening and infection as endpoints was 96.7%. Using the Natural Knee

(Intermedics Orthopaedics, Inc., Austin, Texas), Hofmann (85) reported an overall patellar survivorship of 96% at 6 to 10 year follow-up, which he attributed to its design (countersunk metal-backed) and surgical technique leading to superior patellar tracking. The same group of investigators, reporting on the same knee system and using loose components, revision, or both as failure criteria, found implant survival to be 95.1% (excluding infection and simple polyethylene exchanges) at 10 years when applying the Kaplan-Meier survival analysis (105). When analyzing their results of cementless total knee arthroplasties in patients 50 years or younger, this group also found good clinical and radiographic results (106). Although several other centers have also reported acceptable clinical and radiographic results of cementless knee arthroplasties (37,127,142) and support their use, others have not (15,162). Whereas intially, a comparison of 132 cementless and 139 cemented Miller-Galante (Zimmer, Warsaw, Indiana) did not show significant differences at a mean of 42 to 43 months (199), at a mean 132 months there were significant problems (15). Whereas cementless femoral fixation was excellent in these patients, metal-backed patellar components had a 48% patellar revision rate. Cementless tibial components had an 8% aseptic loosening rate and a 12% incidence of small osteolytic lesions. Based on these results, this group has abandoned cementless fixation in total knee arthroplasty. Fehring et al. (86) analyzed the mechanisms of failure in patients who had revision surgery within five years of their index arthroplasty. Of the 63% of patients in their database that had a knee revision within five years of their index procedure, 13% had revision surgery because of failure of ingrowth of a porous-coated implant. Clearly, further basic science, retrieval, and clinical studies are necessary to further our understanding of the role of biological fixation in total knee arthroplasty.

Revision Arthroplasty

The role of cementless implants in the revision setting is best understood by reviewing the poor results of cemented revisions. After component and cement removal during revision surgery, the bone stock left is often greatly compromised, making cement interdigitation extremely difficult. Acetabular cemented revisions in particular lead to very poor results, and reports of cemented femoral revisions are disappointing as well (123,125,170,174, 179,192). Although modern cementing techniques have improved some of these results, as they have in primary cemented arthroplasties, cemented revisions generally do not fare as well as cementless ones. On the femoral side, several reports of relatively successful results of cementless fixation can be found in the literature. Of these, distal cementless fixation (80,169,256) appears to be superior to proximal (43,50,181) fixation. The success of cementless fixation is even more pronounced on the acetabular side (68,91,118,145,239). Most revision knee replacements by far are cemented

(175,180), although bone grafts and their substitutes and metal augments are often used for filling defects. Press-fit stem extensions are often used in this setting for supplemental support. As implants made of more porous materials such as tantalum are becoming more widely used, clinical results of revision surgery are expected to improve. Adding to this exciting area of innovations is the use of osteoinductive substances in promoting bone ingrowth in the face of compromised host bone.

ANIMAL STUDIES

The basis for a large body of information on the science of implant fixation stems from studies done on animal models (8). The fields of fracture healing and spinal fusion have flourished in part due to the use of animal studies (5,100). As more and more joint replacements are now relying on biological fixation, the need for in vivo analyses is becoming more important. This section is aimed at reviewing some of the basic principles involved in using animal models to study implant fixation, including species selection, implant design and placement, and experimental endpoints. Other issues important to animal studies in this field are discussed elsewhere (233).

Animal studies so far have focused on answering questions related to implant surface properties (chemistry, roughness, and porous microarchitecture), the effects of motion and interface gaps, and the effects of factors leading to inhibition or enhancement of ingrowth. Changes in bone mass and geometry in response to various implants may also be studied with animal models, as they allow investigators to separate and study one variable at a time. Excellent reviews of these studies are available elsewhere (41,113, 128,129,185,223,224,227,233).

The choice of animal species to be used in a study is highly dependent upon the research question. If one were interested in studying the molecular basis of bone ingrowth, for instance, models using rodents would be advantageous, as molecular probes and transgenic animals are more readily available for these species. As bone formation rates of dogs and rabbits resemble human rates more closely than rodent species do, these animals are more commonly used to study fixation in the presence of implant weight bearing. Goats, sheep, and on occasion, primate models are also used. A comparison of primate and canine models for bone ingrowth has verified the applicability of using dogs to study implant fixation (210). Human prospective investigational histological studies are rarely done (104).

Animal studies can be either non-weight-bearing or weight-bearing (Fig. 3). Non-weight-bearing models are useful in studying the biological interaction of the implant material with the host bone in a nonloading environment. Initial studies of factors that enhance or inhibit ingrowth are often done on non-weight-bearing models. Examples of such studies include the effect of radiation (231) or osteoconductive substances (130) on bone ingrowth.

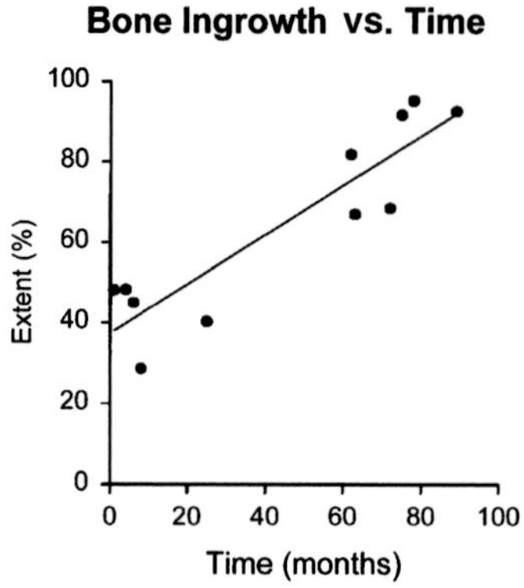

Bone Ingrowth vs. Time

Figure 3 Graph showing the increase with time in the extent of bone ingrowth in 11 porous coated hip replacement femoral stems retrieved postmortem ($r^2 = 0.64$, $p = 0.003$). *Source*: From Ref. 249.

Non-weight-bearing implants may be inserted either with an interface gap or in a press-fit manner (233). Whereas the former method would be a model of implant fixation under ideal mechanical support, the latter could be used as a model of suboptimal environment. Implants can be placed in either an axial or transcortical fashion, both through metaphyseal or dia-physeal bone. Axial metaphyseal implants mimic most human joint replacements that are placed within a trabecular bone bed (e.g., the acetabular component in total hip replacements and the tibial and femoral components in total knee replacements) or within the medullary cavity (e.g., the femoral component in a total hip arthroplasty).

Bone chamber models have the added advantage of performing vital microscopy and making repeated tissue harvests over time (9,93,141,233,237, 260,261). These devices may be implanted into an animal's bone. Once healed, a specimen can be removed from the center chamber. The factor being studied is then delivered to the core of the device, and at various time points, the device is disassembled and bone is removed for analysis. Bone images can be videotaped or photographed and studied in great detail using histomorphometric analysis.

Controlled-motion models enable researchers to test specific hypotheses about interface motion and biological fixation. These types of experiments (29,148,218) eliminate one of the major limitations of non-weight-bearing models, namely the lack of replication of load distribution from a weight-bearing device to the bone. Devices that communicate with the joint (25,109) may also be useful to eliminate the effects of weight-bearing and component movement while studying the role of particulate debris on bone-implant interfaces. As a means of studying "mechano-regulatory path-ways" of tissue differentiation, animal models have been devised that can create controlled micromotions (189).

Critical-sized diaphyseal defect models mimic a clinical situation where bone loss is so massive that normal fracture healing would not occur. Used by many researchers studying fracture healing enhancement (171), similar models also serve as weight-bearing devices relevant to total joint replacement (7,102,252). A more reliable weight-bearing model is hip replacement in the dog (233). These implants can be cemented or cementless, and similar to arthroplasties performed in humans, they allow the components to experience cyclic loading. When placed in a cementless fashion, these implants too can be inserted in a variety of ways, including press fit, "line-to-line," or in an over-reamed fashion creating measurable interface motion. The efficacy of both osteoinductive and osteoconductive factors can be tested using these models. Expanding the utility of such models, Turner et al. (246) created a model that replicated the radiographic and histological features of aseptic loosening of the femoral component of a total hip replacement that had been done with cement.

Either morphological or mechanical endpoints can be used in these studies. The volume fraction of bone ingrowth into a porous prosthesis is an example of a morphological endpoint (226). Other markers of osseointegration may also be developed. Interface soft-tissue characteristics (217) as well as bone tissue kinetics (39) may also serve as endpoints, as can bone formed in proximity to the implant (232). Host bone adaptive changes (244) to the implant may also serve as a morphological endpoint. Molecular markers as measured through in situ hybridization or immunohistochemical studies may also serve as endpoints. Strength of fixation (16) of an implant to the host bone and implant stability (17) have been used as mechanical endpoints in animal studies.

Knee replacement animal models are not as widely used. A study on the fibrous tissue at the bone–cement interface of a canine knee arthroplasty model has been described (108). Several other investigators have proposed canine cementless knee arthroplasty experiments (23,220,221,247,253). Knee implant stability (13,159,218,225,230), bone grafting (251), articular cartilage wear (140), embolism (158), hemorrhage control (63), wear debris (203), and infection (14) have all been studied in animal models.

Once a study question is appropriately formulated, the investigator needs to decide on a suitable model that will address it. More often than not, the most appropriate scientific pathway is to proceed with a simple model before advancing to a more complex one. Careful experimental design and selection of the appropriate model system will enhance scientific efforts in implant fixation research.

RETRIEVAL STUDIES

Several academic centers currently have active implant retrieval programs, and over the past decade, data disseminated from these studies has led to a much better understanding of the basic science of biological fixation. Some of these histological studies of porous-coated implants are based on components retrieved at revision surgery. As most of these were clinical failures, their findings must be interpreted with some caution. These implants may not have experienced normal loads, and as such, may not accurately reflect the quantity and quality of bone ingrowth that implants found in patients with well-functioning implants may demonstrate. Autopsy studies, on the other hand, provide the unique opportunity to analyze devices that have been clinically successful. All of these studies, however, are of utmost importance, as they tend to confirm and/or refute information gained from animal experimental studies. More importantly, these studies, unlike radiographic and clinical follow-ups, provide complete three-dimensional examination of histologic features. Special staining techniques as well as backscattered scanning electron microscopy and computer-assisted image analyses have enabled researchers to meticulously examine these samples. As cementless fixation is most commonly used in hip arthroplasties, most retrieval studies have been on femoral and acetabular components.

Cameron's (44) report of PCA stems having pore widths averaging 50 μm revised up to six years postimplantation confirmed other reports that pore sizes this small are suboptimal (197,257). None of these stems had ingrowth. Bobyn et al. (24), noting observations on a retrieved microporous-coated femoral prosthesis revised seven years after implantation, noted progressive bone resorption in the proximal femur, minimal overall ingrowth, and a sizable posterior pocket of granulation tissue containing chronic inflammatory round cells (most likely associated to the failed acetabular component). In a subsequent study (75), histological analysis of 11 retrieved AML femoral specimens showed bone ingrowth in nine and fibrous tissue fixation in two. Fixation by bone ingrowth occurred in 93% of the cases in which a press fit of the stem at the isthmus was achieved, but in only 69% of those without a press fit. Fixation by the ingrowth of bone or of fibrous tissue both appeared to be stable, but bone ingrowth appeared to lead to better clinical results. In further studies (77) substantiating these early reports, bone ingrowth has been shown to occur over a mean $35 \pm 5\%$ of the porous-coated surface of a femoral component in a quite consistent manner, ranging between 25% and 43%. Proximally coated stems appear to have slightly less ingrowth than extensively coated ones (30% vs. 37%). Regardless of stem type, bone ingrowth occurs most consistently in a circumferential pattern around the termination of the porous coating, and this tends to be cortical bone. In areas where there is a gap between the implant and the cortex, hypertrophied cancellous trabeculae are most commonly observed.

Examining cementless implants from 62 total knee arthroplasties and 28 total hip arthroplasties revised for reasons other than aseptic loosening or infection. Cook et al. (61) showed that approximately one-third of all components had no bone ingrowth or apposition of bone and the porous coating contained only fibrous tissue. In another one-third, ingrowth or apposition of bone was limited to less than 2% of the available porous coating. In the remaining one-third, only 2–10% of the porous structure contained ingrown bone. Notably, implants contained porous coatings of both the spherical-bead and fiber-metal types. No relationship between the degree of bone ingrowth and the length of time in situ was noted. The adherence of bony tissue at the time of removal, a positive roentgenographic evaluation, or a positive clinical presentation was not found to be a definite prognosticator of bone ingrowth. These investigators suggested that the combination of limited bone ingrowth and extensive fibrous tissue ingrowth is adequate for implant fixation. This would certainly be clinically relevant since it has been shown that bone ingrowth into cementless femoral revision stems is even less than that found in the primary setting (59). Although still highly controversial based on clinical and animal experiments, a stem retrieval case report did show that hydroxyapatite may enhance fixation (21).

Urban et al. (249) studied the bone–implant interface of 15 autopsy-retrieved cementless titanium–alloy femoral stems with porous coating limited to three proximal areas that did not cover the full circumference of the device. Eleven of the 15 stems had bone within the porous coating that was

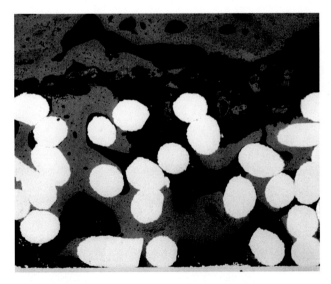

Figure 4 Transverse section of the porous coating of a hip replacement femoral stem retrieved postmortem after 28 months. The patient had osteomalacic renal osteodystrophy with areas of woven bone, which may have failed because of mechanical inadequacy. The histologic appearance of bone ingrowth without continuity with the surrounding trabecular bone bed suggested late failure of fixation of the trabecular bone (backscattered-electron scanning electron micrograph).

in continuity with the surrounding medullary bone (Fig. 4). The mean volume fraction of bone ingrowth in these specimens was 26.9% (range, 12.2–61.0%), and the mean extent of bone ingrowth was 64.3% (range, 28.6–95.2%). Both of these parameters increased with time (Fig. 3), unlike what was reported by Cook. (61) In the other four stems, the bone lacked continuity with the surrounding trabecular bed (Fig. 4). Two of these stems had a limited amount of bone within the porous coating, and two stems (from one patient) had no bone ingrowth. Periprosthetic membranes surrounded by a shell of trabecular bone covered the uncoated surfaces of the stems. The membranes of implants that had been in situ for eight months or more demonstrated polyethylene wear debris, and other particles generated at the level of the joint. The authors concluded that a circumferential coating might hinder particle access into the diaphysis and possibly decrease the incidence of osteolysis (Fig. 5).

Several retrieval studies have analyzed the relationship between cementless fixation and adaptive bone remodeling. Engh et al. (81,235,236), using dual energy X-ray absorptiometry analysis to measure periprosthetic bone-mineral content, evaluated femora of patients who had a cementless AML prostheses implanted. The mean reported bone loss was 23% (range 5.4–47.4%). Females, on average, experienced a greater decrease in mineral content

(A)   **(B)**

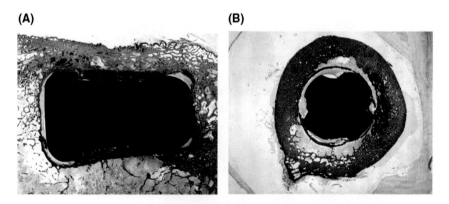

Figure 5 Histologic sections from a hip replacement femoral stem retrieved postmortem after 78 months. (**A**) Transverse, stained section through the proximal portion of the stem, showing extensive bone ingrowth into the anterior, posterior, and lateral porous surfaces. In contrast, the uncoated surfaces of the stem where the porous coating had not been applied are surrounded by particulate-laden fibrous membranes, demonstrating a pathway for distal migration of particulates generated at the bearing surface. (**B**) Transverse, stained section of the distal portion of the stem and femur. Fibrous membranes containing particles generated at the bearing surfaces are interposed between the stem and a shell of trabecular bone, suggesting the mechanism of distal particle-induced endosteal osteolysis. *Source*: From Ref. 249.

(31%) than males (12%, $p < 0.05$). Bone loss was noted to occur on a gradient, with the greatest loss occurring proximally and the least occurring distally (236). Lastly, the extent of bone loss correlated highly with the bone mineral content of the contralateral, normal hip ($r^2 = 0.94$) (236). Stem size, duration of implantation, patient weight, or patient age did not predict bone loss after arthroplasty (236).

Noting some of the limitations of dual energy X-ray absorptiometry analysis, Maloney et al. (154) reported on 13 cemented and 11 cementless retrieved hip prostheses. Cortical thickness, cortical bone area, and bone mineral density were assessed in four quadrants at five discrete levels. The maximum cortical bone loss by level was at the middle section for the cemented femora and at the midproximal and middle sections for the cementless femora. They concluded that the less dense the bone before hip-replacement surgery, the greater the extent of bone loss after total hip arthroplasty, regardless of fixation type. In comparing proximally coated stems with extensively coated stems (161), bone loss appears to occur more with the former (38.6%) than with the latter (18.4%) types of stems; this difference, however, was not found to be statistically significant ($p = 0.13$). Although "stress shielding," the name given to the bone loss phenomenon described in these studies, may complicate revision surgery, it has not appeared to be clinically relevant (71). Limb usage, an implant's modulus of elasticity and its position in the medullary canal are just a few of many other factors that may affect the degree and type of bone "remodeling" that occurs. Differences between true measurements of bone density and bone mineral content, two distinctly different parameters, as measured by current techniques also needs to be further studied such that the phenomenon of "stress shielding" is better understood.

Retrieval studies on femoral stability and micromotion are somewhat lacking. In one group of radiographically ingrown implants, the authors found that relative motion at ingrown areas was generally less than 20 μm and never in excess of 40 μm (82). At the tip of the prostheses, where no ingrowth had occurred, micromotion was inversely proportional to the extent of the porous coating. For proximally coated stems, maximum tip motion was 210 μm as compared to extensively coated stems where tip motion was recorded to be 120 μm. In one implant deemed to be radiographically stable by fibrous tissue, micromotion was 150 μm at the porous area and 350 μm at the tip.

Several retrieval studies have reported on the pattern of bone ingrowth into cementless acetabular components. Engh et al. (83) histologically and radiographically assessed nine well functioning porous coated acetabular components (three types) retrieved postmortem at a mean of 50 months postimplantation. Although highly variable, with a range of 3% to 84%, on average, $32 \pm 27\%$ of the porous coated surface was ingrown. Bone apposition and ingrowth appeared to be random and irregular, but where it did occur, an average of 48% (range, 26–65%) of the available pore space was filled with bone. Interestingly, in areas devoid of bone ingrowth, the fibrous pattern noted appeared to be dense and well organized. Radiographically and clinically, all cups were well fixed. Sumner et al. (228) reported on 25 consecutively retrieved Harris-Galante titanium fiber metal porous acetabular components removed for reasons other than loosening or infection. Eighteen shells had been placed in primary arthroplasties and seven in revision cases. All were implanted with adjuvant screw fixation. After being in place for an average of 30 weeks, 18 cups had bone ingrowth into the porous coating. Up to one-third of the available void space within the porous coating was occupied by bone, while the maximal proportion of the area of the bone-implant interface with bone ingrowth was over 80%. Bone ingrowth was most consistently observed at the dome and in the vicinity of sites of screw fixation. As compared to the implants that had been in place for shorter periods, the long-term cases had more bone ingrowth and more metallic debris observed within histiocytes adjacent to screw holes. Pidhorz et al. (183) reported an autopsy retrieval cohort of 11 cementless Harris-Galante acetabular components implanted with screws and in situ for an average of 41 months (range, 5 weeks to 75 months). Ten of the cups had bone ingrowth, with the average volume fraction being $12.1 \pm 8.2\%$. Interestingly, no differences in the amount of bone ingrowth were found when the component was partitioned into nine anatomic regions. There was more bone adjacent to screw holes through which screws were inserted compared with empty screw holes, however (Fig. 6A). Additionally, as the number of radiolucent zones increased on the clinical radiographs less bone ingrowth was observed histologically. The amount of metal debris in holes with screws and holes without screws was similar (Fig. 6B). In the longest term cases, polyethylene debris was noted within empty screw holes, but no granulomatous reactions or osteolytic processes were observed (Fig. 6C). Bloebaum et al. (19), reporting on bone ingrowth into a porous coated acetabular component, found that an average of $12 \pm 6\%$ (range 4% to 21%) of the porous surface had ingrown bone. Confirming the study by Pidhorz et al. (183), there were no differences observed in the amount of bone ingrowth among the DeLee and Charnley zones (70), suggesting that variances in bone loading do not affect bone ingrowth. Cook et al. (60) examined 42 uncemented, porous-coated acetabular components removed for reasons not related to fixation. Initial fixation in all the components consisted of fixed pegs, spikes, or screws. Bone ingrowth occurred more frequently, in greater amounts and was more evenly distributed anatomically in cups using screws for initial adjunct fixation than in those with pegs or spikes. Although several investigators have questioned the use of screws to supplement a press-fit socket (139), most implant retrieval studies to date are on shells placed with screws. Further postmortem studies on the histological

(A)   **(B)**

(C)

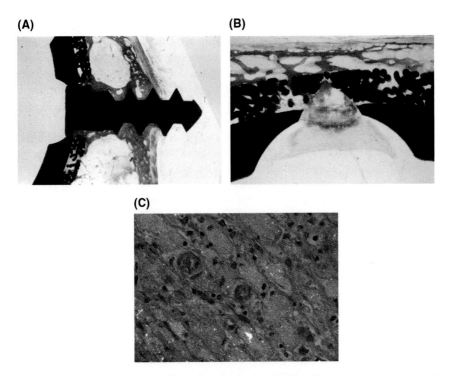

Figure 6 Histologic sections from hip replacement acetabular components retrieved postmortem. (**A**) This specimen was obtained postmortem after 71 months in situ. There is condensation of bone around the threads of the fixation screw with extensive bone ingrowth into the porous coating immediately adjacent to the screw. (**B**) A section of the same acetabular component shown in (**A**), demonstrating metal particulate debris within an unfilled screw hole and adjacent porous coating. (**C**) This specimen was obtained postmortem after 78 months in situ. Soft tissue removed from an unfilled screw hole shows a multitude of polyethylene particles within histiocytes under partially polarized light. *Source*: From Ref. 183.

differences observed between press-fit cups with and without adjuvant screw fixation are awaited.

As compared to hip devices, much fewer retrieved knee implants are available for examination. Sumner et al. (229) looked at 13 primary cementless pegged titanium fiber-metal porous-coated tibial components removed at an average of 15.3 months postimplantation for reasons unrelated to fixation or infection. Supplemental screw fixation was used in all but one component. The average extent of bone ingrowth within the tray was $27.1 \pm 16.1\%$, and the average volume fraction was $9.5 \pm 7.5\%$. There was significantly more bone ingrowth within the fixation pegs than within the tray and also more bone ingrowth in the anterior half of the tray than posteriorly. There was no correlation between the amount of bone ingrowth and the length of implantation, age, or sex of the patient; the depth and orientation of the resection plane, however, were found to correlate with the topographic distribution of bone ingrowth. Particulate debris appeared to gain access to the interface via both the periphery and through the screw fixation holes. A more recent study by investigators from the same center used autopsy-retrieved tibial components retrieved postmortem at an average 51 months postsurgery to examine the relationship between mechanical stability as it relates to fixation type (18). When the adjuvant fixation screws were left in place, they found that the "average" inducible motion, as determined from six-degree-of-freedom measurements, was 25 ± 19 μm for cemented specimens versus 54 ± 31 μm for cementless components ($p = 0.08$). The maximum inducible motion, however, was two-fold higher in the cementless components ($p = 0.05$). Although removal of the screws in the cementless components did not lead to a significant increase in motion, it did reveal a strong correlation between the average motion and the extent of bone ingrowth into the lateral pegs ($R^2 = 0.936$, $p = 0.007$).

Bloebaum et al. (22) analyzed 10 asymmetric porous-coated tibial knee components from nine patients with implantation times ranging from 1 week to 48 months. Morselized autograft bone chips had been applied to the resected surface of the tibia prior to component implantation. Bone appeared to be "in contact" with $64 \pm 10\%$ of the porous-coated interface. Backscattered electron imaging of the bone–implant interface revealed bone within 8–22% of the porous coating. Although bone in the form of autograft bone chips was observed in the porous coating of the one and three week specimens, it was not connected to the host bone. By three and six months, the bone chips were integrated and connected to the host bone providing osseous continuity from the porous coating to the host bone. The authors concluded that reproducible bone ingrowth into porous-coated tibial components is achievable using autograft bone chips to promote bone fixation. This study complemented other reports on cementless knee fixation from the same institution (20,104).

A study by Wasielewski et al. (255) warrants a review. Sixty-seven ultra-high-molecular-weight polyethylene (UHMWPE) tibial inserts from cementless total knee arthroplasties were retrieved at autopsy and revision surgery and analyzed for evidence of articular and nonarticular surface wear after a mean implantation time of 62.8 months (range, 4–131 months). Corresponding prerevision radiographs were evaluated for evidence of tibial metaphyseal osteolysis and osteolysis around tibial fixation screws. Severe wear of the tibial insert undersurface was associated with tibial metaphyseal osteolysis or osteolysis around fixation screws. Time in situ was statistically related to severe undersurface wear and tibial metaphyseal osteolysis. The occurrence of tibial osteolysis was not related statistically to articular wear severity, insert thickness, or implant type. The study concluded that the undersurface of the insert is an additional source of polyethylene debris contributing to tibial metaphyseal osteolysis. The relationship between screws and tibial metaphyseal osteolysis confirms previous reports suggesting possible mechanisms leading to osteolytic lesions in cementless knee arthroplasties (182).

Investigations based on implant retrieval registries have contributed immensely to our understanding of implant fixation. Certainly, as this method of study becomes more refined, more questions will be answered. Some of the issues still considered controversial with regard to this topic include the roles of the federal government, manufacturers, and clinicians in promoting, maintaining, and financing implant retrieval programs. Under the auspices of the National Institute of Health, The National Institute of Biomedical Imaging and Bioengineering has assigned a committee entitled the Bioengineering Materials and Implant Science (BMIS) Group. This committee has already become quite involved with implant retrieval studies. Manufacturers have also become interested in supporting implant retrieval centers, as maintaining these programs can be quite expensive. Another important consideration that still needs to be addressed is determining the ideal pathways of educating the public on the scientific and personal aspects of implant retrieval.

CONCLUSION

The basic science of implant fixation continues to be an emerging field. Implant factors, host bone environment, systemic status of the patient and surgical technique can all affect the ultimate result of an implant that relies on biological fixation. Whereas the fundamental requirements of bony ingrowth are well understood, enhancing fixation of implants placed under suboptimal conditions, such as in the revision setting, requires further research. By enhancing bony fixation in both primary and revision surgeries, conduits for the dissemination of particles leading to osteolysis may be eliminated. Using osteoinductive agents may be one of facilitating osteogenesis into porous structures, although the delivery systems for many of these substances are still being investigated. Gene therapy may be an effective strategy for enhancing delivery of many of these molecules. These and other methods of promoting ingrowth and preventing osteolysis are the topics of several of the chapters in this text.

ACKNOWLEDGMENTS

Inspiration and leadership from J.O. Galante, M.D., technical assistance from Deborah Hall, Susan Infanger and Leslie Manion, support from NIH Grants AR042862 and AR039310 and Zimmer.

REFERENCES

1. Aarden EM, Nijweide PJ, van der Plas A, Alblas MJ, Mackie EJ, Horton MA, Helfrich MH. Adhesive properties of isolated chick osteocytes in vitro. Bone 1996; 18(4):305–313.

2. Aigner C. [10 years results with the corund–blasted Zweymuller titanium alloy threaded acetabular cup]. Z Orthop Ihre Grenzgeb 1998; 136(2):110–114.

3. Albrektsson T, Hansson HA. An ultrastructural characterization of the interface between bone and sputtered titanium or stainless steel surfaces. Biomaterials 1986; 7(3):201–205.

4. An YH, Friedman RJ, eds. Animal models in orthopedic research. Boca Raton, FL: CRC Press, 1999.

5. An YH, Friedman RJ, Draughn RA. Animal models of fracture or osteotomy. In: An YH, Friedman RJ, eds. Animal Models in Orthopaedic Research. Boca Raton: CRC Press, 1999:197–217.

6. Andersen HN, Ernst C, Frandsen PA. Polyethylene failure of metal-backed patellar components. 111 AGC total knees followed for 7–22 months. Acta Orthop Scand 1991; 62(1):1–3.

7. Andersson GB, Gaechter A, Galante JO, Rostoker W. Segmental replacement of long bones in baboons using a fiber titanium implant. J Bone Joint Surg Am 1978; 60(1):31–40.

8. Archibeck MJ, Berger RA, Jacobs JJ, Quigley LR, Gitelis S, Rosenberg AG, Galante JO. Second-generation cementless total hip arthroplasty. Eight to eleven-year results. J Bone Joint Surg Am 2001; 83-A(11):1666–1673.

9. Aufdemorte TB, Fox WC, Holt GR, McGuff HS, Ammann AJ, Beck LS. An intraosseous device for studies of bone-healing. The effect of transforming growth-factor beta. J Bone Joint Surg Am 1992; 74(8):1153–1161.

10. Baech J, Kofoed H. Failure of metal-backed patellar arthroplasty. 47 AGC total knees followed for at least 1 year. Acta Orthop Scand 1991; 62(2):166–168.

11. Bayley JC, Scott RD, Ewald FC, Holmes GB Jr. Failure of the metal-backed patellar component after total knee replacement. J Bone Joint Surg Am 1988; 70(5):668–674.

12. Beckenbaugh RD, Ilstrup DM. Total hip arthroplasty. J Bone Joint Surg Am 1978; 60(3):306–313.

13. Bellemans J. Osseointegration in porous coated knee arthroplasty. The influence of component coating type in sheep. Acta Orthop Scand Suppl 1999; 288:1–35.

14. Belmatoug N, Cremieux AC, Bleton R, Volk A, Saleh-Mghir A, Grossin M, Garry L, Carbon C. A new model of experimental prosthetic joint infection due to methicillin-resistant *Staphylococcus aureus*: a microbiologic, histopathologic, and magnetic resonance imaging characterization. J Infect Dis 1996; 174(2):414–417.

15. Berger RA, Lyon JH, Jacobs JJ, Barden RM, Berkson EM, Sheinkop MB, Rosenberg AG, Galante JO. Problems with cementless total knee arthroplasty at 11 years followup. Clin Orthop 2001; (392):196–207.

16. Berzins A, Sumner DR. Implant pushout and pullout tests. In: An YH, Draughn RA, eds. Mechanical Testing of Bone and the Bone–Implant Interface. Boca Raton: CRC Press, 2000:463–476.

17. Berzins A, Sumner DR. In vitro measurements of implant stability. In: An YH, Draughn RA, eds. Mechanical Testing of Bone and the Bone–Implant Interface. Boca Raton: CRC Press, 2000:515–526.
18. Berzins A, Sumner DR, Igloria R, Jacobs JJ, Urban RM, Galante JO. Trans ORS 1994; 19:247.
19. Bloebaum RD, Bachus KN, Jensen JW, Hofmann AA. Postmortem analysis of consecutively retrieved asymmetric porous-coated tibial components. J Arthroplasty 1997; 12(8):920–929.
20. Bloebaum RD, Bachus KN, Jensen JW, Scott DF, Hofmann AA. porous-coated metal-backed patellar components in total knee replacement. A postmortem retrieval analysis. J Bone Joint Surg Am 1998; 80(4):518–528.
21. Bloebaum RD, Bachus KN, Rubman MH, Dorr LD. Postmortem comparative analysis of titanium and hydroxyapatite porous-coated femoral implants retrieved from the same patient. A case study. J Arthroplasty 1993; 8(2):203–211.
22. Bloebaum RD, Rubman MH, Hofmann AA. Bone ingrowth into porous-coated tibial components implanted with autograft bone chips. Analysis of ten consecutively retrieved implants. J Arthroplasty 1992; 7(4):483–493.
23. Bobyn JD, Cameron HU, Abdulla D, Pilliar RM, Weatherly GC. Biologic fixation and bone modeling with an unconstrained canine total knee prosthesis. Clin Orthop 1982; (166):301–312.
24. Bobyn JD, Engh CA, Glassman AH. Histologic analysis of a retrieved micro-porous-coated femoral prosthesis. A seven-year case report. Clin Orthop 1987; (224):303–310.
25. Bobyn JD, Jacobs JJ, Tanzer M, Urban RM, Aribindi R, Sumner DR, Turner TM, Brooks CE. The susceptibility of smooth implant surfaces to periimplant fibrosis and migration of polyethylene wear debris. Clin Orthop 1995; (311): 21–39.
26. Bobyn JD, Pilliar RM, Cameron HU, Weatherly GC. The optimum pore size for the fixation of porous-surfaced metal implants by the ingrowth of bone. Clin Orthop 1980; (150):263–270.
27. Bobyn JD, Pilliar RM, Cameron HU, Weatherly GC. Osteogenic phenomena across endosteal bone–implant spaces with porous surfaced intramedullary implants. Acta Orthop Scand 1981; 52(2):145–153.
28. Bobyn JD, Stackpool GJ, Hacking SA, Tanzer M, Krygier JJ. Characteristics of bone ingrowth and interface mechanics of a new porous tantalum biomaterial. J Bone Joint Surg Br 1999; 81(5):907–914.
29. Bragdon CR, Burke D, Lowenstein JD, O'Connor DO, Ramamurti B, Jasty M, Harris WH. Differences in stiffness of the interface between a cementless porous implant and cancellous bone in vivo in dogs due to varying amounts of implant motion. J Arthroplasty 1996; 11(8):945–951.
30. Branemark PI. Osseointegration and its experimental background. J Prosthet Dent 1983; 50(3):399–410.
31. Branemark PI, Adell R, Breine U, Hansson BO, Lindstrom J, Ohlsson A. Intra-osseous anchorage of dental prostheses. I. Experimental studies. Scand J Plast Reconstr Surg 1969; 3(2):81–100.

32. Branemark PI, Hansson BO, Adell R, Breine U, Lindstrom J, Hallen O, Ohman A. Osseointegrated implants in the treatment of the edentulous jaw. Experience from a 10-year period. Scand J Plast Reconstr Surg Suppl 1977; 16:1–132.

33. Branson PJ, Steege JW, Wixson RL, Lewis J, Stulberg SD. Rigidity of initial fixation with uncemented tibial knee implants. J Arthroplasty 1989; 4(1):21–26.

34. Britton AR, Murray DW, Bulstrode CJ, McPherson K, Denham RA. Long-term comparison of Charnley and Stanmore design total hip replacements. J Bone Joint Surg Br 1996; 78(5):802–808.

35. Brown CC, McLaughlin RE, Balian G. Intramedullary bone repair and ingrowth into porous coated implants in the adult chicken: a histologic study and biochemical analysis of collagens. J Orthop Res 1989; 7(3):316–325.

36. Bruijn JD, Seelen JL, Feenstra RM, Hansen BE, Bernoski FP. Failure of the Mecring screw-ring acetabular component in total hip arthroplasty. A three to seven-year follow-up study. J Bone Joint Surg Am 1995; 77(5):760–766.

37. Buechel FF Sr. Long-term followup after mobile-bearing total knee replacement. Clin Orthop 2002; (404):40–50.

38. Burke DW, O'Connor DO, Zalenski EB, Jasty M, Harris WH. Micromotion of cemented and uncemented femoral components. J Bone Joint Surg Br 1991; 73(1):33–37.

39. Burr DB, Mori S, Boyd RD, Sun TC, Blaha JD, Lane L, Parr J. Histomorphometric assessment of the mechanisms for rapid ingrowth of bone to HA/TCP coated implants. J Biomed Mater Res 1993; 27(5):645–653.

40. Burt CF, Garvin KL, Otterberg ET, Jardon OM. A femoral component inserted without cement in total hip arthroplasty. A study of the Tri-Lock component with an average ten-year duration of follow-up. J Bone Joint Surg Am 1998; 80(7):952–960.

41. Callaghan JJ. The clinical results and basic science of total hip arthroplasty with porous-coated prostheses. J Bone Joint Surg Am 1993; 75(2):299–310.

42. Callahan BC, Lisecki EJ, Banks RE, Dalton JE, Cook SD, Wolff JD. The effect of warfarin on the attachment of bone to hydroxyapatite-coated and uncoated porous implants. J Bone Joint Surg Am 1995; 77(2):225–230.

43. Cameron H. Experience with proximal ingrowth implantation in hip revision surgery. Acta Orthop Belg 1997; 63(suppl 1):66–68.

44. Cameron HU. Six-year results with a microporous-coated metal hip prosthesis. Clin Orthop 1986; (208):81–83.

45. Cameron HU, Pilliar RM, Macnab I. The rate of bone ingrowth into porous metal. J Biomed Mater Res 1976; 10(2):295–302.

46. Campbell AC, Rorabeck CH, Bourne RB, Chess D, Nott L. Thigh pain after cementless hip arthroplasty. Annoyance or ill omen. J Bone Joint Surg Br 1992; 74(1):63–66.

47. Capello WN, Colyer RA, Kernek CB, Carnahan JV, Hess JJ. Failure of the Mecron screw-in ring. J Bone Joint Surg Br 1993; 75(5):835–836.

48. Capello WN, D'Antonio JA, Manley MT, Feinberg JR. Hydroxyapatite in total hip arthroplasty. Clinical results and critical issues. Clin Orthop 1998; 355:200–211.

49. Carter DR, Beaupre GS, Giori NJ, Helms JA. Mechanobiology of skeletal regeneration. Clin Orthop 1998; (355 suppl):S41–55.

50. Chandler HP, Ayres DK, Tan RC, Anderson LC, Varma, AK. Revision total hip replacement using the S-ROM femoral component. Clin Orthop 1995; (319):130–140.
51. Charnley J. The lubrication of animal joints. New Scientist 1959; 6:60.
52. Cheng SL, Davey JR, Inman RD, Binnington AG, Smith TJ. The effect of the medial collar in total hip arthroplasty with porous-coated components inserted without cement. An in vivo canine study. J Bone Joint Surg Am 1995; 77(1):118–123.
53. Chin HC, Frassica FJ, Markel MD, Frassica DA, Sim FH, Chao EY. The effects of therapeutic doses of irradiation on experimental bone graft incorporation over a porous-coated segmental defect endoprosthesis. Clin Orthop 1993; (289):254–266.
54. Clemow AJ, Weinstein AM, Klawitter JJ, Koeneman J, Anderson J. Interface mechanics of porous titanium implants. J Biomed Mater Res 1981; 15(1):73–82.
55. Clohisy JC, Harris WH. The Harris–Galante porous-coated acetabular component with screw fixation. An average ten-year follow-up study. J Bone Joint Surg Am 1999; 81(1):66–73.
56. Clohisy JC, Harris WH. The Harris–Galante uncemented femoral component in primary total hip replacement at 10 years. J Arthroplasty 1999; 14(8):915–917.
57. Clohisy JC, Harris WH. Matched-pair analysis of cemented and cementless acetabular reconstruction in primary total hip arthroplasty. J Arthroplasty 2001; 16(6):697–705.
58. Cook SD, Barrack RL, Dalton JE, Thomas KA, Brown TD. Effects of indomethacin on biologic fixation of porous-coated titanium implants. J Arthroplasty 1995; 10(3):351–358.
59. Cook SD, Barrack RL, Thomas KA, Haddad RJ Jr. Tissue growth into porous primary and revision femoral stems. J Arthroplasty 1991; 6(suppl):S37–46.
60. Cook SD, Thomas KA, Barrack RL, Whitecloud TS III. Tissue growth into porous-coated acetabular components in 42 patients. Effects of adjunct fixation. Clin Orthop 1992; (283):163–170.
61. Cook SD, Thomas KA, Haddad RJ Jr. Histologic analysis of retrieved human porous-coated total joint components. Clin Orthop 1988; (234):90–101.
62. Cook SD, Walsh KA, Haddad RJ Jr. Interface mechanics and bone growth into porous Co–Cr–Mo alloy implants. Clin Orthop 1985; (193):271–280.
63. Curtin WA, Wang GJ, Goodman NC, Abbott RD, Spotnitz WD. Reduction of hemorrhage after knee arthroplasty using cryo-based fibrin sealant. J Arthroplasty 1999; 14(4):481–487.
64. Daculsi G, LeGeros RZ, Deudon C. Scanning and transmission electron microscopy, and electron probe analysis of the interface between implants and host bone. Osseo-coalescence versus osseo-integration. Scanning Microsc 1990; 4(2):309–314.
65. Dalton JE, Cook SD, Thomas KA, Kay JF. The effect of operative fit and hydroxyapatite coating on the mechanical and biological response to porous implants. J Bone Joint Surg Am 1995; 77(1):97–110.
66. de Nies F, Fidler MW. The Harris–Galante cementless femoral component: poor results in 57 hips followed for 3 years. Acta Orthop Scand 1996; 67(2):122–124.

67. Dean JC, Tisdel CL, Goldberg VM, Parr J, Davy D, Stevenson S. Effects of hydroxyapatite tricalcium phosphate coating and intracancellous placement on bone ingrowth in titanium fibermetal implants. J Arthroplasty 1995; 10(6):830–838.
68. Dearborn JT, Harris WH. Acetabular revision arthroplasty using so-called jumbo cementless components: an average 7-year follow-up study. J Arthroplasty 2000; 15(1):8–15.
69. Delaunay CP, Kapandji AI. Primary total hip arthroplasty with the Karl Zweymuller first-generation cementless prosthesis. A 5- to 9-year retrospective study. J Arthroplasty 1996; 11(6):643–652.
70. DeLee JG, Charnley J. Radiological demarcation of cemented sockets in total hip replacement. Clin Orthop 1976; (121):20–32.
71. Della Valle CJ, Paprosky WG. The middle-aged patient with hip arthritis: the case for extensively coated stems. Clin Orthop 2002; (405):101–107.
72. Dorr LD, Lewonowski K, Lucero M, Harris M, Wan Z. Failure mechanisms of anatomic porous replacement I cementless total hip replacement. Clin Orthop 1997; (334):157–167.
73. Einhorn TA, Bonnarens F, Burstein AH. The contributions of dietary protein and mineral to the healing of experimental fractures. A biomechanical study. J Bone Joint Surg Am 1986; 68(9):1389–1395.
74. Emerson RH Jr, Sanders SB, Head WC, Higgins L. Effect of circumferential plasma-spray porous coating on the rate of femoral osteolysis after total hip arthroplasty. J Bone Joint Surg Am 1999; 81(9):1291–1298.
75. Engh CA, Bobyn JD, Glassman AH. Porous-coated hip replacement. The factors governing bone ingrowth, stress shielding, and clinical results. J Bone Joint Surg Br 1987; 69(1):45–55.
76. Engh CA, Griffin WL, Marx CL. Cementless acetabular components. J Bone Joint Surg Br 1990; 72(1):53–59.
77. Engh CA, Hooten JP Jr, Zettl-Schaffer KF, Ghaffarpour M, McGovern TF, Bobyn JD. Evaluation of bone ingrowth in proximally and extensively porous-coated anatomic medullary locking prostheses retrieved at autopsy. J Bone Joint Surg Am 1995; 77(6):903–910.
78. Engh CA, Hooten JP Jr, Zettl-Schaffer KF, Ghaffarpour M, McGovern TF, Macalino GE, Zicat BA. Porous-coated total hip replacement. Clin Orthop 1994; (298):89–96.
79. Engh CA Jr, Culpepper WJ II, Engh CA. Long-term results of use of the anatomic medullary locking prosthesis in total hip arthroplasty. J Bone Joint Surg Am 1997; 79(2):177–184.
80. Engh CA Jr, Ellis TJ, Koralewicz LM, McAuley JP, Engh CA Sr. Extensively porous-coated femoral revision for severe femoral bone loss: minimum 10-year follow-up. J Arthroplasty 2002; 17(8):955–960.
81. Engh CA, McGovern TF, Bobyn JD, Harris WH. A quantitative evaluation of periprosthetic bone-remodeling after cementless total hip arthroplasty. J Bone Joint Surg Am 1992; 74(7):1009–1020.
82. Engh CA, O'Connor D, Jasty M, McGovern TF, Bobyn JD, Harris WH. Quantification of implant micromotion, strain shielding, and bone resorption with porous-coated anatomic medullary locking femoral prostheses. Clin Orthop 1992; (285):13–29.

83. Engh CA, Zettl-Schaffer KF, Kukita Y, Sweet D, Jasty M, Bragdon C. Histological and radiographic assessment of well functioning porous-coated acetabular components. A human postmortem retrieval study. J Bone Joint Surg Am 1993; 75(6):814–824.

84. Epinette JA, Manley MT, D'Antonio JA, Edidin AA, Capello WN. A 10-year minimum follow-up of hydroxyapatite-coated threaded cups: clinical, radiographic and survivorship analyses with comparison to the literature. J Arthroplasty 2003; 18(2):140–148.

85. Evanich CJ, Tkach TK, von Glinski S, Camargo MP, Hofmann AA. 6- to 10-year experience using countersunk metal-backed patellas. J Arthroplasty 1997; 12(2):149–154.

86. Fehring TK, Odum S, Griffin WL, Mason JB, Nadaud M. Early failures in total knee arthroplasty. Clin Orthop 2001; (392):315–318.

87. Frosch KH, Barvencik F, Lohmann CH, Viereck V, Siggelkow H, Breme J, Dresing K, Sturmer KM. Migration, matrix production and lamellar bone formation of human osteoblast-like cells in porous titanium implants. Cells Tissues Organs 2002; 170(4):214–227.

88. Galante J, Rostoker W, Lueck R, Ray RD. Sintered fiber metal composites as a basis for attachment of implants to bone. J Bone Joint Surg Am 1971; 53(1):101–114.

89. Garcia-Cimbrelo E, Munuera, L. Early and late loosening of the acetabular cup after low–friction arthroplasty. J Bone Joint Surg Am 1992; 74(8):1119–1129.

90. Giancotti FG. A structural view of integrin activation and signaling. Dev Cell 2003; 4(2):149–151.

91. Goldberg VM. Revision of failure acetabular components with cementless acetabular components. Am J Orthop 2002; 31(4):206–207.

92. Goodman S. et al. COX-2 selective NSAID decreases bone ingrowth in vivo. J Orthop Res 2002; 20(6):1164–1169.

93. Goodman SB, Song Y, Chun L, Regula D, Aspenberg P. Effects of TGFbeta on bone ingrowth in the presence of polyethylene particles. J Bone Joint Surg Br 1999; 81(6):1069–1075.

94. Gortz W, Nagerl UV, Nagerl H, Thomsen M. Spatial micromovements of uncemented femoral components after torsional loads. J Biomech Eng 2002; 124(6):706–713.

95. Groessner-Schreiber B, Tuan RS. Enhanced extracellular matrix production and mineralization by osteoblasts cultured on titanium surfaces in vitro. J Cell Sci 1992; 101(Pt 1):209–217.

96. Haboush EJ. A new operation for arthroplasty of the hip based on biomechanics, photoelasticity, fast-setting dental acrylic, and other considerations. Bull Hosp Joint Dis 1953; 14:242–277.

97. Haddad RJ, Cook SD, Brinker MR. A comparison of three varieties of noncemented porous-coated hip replacement. J Bone Joint Surg Br 1990; 72(1):2–8.

98. Harris WH, Jasty M. Bone ingrowth into porous coated canine acetabular replacements: the effect of pore size, apposition, and dislocation. Hip 1985:214–234.

99. Harris WH, Mulroy RD Jr, Maloney WJ, Burke DW, Chandler HP, Zalenski EB. Intraoperative measurement of rotational stability of femoral components of total hip arthroplasty. Clin Orthop 1991; (266):119–126.

100. Harvinder SS, Kanim LEA, Girardi F, Cammisa FP, Dawson ED. Animal models of spinal instability and spinal fusion. In: An YH, Friedman RJ, eds. Animal Models in Orthopaedic Research. Boca Raton: CRC Press, 1999:505–526.

101. Hastings DE, Tobin H, Sellenkowitsch M. Review of 10-year results of PCA hip arthroplasty. Can J Surg 1998; 41(1):48–52.

102. Heck DA, Nakajima I, Kelly PJ, Chao EY. The effect of load alteration on the biological and biomechanical performance of a titanium fiber-metal segmental prosthesis. J Bone Joint Surg Am 1986; 68(1):118–126.

103. Hodgkinson JP, Shelley P, Wroblewski BM. The correlation between the roentgenographic appearance and operative findings at the bone–cement junction of the socket in Charnley low friction arthroplasties. Clin Orthop 1988; (228):105–109.

104. Hofmann AA, Bloebaum RD, Rubman MH, Bachus KN, Plaster RL. Microscopic analysis of autograft bone applied at the interface of porous-coated devices in human cancellous bone. Int Orthop 1992; 16(4):349–358.

105. Hofmann AA, Evanich JD, Ferguson RP, Camargo MP. Ten- to 14-year clinical followup of the cementless natural knee system. Clin Orthop 2001(388):85–94.

106. Hofmann AA, Heithoff SM, Camargo M. Cementless total knee arthroplasty in patients 50 years or younger. Clin Orthop 2002; (404):102–107.

107. Hoogendoorn HA, Renooij W, Akkermans LM, Visser W, Wittebol P. Long-term study of large ceramic implants (porous hydroxyapatite) in dog femora. Clin Orthop 1984; (187):281–288.

108. Hori RY, Lewis JL. Mechanical properties of the fibrous tissue found at the bone–cement interface following total joint replacement. J Biomed Mater Res 1982; 16(6):911–927.

109. Howie DW, Vernon-Roberts B, Oakeshott R, Manthey B. A rat model of resorption of bone at the cement–bone interface in the presence of polyethylene wear particles. J Bone Joint Surg Am 1988; 70(2):257–263.

110. Hozack W, Gardiner R, Hearn S, Eng K, Rothman R. Taperloc femoral component. A 2–6-year study of the first 100 consecutive cases. J Arthroplasty 1994; 9(5):489–493.

111. Hozack WJ, Rothman RH, Eng K, Mesa J. Primary cementless hip arthroplasty with a titanium plasma sprayed prosthesis. Clin Orthop 1996; (333):217–225.

112. Itala AI, Ylanen HO, Ekholm C, Karlsson KH, Aro HT. Pore diameter of more than 100 micron is not requisite for bone ingrowth in rabbits. J Biomed Mater Res 2001; 58(6):679–683.

113. Jacobs JJ, Goodman SB, Sumner DR, Hallab NJ. Biological response to orthopaedic implants. In: Buckwalter JA, Einhorn TA, Simon SR, eds. Orthopaedic Basic Science. Rosemont: American Academy of Orthopaedic Surgeons, 2000:401–426.

114. Jacobs JJ, Kull LR, Frey GA, Gitelis S, Sheinkop MB, Kramer TS, Rosenberg AG. Early failure of acetabular components inserted without cement after previous pelvic irradiation. J Bone Joint Surg Am 1995; 77(12):1829–1835.

115. Jarcho M. Biomaterial aspects of calcium phosphates. Properties and applications. Dent Clin North Am 1986; 30(1):25–47.

116. Jarcho M. Calcium phosphate ceramics as hard tissue prosthetics. Clin Orthop 1981; (157):259–278.

117. Jarcho M, Kay JF, Gumaer KI, Doremus RH, Drobeck HP. Tissue, cellular and subcellular events at a bone–ceramic hydroxylapatite interface. J Bioeng 1977; 1(2):79–92.
118. Jasty M. Jumbo cups and morsalized graft. Orthop Clin North Am 1998; 29(2):249–254.
119. Jasty M, Bragdon CR, Schutzer S, Rubash H, Haire T, Harris WH. Bone ingrowth into porous coated canine total hip replacements. Quantification by backscattered scanning electron microscopy and image analysis. Scanning Microsc 1989; 3(4):1051–1056; discussion 1056–1057.
120. Johnson RW. A physiological study of the blood supply of the diaphysis. J Bone Joint Surg Am 1927; 9:153–184.
121. Karrholm J, Malchau H, Snorrason F, Herberts P. Micromotion of femoral stems in total hip arthroplasty. A randomized study of cemented, hydroxyapatite-coated, and porous-coated stems with roentgen stereophotogrammetric analysis. J Bone Joint Surg Am 1994; 76(11):1692–1705.
122. Karrholm J, Snorrason F. Migration of porous coated acetabular prostheses fixed with screws: roentgen stereophotogrammetric analysis. J Orthop Res 1992; 10(6):826–835.
123. Katz RP, Callaghan JJ, Sullivan PM, Johnston RC. Long-term results of revision total hip arthroplasty with improved cementing technique. J Bone Joint Surg Br 1997; 79(2):322–326.
124. Kavanagh BF, Dewitz MA, Ilstrup DM, Stauffer RN, Coventry MB. Charnley total hip arthroplasty with cement. Fifteen-year results. J Bone Joint Surg Am 1989; 71(10):1496–1503.
125. Kavanagh BF, Ilstrup DM, Fitzgerald RH Jr. Revision total hip arthroplasty. J Bone Join Surg Am 1985; 67(4):517–526.
126. Kavanagh BF, Wallrichs S, Dewitz M, Berry D, Currier B, Ilstrup D, Coventry MB. Charnley low-friction arthroplasty of the hip. Twenty-year results with cement. J Arthroplasty 1994; 9(3):229–234.
127. Khaw FM, Kirk LM, Morris RW, Gregg PJ. A randomised, controlled trial of cemented versus cementless press-fit condylar total knee replacement. Ten-year survival analysis. J Bone Joint Surg Br 2002; 84(5):658–666.
128. Kienapfel H, Griss P. Fixation by ingrowth. In: Rubash H, ed. The Adult Hip. Philadelphia: Lippincott–Raven, 1998:201–209.
129. Kienapfel H, Sprey C, Wilke A, Griss P. Implant fixation by bone ingrowth. J Arthroplasty 1999; 14(3):355–368.
130. Kienapfel H, Sumner DR, Turner TM, Urban RM, Galante JO. Efficacy of autograft and freeze-dried allograft to enhance fixation of porous coated implants in the presence of interface gaps. J Orthop Res 1992; 10(3):423–433.
131. Kim YH, Kim JS, Cho SH. Primary total hip arthroplasty with a cementless porous-coated anatomic total hip prosthesis: 10- to 12-year results of prospective and consecutive series. J Arthroplasty 1999; 14(5):538–548.
132. Kim YH, Kim JS, Cho SH. Primary total hip arthroplasty with the AML total hip prosthesis. Clin Orthop 1999; (360):147–158.
133. Kim YH, Kook HK, Kim JS. Total hip replacement with a cementless acetabular component and a cemented femoral component in patients younger than fifty years of age. J Bone Joint Surg Am 2002; 84-A(5):770–774.

134. Kim YH, Oh SH, Kim JS. Primary total hip arthroplasty with a second-generation cementless total hip prosthesis in patients younger than fifty years of age. J Bone Joint Surg Am 2003; 85-A(1):109–114.

135. Kitsugi T, Yamamuro T, Nakamura T, Oka M. Influence of disodium (1-hydroxythylidene) diphosphonate on bone ingrowth into porous, titanium fiber-mesh implants. J Arthroplasty 1995; 10(2):245–253.

136. Kody MH, Kabo JM, Markolf KL, Dorey FJ, Amstutz HC. Strength of initial mechanical fixation of screw ring acetabular components. Clin Orthop 1990; (257):146–153.

137. Kronick JL, Barba ML, Paprosky WG. Extensively coated femoral components in young patients. Clin Orthop 1997; (344):263–274.

138. Kurz LT, Garfin SR, Booth RE Jr. Harvesting autogenous iliac bone grafts. A review of complications and techniques. Spine 1989; 14(12):1324–1331.

139. Kwong LM, O'Connor DO, Sedlacek RC, Krushell RJ, Maloney WJ, Harris WH. A quantitative in vitro assessment of fit and screw fixation on the stability of a cementless hemispherical acetabular component. J Arthroplasty 1994; 9(2):163–170.

140. LaBerge M, Bobyn JD, Drouin G, Rivard CH. Evaluation of metallic personalized hemiarthroplasty: a canine patellofemoral model. J Biomed Mater Res 1992; 26(2):239–254.

141. Lamerigts NM, Buma P, Aspenberg P, Schreurs BW, Slooff TJ. Role of growth factors in the incorporation of unloaded bone allografts in the goat. Clin Orthop 1999; (368):260–270.

142. Laskin RS. Tricon-M uncemented total knee arthroplasty. A review of 96 knees followed for longer than 2 years. J Arthroplasty 1988; 3(1):27–38.

143. Lee TM, Wang BC, Yang YC, Chang E, Yang CY. Comparison of plasma-sprayed hydroxyapatite coatings and hydroxyapatite/tricalcium phosphate composite coatings: in vivo study. J Biomed Mater Res 2001; 55(3): 360–367.

144. Lembert E, Galante J, Rostoker W. Fixation of skeletal replacement by fiber metal composites. Clin Orthop 1972; 87:303–310.

145. Leopold SS, Rosenberg AG, Bhatt RD, Sheinkop MB, Quigley LR, Galante JO. Cementless acetabular revision. Evaluation at an average of 10.5 years. Clin Orthop 1999; (369):179–186.

146. Lewis CG, Jones LC, Hungerford DS. Effects of grafting on porous metal ingrowth. A canine model. J Arthroplasty 1997; 12(4):451–460.

147. Lind M, Overgaard S, Bunger C, Soballe K. Improved bone anchorage of hydroxypatite coated implants compared with tricalcium-phosphate coated implants in trabecular bone in dogs. Biomaterials 1999; 20(9):803–808.

148. Lind M, Overgaard S, Ongpipattanakul B, Nguyen T, Bunger C, Soballe K. Transforming growth factor-beta 1 stimulates bone ongrowth to weight-loaded tricalcium phosphate coated implants: an experimental study in dogs. J Bone Joint Surg Br 1996; 78(3):377–382.

149. Lisecki EJ, Cook SD, Dalton JE. Attachment of HA coated and uncoated porous implants is influenced by methotrexate and coumadine [abstract]. Trans Orthop Res Soc 1992; 17:368.

150. Lombardi AV Jr, Engh GA, Volz RG, Albrigo JL, Brainard BJ. Fracture/dissociation of the polyethylene in metal-backed patellar components in total knee arthroplasty. J Bone Joint Surg Am 1988; 70(5):675–679.

151. Macey LR, Kana SM, Jingushi S, Terek RM, Borretos J, Bolander ME. Defects of early fracture-healing in experimental diabetes. J Bone Joint Surg Am 1989; 71(5):722–733.

152. Malchau H, Herberts P, Ahnfelt L. Prognosis of total hip replacement in Sweden. Follow-up of 92,675 operations performed 1978–1990. Acta Orthop Scand 1993; 64(5):497–506.

153. Maloney WJ, et al. Fixation, polyethylene wear, and pelvic osteolysis in primary total hip replacement. Clin Orthop 1999; (369):157–164.

154. Maloney WJ, Sychterz C, Bragdon C, McGovern T, Jasty M, Engh CA, Harris WH. The Otto Aufranc Award. Skeletal response to well fixed femoral components inserted with and without cement. Clin Orthop 1996; (333):15–26.

155. Maloney WJ, Woolson ST. Increasing incidence of femoral osteolysis in association with uncemented Harris–Galante total hip arthroplasty. A follow-up report. J Arthroplasty 1996; 11(2):130–134.

156. Manley MT, Capello WN, D'Antonio JA, Edidin AA, Geesink RG. Fixation of acetabular cups without cement in total hip arthroplasty. A comparison of three different implant surfaces at a minimum duration of follow-up of five years. J Bone Joint Surg Am 1998; 80(8):1175–1185.

157. Maric Z, Karpman RR. Early failure of noncemented porous coated anatomic total hip arthroplasty. Clin Orthop 1992; (278):116–120.

158. Markel DC, Femino JE, Farkas P, Markel SF. Analysis of lower extremity embolic material after total knee arthroplasty in a canine model. J Arthroplasty 1999; 14(2):227–232.

159. Matthews LS, Goldstein SA. The prosthesis–bone interface in total knee arthroplasty. Clin Orthop 1992; (276):50–55.

160. McAuley JP, Culpepper WJ, Engh CA. Total hip arthroplasty. Concerns with extensively porous coated femoral components. Clin Orthop 1998; (355): 182–188.

161. McAuley JP, Sychterz CJ, Engh CA Sr. Influence of porous coating level on proximal femoral remodeling. A postmortem analysis. Clin Orthop 2000; (371):146–153.

162. McCaskie AW, Deehan DJ, Green TP, Lock KR, Thompson JR, Harper WM, Gregg PJ. Randomised, prospective study comparing cemented and cementless total knee replacement: results of press-fit condylar total knee replacement at five years. J Bone Joint Surg Br 1998; 80(6):971–975.

163. McCracken M, Lemons JE, Rahemtulla F, Prince CW, Feldman D. Bone response to titanium alloy implants placed in diabetic rats. Int J Oral Maxillofac Impl 2000; 15(3):345–354.

164. McDonald DJ, Fitzgerald RH Jr, Chao EY. The enhancement of fixation of a porous-coated femoral component by autograft and allograft in the dog. J Bone Joint Surg Am 1988; 70(5):728–737.

165. McKibbin B. The biology of fracture healing in long bones. J Bone Joint Surg Br 1978; 60-B(2):150–162.

166. McLaughlin JR, Lee KR. Total hip arthroplasty in young patients. 8- to 13-year results using an uncemented stem. Clin Orthop 2000; (373):153–163.
167. McLaughlin JR, Lee KR. Total hip arthroplasty with an uncemented femoral component. Excellent results at ten-year follow-up. J Bone Joint Surg Br 1997; 79(6):900–907.
168. Mittelmeier H. Report on the first decennium of clinical experience with a cementless ceramic total hip replacement. Acta Orthop Belg 1985; 51(2–3): 367–376.
169. Moreland JR, Moreno MA. Cementless femoral revision arthroplasty of the hip: minimum 5 years followup. Clin Orthop 2001; (393):194–201.
170. Morrey BF, Kavanagh BF. Complications with revision of the femoral component of total hip arthroplasty. Comparison between cemented and uncemented techniques. J Arthroplasty 1992; 7(1):71–79.
171. Moucha CS, Einhorn TA. Enhancement of sketal repair. In: Trafton PG, ed. Skeletal Trauma: Basic Science, Management, and Reconstruction. Philadelphia: Saunders, 2003:639–659.
172. Muller-Mai C, Schmitz HJ, Strunz V, Fuhrmann G, Fritz T, Gross UM. Tissues at the surface of the new composite material titanium/glass-ceramic for replacement of bone and teeth. J Biomed Mater Res 1989; 23(10):1149–1168.
173. Mulroy RD Jr, Harris WH. The effect of improved cementing techniques on component loosening in total hip replacement. An 11-year radiographic review. J Bone Joint Surg Br 1990; 72(5):757–760.
174. Mulroy WF, Harris WH. Revision total hip arthroplasty with use of so-called second-generation cementing techniques for aseptic loosening of the femoral component. A fifteen-year-average follow-up study. J Bone Joint Surg Am 1996; 78(3):325–330.
175. Nelson CL, Gioe TJ, Cheng EY, Thompson RC Jr. Implant selection in revision total knee arthroplasty. J Bone Joint Surg Am 2003; 85-A(suppl 1):S43–51.
176. Nilsson KG, Karrholm J, Ekelund L, Magnusson P. Evaluation of micromotion in cemented vs uncemented knee arthroplasty in osteoarthrosis and rheumatoid arthritis. Randomized study using roentgen stereophotogrammetric analysis. J Arthroplasty 1991; 6(3):265–278.
177. Onsten I, Berzins A, Shott S, Sumner DR. Accuracy and precision of radiostereometric analysis in the measurement of THR femoral component translations: human and canine in vitro models. J Orthop Res 2001; 19(6):1162–1167.
178. Owen TD, Moran CG, Smith SR, Pinder IM. Results of uncemented porous-coated anatomic total hip replacement. J Bone Joint Surg Br 1994; 76(2):258–262.
179. Pellicci PM, Wilson PD Jr, Sledge CB, Salvati EA, Ranawat CS, Poss R, Callaghan JJ. Long-term results of revision total hip replacement. A follow-up report. J Bone Joint Surg Am 1985; 67(4):513–516.
180. Peters CL, Hennessey R, Barden RM, Galante JO, Rosenberg AG. Revision total knee arthroplasty with a cemented posterior-stabilized or constrained condylar prosthesis: a minimum 3-year and average 5-year follow-up study. J Arthroplasty 1997; 12(8):896–903.
181. Peters CL, Rivero DP, Kull LR, Jacobs JJ, Rosenberg AG, Galante JO. Revision total hip arthroplasty without cement: subsidence of proximally porous-coated femoral components. J Bone Joint Surg Am 1995; 77(8):1217–1226.

182. Peters PC Jr, Engh GA, Dwyer KA, Vinh TN. Osteolysis after total knee arthroplasty without cement. J Bone Joint Surg Am 1992; 74(6):864–876.
183. Pidhorz LE, Urban RM, Jacobs JJ, Sumner DR, Galante JO. A quantitative study of bone and soft tissues in cementless porous-coated acetabular components retrieved at autopsy. J Arthroplasty 1993; 8(2):213–225.
184. Pierschbacher MD, Hayman EG, Ruoslahti E. Location of the cell-attachment site in fibronectin with monoclonal antibodies and proteolytic fragments of the molecule. Cell 1981; 26(2 Pt 2):259–267.
185. Pilliar RM. Porous-surfaced metallic implants for orthopedic applications. J Biomed Mater Res 1987; 21(A1 suppl):1–33.
186. Pilliar RM, Lee JM, Maniatopoulos C. Observations on the effect of movement on bone ingrowth into porous-surfaced implants. Clin Orthop 1986; (208):108–113.
187. Piraino D, Richmond B, Freed H, Belhobek G, Schils J, Stulberg B. Total knee replacement: radiologic findings in failure of porous-coated metal-backed patellar component. AJR Am J Roentgenol 1990; 155(3):555–558.
188. Poss R, Brick GW, Wright RJ, Roberts DW, Sledge CB. The effects of modern cementing techniques on the longevity of total hip arthroplasty. Orthop Clin North Am 1988; 19(3):591–598.
189. Prendergast PJ, Huiskes R, Soballe K. ESB Research Award 1996. Biophysical stimuli on cells during tissue differentiation at implant interfaces. J Biomech 1997; 30(6):539–548.
190. Pupparo F, Engh CA. Comparison of porous-threaded and smooth-threaded acetabular components of identical design. Two- to four-year results. Clin Orthop 1991; (190):201–206.
191. Ranawat CS, Peters LE, Umlas ME. Fixation of the acetabular component. The case for cement. Clin Orthop 1997; (344):207–215.
192. Raut VV, Siney PD, Wroblewski BM. Revision of the acetabular component of a total hip arthroplasty with cement in young patients without rheumatoid arthritis. J Bone Joint Surg Am 1996; 78(12):1853–1856.
193. Rhinelander FW. The normal circulation of bone and its response to surgical intervention. J Biomed Mater Res 1974; 8(1):87–90.
194. Rhinelander FW, Nelson CL, Stewart RD, Stewart CL. Experimental reaming of the proximal femur and acrylic cement implantation: vascular and histologic effects. Clin Orthop 1979; (141):74–89.
195. Rhinelander FW, Rouweyha M, Milner JC. Microvascular and histogenic responses to implantation of a porous ceramic into bone. J Biomed Mater Res 1971; 5(1):81–112.
196. Ritter MA, Keating EM, Faris PM, Brugo G. Metal-backed acetabular cups in total hip arthroplasty. J Bone Joint Surg Am 1990; 72(5):672–677.
197. Robertson DM, Pierre L, Chahal R. Preliminary observations of bone ingrowth into porous materials. J Biomed Mater Res 1976; 10(3):335–344.
198. Rosenberg AG, Andriacchi TP, Barden R, Galante JO. Patellar component failure in cementless total knee arthroplasty. Clin Orthop 1988; (236):106–114.
199. Rosenberg AG, Barden RM, Galante JO. Cemented and ingrowth fixation of the Miller–Galante prosthesis. Clinical and roentgenographic comparison after three- to six-year follow-up studies. Clin Orthop 1990; (260):71–79.

200. Rothman RH, Klemek JS, Toton JJ. The effect of iron deficiency anemia on fracture healing. Clin Orthop 1971; 77:276–283.

201. Ruoslahti E. Integrins. J Clin Invest 1991; 87(1):1–5.

202. Russotti GM, Okada Y, Fitzgerald RH Jr, Chao EY, Gorski JP. The John Charnley Award paper. Efficacy of using a bone graft substitute to enhance biological fixation of a porous metal femoral component. Hip 1987; 120–154.

203. Sacomen D, Smith RL, Song Y, Fornasier V, Goodman SB. Effects of polyethylene particles on tissue surrounding knee arthroplasties in rabbits. J Biomed Mater Res 1998; 43(2):123–130.

204. Sakalkale DP, Eng K, Hozack WJ, Rothman RH. Minimum 10-year results of a tapered cementless hip replacement. Clin Orthop 1999; (362):138–144.

205. Sandborn PM, Cook SD, Spires WP, Kester MA. Tissue response to porous-coated implants lacking initial bone apposition. J Arthroplasty 1988; 3(4): 337–346.

206. Schmalzried TP, Harris WH. The Harris–Galante porous-coated acetabular component with screw fixation. Radiographic analysis of eighty-three primary hip replacements at a minimum of five years. J Bone Joint Surg Am 1992; 74(8):1130–1139.

207. Schreurs BW, Huiskes R, Buma P, Slooff TJ. Biomechanical and histological evaluation of a hydroxyapatite-coated titanium femoral stem fixed with an intramedullary morsellized bone grafting technique: an animal experiment on goats. Biomaterials 1996; 17(12):1177–1186.

208. Schulte KR, Callaghan JJ, Kelley SS, Johnston RC. The outcome of Charnley total hip arthroplasty with cement after a minimum twenty-year follow-up. The results of one surgeon. J Bone Joint Surg Am 1993; 75(7):961–975.

209. Shah AK, Sinha RK, Hickok NJ, Tuan RS. High-resolution morphometric analysis of human osteoblastic cell adhesion on clinically relevant orthopedic alloys. Bone 1999; 24(5):499–506.

210. Shaw JA, Wilson SC, Bruno A, Paul EM. Comparison of primate and canine models for bone ingrowth experimentation, with reference to the effect of ovarian function on bone ingrowth potential. J Orthop Res 1994; 12(2):268–273.

211. Shimagaki H, Bechtold JE, Sherman RE, Gustilo RB. Stability of initial fixation of the tibial component in cementless total knee arthroplasty. J Orthop Res 1990; 8(1):64–71.

212. Shimazaki K, Mooney V. Comparative study of porous hydroxyapatite and tricalcium phosphate as bone substitute. J Orthop Res 1985; 3(3):301–310.

213. Shimizu T, Mehdi R, Yoshimura Y, Yoshikawa H, Nomura S, Miyazono K, Takaoka K. Sequential expression of bone morphogenetic protein, tumor necrosis factor, and their receptors in bone-forming reaction after mouse femoral marrow ablation. Bone 1998; 23(2):127–133.

214. Smith SE, Estok DM II, Harris WH. 20-year experience with cemented primary and conversion total hip arthroplasty using so-called second-generation cementing techniques in patients aged 50 years or younger. J Arthroplasty 2000; 15(3):263–273.

215. Smith SE, Estok DM II, Harris WH. Average 12-year outcome of a chrome–cobalt, beaded, bony ingrowth acetabular component. J Arthroplasty 1998; 13(1):50–60.

216. Smith SW, Estok DM II, Harris WH. Total hip arthroplasty with use of second-generation cementing techniques. An eighteen-year-average follow-up study. J Bone Joint Surg Am 1998; 80(11):1632–1640.

217. Soballe K, Hansen ES, Brockstedt-Rasmussen H, Bunger C. Hydroxyapatite coating converts fibrous tissue to bone around loaded implants. J Bone Joint Surg Br 1993; 75(2):270–278.

218. Soballe K, Hansen ES, Rasmussen H, Jorgensen PH, Bunger C. Tissue ingrowth into titanium and hydroxyapatite-coated implants during stable and unstable mechanical conditions. J Orthop Res 1992; 10(2):285–299.

219. Stauffer RN. Ten-year follow-up study of total hip replacement. J Bone Joint Surg Am 1982; 64(7):983–990.

220. Stulberg BN, Watson JT, Stulberg SD, Bauer TW, Manley MT. A new model to assess tibial fixation in knee arthroplasty. I. Histologic and roentgenographic results. ClinOrthop 1991; (263):288–302.

221. Stulberg BN, Watson JT, Stulberg SD, Bauer TW, Manley MT. A new model to assess tibial fixation. II. Concurrent histologic and biomechanical observations. Clin Orthop 1991; (263):303–309.

222. Stulberg SD, Stulberg BN, Hamati Y, Tsao A. Failure mechanisms of metal-backed patellar components. Clin Orthop 1988; (236):88–105.

223. Sumner DR. Bone ingrowth implications for establishment and maintenance of cementless porous-coated interfaces. In: Rosenberg AG, ed. Orthopaedic Knowledge Update: Hip and Knee Reconstruction. Rosemont: American Academy of Orthopaedic Surgeons, 1995:57–68.

224. Sumner DR. Bone remodeling of the proximal femur. In: Rubash H, ed. The Adult Hip. New York: Lippincott-Raven, 1998:211–216.

225. Sumner DR, Berzins A, Turner TM, Igloria R, Natarajan RN. Initial in vitro stability of the tibial component in a canine model of cementless total knee replacement. J Biomech 1994; 27(7):929–939.

226. Sumner DR, Bryan JM, Urban RM, Kuszak JR. Measuring the volume fraction of bone ingrowth: a comparison of three techniques. J Orthop Res 1990; 8(3):448–452.

227. Sumner DR., Galante JO. Bone ingrowth. In: Envarls CM, ed. Surgery of the Musculoskeletal System. New York: Churchill Livingstone, 1990:151–176.

228. Sumner DR, Jasty M, Jacobs JJ, Urban RM, Bragdon CR, Harris WH, Galante JO. Histology of porous-coated acetabular components. 25 cementless cups retrieved after arthroplasty. Acta Orthop Scand 1993; 64(6): 619–626.

229. Sumner DR, Kienapfel H, Jacobs JJ, Urban RM, Turner TM, Galante JO. Bone ingrowth and wear debris in well–fixed cementless porous-coated tibial components removed from patients. J Arthroplasty 1995; 10(2):157–167.

230. Sumner DR, Turner TM, Dawson D, Rosenberg AG, Urban RM, Galante JO. Effect of pegs and screws on bone ingrowth in cementless total knee arthroplasty. Clin Orthop 1994; (309):150–155.

231. Sumner DR, Turner TM, Pierson RH, Kienapfel H, Urban RM, Liebner EJ, Galante JO. Effects of radiation on fixation of non-cemented porous-coated implants in a canine model. J Bone Joint Surg Am 1990; 72(10): 1527–1533.

232. Sumner DR, Turner TM, Purchio AF, Gombotz WR, Urban RM, Galante JO. Enhancement of bone ingrowth by transforming growth factor-beta. J Bone Joint Surg Am 1995; 77(8):1135–1147.

233. Sumner DR, Turner TM, Urban RM. Animal models of bone ingrowth and joint replacement. In: An YH, Friedman RJ, eds. Animal models in Orthopaedic Research. Boca Raton: CRC Press, 1999:407–425.

234. Suva LJ, Seedor JG, Endo N, Quartuccio HA, Thompson DD, Bab I, Rodan G. Pattern of gene expression following rat tibial marrow ablation. J Bone Miner Res 1993; 8(3):379–388.

235. Sychterz CJ, Claus AM, Engh CA. What we have learned about long-term cementless fixation from autopsy retrievals. Clin Orthop 2002; (405):79–91.

236. Sychterz CJ, Engh CA. The influence of clinical factors on periprosthetic bone remodeling. Clin Orthop 1996; (322):285–292.

237. Tagil M, Jeppsson C, Aspenberg P. Bone graft incorporation. Effects of osteogenic protein-1 and impaction. Clin Orthop 2000; (371):240–245.

238. Tanaka H, Barnes J, Liang CT. Effect of age on the expression of insulin-like growth factor-I, interleukin-6, and transforming growth factor-beta mRNAs in rat femurs following marrow ablation. Bone 1996; 18(5):473–478.

239. Templeton JE, Callaghan JJ, Goetz DD, Sullivan PM, Johnston RC. Revision of a cemented acetabular component to a cementless acetabular component. A ten to fourteen-year follow-up study. J Bone Joint Surg Am 2001; 83–A(11): 1706–1711.

240. Thanner J, Karrholm J, Herberts P, Malchau H. Porous cups with and without hydroxylapatite–tricalcium phosphate coating: 23 matched pairs evaluated with radiostereometry. J Arthroplasty 1999; 14(3):266–271.

241. Thompson Z, Miclau T, Hu D, Helms JA. A model for intramembranous ossification during fracture healing. J Orthop Res 2002; 20(5):1091–1098.

242. Tooke SM, Nugent PJ, Chotivichit A, Goodman W, Kabo JM. Comparison of in vivo cementless acetabular fixation. Clin Orthop 1988; (235):253–260.

243. Trancik T, Mills W, Vinson N. The effect of indomethacin, aspirin, and ibuprofen on bone ingrowth into a porous-coated implant. Clin Orthop 1989; (249):113–121.

244. Turner TM, Sumner DR, Urban RM, Igloria R, Galante JO. Maintenance of proximal cortical bone with use of a less stiff femoral component in hemiarthroplasty of the hip without cement. An investigation in a canine model at six months and two years. J Bone Joint Surg Am 1997; 79(9): 1381–1390.

245. Turner TM, Sumner DR, Urban RM, Rivero DP, Galante JO. A comparative study of porous coatings in a weight-bearing total hip-arthroplasty model. J Bone Joint Surg Am 1986; 68(9):1396–1409.

246. Turner TM, Urban RM, Sumner DR, Galante JO. Revision, without cement, of aseptically loose, cemented total hip prostheses. Quantitative comparison of the effects of four types of medullary treatment on bone ingrowth in a canine model. J Bone Joint Surg Am 1993; 75(6):845–862.

247. Turner TM, Urban RM, Sumner DR, Skipor AK, Galante JO. Bone ingrowth into the tibial component of a canine total condylar knee replacement prosthesis. J Orthop Res 1989; 7(6):893–901.

248. Uchida A, Nade S, McCartney E, Ching W. Bone ingrowth into three different porous ceramics implanted into the tibia of rats and rabbits. J Orthop Res 1985; 3(1):65–77.
249. Urban RM, Jacobs JJ, Sumner DR, Peters CL, Voss FR, Galante JO. The bone–implant interface of femoral stems with non-circumferential porous coating. J Bone Joint Surg Am 1996; 78(7):1068–1081.
250. Urist MR. Bone: formation by autoinduction. Science 1965; 150(698):893–899.
251. van Loon CJ, de Waal Malefijt MC, Buma P, Stolk T, Verdonschot N, Tromp AM, Huiskes R, Barneveld A. Autologous morsellised bone grafting restores uncontained femoral bone defects in knee arthroplasty. An in vivo study in horses. J Bone Joint Surg Br 2000; 82(3):436–444.
252. Virolainen P, Inoue N, Nagao M, Ohnishi I, Frassica F, Chao EY. Autogenous onlay grafting for enhancement of extracortical tissue formation over porous-coated segmental replacement prostheses. J Bone Joint Surg Am 1999; 81(4):493–499.
253. Walker PS, Rodger RF, Miegel RE, Schiller AL, Deland JT, Robertson DD. An investigation of a compliant interface for press-fit joint replacement. J Orthop Res 1990; 8(3):453–463.
254. Walsh WR, Sherman P, Howlett CR, Sonnabend DH, Ehrlich MG. Fracture healing in a rat osteopenia model. Clin Orthop 1997; (342):218–227.
255. Wasielewski RC, Parks N, Williams I, Surprenant H, Collier JP, Engh G. Tibial insert undersurface as a contributing source of polyethylene wear debris. Clin Orthop 1997; (345):53–59.
256. Weeden SH, Paprosky WG. Minimal 11-year follow-up of extensively porous-coated stems in femoral revision total hip arthroplasty. J Arthroplasty 2002; 17(4suppl 1):134–137.
257. Welsh RP, Pilliar RM, Macnab I. Surgical implants. The role of surface porosity in fixation to bone and acrylic. J Bone Joint Surg Am 1971; 53(5):963–977.
258. Whiteside LA. Cementless total knee replacement. Nine- to 11-year results and 10-year survivorship analysis. Clin Orthop 1994; (309):185–192.
259. Wilke A, Orth J, Lomb M, Fuhrmann R, Kienapfel H, Griss P, Franke RP. Biocompatibility analysis of different biomaterials in human bone marrow cell cultures. J Biomed Mater Res 1998; 40(2):301–306.
260. Winet H, Bao JY. Fibroblast growth factor-2 alters the effect of eroding polylactide–polyglycolide on osteogenesis in the bone chamber. J Biomed Mater Res 1998; 40(4):567–576.
261. Winet H, Bao JY, Moffat R. Neo-osteogenesis of haversian trabeculae through a bone chamber implanted in a rabbit tibial cortex: a control model. Calcif Tissue Int 1990; 47(1):24–34.
262. Wise MW III, Robertson ID, Lachiewicz PF, Thrall DE, Metcalf M. The effect of radiation therapy on the fixation strength of an experimental porous-coated implant in dogs. Clin Orthop 1990; (261):276–280.
263. Woolson ST, Adler NS. The effect of partial or full weight bearing ambulation after cementless total hip arthroplasty. J Arthroplasty 2002; 17(7):820–825.
264. Wroblewski BM. 15–21-year results of the Charnley low–friction arthroplasty. Clin Orthop 1986; (211):30–35.

265. Wykman A, Lundberg A. Subsidence of porous coated noncemented femoral components in total hip arthroplasty. A roentgen stereophotogrammetric analysis. J Arthroplasty 1992; 7(2):197–200.
266. Yamada KM. Adhesive recognition sequences. J Biol Chem 1991; 266(20):12,809–12,812.
267. Younger EM, Chapman MW. Morbidity at bone graft donor sites. J Orthop Trauma 1989; 3(3):192–195.

3

Fixation of Implants with Bone Cement

Hans Georg Willert and Georg Köster

University of Göttingen, Göttingen, Germany

INTRODUCTION TO THE USE OF POLYMETHYLMETHACRYLATE AS BONE CEMENT

During the first half of the 20th century, orthopaedic surgeons attempted to replace destroyed or worn-out sections of diseased articulating joints with prosthetic implants made of metal or plastic and thus to improve the functional mobility. Examples include the hip endoprostheses of Wiles, McKee, Moore, or Thompson and the femoral head cups of Smith-Petersen or Judet. Often however, these implants still caused pain because they could not be anchored firmly enough in the bone.

It was thanks to Charnley (1) that polymer cement came to be recommended as a new method of fixing hip joint endoprostheses in the bone. At this time various investigators had already tested this cement in animal experiments (2,3) and in clinical practice (4), but it was Charnley who first used it routinely in patients in the late 1950s (5,6). Chemically, the polymer cement is [poly-] methyl- or butylmethacrylate (PMMA) and is now available from various manufacturers as *bone cement* (e.g., CMW®, Palacos®, Simplex®, Sulfix®). The ingredients are two separately provided components: a powder consisting of tiny beads of completely polymerized PMMA, a radiographic contrast medium such as barium sulfate or zirconia, and a starter to initiate the polymerization process. The second component is the liquid monomer, which also contains a stabilizer. In the operating room a few minutes before implantation into the bone, the polymer powder and liquid monomer are mixed together and stirred to form a paste. The liquid monomer partially dissolves the surface of the powder beads; at the same time, it starts to polymerize and binds the beads together, embedding them in the matrix as it forms.

This yields a composite material. As the polymerization of the monomer progresses, the consistency of the cement paste becomes even thicker until it completely hardens. The bone cements currently used need about 12–15 minutes to harden completely (from stirring to complete hardening). The "processing time" is in the middle section of this period. To guarantee optimal anchorage of the prostheses in bone, the cement paste must be inserted into the implant bed in a malleable consistency, i.e., it should neither be too runny nor too thick. At the right consistency, the polymerizing bone cement can adapt to the irregularities of the bone, penetrate the opened medullary cavities, and then receive the prosthetic component. Once the prosthesis has been inserted, and the processing time ended, the cement then still needs a few more minutes to harden completely.

Once Charnley had laid the foundation for using the bone cement (1,5,6), both the bone cements and their use, including the preparation of the bony implant bed, were progressively modified and improved right up to today's fourth generation of cementing technology. To ensure that air bubbles are not created during the mixing step, the cement components are mixed in special containers, some even using vacuum to evacuate the air. The doughy form of the paste is packed into the implant bed, not using fingers, but by a syringe-like device. This together with the insertion of a drain is intended to prevent the cement paste from mixing with the blood. Prior to cementing, the implant bed is cleaned of residual blood and bone marrow by means of irrigation, brushing, and the distal end of the femoral medullary cavity is sealed with a metal or polymer stopper. A lower viscosity cement is also used which, when placed under pressure, penetrates the medullary cavities more effectively. A uniformly thick cement mantle around the prosthesis is achieved by, for example, centralizing the stem of the femoral prosthesis.

These evolutionary modifications and improvements undoubtedly help to avoid errors in using the bone cement and to increase the life span of stably anchored cemented prostheses. Two main disadvantages associated with the PMMA bone cement, however could neither be removed nor replaced easily.

DISADVANTAGES OF PMMA BONE CEMENT AND RESULTANT ISSUES FOR CLINICAL USE

There are primarily two deficiencies of this biomaterial which relate to the way the bone cement is prepared in the operating room, and its structure:

1. The end product is formed as a composite material only at the site of implantation, amidst the living tissue where it is subject to interactions that are difficult to control.
2. The rigidity of the composite bone cement is particularly inadequate for tensile stresses.

Regarding 1: What Effect Does the Formation of the Definitive Composite Material Have at the Site of Implantation?

Disruption of the Surface Structure of the Cement Implant by Monomer Depletion

Once the bone cement paste has been stirred, it must be inserted into the bony bed while it is still easily malleable in a doughy state. Polymerization of the monomer has not yet been completed. Some free monomer is thus still present. This has a great affinity for fats or fat-containing organic material in particular, and is dissolved out of the surface layers of the cement paste by that material. The layer of cement that comes into contact with tissue is thereby depleted of monomer and there is no longer sufficient monomer to bind the polymer beads tightly together. The beads are thus left isolated, or remain in contact with the main mass of the cement, only by means of narrow cement bridges (Fig. 1) (7). The result is disruption of the surface structure of the implanted cement, which is equivalent to mechanical weakening. Under functional loading of the cement–bone interface, individual beads or their aggregates can break off and initiate fragmentation of the bone–cement surface.

Necrosis of Bone and Bone Marrow Adjacent to the Bone Cement

Heat generated during polymerization of the monomer is conducted into the surrounding tissue. Temperatures as high as 56°C are not uncommon. The unused monomer is also released to the tissue and is cytotoxic. In addition to the unavoidable disturbance of the blood circulation as a result of surgically preparing the implant bed, the heat of polymerization and the toxicity of the monomer contribute to necroses of the adjacent bone marrow and bone at the interface with the cement.

Polymerization Shrinkage

Contrary to the assertion originally made by Charnley that the cement expands in the implant bed, it is actually subject to some shrinkage as the monomer component hardens by polymerization. This shrinkage is relatively small but can lead to the formation of a narrow crack at the bone–cement interface and reduce the hoped-for intimate contact.

(A) **(B)** **(C)**

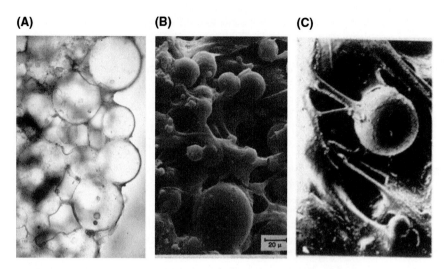

Figure 1 Fully polymerized PMMA bone cement. (**A**) Microphotograph of a cross section through a specimen through a piece of bone cement polymerized in air. The spheres of the prepolymerized powder are completely bound together by monomer which polymerized after mixing. (**B** and **C**) Scanning electron microscopic photograph of the surface of bone cement implanted in a human femur. The spheres at the surface of the implant are only incompletely connected or stay isolated due to the release of monomer into the surrounding tissue.

Regarding 2: What Are the Effects of Inadequate Rigidity of the Composite Bone Cement Material?

Air, Blood, and Liquid Inclusions in the Cement

Whereas folding and laminations with the admixture of blood do not adversely affect the bending strength and compressive strength of the implanted cement, larger inclusions of air, blood, and other liquids reduce the mechanical strength of the cement if they cannot escape. This can be prevented by effective drainage from the implant bed.

Conversion of the Implant Bed

The repair process of the damaged tissue directly adjoining the cement starts immediately after implantation, and resembles fracture healing. The necrotic tissues are progressively replaced by vital tissues, and the medullary cavities are again filled with blood-forming bone marrow. Necrotic bone is broken down and new bone is formed in its place, but only reaches the cement interface in places, so that once bone conversion has been completed, the support provided for the cement by bone is less extensive than immediately after implantation. Instead, bone marrow and bone are often separated from the cement by a connective tissue membrane that is intermittently thick, and in many places permeated with foreign-body giant cells (8).

Fissuring of the Cement

Micro-fissures starting from the periphery of individual polymer beads more or less well integrated into the compound, air bubbles or contrast medium inclusions, or from the interface between the cement and the tissue, may be formed under functional loading (Fig. 2). These fissures propagate by running primarily in the network of the secondarily polymerized matrix. The result is fragmentation of the cement, which only increases over time. Cells and connective tissues grow into the emerging cracks and the supporting function of the cement for the prosthesis which it anchors, is lost. Further fragmentation can even trigger a foreign-body reaction to the released particles at the bone–cement interface. This reaction is then accompanied by granuloma formation and the development of osteolysis.

Debonding and Fractures of the Cement Socket

The cement mantle around the metal stem of the femoral component, for example, is more elastic than the metal of the prosthesis. Muscle tension and functional loading tend to displace the prosthetic stem, especially

(A)   **(B)**   **(C)**

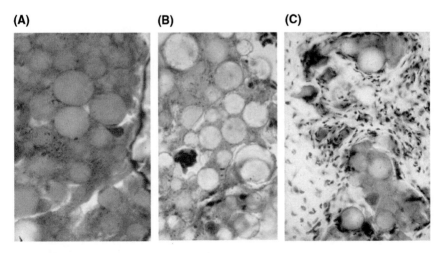

Figure 2 Microfissures in PMMA bone cement, implants and disintegration of the cement implant. (**A** and **B**) Microphotograph of a cross section through a specimen of bone cement which had been implanted in a human femur: Cells are invading several fissures which run between the spheres in the "matrix," formed by the in situ polymerized monomer. (**C**) Disintegration of the bone cement implant into small pieces gives rise to foreign body granulomas at the interface between bone and bone cement. (*See color insert.*)

proximally in the region of the greater trochanter, by means of loading the calcar and in torsion. While this may lead to minimal displacements at the interface between cement and prosthesis, the prosthesis loses its bond with the cement, resulting in debonding. Displacement of the prosthesis vis-à-vis the proximal end of the femur results in rubbing of the prosthetic stem against the bone cement. The abrasion results in polishing of the metal surface and the PMMA, yielding tiny particles. Mechanically it is not only the pressure but also tensile forces that act on the cement in the proximal femur, i.e., loading, for which the cement has very little strength.

Under functional loading there are axial forces on the prosthesis, which presses the generally conical prosthetic component into the cement mantle in an axial direction. This results in hoop stresses in the cement, and in turn acts as tensile forces in the cement mantle (9,10).

As long as the outer surface of the cement mantle is firmly contained and supported by the bone bed, these forces can be directed into the bone and can compensate for the tensile stresses in the cement. However, if the normally stiff bone surrounding the cement in the implant bed is replaced by softly yielding connective tissue, the cement cannot withstand the tensile stress and breaks. Fractures occur in the cement mantle and the component is loosened. Using an endoscope specially developed for this purpose, Köster et al. (11), examined the cement sockets of 72 femoral prostheses (24 autopsy specimens and 48 revisions). They reported that irrespective of prosthesis design, clefts in the form of fissures and fractures in the cement mantle were visible in all the autopsy cases and in 92% of the revisions. While the signs of debonding were predominantly longitudinal, horizontal clefts were also observed in nearly half the patients. The clefts were connected with cement defects and/or the proximal end of the cement socket and were of differing lengths. From the age of the fissures and fractures it could be seen whether and to what extent connective tissue had grown into the clefts as a biological reaction emanating from the bony implant bed. In 75% of the autopsy cases and 81% of the revisions, the connective tissue had already spread to large areas of the interface between stem and cement. In 75% of the revision cases, loosening of the stem in the cement socket had also affected its anchorage in the bony bed and the cemented femoral component as a whole had loosened (9).

The loosening cascade: From his findings, Köster et al. reconstructed the time course of the incessant progressive loosening of the femoral prosthesis, the stages of which he called the "loosening cascade" and defined as follows: (1) debonding, (2) development of fissures and fractures in the cement socket, (3) growth of connective tissue from the bony implant bed into the clefts and spread in the interface between prosthesis stem and cement, and (4) loss of anchorage by the cement socket in the bone and thus failure of the implants in the form of prosthesis loosening (Fig. 3).

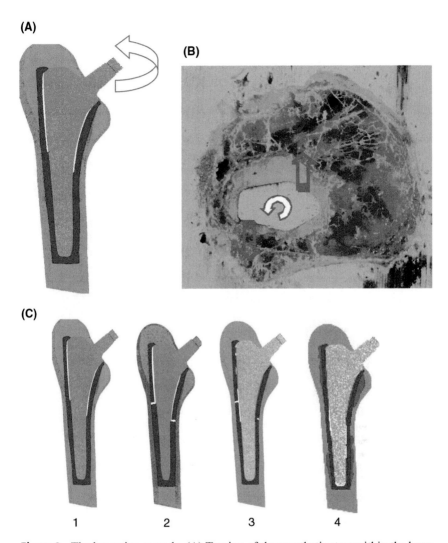

Figure 3 The loosening cascade. (**A**) Torsion of the prosthetic stem within the bone cement cuff causes debonding. (**B**) Torsion of the prosthetic stem puts the bone cement cuff under tensile stress. (**C**) Cascade of loosening: 1, debonding; 2, development of fissures and fractures in the bone cement mantle; 3, ingrowth of connective tissue in fissures and fractures and the interface between stem and bone; 4, loss of fixation of the bone cement cuff to the bone of the implant bed leads to a complete loosening of the femoral prosthesis. (*See color insert.*)

QUESTION OF THE GOLD STANDARD

Gold Standard of Hip Prostheses Fixed with Bone Cement

The anchorage of hip prostheses with bone cement is still a widespread, commonly used procedure. In the hands of experienced surgeons, cementing components produce reliable and very reproducible results. Cementing has also been aided by numerous modifications of the cements available from manufacturers, plus improvements in their use and in implantation techniques. However, there are inherent inadequacies in using bone cement as a biomaterial, specifically because of its chemistry, and thus it still has detrimental effects especially in the long term. The cemented implant is subject to irreversible structural changes, both in contact with the tissue and in contact with the prosthesis and these ultimately lead, more or less inevitably, to the failure of its function as an anchoring medium. The period over which the "loosening cascade" develops is, however, very variable.

Prostheses anchored with bone cement can achieve long-term stability with good function. In the literature, for example, the Müller straight-stem prosthesis is reported to have average 10-year survival rates of 73–98% and 15-year survival rates of 82–88%. This does not, however, alter the problems presented here which are further complicated by numerous other factors such as individual surgeon operating technique and the handling of cement in surgical practice, the design of the prosthesis, and the age and gender of the patient. For this reason, cemented prostheses cannot all be expected to have the same service life. In autopsy cases examined by Köster et al. (11), the average time in situ was 8.2 years (range 2 months to 18 years) and with the revisions 8.3 years (range 2 months to 20 years). For cemented hip prostheses, 10-year survival rates of about 98% are regarded as the gold standard.

Gold Standard for Hip Prostheses Fixed Without Bone Cement

Joint replacement prostheses fixed without bone cement, specifically those made from titanium or titanium alloys, allow the bone to grow directly onto the anchoring surfaces of the prosthetic components; titanium combined with a degree of roughness can to some extent even have an "osteo-inductive" effect. The modern implantation technique of prosthesis stabilization without cement was, however, developed much later and also gained general acceptance later than the method of cement fixation introduced by Charnley. It was thus possible to report longer term results for cemented arthroplasties much earlier than for noncemented ones.

Follow-up results are also now available for cement-free prosthesis anchorage which impressively demonstrate performance as regards function and stability. Thus, the Zweymüller SL stem has average 10-year survival rates of 91.5–99% and 12-year survival rates of 98.4%. The 10-year results are thus even better than those for cemented prostheses. Thus, at the 10–12 year interval, the results for cement-free prostheses set a higher standard and could thus in the future replace the gold standard which has hitherto applied to cemented fixation.

REFERENCES

1. Charnley J. Anchorage of the femoral head prosthesis to the shaft of the femur. J Bone Joint Surg 1960; 42-B:28–30.
2. Henrichsen E, Jansen K, Krough-Poulsen W. Experimental investigation of the tissue reaction to acrylic plastics. Acta Orthop Scand 1952; 22(2):141–146.
3. Wiltse LL, Hall RH, Stenehjem JC. Experimental studies regarding the possible use of self-curing acrylic in orthopedic surgery. J Bone Joint Surg Am 1957; 39-A(4):961–972.
4. Haboush EJ. A new operation for arthroplasty of the hip based on biomechanics, photoelasticity, fast-setting dental acrylic, and other considerations. Bull Hosp Joint Dis 1953; 14(2):242–277.
5. Charnley J. Arthroplasty of the hip. Lancet 1961; 1129–1132.
6. Charnley J. The bonding of prostheses to bone by cement. J Bone Joint Surg 1964; 46-B:518–529.
7. Willert HG, Mueller K, Semlitsch M. The morphology of polymethylmethacrylate (PMMA) bone cement: surface structures and causes of their origin. Arch Orthop Trauma Surg 1979; 94(4):265–292.
8. Willert HG, Ludwig J, Semlitsch M. Reaction of bone to methacrylate after hip arthroplasty: a long-term gross, light microscopic, and scanning electron microscopic study. J Bone Joint Surg Am 1974; 56(7):1368–1382.
9. Lee AJ. The effect of mixing technique and surgical technique on the properties of bone cement. Aktuelle Probl Chir Orthop 1987; 31:145–150.
10. Lee AJ. Revision of total hips using bone cement: improvement of materials and operative technique. Acta Orthop Belg 1986; 52(3):263–270.
11. Köster G, Willert H, Buchhorn GH. Endoscopy of the femoral canal in revision arthroplasty of the hip. A new method for improving the operative technique and analysis of implant failure. Arch Orthop Trauma Surg 1999; 119(5–6): 245–252.

4

Total Hip Replacement: Incidence of Osteolysis and Clinical Presentation

Rajiv K. Sethi, Sanjeev Agarwal, Harry E. Rubash, and Arun Shanbhag

Department of Orthopaedic Surgery, Massachusetts General Hospital, Harvard Medical School, Boston, Massachusetts, U.S.A.

INTRODUCTION

Osteolysis is a result of a particle-induced biologic process at the metal–bone or cement–bone interface, resulting in bone loss. Manifestations of this type of bone loss in patients range from new radiolucency around previously well-fixed implants, which usually progress and may result in loosening, to rapidly expanding focal lesions that may result in mechanical instability or pathologic fracture. Among orthopaedic surgeons, for ease of description, the former process is generally termed aseptic loosening and the latter is widely known as "osteolysis." Due to the popular usage of these two terms, a common misconception is that each phenomenon represents a distinct clinical entity with dissimilar implications. However, it is important to appreciate that the radiological appearance of osteolysis or aseptic loosening depends on the access of the particulate debris to the metal–bone or cement–bone interface and that the underlying biologic process is the same in both instances.

The loosening of prosthetic components in the absence of infection has been a known clinical entity since the inception of joint replacement in the early 1960s. During the revision of loose cemented cups, the implant is invariably surrounded by macrophage-laden fibrous tissue at the cement–bone interface (1–5). Initially, this interfacial membrane was believed to form in response to the curing of acrylic bone cement. However, after evaluating tissues around failed prostheses, Willert and Semlitsch (6,7) demonstrated the presence of macrophage response to wear debris and concluded that the particles accumulate when pericapsular lymph drainage is overwhelmed by the particle load, and this leads to a foreign-body response and eventual loosening of the implant. Goldring et al. (8) described the synovial- like character of the interfacial membrane. Wear particles are generated within the joint space from the relative motion between intended articulating surfaces as well as unintended interfaces such as the contact of femoral prosthesis neck against the polyethylene insert, and the contact of the femoral collar against the acetabular margin. Smaller particles ($<7\,\mu$m) are generally retained within macrophages (9) and lead to production of inflammatory cytokines such as tumor necrosis factor and interleukin 1, whereas foreign-body giant cells encapsulate larger nonphagocytosable particles (10). Depending on the biocompatibility and toxicity of the debris material, there is a variable amount of cellular necrosis and associated infiltration by inflammatory cells. Particulate debris, cleared from the local area by lymphatic drainage, has been recovered from regional lymph nodes (11,12) as well as lungs and spleen.

With progressive wear, the capacity of the capsule to clear or store the wear particles is overwhelmed. In this case, all periprosthetic interfaces may be susceptible to infiltration by wear debris and granulation tissue (7,13). The associated inflammation and interfacial bone loss can compromise bony fixation of the implant, resulting in loosening (7,13). One manifestation of interfacial bone loss is a linear radiolucency about the implant that may progress to circumferential canal enlargement and endosteal bone lysis. Alternately, the bone loss may appear to be focal, manifesting as a lytic, expansile lesion (Fig. 1) (14–16). These focal lesions are associated with both stable and loose components, and may progress in size (14,17). If this process compromises the stability of the component, revision may be required. Revision may also be required for progressive bone loss leading to fracture with or without component instability (Fig. 2).

Although Willert and Semlitch's original observations involved cemented components, others have described a similar process adjacent to uncemented implants (9,13,18,19). Schmalzried et al. (13) suggested that particulate wear debris generated at the new joint surface can be carried to all periprosthetic regions that are accessible to joint fluid. It has been further suggested that the flow pattern of wear debris is determined by the degree of access to the interfaces (20–22). Dispersion of particles along the interface results in linear osteolysis (Fig. 3), whereas accumulation in discrete areas is thought to lead to focal osteolysis. The pathology of the interfacial membrane has been extensively studied. Periprosthetic membranes with sheets of macrophages in a fibrous stroma intermingled with multinucleated giant cells, polymethylmethacrylate (PMMA) particles, and metallic wear debris are a common

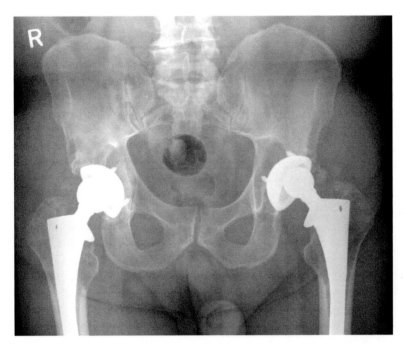

Figure 1 A 59-year-old male, 12 years following total hip arthroplasty presented with extensive pelvic osteolysis. There is eccentric wear of the polyethylene insert on the left side which is a particle generator.

finding (3,4,23,24). When interfacial tissues are placed in organ culture, they produce collagenase and prostaglandin E_2 (PGE_2), both stimulators of osteoclastic bone resorption and matrix degradation in vivo. These data support the hypothesis of Willert and Semlitsch that the interface tissue actively participates in bone resorption, possibly leading to loosening of the components (7). Since this hypothesis was first proposed, numerous investigators have shown that cellular activity within the membrane produces a variety of enzymes such as gelatinase, stromelysin and other metalloproteinases, prostaglandins, and cytokines such as interleukin-1 (IL-1α, IL-1β), IL-6, and tumor necrosis factor α (TNF-α) (25–33).

INCIDENCE

Osteolysis is the foremost long-term complication of total hip arthroplasty and in most studies evaluating long-term follow-up, it is the predominant cause of failure (34,35). There is a well-recognized direct correlation of osteolysis and wear (36) and this has important implications on the incidence of osteolysis and the bearing surface employed in hip arthroplasty.

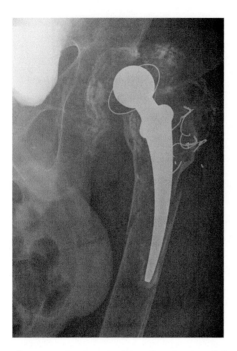

Figure 2 A 72-year-old male, 29 years following a total hip arthroplasty presented with a grossly loose femoral component, gross lysis, and periprosthetic femoral fracture. The acetabular component was loose and was exchanged to a constrained liner. The femoral reconstruction was done by proximal femoral replacement prosthesis.

Osteolysis is rarely seen with linear wear rates less than 50 μm/yr in polyethylene bearings (37). Manley et al. (38) demonstrated the importance of particle access to the bone in the development of osteolysis. Van der Vis (39) showed that fluctuating pressure applied to bone could result in osteolysis even in the absence of significant particle load.

The incidence of osteolysis in hip replacement is most easily described in terms of the components and their mode of fixation. For cemented cups, the incidence of focal osteolysis has been reported from 0% to 19%, with loss of fixation occurring at rates between 0% and 44% (15,40–49). Salvati and associates reported on 100 consecutive polyethylene cups implanted using first-generation cementing techniques. At an average follow-up of 10 years, two of the patients (3.7%) demonstrated linear osteolysis at the cement–bone interface that led to component loosening and migration. One of these was revised for progressive bone loss. No patient had expansile osteolysis. Others have reported loosening rates due to linear osteolysis of 11–23% for first-generation cemented polyethylene cups after a minimum of 10 years (40,48). At 20 year follow-up, no difference in aseptic loosening was noted

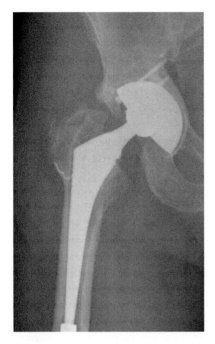

Figure 3 A 63-year-old male, 12 years following a revision of right hip presented with a loose femoral component. A linear radiolucency is seen around the femoral stem. At surgery, the femoral component was grossly loose and was revised. The acetabulum showed lucency in zone 2 and 3 but was found to be stable.

between patients younger than 55 years and patients over the age of 55 years at the time of surgery (48). Another long-term follow-up over 20 years showed a 6% overall revision rate for aseptic loosening of the acetabular component after 20 years (50). Ten percent of the patients living over 20 years had a revision for aseptic loosening. MacKenna et al. used all-polyethylene cups implanted with second-generation cementing technique in patients with developmental dysplasia or chronic dislocation of the hip. They found focal osteolysis in seven of 37 patients (19%), and in 16 of 59 patients (27%), linear osteolysis resulted in loosening after an average of 192 months. Ranawat et al. (51,52) reported two revisions for loose acetabular cups at an average eight year follow-up in 236 patients using second-generation cementing techniques and hypotensive anaesthesia. However, the overall failure rate was 7.2% and radiographic loosening was 6%. Most of the failures were in patients with rheumatoid arthritis and hip dysplasia, and radiographic loosening was present in 2.3% of patients with primary osteoarthritis after an average eight year follow-up. Second-generation cementing techniques did not show any improvement in a study by Mulroy et al. (41), with linear osteolysis leading to loosening in 44% of patients, a minimum of 14 years after implantation. Some authors believe the rates of osteolysis will increase with longer follow-up, thus warranting a repeat evaluation of results (53).

Acetabular components inserted without cement have shown encouraging results in short-and medium-term follow-up. The Harris-Galante Porous (HGP) cup consistently has achieved very low intermediate and long-term rates of osteolysis and loosening (0–2 %) (17,47,54–61). This is dependent on age of the patient and duration since surgery. Maloney et al. (62), have shown with an 81-month follow-up of Harris-Galante-I cementless acetabular components with screw fixation that 22% of hip replacements in patients younger than 50 years of age at the time of their index operation had evidence of osteolysis. In contrast, for patients older than 50 years of age at the time of surgery, only 7.8% (8 hips) had osteolysis of the pelvis. Another study (61) of 264 consecutive primary total hip replacements using the Harris–Galante I porous coated acetabular components showed no revision for aseptic loosening and only one patient had focal pelvic osteolysis. The average age of the patients was 56.8 years. In a 7- to 11-year follow-up of the Harris-Galante I acetabular cup in 79 consecutive young people with average age of 37 years, there were no revisions for loosening (63). Five patients (7.4%) had acetabular osteolysis which developed between 7 and 9 years after surgery. It is important to realize that incidence of radiological osteolysis is far more than the revision rate in most series. In 121 hybrid primary hip replacements using the Harris-Galante acetabular component, one was revised and five had radiological evidence of osteolysis at average 10-year follow-up (64). One of these five was bone grafted, but the shell was not considered loose in any of them.

However, different cementless cups have varying track records. For the porous coated anatomic (PCA) cup, rates of focal osteolysis have ranged from 1% at four years to 36% after more than five years (59,65–67). The same reports noted that loosening had an incidence of between 0% and 11%, but it was not attributed to osteolysis. However, certain variables in these studies have been implicated in the high rates of osteolysis. The patients tended to be younger with higher activity levels and 32 mm heads were commonly used. In addition, shedding of the porous coating can lead to accelerated third-body wear. Mont et al. (68) reported one revision for loose acetabular component at a mean follow-up of 72 months using the PCA acetabular cup in 109 hips. Engh et al. (69) and Zicat et al. (70) reported that focal osteolysis occurred in 20% of the patients 84–102 months after receiving nonmodular anatomic medullary locking (AML) cups with 32 mm heads, and the loosening rate was 4%. A comparison of 126 AML cups having no holes with 112 Arthropor cups having multiple holes at a minimum 10-year follow-up showed 47.6% and 47.3% osteolysis, respectively. The time of onset of osteolysis was also similar—7.5 years in Arthropor and 7.4 years in the AML cup (71).

Threaded cups such as T-TAP (Biomet, Warsaw, Indiana) have also produced high rates of osteolysis (59 of 68 patients, 87%) and osteolysis-associated loosening (26 of 68, 38%) after only six years post implantation (72). Similarly, 95 of 378 (25%) threaded Mecring (Mecron, Berlin, Germany) cups were found to be radiologically loose only 4.5 years after implantation (73). Although initially stable, screw-in cups cause a high concentration of local stress and possibly pressure necrosis. Brujin et al. (73) also suggested that such stress causes bone resorption, decreased stability, increased micromotion, and greater access of wear particles to the metal–bone interface, resulting in rapidly progressive osteolysis. Regardless of the mechanism of failure, most studies have found that threaded acetabular cups fail at sufficiently high rates to preclude their continued use.

Whereas femoral components inserted with first-generation cementing techniques loosened at rates between 11% and 30% (40,42,48), those inserted using second- or third-generation cementing techniques have enjoyed excellent results in terms of osteolysis, loosening, and revision rates. Several authors have reported the long-term incidence of focal osteolysis to be less than 8%, even in difficult reconstructions (15,41,47,49,74,75). The age at surgery has not been a significant determining factor for stem survival. Mulroy and Harris (76) reported 95% survival at 18 years using revision of the stem as the end point. Radiographic evaluation revealed no additional loose stems. Intermediate to long-term rates of loosening associated with osteolysis have increased from 1.5% to 7% at latest follow-up (15,41,47,53).

On the other hand, the incidence of osteolysis in femurs that received uncemented stems is unacceptably high. The HGP prosthesis was associated with focal osteolysis rates of 13–52% over short to intermediate follow-up periods (17,54–57,77,78). The incidence of loosening of these components is between 8% and 32%. With the PCA stem (58,65–67), the incidence of osteolysis was also quite high (13–25%) at 50- to 84-month follow-up. At 11-years follow-up with the PCA stem, Kim et al. (79) showed femoral osteolysis in 69 hips (59%) and acetabular osteolysis in 65 hips (56%). Osteolytic lesions occurred in periarticular Gruen zones 1, 2, and 7, and were not the cause of loosening. Rather, implant micromotion and shedding of the porous coating appeared to be responsible (65,80). Although studies suggested high rates (32–34%) of osteolysis with the AML stem (69,70), these lesions were also confined to Gruen zones 1 and 7, were small in size, and according to the authors conclusions, did not result in loosening. In a cohort of 348 hips in 304 patients followed for an average of 14.2 years with an AML extensively coated stem, there was no osteolysis distal to Gruen zone 1 or 7 in any case and only two stems were revised for loosening (81). Kim et al. (82) have recently demonstrated with a 11.3-year follow-up of the AML prosthesis that 38% of their hips had acetabular and femoral osteolysis and 17% had femoral osteolysis. Fractures of the greater trochanter secondary to osteolysis have been reported in 4.3% of 208 hips with AML stems followed for a mean of 12.2 years (83). Nashed et al. (59) reported that osteo-lysis occurred in 13 of 15 (87%) hip arthroplasties using a BIAS (Zimmer, Warsaw, Indiana) stem with a titanium head and in 16 of 74 (22%) arthroplasties using a cobalt–chrome femoral head. Loosening associated with osteolysis occurred in 40% and 14% of these patients, respectively. The incidence of osteolysis was 9% for the Identifit (Thackeray, Leeds, England) stem without porous coating, although loosening was more fre-quent (28%) and was not entirely the result of osteolysis (84).

In a recent study of a primary hybrid total hip replacement with an average 10-year follow-up, performed with insertion of the acetabular com-ponent without cement and a precoated femoral component with cement, seven out of 86 hips had osteolytic areas located in the proximal aspect of the most proximal Gruen zone, and five had small osteolytic lesions in more distal areas (85). Smith et al. (86) have reported a 10- to 13-year follow-up study with the insertion of a hemispherical porous-coated acetabular component, inserted without cement and the use of screws, and a femoral component, inserted with second-generation cementing technique. They reported development of pelvic osteolysis in one hip (2%), femoral osteolysis in eight hips (1%), and distal femoral osteolysis in three hips (6%).

Hydroxyapatite coated stems are being used to enhance fixation and longevity. A minimum 10-year follow-up study of 270 hips with a proximally hydroxyapatite coated stem showed only one stem revised for loosening and no radiologically loose stems. However, 48% of the patients less than 45 years old and 38% of the patients older that 45 years had proximal osteolysis. Six stems in the young cohort were revised for wear or osteolysis (87).

Yoon et al. (88) reported 103 hip arthroplasties in 96 patients with a ceramic femoral head and a ceramic acetabular component. Progressive femoral osteolysis was observed in 22% in Gruen zones 1 and 7 at a mean follow-up of 92 months. None of the stable acetabular components were associated with pelvic osteolysis. Ten cups were revised for loosening and migration. Ceramic particles were found in the periarticular tissue. The long-term in vivo performance of third-generation ceramics are awaited (89). There has been a recent resurgence of interest in the metal-on-metal articulation hips. A recent study reported 84.4% implant survivorship prob-ability after 20 years with the McKee-Farrar prosthesis (90). Fourteen implants out of 123 were revised for aseptic loosening over a follow-up of 28 years. The low wear rate has been shown in laboratory studies, although some clinical data on the currently available implants (91) have reported sig-nificantly high levels of metal ions in the blood and urine of patients. Longer-term follow-up would be needed to evaluate the safety potential for lytic lesions with the contemporary prostheses.

The highly cross linked polyethylene has been developed to reduce the wear and this has been substantiated in laboratory studies (92). The femoral head size was not found to affect the magnitude of wear. Two of these electron beam irradiated polyethylenes have been approved by the Food and Drug Administration (93) and clinical results are forthcoming.

DIAGNOSIS AND CLINICAL SYMPTOMS

Osteolysis per se is asymptomatic (35). The accompanying phenomena and secondary developments may draw the attention of the patient or the physician to the underlying process. Some patients may have groin pain from particle debris induced synovitis. The secondary processes may be loosening of a component or fracture. Lysis involving the greater trochanter may lead to pathologic fracture and escape of the trochanter resulting in abductor insufficiency and late onset of Trendelenburg gait.

Extensive bone loss can occur with focal osteolysis in the absence of symptoms. Cemented components can cause increasing pain, which is suggestive of loosening but which may not be apparent until the osteolysis has caused severe bone loss (94). Uncemented components may present initially with pain secondary to wear-debris induced synovitis or after periprosthetic fracture through the site of the lesion (95,96). Osteolysis has been reported to occur as early as 12 months after implantation (97). Once osteolysis has developed, it is likely to progress. If components become loose, bone loss progresses more rapidly resulting in defects larger than those seen with well-fixed components (17). Therefore, most clinicians recommend routine serial radiographic follow-up once osteolysis is identified.

In patients who have undergone total joint replacement, the implication of radiographic osteolysis largely depends on the surgeon's point of view. Based on radiographic appearance, aseptic loosening was first identified around cemented components, and subsequently was defined as the development of a radiolucent line around a previously well-fixed prosthesis (Fig. 1) (98). The natural history of this radiolucency with cemented components is slow progression (40). When the zone of radiolucency is wider than 2 mm, or becomes circumferential, the prosthesis is considered to be at risk for loosening and may be clinically loose (99). The radiolucency appears to progress from the intra-articular margin of the interface until it extends circumferentially. Alternatively, aseptic loosening may manifest as a circumferential periprosthetic endosteal scalloping of bone at the implant–bone or cement–bone interface. In addition to the thin zone of circumferential radiolucency, certain regions of the interface exhibit greater bone loss. It is possible that such focal areas of bone loss are more accessible to, or have a higher concentration of particles (31). Regardless, aseptic loosening may appear as either a linear or expansile radiolucency. Once the component is loose, interfacial bone loss is progressive (100).

Osteolysis is generally defined as a focal, often rapidly expanding radiolucency at the implant–bone or cement–bone interface (Fig. 1) (101).

Such radiolucencies can represent small, clinically insignificant lesions that may not lead to loosening of the implant, such as with well-fixed, uncemented, extensively porous-coated stems (69). On the other hand, lytic lesions may progress leading to loss of fixation of cemented and uncemented implants (102). Although the latter phenomenon is rarely reported, the failure of the component is catastrophic. In addition, a common appearance of pelvic osteolysis in uncemented cups is that of a ballooning lesion that extends away from the component (94). Despite interfacial bone loss, osteolysis results in loosening only when a large amount of structural bone loss occurs.

In patients with aseptic loosening described as a linear pattern of radiolucency typically associated with cemented components, a previously well-fixed implant has become loose. In patients with osteolysis (i.e., the radiographic appearance of an expansile lytic lesion), there is focal loss of bone but the implant is stable. However in some patients, osteolysis may result in loosening (Fig. 2). Nevertheless, despite the different radiographic appearances, the same pathologic phenomena occur in both sets of patients. This implies that both osteolysis and aseptic loosening are terms that merely describe different manifestations of the same disease process. Therefore, it is important to realize that both manifestations represent interfacial bone resorption.

RADIOGRAPHIC APPEARANCE

Osteolysis is commonly described in characteristic patterns. On the acetabular side, osteolytic regions may appear linear, focal, or expansile with both cemented and uncemented components (13,65–67,69,70,94,97,99,103–105). Osteolysis has also been associated with both stable and unstable components (94–97,103). Quite commonly, both the location and volume of bone loss will progress, resulting in extensive expansile lesions involving the pelvis and femur (17,77,106,107). The site of osteolysis is determined by the access of the particulate debris to the bone surfaces and the effective joint space. Although in clinical practice, plain radiographs are the most frequently employed investigative modality to determine osteolysis, an important caveat is that radiographs consistently underestimate the size of osteolytic lesions. In addition, the radiographic appearance differs depending on the mode of fixation. Significant interobserver variability has been reported in the radiological evaluation of osteolysis (108). Helical computed tomography is a more reliable tool to assess the extent and location of lytic lesions as compared to plain radiographs (Fig. 4) (109).

Cemented Sockets

With cemented acetabular components, the path of least resistance for joint fluid and wear particles is at the cement–bone interface. As demonstrated in autopsy studies by Schmalzried et al. (110), after the implantation of a

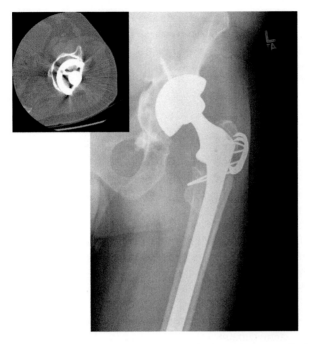

Figure 4 AP view showing gross lysis around the acetabular component, two years following third revision of the cup in a 60-year-old male; (*inset*): Cross sectional CT scan of the same patient showing the extent of acetabular lysis.

cemented socket, the subchondral bone reconstitutes and acts as a partial barrier that prevents joint fluid and particles from gaining access to the trabecular bone of the ilium. The soft tissue membrane created by the biologic reaction to wear particles dissects circumferentially along the cement–bone interface, leading to disruption of this interface. As the interfacial disruption progresses to the acetabular dome, fixation is lost. Radiographically, the osteolytic pattern is linear, and the radiolucency occurs at the cement–bone junction (Fig. 3). The component tends to migrate into the radiolucent areas in the superior and medial aspects of the acetabulum. Although cystic lesions are uncommon, bone loss can still be extensive, especially if the disease has been long standing and untreated.

Zicat et al. (70) described patterns of osteolysis around all polyethylene cemented components. In 12 of 63 patients, loosening necessitated revision of the cups within seven years of implantation. Eight of these 12 cases (75%) had a circumferential linear pattern. Although 51 patients did not require revision of the acetabular component, 19 had unstable cups. Of these 19, four (22%) had a progressive linear pattern present in all three zones, and three (18%) had focal expansile lesions at the superolateral or the inferomedial margin of the cup. As expected, the expansile lesions occurred predominantly in zone III (111) with greater contact with the joint fluid. Failure of the cemented cups requiring revision was more often associated with a higher patient weight (66 vs. 55 kg) and younger age at the time of implantation (44 vs. 60 years).

Cemented Stems

The appearance of osteolysis in cemented femoral stems can be in the form of a radiolucent line at the cement–bone interface or as focal lesions. When linear, this has to be differentiated from the radiolucent line present on the early postoperative radiographs which is likely to represent nonfilling of the canal with cement. Adaptive remodeling is also an early feature with similar appearance but it would not be present on the first postoperative radiograph (35). The progression of a line noted initially could point towards an osteolytic process. In arthroplasties with a cemented femoral component, the path of least resistance for particle migration on the femoral side is along the cement–metal or the cement–bone interface. Linear, expansile, and focal lesions all have been seen with both the stable and unstable stems (14,70,84,101,112). Several authors have demonstrated the potential for a passage to form at the stem–cement interface (14,112). Anthony et al. (112) postulated that the formation of a membrane within the passage may be a causative factor for the focal lytic lesions that develop around the distal aspect of an otherwise well-fixed cemented femoral component. They suggested that fluid and particles are driven along the interface by the high intra-articular pressures generated during normal gait and reach the cement–bone interface via defects in the cement mantle. The resulting biologic reaction can lead to focal osteolysis in the presence of a well-fixed cemented stem.

As with cemented acetabular components, particles can migrate along the cement–bone interface of femoral components. However, the consequences are quite different. In the absence of cement fracture or debonding at the cement–metal interface, the femoral component usually does not loosen, probably because surface area for fixation is much larger than that of the acetabular component (22). The 2–3 cm disruption of the proximal cement–bone interface due to linear osteolysis (i.e., membrane formation) will not significantly compromise femoral component stability. In contrast, any disruption at the cement–metal interface is likely to have a significant effect on implant stability. Osteolysis around the proximal femur thus can result in progressive bone loss. With modern cementing techniques though, it is rarely the primary cause of loosening (41,53). However, with stem debonding or cement fracture, cement debris is produced. With adequate access to the cement–bone interface, the debris leads to the development of osteolysis as a secondary phenomenon.

Clinical studies of stems inserted using first-generation cementing techniques found osteolysis in all Gruen zones (18,103). Callaghan et al. (113) reported the results of a 25 year experience with the use of Charnley total hip arthroplasty with cement and reported osteolysis in 33/295 hips in Gruen zones 1 or 7 and in Gruen zones 2 through 6 in two hips. With second- and third-generation cementing techniques, radiolucencies at the cement–bone interface are primarily linear and are located in Gruen zones 1, 7, 8, and 14 (41). In addition, although the incidence of osteolysis in cemented stems is quite low, an increase from 3% to 9% has been reported for the same patients between the 11- and 15-year follow-up.

Cemented stems are definitely loose when the component has migrated, a new radiolucency at the cement–metal interface has developed, the stem is deformed or fractured, or when the cement mantle is fractured (98,101). A complete radiolucency at the cement–bone interface suggests probable loosening, whereas 50–99% radiolucency suggests possible loosening. Significantly, interpretation of the radiolucent line is critical in determining whether the radiographic manifestations are suggestive of linear osteolysis or remodeling (114). Serial radiographs over a period of time are often helpful.

Cementless Sockets

The pattern of osteolysis around cementless sockets is a function of extent of bone ingrowth. If the socket is stable and bone-ingrown, the path of least resistance is via noningrown areas and screw areas, which allow particles to migrate into the trabecular bone of the ilium, ischium, and pubis. This results in two patterns of osteolysis in bone-ingrown cups that may be related to the local particle concentration (Fig. 4). High particle loads may be more likely to result in the first pattern, which is rapidly growing expansile lesions with indirect margins. The consequence of osteolysis in these cases is progressive bone loss. Loosening does not result until bone loss is extensive, and failure is usually acute and catastrophic. Reiterating, patients usually remain clinically asymptomatic until the components loosen.

The second pattern of osteolysis is a more slowly growing lesion that has sclerotic margins. Sclerotic bone often forms at the implant–bone interface, probably as a result of micromotion. The pattern of osteolysis in this case is quite similar to that seen with cemented sockets. Linear osteolysis occurs with the implant migrating into the radiolucent area. In addition, if late migration of the component is noted in the absence of previous radiolucency, then fibrous fixation with progressive osteolysis should be assumed to have developed. The consequences of osteolysis in this case are progressive bone loss and clinical loosening.

The radiographic determination of whether a socket has bone ingrowth may be fallacious. Ingrowth can be suggested but cannot be proven on radiographs. Radiographic criteria of the type described for bone ingrown porous-coated cementless stems have not been delineated for cementless cups. A cementless socket that is radiographically stable is often presumed to be bone-ingrown, although that may not be the case. Cementless sockets in which bone ingrowth does not occur are predisposed to late migration. In a study by Zicat et al. (70), 71 of 74 one-piece metal-backed anatomic medullary locking (AML, DePuy, Warsaw, Indiana) sintered-bead porous coated cups, inserted with cementless techniques with three spikes and no screw holes, were well-functioning after seven years. Fourteen (20%) had radiolucent lines in at least one zone, most commonly zone III. No component had circumferential linear osteolysis. One or more periarticular focal lesions occurred in 18% of the cups. Two cups (3%) also had osteolytic areas remote from the joint. Similarly, porous coated anatomic (PCA, Howmedica, East Rutherford, New Jersey) cups have been associated with an equal incidence of focal osteolysis in all three zones (65,66). Reports have noted the occurrence of nonprogressive radiolucent lines around Harris Galante (HG-I, Zimmer, Warsaw, Indiana) cups, but no focal osteolysis has been noted at 7- to 11-years of follow-up (15,54). Studies have shown that with screw-in cups, osteolysis occurs rapidly in a linear circumferential pattern with catastrophic migration of the components (72,73). In addition, regardless of cup type, both linear and expansile osteolysis have been noted around the fixation screws (72,104). With the HG cups after five years, the use of screws for internal fixation showed one lesion in 83 cups (1.2%) (78); no osteolysis was identified in the same cup fixed without screws in 122 hips (115). Soto et al. (116) showed with HG cups and a mean follow-up period of 87 months, that 22 (24%) hips had periacetabular osteolysis, and 16 of these 22 (73%) were associated with screws. Clohisy and Harris (64) have reported a recent 10-year follow-up study with HG cups with screw fixation that showed osteolytic lesions associated with 5% of the acetabular components. Thus, the patterns of osteolysis around uncemented cups depend on the cup design.

When cemented cups are used, migration greater than 5 mm is consistent with definite loosening. Migration may be difficult to detect because of the variation in imaging planes of radiographs. Roentgenographic stereophotogrammeteric analysis is more accurate (117) but is not widely used. Migration may occur with associated fracture of trans-acetabular screws, shedding of porous coating, or implant fracture. Progressive radiolucent lines suggest imminent loosening, whereas static lines are of less concern.

Cementless Stems

As with the cementless sockets, the pattern of osteolysis with cementless stems depends on whether bone ingrowth has occurred. In addition, the implant design is a major factor in the location of osteolytic lesions. With patch-porous coated implants, the path of least resistance is often along the smooth portion of the stem into the diaphysis of the femur. Thus, these types of stems are prone to diaphyseal osteolysis, as demonstrated in studies in which partially porous-coated cylinders were implanted into the distal femur of rabbits (21). Polyethylene particles were then injected into the joint, and the femora were harvested several weeks after surgery. Histological analysis demonstrated that the bone-ingrowth areas were relative barriers to the ingress of joint fluid and polyethylene debris. In contrast, a periprosthetic cavity with a membrane formed around the smooth portion of the stem. Polarized light microscopy demonstrated that this soft-tissue membrane contained abundant polyethylene particles. Similar findings have been noted in studies examining patch-porous coated stems that were implanted in humans (14,17,54,55,103).

With circumferential porous-coated stems such as the AML or the PCA, focal osteolytic lesions occur most commonly in the proximal aspect of the femur. Occasionally, these lesions are presented as spontaneous fractures of the greater and lesser trochanter (96). With AML femoral components, Zicat et al. (70) and Engh et al. (69) described primarily periarticular lesions occurring in zones 1 and 7 (greater and lesser trochanter, respectively). In these two studies, the clinical significance of the osteolysis was minimal. Osteolysis around the PCA stem also occurred in zones 1, 7 or both in some studies (65,80) and in zones 1, 2, 3, and 7 in another study (96). A five-year study of the PCA stem by Sharkey et al. (118) revealed that acetabular osteolysis was present in 7 of 39 hips, with four of the seven centered around acetabular fixation screws. A five- to nine-year prospective study of the PCA stem showed 2.8% rate of endosteal osteolysis and this osteolysis was benign in appearance (119). A recent 10-year follow-up study of the PCA stem by Xenos et al. (58) reveals that acetabular osteolysis occurred in 17 hips (17/77). Femoral osteolysis occurred in 39 hips: in the proximal aspect of 31 hips, in the distal aspect of four, and in both the proximal and distal aspect of four (120).

In contrast, diaphyseal expansile osteolysis is much more common in patch-porous coated implants such as the original Harris Galante porous-coated stem (HGP, Zimmer, Warsaw, Indiana) (55), the anatomic porous replacement (APR-I, Intermedics Orthopaedics, Austin, Texas) stem, and the initial S-ROM (Joint Medical Products, Stamford, Connecticut) implant, which had a seam that allowed joint fluid to reach the diaphysis. The S-ROM modular femoral stem in a seven year follow-up study has noted periprosthetic osteolytic lesions in 12 hips (7%). The lesions were observed in the femur in eight hips, in the acetabulum in two hips, and in both the femur and the acetabulum in two hips (121). In a five-year follow-up study of the HGP stem, Maloney and Woolson (77) reported a 52% incidence of femoral osteolysis. Sixty-seven percent of these lesions were in the diaphysis in Gruen zones 3, 4, and 5. Many other reports indicate a high incidence of osteolysis in all periprosthetic femoral zones of patients who received the HGP stem (17,54,55). Clohisy et al. (122) have shown osteolysis in 60% of their cases with the HGP stem. The consequence of osteolysis in these cases is progressive diaphyseal bone loss. Loosening can occur when significant support for the implant is lost along the smooth portion of the stem. Because loads then transferred across a small area of bone ingrowth, stress fractures of the ingrown area leading to implant loosening can occur and has been reported (102,123). Thus, it is possible for the surgeon to predict the location, appearance, and prevalence of osteolysis as a function of the implant design. McLaughlin and Lee (124) have shown at 10-year follow-up with the uncemented Taperloc femoral component a rate of femoral osteolysis to be 6%.

If bone ingrowth does not occur in a porous-coated cementless stem, a fibrous interface develops. Radiographically, sclerotic lines adjacent to the fibrous tissue suggest the presence of a partial barrier obstructing the access of fluid and particle to the endosteal surface of the femur. In these cases, linear osteolysis described as a "windshield wiper" pattern is often noted. Progressive loss of diaphyseal bone may occur, leading to expansion of the endosteal canal. These patients often have pain from the time of surgery that progressively worsens. Implant migration also suggests unstable fibrous ingrowth.

Uncemented stems are definitely loose if migration and subsidence are evident. Radiographic criteria for uncemented stems are in a state of evolution, but particular findings for individual implants have been described to help determine whether specific implants may be loose. Unstable PCA components demonstrate subsidence of greater than 2 mm, cortical hypertrophy, or cancellous hypertrophy at the stem tip (i.e., pedestal formation) (125). Similarly possible loosening of AML femoral components is indicated radiographically by widening circumferential lucencies adjacent to the porous surface, divergent lines of demarcation, shedding of the porous coating, absence of proximal stress shielding, or cortical hypertrophy with pedestal formation (126). In addition, dynamic rotational computed tomography has been used to determine whether uncemented femoral components are loose (127). In this technique, femoral component version is measured in maximal internal and external rotation. The component is considered loose if there is a difference of 2 degrees or more between these angles.

Ragab et al. (128) recently reported a study with a minimum of six-year follow-up of the clinical and radiographic outcomes of total hip arthroplasty with insertion of an anatomically designed femoral component without cement for the treatment of primary osteoarthritis. Their radiographic assessment revealed consistent evidence of proximal bone ingrowth. No complete radiolucent line was identified, except around the one stem that loosened. Twenty-seven femoral components (27/88) were associated with incomplete pedestal formation. No osteolytic lesion of the femur was identified. Nonprogressive pelvic osteolysis was identified in four hips but none of the lesions were more than 2 mm in diameter. None of the acetabular components migrated, and no radiolucent line of more than 2 mm in thickness was seen around any acetabular cup.

ACKNOWLEDGMENTS

The authors thank Andrew Freiberg, MD, for academic discussions and providing Figures 1–3.

REFERENCES

1. Charnley J. The bonding of prostheses to bone by cement. J Bone Joint Surg 1964; 46-B:518–529.
2. Charnley J, Follacci FM, Hammond BT. The long-term reaction of bone to self-curing acrylic cement. J Bone Joint Surg 1968; 50-B:822–829.
3. Mirra JM, Amstutz HC, Matos M, Gold R. The pathology of the joint tissues and its clinical relevance in prosthesis failure. Clin Orthop 1976; 117:221–240.
4. Mirra JM, Marder RA, Amstutz HC. The pathology of failed total joint arthroplasty. Clin Orthop 1982; 170:175–183.
5. Bullough PG, DiCarlo EF, Hansraj KK, Neves MC. Pathologic studies of total joint replacement. Orthop Clin North Am 1988; 19:611–625.
6. Willert HG, Semlitsch M. Tissue reactions to plastic and metallic wear products of joint endoprostheses. In: Gschwend N, Debrunner HU, eds. Total Hip Prosthesis. Baltimore: Williams & Wilkins, 1976:205–239.
7. Willert HG, Semlitsch M. Reactions of the articular capsule to wear products of artificial joint prostheses. J Biomed Mater Res 1977; 11:157–164.
8. Goldring SR, Schiller AL, Roelke M, Rourke CM, O'Neill DA, Harris WH. The synovial-like membrane at the bone–cement interface in loose total hip replacements and its proposed role in bone lysis. J Bone Joint Surg 1983; 65A:575–584.
9. Horowitz SM, Doty SB, Lane JM, Burstein AH. Studies of the mechanism by which the mechanical failure of polymethylmethacrylate leads to bone resorption. J Bone Joint Surg 1993; 75-A:802–813.
10. Goodman SB, Fornasier VL, Lee J, Kei J. The histological effects of the implantation of different sizes of polyethylene particles in the rabbit tibia. J Biomed Mater Res 1990; 24(4):517–524.
11. Gray MH, Talbert ML, Talbert WM, Bansal M, Hsu A. Changes seen in lymph nodes draining the sites of large joint prostheses. Am J Surg Path 1989; 13:1050–1056.
12. Urban RM, Jacobs JJ, Gilbert JL, Galante JO. Migration of corrosion products from modular hip prostheses. J Bone Joint Surg Am 1994; 76-A: 1345–1359.
13. Schmalzried TP, Jasty M, Harris WH. Periprosthetic bone loss in total hip arthroplasty. Polyethylene wear debris and the concept of the effective joint space. J Bone Joint Surg Am 1992; 74(6):849–863.
14. Maloney WJ, Jasty M, Harris WH, Galante JO, Callaghan JJ. Endosteal erosion in association with stable uncemented femoral components. J Bone Joint Surg Am 1990; 72(7):1025–1034.

15. Mohler CG, Callaghan JJ, Collis DK, Johnston RC. Early loosening of the femoral component at the cement–prosthesis interface after total hip replacement [see comments]. J Bone Joint Surg Am 1995; 77(9):1315–1322.

16. Jacobs JJ, Kull LR, Frey GA, Gitelis S, Sheinkop MB, Kramer TS et al. Early failure of acetabular components inserted without cement after previous pelvic irradiation. J Bone Joint Surg Am 1995; 77(12):1829–1835.

17. Tanzer M, Maloney WJ, Jasty MJ, Harris WH. The progression of femoral cortical osteolysis in association with total hip arthroplasty without cement. J Bone Joint Surg Am 1992; 74-A:404–410.

18. Willert HG, Bertram H, Buchhorn GH. Osteolysis in alloarthroplasty of the hip. The role of bone cement fragmentation. Clin Orthop 1990; 258:108–121.

19. Willert HG, Bertram H, Buchhorn GH. Osteolysis in alloarthroplasty of the hip. The role of ultra-high molecular weight polyethylene wear particles. Clin Orthop 1992; 258:95–107.

20. Urban RM, Jacobs JJ, Sumner DR, Peters CL, Voss FR, Galante JO. The bone–implant interface of femoral stems with non-circumferential porous coating. J Bone Joint Surg Am 1996; 78(7):1068–1081.

21. Bobyn JD, Jacobs JJ, Tanzer M, Urban RM, Aribindi R, Sumner DR, et al. The susceptibility of smooth implant surfaces to perimplant fibrosis and migration of polyethylene wear debris. Clin Orthop 1995; 311:21–39.

22. Horikoshi M, Macaulay W, Booth RE, Crossett LS, Rubash HE. Comparison of interface membranes obtained from failed cemented cementless hip and knee prostheses. Clin Orthop 1994; 309:69–87.

23. Vernon-Roberts B, Freeman MAR. Morphological and analytical studies of the tissues adjacent to joint prostheses: investigations into the causes of loosening prostheses. In: Schaldach M, Hohmann D, eds. Advances in Artificial Hip and Knee Joint Technology. Berlin: Springer, 1976:148–186.

24. Vernon-Roberts B, Freeman MAR. The tissue response to total joint replacement prostheses. In: Swanson SAV, Freeman MAR, eds. The Scientific Basis of Joint Replacement. New York: Wiley, 1977:86–129.

25. Goodman SB, Chin RC, Chiou SS, Schurman DJ, Woolson ST, Masada MP. A clinical-pathologic-biochemical study of the membrane surrounding loosened and nonloosened total hip arthroplasties. Clin Orthop 1989; 244:182–187.

26. Howie DW. Tissue response in relation to type of wear particles around failed hip arthroplasties. J Arthroplasty 1990; 5:337–348.

27. Thornhill TS, Ozuna RM, Shortkroff S, Keller K, Sledge CB, Spector M. Biochemical and histological evaluation of the synovial-like tissue around failed (loose) total joint replacement prostheses in human subjects and a canine model. Biomaterials 1990; 11:69–72.

28. Kim KJ, Rubash HE. Large amounts of polyethylene debris in the interface tissue surrounding bipolar endoprostheses. Comparison to total hip prostheses. J Arthroplasty 1997; 12(1):32–39.

29. Jiranek WA, Machado M, Jasty M, Jevsevar D, Wolfe HJ, Goldring SR et al. Production of cytokines around loosened cemented acetabular components. Analysis with immunohistochemical techniques and in situ hybridization. J Bone Joint Surg Am 1993; 75(6):863–879.

30. Kim KJ, Rubash HE, Wilson SC, D'Antonio JA, McClain EJ. A histological and biochemical comparison of the interface tissues in cementless and cemented hip prosthesis. Clin Orthop 1993; 287:142–152.
31. Chiba J, Rubash HE, Kim KJ, Iwaki Y. The characterization of cytokines in the interface tisssue obtained from failed cementless total hip arthroplasty with and without femoral osteolysis. Clin Orthop 1994; 300:304–312.
32. Gelb H, Schumacher HR, Cuckler J, Baker DG. In vivo inflammatory response to polymethylmethacrylate particulate debris: Effect of size, morphology, and surface area. J Orthop Res 1994; 12:83–92.
33. Shanbhag AS, Jacobs JJ, Black J, Galante JO, Glant TT. Cellular mediators secreted by interfacial membranes obtained at revision total hip arthroplasty. J Arthroplasty 1995; 10(4):498–506.
34. Harris WH. The problem is osteolysis. Clin Orthop 1995; 311:46–53.
35. Harris WH. Wear and periprosthetic osteolysis: the problem. Clin Orthop 2001; 393:66–70.
36. Dowd JE, Sychterz CJ, Young AM, Engh CA. Characterization of long-term femoral-head-penetration rates. Association with and prediction of osteolysis. J Bone Joint Surg Am 2000; 82-A(8):1102–1107.
37. Dumbleton JH, Manley MT, Edidin AA. A literature review of the association between wear rate and osteolysis in total hip arthroplasty. J Arthroplasty 2002; 17(5):649–661.
38. Manley MT, D'Antonio JA, Capello WN, Edidin AA. Osteolysis: a disease of access to fixation interfaces. Clin Orthop 2002; 405:129–137.
39. Van d Vis, Aspenberg P, de Kleine R, Tigchelaar W, Van Noorden CJ. Short periods of oscillating fluid pressure directed at a titanium–bone interface in rabbits lead to bone lysis. Acta Orthop Scand 1998; 69(1):5–10.
40. Stauffer RN. Ten-year follow-up study of total hip replacement. J Bone Joint Surg 1982; 64-A:983–990.
41. Mulroy WF, Estok DM, Harris WH. Total hip arthroplasty with use of so-called second-generation cementing techniques. J Bone Joint Surg 1995; 77-A(December):1845–1852.
42. Salvati EA, Wilson PD Jr, Jolley MN, Vakili F, Aglietti P, Brown GC. A ten-year follow-up study of our first one hundred consecutive Charnley total hip replacements. J Bone Joint Surg 1981; 63-A:753–767.
43. Sutherland CJ, Wilde AH, Borden LS, Marks KE. A ten-year follow-up of one hundred consecutive muller curved-stem total hip-replacement arthroplasties. J Bone Joint Surg 1982; 64-A:970–982.
44. Bosco JA, Lachiewicz PF, DeMasi R. Survivorship analysis of cemented high modulus total hip arthroplasty. Clin Orthop 1993; 294:131–139.
45. Hozack WJ, Rothman RH, Booth RE Jr, Balderston RA. Cemented versus cementless total hip arthroplasty. A comparative study of equivalent patient populations. Clin Orthop 1993; (289):161–165.
46. Havelin LI, Espehaug B, Vollset SE, Engesaeter LB. The effect of the type of cement on early revision of Charnley total hip prostheses. A review of eight thousand five hundred and seventy-nine primary arthroplasties from the Norwegian Arthroplasty Register. J Bone Joint Surg Am 1995; 77(10): 1543–1550.

47. Mohler CG, Kull LR, Martell JM, Rosenberg AG, Galante JO. Total hip replacement with insertion of an acetabular component without cement and a femoral component with cement. J Bone Joint Surg 1995; 77-A(January):86–96.

48. Neumann L, Freund KG, Sorensen KH. Total hip arthroplasty with the Charnley prosthesis in patients fifty-five years old and less. J Bone Joint Surg 1996; 78-A(1):73–79.

49. MacKenzie JR, Kelley SS, Johnston RC. Total hip replacement for coxarthrosis secondary to congenital dysplasia and dislocation of the hip. Long-term results. J Bone Joint Surg Am 1996; 78(1):55–61.

50. Schulte KR, Callaghan JJ, Kelley SS, Johnston RC. The outcome of Charnley total hip arthroplasty with cement after a minimum twenty-year follow-up. The results of one surgeon. J Bone Joint Surg Am 1993; 75(7):961–975.

51. Ranawat CS, Rawlins BA, Harju VT. Effect of modern cement technique on acetabular fixation total hip arthroplasty. A retrospective study in matched pairs. Orthop Clin North Am 1988; 19(3):599–603.

52. Ranawat CS, Peters LE, Umlas ME. Fixation of the acetabular component: the case for cement. J Arthroplasty 1996; 11(1):1–3.

53. Mulroy RD Jr, Harris WH. The effect of improved cementing techniques on component loosening in total hip replacement. J Bone Joint Surg 1990; 72-B:757–760.

54. Moyle DD, Klawitter JJ, Hulbert SF. Mechanical properties of the bone-porous biomaterial interface: elastic behaviour. J Biomed Mater Res 1973; Symp. 4:363–382.

55. Goetz DD, Smith EJ, Harris WH. The prevalence of femoral osteolysis associated with components inserted with or without cement in total hip replacements. J Bone Joint Surg 1994; 76–A(August):1121–1129.

56. Woolson ST, Maloney WJ. Cementless total hip arthroplasty using a porous-coated prosthesis for bone ingrowth fixation. 3 1/2-year follow-up. J Arthroplasty 1992; 7 suppl:381–388.

57. Smith E, Harris WH. Increasing prevalence of femoral lysis in cementless total hip arthroplasty. J Arthroplasty 1995; 10(4):407–412.

58. Xenos JS, Hopkinson WJ, Callaghan JJ, Heekin RD, Savory CG. Osteolysis around an uncemented cobalt chrome total hip arthroplasty. Clin Orthop 1995; 317:29–36.

59. Nashed RS, Becker DA, Gustilo RB. Are cementless acetabular components the cause of excess wear and osteolysis in total hip arthroplasty?. Clin Orthop 1995; 317:19–28.

60. Lecog C, Rochwerger A, Curvale G, Groulier P. Complications associated with the use of first generation Harris–Galante porous-coated acetabular component after a mean followup of 7 years. Rev Chir Orthop Reparatrice Appar Mot 1999; 85(7):689–697.

61. Bohm P, Bosche R. Survival analysis of the Harris–Galante I acetabular cup. J Bone Joint Surg 1998; 80B(3):396–403.

62. Maloney WJ, Galante JO, Anderson M, Goldberg V, Harris WH, Jacobs JJ, et al. Fixation, polyethylene wear, and pelvic osteolysis in primary total hip replacement. Clin Orthop 1999; 369:157–164.

63. Berger RA, Jacobs JJ, Quigley LR, Rosenberg AG, Galante JO. Primary cementless acetabular reconstruction in patients younger than 50 years old. 7- to 11-year results. Clin Orthop 1997; 344:216–226.

64. Clohisy JC, Harris WH. The Harris–Galante porous-coated acetabular component with screw fixation. An average ten-year follow-up study. J Bone Joint Surg 1999; 81A(1):66–73.

65. Kim YH, Kim VE. Cementless porous-coated anatomic medullary locking total hip prostheses. J Arthroplasty 1994; 9(3):243–252.

66. Owen TD, Moran CG, Smith SR, Pinder IM. Results of uncemented porous-coated anatomic total hip replacement. J Bone Joint Surg Br 1994; 76(2): 258–262.

67. Learmonth ID, Grobler GP, Dall DM, Jandera V. Loss of bone stock with cementless hip arthroplasty. J Arthroplasty 1995; 10(3):257–263.

68. Mont MA, Yoon TR, Krackow KA, Hungerford DS. Clinical experience with a proximally porous-coated second-generation cementless total hip prosthesis: minimum 5-year follow-up. J Arthroplasty 1999; 14(8):930–939.

69. Engh CA, Hooten JP Jr, Zettl-Schaffer KF, Ghaffarpour M, McGovern TF, Macalino GE, et al. Porous-coated total hip replacement. Clin Orthop 1994; 298:89–96.

70. Zicat B, Engh CA, Gokcen E. Patterns of osteolysis around total hip components inserted with and without cement. J Bone Joint Surg Am 1995; 77(3):432–439.

71. Claus AM, Sychterz CJ, Hopper RH Jr, Engh CA. Pattern of osteolysis around two different cementless metal-backed cups: retrospective, radiographic analysis at minimum 10-year follow-up. J Arthroplasty 2001; 16(8 suppl 1): 177–182.

72. Fox GM, McBeath AA, Heiner JP. Hip replacement with a threaded acetabular cup. A follow-up study. J Bone Joint Surg Am 1994; 76(2):195–201.

73. Bruijn JD, Seelen JL, Feenstra RM, Hansen BE, Bernoski FP. Failure of the Mecring screw-ring acetabular component in total hip arthroplasty. A three to seven-year follow-up study. J Bone Joint Surg Am 1995; 77(5):760–766.

74. Smith SE, Estok DM, Harris WH. 20-year experience with cemented primary and conversion total hip arthroplasty using so-called second generation cementing techniques in patients aged 50 years or younger. J Arthroplasty 2000; 15(3):263–273.

75. Kale AA, Della Valle CJ, Frankel VH, Stuchin SA, Zuckerman JD, Di Cesare PE. Hip arthroplasty with a collared straight cobalt–chrome femoral stem using second-generation cementing technique: a 10-year-average follow-up study. J Arthroplasty 2000; 15(2):187–193.

76. Mulroy WF, Harris WH. Acetabular and femoral fixation 15 years after cemented total hip surgery. Clin Orthop 1997; (337):118–128.

77. Maloney WJ, Woolson ST. Increasing incidence of femoral in association with uncemented Harris-Galante total hip arthroplasty. J Arthroplasty 1996; 11:130–134.

78. Schmalzried TP, Harris WH. The Harris–Galante porous-coated acetabular component with screw fixation. Radiographic analysis of eighty-three primary hip replacements at a minimum of five years. J Bone Joint Surg Am 1992; 74(8):1130–1139.

79. Kim Y-H, Kim JS, Cho SH. Primary total hip arthroplasty with a cementless porous-coated anatomic total hip prosthesis: 10- to 12-year results of prospective and consecutive series. J Arthroplasty 1999; 14(5):538–548.

80. Heekin RD, Callaghan JJ, Hopkinson WJ, Savory CG, Xenos JS. The porous-coated anatomic total hip prosthesis, inserted without cement. J Bone Joint Surg 1993; 75-A:77–91.

81. Della Valle CJ, Paprosky WG. The middle-aged patient with hip arthritis: the case for extensively coated stems. Clin Orthop 2002; 405:101–107.

82. Kim Y-H, Kim JS, Cho SH. Primary total hip arthroplasty with the AML total hip prosthesis. Clin Orthop 1999; 360:147–158.

83. Claus AM, Hopper RH Jr, Engh CA. Fractures of the greater trochanter induced by osteolysis with the anatomic medullary locking prosthesis. J Arthroplasty 2002; 17(6):706–712.

84. Lombardi AV Jr, Mallory TH, Eberle RW, Mitchell MB, Lefkowitz MS, Williams JR. Failure of intraoperatively customized non-porous femoral components inserted without cement in total hip arthroplasty. J Bone Joint Surg Am 1995; 77(12):1836–1844.

85. Clohisy JC, Harris WH. Primary hybrid total hip replacement, performed with insertion of the acetabular component without cement and a precoat femoral component with cement. An average ten-year follow-up study. J Bone Joint Surg Am 1999; 81A(2):247–255.

86. Smith SE, Harris WH. Total hip arthroplasty performed with insertion of the femoral component with cement and the acetabular component without cement. Ten to thirteen-year results. J Bone Joint Surg 1997; 79(12): 1827–1833.

87. Capello WN, D'Antonio JA, Feinberg JR, Manley MT. Hydroxyapatite coated stems in younger and older patients with hip arthritis. Clin Orthop 2002; (405):92–100.

88. Yoon TR, Rowe SM, Jung ST, Seon KJ, Maloney WJ. Osteolysis in association with a total hip arthroplasty with ceramic bearing surfaces. J Bone Joint Surg Am 1998; 80(10):1459–1468.

89. Bierbaum BE, Nairus J, Kuesis D, Morrison JC, Ward D. Ceramic-on-ceramic bearings in total hip arthroplasty. Clin Orthop 2002; 405:158–163.

90. Brown SR, Davies WA, DeHeer DH, Swanson AB. Long-term survival of McKee–Farrar total hip prostheses. Clin Orthop 2002; 402:157–163.

91. MacDonald SJ, McCalden RW, Chess DG, Bourne RB, Rorabeck CH, Cleland D, et al. Metal-on-metal versus polyethylene in hip arthroplasty: a randomized clinical trial. Clin Orthop 2003; 406:282–296.

92. Muratoglu OK, Bragdon CR, O'Connor DO, Jasty M, Harris WH. A novel method of cross-linking ultra-high-molecular-weight polyethylene to improve wear, reduce oxidation, and retain mechanical properties. Recipient of the 1999 HAP Paul Award. J Arthroplasty 2001; 16(2):149–160.

93. Burroughs BR, Rubash HE, Harris WH. Femoral head sizes larger than 32 mm against highly cross-linked polyethylene. Clin Orthop 2002; 405:150–157.

94. Maloney WJ, Peters P, Engh CA, Chandler H. Severe osteolysis of the pelvic in association with acetabular replacement without cement. J Bone Joint Surg Am 1993; 75(11):1627–1635.

95. Pazzaglia UE, Byers PD. Fractured femoral shaft through an osteolytic lesion resulting from the reaction to a prosthesis: a case report. J Bone Joint Surg 1984; 66-B(May):337–339.

96. Heekin RD, Engh CA, Herzwurm PJ. Fractures through cystic lesions of the greater trochanter. A cause of late pain after cementless total hip arthroplasty. J Arthroplasty 1996; 11(6):757–760.

97. Buechel FF, Drucker D, Jasty M, Jiranek WA, Harris WH. Osteolysis around uncemented acetabular components of cobalt–chrome surface replacement hip arthroplasty. Clin Orthop 1994; 298:202–211.

98. Gruen TA, McNeice GM, Amstutz HC. "Modes of Failure" of cemented stem-type femoral components. Clin Orthop 1979; 141:17–27.

99. Kim YH, Kim VE. Uncemented porous-coated anatomic total hip replacement. Results at six years in a consecutive series. J Bone Joint Surg Br 1993; 75(1):6–13.

100. Hodgkinson JP, Shelley P, Wroblewski BM. The correlation between the roentgenographic appearance and operative findings at the bone–cement junction of the socket in Charnley low friction arthroplasties. Clin Orthop 1988; 228:105–109.

101. Harris WH, Schiller AL, Scholler J-M, Freiberg RA, Scott R. Extensive localized bone resorption in the femur following total hip replacement. J Bone Joint Surg 1976; 58A:612–618.

102. Jasty M, Maloney WJ, Bragdon CR, Haire T, Harris WH. Histomorphological studies of the long-term skeletal responses to well fixed cemented femoral components. J Bone Joint Surg Am 1990; 72(8):1220–1229.

103. Jasty MJ, Floyd WE, Schiller AL, Goldring SR, Harris WH. Localized osteolysis in stable, non-septic total hip replacement. J Bone Joint Surg 1986; 68A: 912–919.

104. Santavirta S, Konttinen YT, Bergroth V, Eskola A, Tallroth K, Lindholm TS. Aggressive granulomatous lesions associated with hip arthroplasty. J Bone Joint Surg 1990; 72-A:252–258.

105. Schmalzried TP, Guttman D, Grecula M, Amstutz HC. The relationship between the design, position and articular wear of acetabular components inserted without cement and the development of pelvic osteolysis. J Bone Joint Surg 1994; 76-A:677–688.

106. D'Antonio JA, Capello WN, Borden LS, Bargar WL, Bierbaum BF, Boettcher WG, et al. Classification and management of acetabular abnormalities in total hip arthroplasty. Clin Orthop 1989; 243:126–137.

107. Paprosky WG, Perona PG, Lawrence JM. Acetabular defect classification and surgical reconstruction in revision arthroplasty. A 6-year follow-up evaluation. J Arthroplasty 1994; 9(1):33–44.

108. Engh CA Jr, Sychterz CJ, Young AM, Pollock DC, Toomey SD, Engh CA Sr. Interobserver and intraobserver variability in radiographic assessment of osteolysis. J Arthroplasty 2002; 17(6):752–759.

109. Puri L, Wixson RL, Stern SH, Kohli J, Hendrix RW, Stulberg SD. Use of helical computed tomography for the assessment of acetabular osteolysis after total hip arthroplasty. J Bone Joint Surg Am 2002; 84-A(4):609–614.

110. Schmalzried TP, Kwong LM, Jasty M, Sedlacek RC, Haire TC, O'Connor DO, et al. The mechanism of loosening of cemented acetabular components in total hip arthroplasty. Analysis of specimens retrieved at autopsy. Clin Orthop 1992; 274:60–78.

111. DeLee JG, Charnley J. Radiological demarcation of cemented sockets in total hip arthroplasty. J Clin Invest 1979; 64:1386–1392.

112. Anthony PP, Gie GA, Howie CR, Ling RS. Localised endosteal bone lysis in relation to the femoral components of cemented total hip arthroplasties. J Bone Joint Surg Br 1990; 72(6):971–979.

113. Callaghan JJ, Albright JC, Goetz DD, Olejniczak JP, Johnston RC. Charnley total hip arthroplasty with cement. Minimum twenty five year followup. J Bone Joint Surg 2000; 82A(4):487–497.

114. Kwong LM, Jasty M, Mulroy RD, Maloney WJ, Bragdon C, Harris WH. The histology of the radiolucent line. J Bone Joint Surg Br 1992; 74(1):67–73.

115. Schmalzried TP, Wessinger SJ, Hill GE, Harris WH. The Harris–Galante porous acetabular component press-fit without screw fixation. Five-year radiographic analysis of primary cases. J Arthroplasty 1994; 9(3):235–242.

116. Soto MO, Rodriguez JA, Ranawat CS. Clinical and radiographic evaluation of the Harris–Galante cup: Incidence of wear and osteolysis at 7 to 9 years follow-up. J Arthroplasty 2000; 15(2):139–145.

117. Onsten I, Carlsson AS, Ohlin A, Nilsson JA. Migration of acetabular components, inserted with and without cement, in one-stage bilateral hip arthroplasty. A controlled, randomized study using roentgenstereophotogrammetric analysis. J Bone Joint Surg Am 1994; 76(2):185–194.

118. Sharkey PF, Barrack RL, Tvedten DE. Five-year clinical and radiographic follow-up of the uncemented long-term stable fixation total hip arthroplasty. J Arthroplasty 1998; 13(5):546–541.

119. Knight JL, Atwater RD, Guo J. Clinical results of the midstem porous-coated anatomic uncemented femoral stem in primary total hip arthroplasty: a five- to nine-year prospective study. J Arthroplasty 1998; 13(5):535–545.

120. Ramaswamy S, Golub TR. DNA microarrays in clinical oncology. J Clin Oncol 2002; 20(7):1932–1941.

121. Christie MJ, DeBoer DK, Trick LW, Brothers JC, Jones RE, Vise GT, et al. Primary total hip arthroplasty with use of the modular S-ROM prosthesis. Four to seven-year clinical and radiographic results. J Bone Joint Surg 1999; 81A(12):1707–1716.

122. Clohisy JC, Harris WH. The Harris–Galante uncemented femoral component in primary total hip replacement at 10 years. J Arthroplasty 1999; 14(8): 915–917.

123. Jasty M, Bragdon C, Jiranek WA, Chandler H, Maloney W, Harris WH. Etiology of osteolysis around porous-coated cementless total hip arthroplasties. Clin Orthop 1994(308):111–126.

124. McLaughlin JR, Lee KR. Total hip arthroplasty with an uncemented femoral component. Excellent results at ten-year follow-up. J Bone Joint Surg 1997; 79(6):900–907.

125. Callaghan JJ, Salvati EA, Pellicci PM, Wilson PD Jr, Ranawat CS. Results of revision for mechanical failure after cemented total hip replacement, 1979

to 1982. A two to five-year follow-up. J Bone Joint Surg Am 1985; 67(7): 1074–1085.

126. Engh CA, Bobyn JD. The influence of stem size and extent of porous coating on femoral bone resorption after primary cementless hip arthroplasty. Clin Orthop 1988; 231:7–28.

127. Berger R, Fletcher F, Donaldson T, Wasielewski R, Peterson M, Rubash HE. Dynamic test to diagnose loose uncemented femoral total hip components. Clin Orthop 1996; 330:115–123.

128. Ragab AA, Kraay MJ, Goldberg VM. Clinical and radiographic outcomes of total hip arthroplasty with insertion of an anatomically designed femoral component without cement for the treatment of primary osteoarthritis. A study with a minimum of six years of follow-up. J Bone Joint Surg Am 1999; 81(2): 210–218.

Total Knee Arthroplasty: Incidence of Osteolysis and Clinical Presentation

Jeffrey Wiley
Concord Orthopaedics, Concord, New Hampshire, U.S.A.

Daniel M. Estok, II
Department of Orthopaedic Surgery, Brigham and Women's Hospital, Harvard Medical School, Boston, Massachusetts, U.S.A.

INTRODUCTION

The search for a reliable and durable prosthesis for knee arthroplasty has been evolving since 1861, when Ferguson (1) reported the first successful arthroplasty. High density polyethylene and ultrahigh molecular weight polyethylene have been used as bearing surfaces since the early 1960s when they were introduced for total hip replacements by Sir John Charnley (2). In 1971, Gunston (3) introduced a prosthesis using a metal femoral condyle articulating with a polyethylene tibial plateau. Today, total knee arthroplasty yields beneficial and predictable results with well over 90% survival at 10-year follow-up (4–10).

Despite the recognized success of hip and knee arthroplasty, wear of materials has become the primary limiting factor in the survival of the implants. Charnley (11) originally described an intense foreign body granulomatous reaction to particles of polytetrafluoroethylene (PTFE) in a letter to the Lancet in 1963. After initially pioneering its use in arthroplasty, he soon abandoned it due to this intense foreign body reaction, which was well encapsulated in the soft tissues but slowly erosive when in contact with bone (11). Interestingly,

Charnley (11) injected himself with PTFE and warned against the use of this substance due to the intense foreign body reaction he observed in his soft tissues. He indicated that a similar injection of high-density polyethylene had not produced any reaction, and he postulated that high-density polyethylene may not produce any soft tissue reaction.

Willert (12) described the process of bone resorption, now known as osteolysis, from his analysis of failed implants. Osteolysis became widely recognized as a concern with both cemented and uncemented total hip arthroplasty, and Jasty et al. (13) described osteolysis in well fixed components as well as loose components. However, early clinical reports did not note this as a complication of total knee arthroplasty, despite retrieval studies demonstrating a greater prevalence of polyethylene wear in knee arthroplasty compared to hip arthroplasty (14).

INCIDENCE

Until the first case report series of osteolysis was reported in 1992, osteolysis was a little recognized complication of total knee arthroplasty. Peters (15) reported 27 cases of osteolysis in 174 consecutive cementless total knee arthroplasties. This equated to a 16% incidence in this series of uncemented implants using cancellous bone screws to obtain tibial fixation. The medial side of the tibial plateau was the most commonly affected site (15).

Initially, osteolysis was associated with cementless techniques. A report by Ezzet et al. (16) showed that osteolysis occurred with a variety of fixation techniques including fixation with cement. However, the incidence varied depending upon fixation technique (16). In this report, the highest incidence of osteolysis, 30%, was seen in the group that had an uncemented femoral component and a cemented tibial component augmented with screws. The group with a cemented tibia without screw fixation and a press fit femur had a 10% incidence of osteolysis. No osteolysis was identified in the patients who had cemented femoral and tibial components without screws (16).

Later reports, however, revealed that osteolysis was not limited to uncemented techniques (17–21). In their report on 17 cases of catastrophic osteolysis, Robinson et al. noted four occurred in fully cemented components. Duffy et al. (21) found that fully cemented components had less revision for osteolysis compared to uncemented techniques. In their study, they discovered a 72% 10-year survival to revision for aseptic failure or loosening for uncemented components compared with a 94% 10-year survival for cemented components (21). Recently, rotational forces from box-post impingement in fully cemented cruciate substituting designs have been postulated to result in rotational forces causing loosening of the implant–cement mantle and subsequent osteolysis (18–20).

Peters (15) speculated that a cement mantle may have been protective of osteolysis by sealing the bony interface. Ezzet's report, however, suggests that this may only be the case when the cement mantle is not violated by screws, therefore sealing the effective joint space (22). Tibial osteolysis may be seen in cases where radiolucent lines are seen on the radiographs of cemented tibial components (23). These radiolucent lines typically correspond to areas of significant preoperative bony sclerosis resulting in poor cement interdigitation to the underlying bony surface. Though they did not observe any progression of these radiolucent lines in their review, they hypothesized that this may allow the synovial fluid and its particulate burden to access the subchondral bone and result in osteolysis in high wear conditions (23).

These reports also revealed that the incidence of osteolysis increases over time, likely correlating with an increasing particle load. No radiographic evidence of lysis was seen before 24 months in the report by Ezzet (16). However, a 25% incidence of osteolysis was seen with follow-up of two to five years and a 39% incidence was noted in patients with follow-up greater than five years (16). Additionally, the average time interval from primary knee replacement to radiographic evidence of osteolysis was 56 months in the report by Robinson (17).

CLINICAL PRESENTATION

Osteolysis around total knee arthroplasty typically goes unnoticed in the early follow-up period and has been described as the "silent disease of orthopaedics" (24). Engh (25) has noted that clinical manifestations of osteolysis are rarely seen in the first five years following total knee arthroplasty. Often, radiographs reveal the osteolytic lesions before symptoms develop, and occasionally these lesions can be large and asymptomatic (25). This emphasizes the need for consistent clinical and radiographic "follow-up on patients that have total knee arthroplasty.

Numerous reports have cited a joint effusion as a presenting clinical feature of osteolysis (15,25,26). This is likely due to the synovial lining being saturated by particulate debris (Fig. 1). The volume of particulate debris increases the synovial pressure in a knee with an intact joint capsule causing the effusion which may be associated with discomfort (25). Additionally, a boggy synovitis induced by the particulate load may be present and cause pain (Fig. 2) (15).

However, when the effective joint space (22) is expanded by a capsular tear or the periprosthetic bone is exposed, the synovial fluid and its particulate debris has access to these extracapsular regions. Painful soft tissue masses have been reported by the formation of extracapsular pseudocysts (27–29). Peters (15) found that pain, which was typically activity related and mild, was most commonly associated with radiographically unstable components.

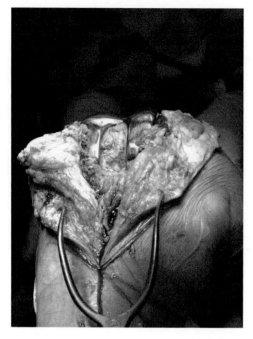

Figure 1   Abundant synovitis and granulation tissue due to polyethylene debris.

Engh (25) also notes that knee flexion is reduced with a long-standing synovitis, which typically presents as a deep ache in the region of the knee aggravated by activity.

In addition to the clinical exam focusing on knee range of motion and the presence of an effusion or synovitis, one should investigate the nature of the pain. A chronic deep ache may be noticed in a synovitic knee with loose components, whereas acute onset of pain may be the result of a periprosthetic fracture through osteolytic lesions (30). A thorough examination of the patient's gait, hip, and back is also indicated. Referred pain to the knee region from an arthritic hip, or from a failing total hip arthroplasty, may be the source of the perceived knee pain. Lumbar spine pathology may also result in referred pain to the region of the knee.

Further clinical findings associated with periprosthetic osteolysis and bone loss include the onset of new or increasing crepitus, as well as a change of axial alignment. Catastrophic failure of the tibial polyethylene by fracture or wear-through may expose the prosthesis to a metal-on-metal articulation resulting in the development of new or increased crepitus or audible metal-on-metal articulation with a clinical change in axial alignment (Figs. 3A–C). This crepitus may represent third body wear associated with increased polyethylene wear and resultant osteolysis as reported by Kloen et al. (31).

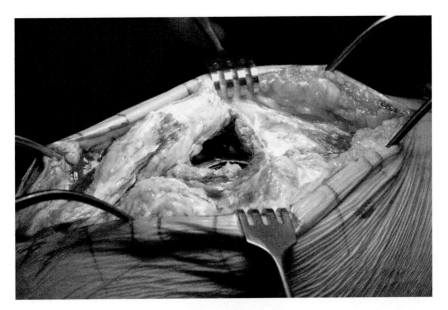

Figure 2 Metallosis in synovial tissue due to polyethylene wear-through resulting in metal-on-metal articulation and the generation of metallic debris.

RADIOGRAPHIC EVALUATION

After the clinical exam, radiographs may be the most easily obtained study in the evaluation of periprosthetic bone loss. As with the clinical exam, however, radiographs may be nonspecific in distinguishing septic from aseptic bone loss. Serial radiographs are most helpful in following the gradual progression of osteolytic lesions over time. On the other hand, the rapid appearance of periprosthetic bone loss without evidence of prosthetic wear is more likely to represent an infectious etiology (33).

Radiographic evaluation is required on an annual or biannual basis to monitor for signs of osteolysis. Peters et al. (15) were unable to predict who would develop osteolysis based on clinical factors such as age, weight, sex, range of motion, clinical scores, and alignment. Additionally, they noted that once it was identified, osteolysis was progressive around both radiographically stable and unstable components in sequential radiographs (15). Three-foot standing anterior posterior radiographs help identify changes in alignment due to eccentric wear of the polyethylene or loss of bony support of the femoral or tibial component due to osteolytic lesions. Standard anterior posterior and lateral radiographs are also helpful in identifying these lesions (Fig. 4).

Osteolysis develops in areas of poor implant bonding and can lead to circumferential radiolucency with loss of component support and eventual

(A)

(B)

(C)

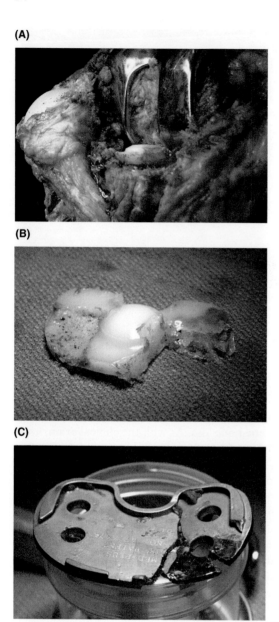

Figure 3 (**A**) Synovitis and metal stained granulation tissue in the face of polyethylene wear-through resulting in metal-on-metal articulation. (**B**) Tibial polyethylene insert retrieved showing delamination damage and wear as well as metal particles imbedded in the articular surface. (**C**) Tibial tray retrieved from the same case showing damage from polyethylene wear-through.

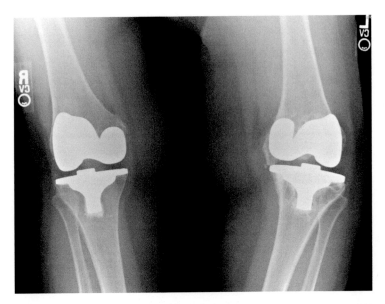

Figure 4 Standing AP radiograph of a 78-year-old, 18 years after bilateral TKA. Osteolysis of the distal femur and proximal tibia has resulted in subsidence of the femoral and tibial components resulting in varus malalignment. *Abbreviations*: AP, anterio-posterior; TKA, total knee arthroplasty.

component migration (32). Engh (32) noted that two types of bone defects can result from the accumulation of wear debris near a stable implant. Focal lesions may develop near components with rigid fixation and are likely to develop borders of sclerotic bone. These focal areas of periprosthetic bone loss typically appear as scalloped defects at the margins of the femoral or tibial components (Fig. 5). The degree of bone loss is outlined by these sclerotic lines of new bone formation and may be the only suggestion of osteolysis (25). In some cases, however, aggressive lesions develop. This may result in expansile lesions with subsequent compromise of the host bone's cortical integrity (Fig. 6) (32).

Osteolysis may be difficult to see on the AP view of the femur due to the prosthesis obscuring the defects. As a result, high-quality radiographs are essential (32) and should include weight bearing AP and true lateral images, as well as standing alignment images. Scalloped borders with sclerotic margins may be present near the condyles when bone loss is evident on the AP view. Additionally, it may present as multiple lobular lesions extending proximally from the prosthesis (32). The most common site for osteolytic lesions to occur in the femur is in the posterior femoral condyles (Fig. 7) (32). These femoral lesions frequently develop as a result of incomplete capping of the condyles by the prosthesis (25). This allows the synovial fluid and its particulate

(A)   **(B)**

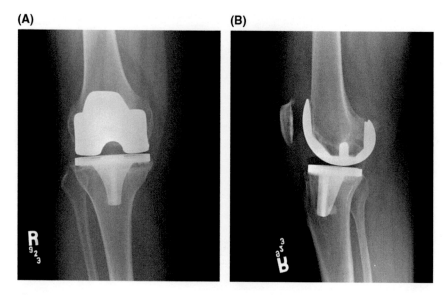

Figure 5 (**A**) Anterio-posterior, and (**B**) lateral X-rays of a 64-year-old man 10 years after primary TKA showing focal osteolytic lesions in the proximal tibia and distal femur. *Abbreviation*: TKA, total knee arthroplasty.

burden to access the femoral bone. As Engh (25) notes, osteolysis in the anterior metaphyseal region may also occur as a result of oversizing of the femoral component in the anterior-posterior dimension. This allows synovial fluid access to this bone when the component does not have an ingrowth surface adjacent to the host bone, or a cement mantle, to seal the bony surface.

The radiographic appearance of aseptic loosening (a gradual breakdown of the cement–bone interface) may have a different radiographic appearance (32). In this case, circumferential radiolucencies develop at the bone–cement interface. The component then migrates into bone, expanding and occasionally fracturing the weakened condyle with resultant component subsidence and instability (32).

Tibial bone loss is easier to see on AP radiographs because the metaphyseal region of the proximal tibia is not hidden by the tibial component (Fig. 5A) (32). Weight bearing films are helpful in revealing polyethylene wear and resulting instability (32). Areas of bone loss may be easier to visualize in an all-polyethylene tibial component (32). When a metal tibial tray has been used, it is important to have the X-ray beam parallel to the tibial tray in order to prevent the tray from obscuring areas of bone loss (32).

Though the clinical history and radiographs are helpful in diagnosing aseptic periprosthetic bone loss or osteolysis, the majority of these findings are nonspecific. Consequently, osteolysis is a diagnosis of exclusion and

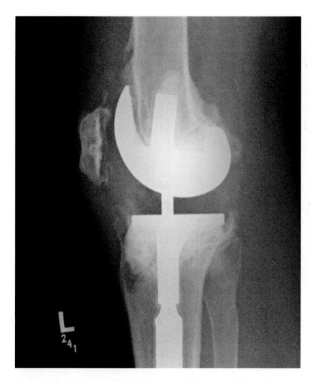

Figure 6   Lateral radiograph of a 64-year-old man 10 years after revision TKA with focal osteolytic lesion in the tibial tubercle as well as subsidence of the tibial component. *Abbreviation*: TKA, total knee arthroplasty.

must be differentiated from infection, and other causes for bone loss, in order to provide appropriate treatment. Dunbar et al. (33) note that radiographic findings of osteolysis are rare within the first two years after surgery and infection should be suspected when these linear or scalloped lesions are present in this time period, and should be considered when these lesions appear at any time. Despite thorough diagnostic evaluation it can often be difficult to distinguish osteolysis from infection.

OTHER IMAGING STUDIES

Specialized radiographic studies may also be helpful in distinguishing aseptic from septic periprosthetic bone loss. Standard Technetium 99 bone scans are of little use in identifying an infectious etiology. Increased uptake can be seen in cases of infection, loosening, tumor, trauma, and may be seen for up to a year following total knee arthroplasty (34). Gallium scans and indium labeled scans are more reliable. Gallium scans have a high sensitivity; therefore, a negative

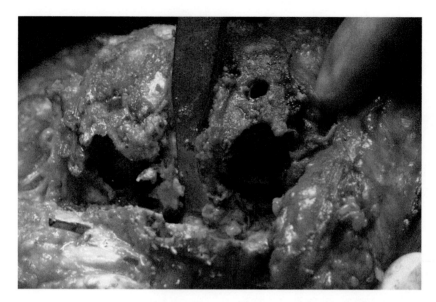

Figure 7   Large osteolytic defects seen in the medial and lateral femoral.

scan can reliably rule out infection (34). Indium-labeled scans have been shown to have an accuracy of 84% in diagnosing periprosthetic infections (35). These studies may be helpful in situations in which serologic studies are confounded by other systemic conditions and aspirates are unreliable due to antibiotic use.

Computerized tomography and magnetic resonance imaging may also have a role in the evaluation of periprosthetic bone loss. Historically, the use of these modalities has been somewhat limited due to scatter from the metallic implants. However, continued improvements in software technology may allow for suppression of the metallic artifact and allow improved visualization of the various interfaces as well as improved evaluation of periprosthetic bone loss. Recent reports using CT and MRI for the evaluation of total hip arthroplasty found both modalities to be more accurate in identifying the presence and extent of osteolysis than standard radiographs (36,37). Most importantly, these improvements in radiographic evaluation influenced patient management and surgical planning.

LABORATORY EVALUATION

Routine blood work including white blood cell count, erythrocyte sedimentation rate (ESR), and c-reactive protein (CRP) also may be helpful when trying to differentiate osteolysis from infection. Care must be taken in the interpretation of these studies, however, for they are not specific. Chronic inflammatory disorders, recent trauma, or surgeries can result in elevated acute phase reactants. In particular, the white blood cell count may not be elevated in chronic infections (33).

The ESR and CRP are much more sensitive studies than the white blood cell count (38). Ruling out infection is the real utility of the ESR and CRP. The negative predictive value has been shown to be 95% for the ESR and 99% for the CRP by Sprangehl et al. (38) in a study investigating the diagnosis of infection in total hip arthroplasties. ESR values of more than 30–35 mm/hr and CRP values over 0.1 mg/L should be considered abnormal and warrant additional investigations (34). Care should be taken when assess"ing these values, however, as normal values are lab-specific. Additionally, "different testing sites may report the results expressed in different units.

Knee aspiration and culture is a valuable tool in differentiating septic from aseptic periprosthetic bone loss. This can be performed as a simple office based procedure; however, false negative aspirations may occur. White blood cell counts of greater than 25,000 mm^{-3} or a differential of greater than 75% polymorphonuclear leukocytes (PMNS) are indicative of infection (34).

Duff et al. (39) reported that preoperative aspiration of a total knee prosthesis was the best method to diagnose or exclude infection in total knee arthroplasties. Aspiration yielded a sensitivity, specificity, and accuracy of 100% in diagnosing infection, while lab values, clinical symptoms, and radiographs were less reliable in diagnosing infection.

Antibiotic use prior to aspiration may result in false negative culture results as reported by Barrack et al. (40). In this report, 58% of patients who were taking antibiotics at the time of aspiration and had a negative culture were ultimately found to have an infected total knee arthroplasty. The authors (40) found that a repeat aspiration after discontinuing antibiotics significantly improved in the results in diagnosing infection. Some authors (34) recommend obtaining three samples for culture. If all three are positive an infection is diagnosed; however, if two cultures are positive in the previous studies, clinical presentation and preoperative suspicion are used to make the diagnosis of infection. When only one sample grows an organism, it is recommended the aspiration be repeated (34).

Occasionally, infection still cannot be excluded as a diagnosis despite using all of the above diagnostic modalities. In this case, intraoperative tests are used to exclude an infectious etiology. Tissue samples obtained from the knee joint, femoral, and tibial canals may be sent for histological analysis. Mirra et al. (41) described submitting five tissue samples for frozen section analysis at the time of revision. The authors found that more than five PMNs per high-powered field were highly correlated with infection. In order to improve test specificity, Lonner et al. (42) recommended a threshold of 10 PMNs per high-powered field for a diagnosis of infection and less than five PMNs to exclude active infection. If infection is ruled out, the surgeon may then address the aseptic periprosthetic bone loss in the course of the revision total knee arthroplasty.

TREATMENT

Routine follow-up is needed following total knee arthroplasties in order to monitor for periprosthetic bone loss as its incidence increases over time (16,17). Once osteolysis is identified and infection is ruled out, the patient is involved in treatment options. Observation of small, stable lesions is a reasonable approach, especially if the patient is asymptomatic and the components are stable without risk of fracture from the lesion (25). Since osteolysis has been reported to be progressive despite initially stable appearing lesions and components (15), biannual radiographs will allow the observation of these lesions and assess progression. Additionally, this allows increased interaction with the patient and helps establish patient concurrence with the treatment plan (25).

When the femoral and tibial components are well fixed in the presence of osteolytic lesions in a symptomatic patient, partial revision surgery may be considered. It should be noted, however, that the extent of the osteolytic lesions is usually grossly underestimated on radiographs (17). When the femoral and tibial components are undamaged, as assessed by visual inspection and palpation of their articulating surfaces, it may be reasonable to perform an isolated polyethylene insert exchange with curettage and bone grafting of the osteolytic defects. However, the cause for failure must be determined before embarking upon this treatment option. Engh (43) has reported that isolated insert exchange for osteolysis with curettage and allograft bone grafting of the osteolytic lesions was most successful in patients who demonstrated acceptable wear of at least 10 years. In patients who had failure of their total knee arthroplasty in less than 10 years, 27% of patients had failure of their isolated insert revision due to accelerated wear of the new insert (43). These instances of early (<10 years) failure and osteolysis are likely due to high wear conditions. Malalignment, backside wear of tibial polyethylene inserts from micromotion in modular tibial trays (44), or postimpingement in cruciate substituting components (16–18), may contribute to increased wear and in these circumstances complete revision is required (25).

When fractures develop through osteolytic lesions, loss of component fixation or subsidence of the components can occur. Patients usually are symptomatic and complete revision is required. Frequently, in cases of complete knee revision for osteolysis, modular systems with allografts or a rotating hinged systems are required (25). Engh (25) describes three principles to follow when performing complete revisions for knees with large osteolytic defects. First, reconstitute the cancellous bone structure in the metaphyseal regions to allow for cement interdigitation and component stability. Second, utilize long stemmed components to engage the diaphysis of the femur and tibia. Third, use the least constraint required for satisfactory knee stability (25). Typically, component selection is chosen after the osteolytic lesions have been curettaged and bony defects and knee stability assessed. In cases of ligamentous instability, linked or rotating hinged components are required.

Smaller, contained bony defects can be managed with local use of cement or prosthetic augments—especially in older, low demand patients. Engh (25) notes that defects up to 12 mm in depth can be managed by prosthetic augments and those larger than this are best managed with allografts. Several studies have reviewed the success of allograft use in total knee revisions for periprosthetic bone loss (45–48). The longest reported follow-up of structural allografts used in revision total knee arthroplasty has been reported by Clatworthy et al. (48). These authors reported on 50 patients who underwent revision arthroplasty with structural allografting for uncontained bony defects (defined as segmental bone loss with no remaining "cortex) with a minimum of five-year follow-up. Seventy-three percent of these patients had whole distal femoral or proximal tibial grafts, with the remainder requiring partial distal femoral, partial proximal tibial, or femoral head graft. They found a 75% success rate and a 72% survival rate of the "allografts at 10 years, and concluded that allografts have an encouraging medium-term survival in these difficult cases of massive bone loss.

Rotating hinge components are an alternative to structural allografting in the setting of massive bone loss. Rand et al. (49) reported higher rates of loosening (13%) and infection (16%) at mean follow-up of 4.2 years after revision arthroplasty. Shaw (50) also reported a higher rate of loosening (20%) using rotating hinged components with two-year follow-up. More recent reports, however, have noted lower rates of loosening and early failure (51,52).

SUMMARY

Osteolysis following total knee arthroplasty has become a recognized entity. Its incidence increases over the lifetime of the components and is related to the manufacturing process of the components as well as surgical technique. Routine clinical and radiographic follow-up is required to monitor the evolution of periprosthetic bone loss following total knee arthroplasty. The clinical and radiographic appearance of osteolysis is nonspecific and must be differentiated from an infectious process. More frequent follow-up is then required in order to form a treatment plan consistent with the patient's needs and possibly limit massive bone loss. Surgical treatment should be individualized on a case-by-case basis. This may involve isolated insert exchange with curettage and grafting for solidly fixed and well-aligned components, full revision, or revision with structural allografts or rotating hinged components in cases of massive bone loss and instability.

REFERENCES

1. Ferguson M. Excision of the knee joint: recovery with a false joint and a useful limb. Med Times Gazette 1861; 1:601.
2. Charnley J. The long-term results of low friction arthroplasty of the hip performed as a primary intervention. JBJS 1972; 54B:61.

3. Riley LH Jr. The evolution of total knee arthroplasty. CORR 1976; 120:7–10.
4. Schai P, Thornhill TS, Scott RD. Total knee arthroplasty with the PFC system, results at a minimum of 10 years and survivorship analysis. JBJS 1998; 80(5): 850–858.
5. Rodriguez JA, Harish B, Ranawat CS. Total condylar knee replacement: a 20-year follow-up study. CORR 2001; 388:10–17.
6. Berger RA, Rosenberg AG, Barden RM, Sheinkop MB, Jacobs JJ, Galante JO. Long Term Follow-up of the Miller-Gallante Total Knee Replacement. CORR 2001; 388:58–67.
7. Laskin RS. The genesis total knee prosthesis: a 10-year follow-up study. CORR 2001; 388:95–102.
8. Buechel FF Sr, Buechel FF Jr, Pappas MJ, D'Alessio J. Twenty-Year Evaluation of Mensiscal Bearing and Rotating Platform Knee Replacements. CORR 2001; 388:41–50.
9. Callaghan JJ, Insall JN, Greenwald AS, Dennis DS, Komistek RD, Murray DW, Bourne RB, Rorabeck CH, Dorr LD. Mobile Bearing Knee Replacements: Concepts and Results. AAOS Inst Course Lec 2001; 50:431–50. AAOS Rosemont, IL. 2001.
10. Brassard MF, Insall JN, Scuderi GR, Colizza W. Does Modularity Affect Clinical Success? A comparison with a minimum 10-year follow-up. CORR 2001; 388:26–32.
11. Charnley J. Letter: Tissue reaction to polytetrafluorethylene. Lancet 1963; 1379.
12. Willert HG, Semlitsch M. Reactions of the articular capsule to wear products of artificial joint prostheses. J Biomed Mater Res 1977; 11:157–164.
13. Jasty MJ, Floyd WE III, Schiller AL, Goldring SR, Harris, WH. Localized Osteolysis in Stable Non-Septic Total Hip Arthroplasty. JBJS 1986; 68-A:912–919.
14. Engh GA, Parks NL, Ammeen DJ. Tibial osteolysis in cementless total knee arthroplasty: a review of 25 cases treated with and without tibial component revision. CORR 1994; 309:33–43.
15. Peters PC Jr, Engh GA, Dwyer KA, Vinh TN. Osteolysis After Total Knee Replacement Without Cement. JBJS 1992; 74-A (6):864–876.
16. Ezzet KA, Garcia R, Barrack RL. Effect of component fixation on osteolysis in total knee arthroplasty. CORR 1995; 321:86–91.
17. Robinson EJ, Mulliken BD, Bourne RB, Rorabeck CH. Catastrophic osteolysis in total knee replacement. CORR 1995; 321:98–105.
18. Mikulak SA, Mahoney OM, dela Rosa MA, Schmalzried TP. Loosening and osteolysis with the press fit condylar posterior cruciate substituting total knee replacement. JBJS 2001; 83-A:398.
19. Pagnano MW, Scuderi GR, Insall JN. Tibial osteolysis associated with the modular tibial tray of a cemented posterior stabilized total knee replacement. A case report. JBJS 2001; 83-A:1545–1548.
20. Puloski SK, McCalden RW, MacDonald SJ, Rorabeck CH, Bourne RB. Tibial Post Wear in Posterior-Stabilized Total Knee Arthroplasty. An unrecognized source of polyethylene debris. JBJS 2001; 83-A(3):390.
21. Duffy GP, Berry DJ, Rand JA. Cement vs cementless fixation in total knee arthroplasty. CORR 1998; 356:66–72.

22. Schmalzried TP, Harris WH. Periprosthetic bone loss in total hip arthroplasty. Polyethylene wear debris and the concept of the effective joint space. JBJS 1992; 74-A(6):849–863.

23. Smith S, Naima VS, Freeman MA. The natural history of tibial radiolucent lines in a proximally cemented stemmed total knee arthroplasty. J Arthroplasty 1999; 14(1):3–8.

24. Engh GA, Ammeen DJ. Clinical manifestations of a sometimes silent disease. Orthopedics 1999; 22:799–801.

25. Engh GA, Ammeen DA. Periprosthetic osteolysis with total knee arthroplasty. AAOS Inst Course Lect. 2001; 50:391–398. AAOS Rosemont, IL, 2001.

26. Berry DJ, Wold LE, Rand JA. Extensive osteolysis around an aseptic, stable, uncemented total knee replacement. CORR 1993; 293:204–207.

27. Yasuda M, Inoue K, Ikawa T, Yukioka M, Shichikawa K. A Giant Thigh Mass in a Patient with Total Knee Arthroplasty for Charcot Joint. CORR 1995; 317:159–161.

28. Chavda DV, Garvin KL. Failure or a polyethylene total knee component presenting as a thigh mass. Report of a rare complication of total knee arthroplasty. CORR 1994; 303:211–216.

29. Dirschl DR, Lachiewicz PF. Dissecting popliteal cyst as a presenting symptom of a malfunctioning total knee arthroplasty. Report of four cases. J Arthroplasty 1992; 7(1):37–41.

30. Rand JA. Supracondylar fracture of the femur associated with polyethylene wear after total knee arthroplasty. A case report. JBJS 1994; 76-A:1389–1393.

31. Kloen P, Burke DW, Chew FS, Mildrum R. Radiographic Pseudochondrocalcinosis in Early Failure of a Cemented Total Knee replacement. J Arthroplasty 1998; 13(8):953–956.

32. Engh GA, Ammeen DJ. Classification and preoperative radiographic evaluation: knee. Orhto Clin N Am 1998; 29(2):205–217.

33. Dunbar MJ, Blackley H, Bourne RB. Osteolysis of the femur: principles of management. AAOS Inst Course Lect 2001; 50:197–209. AAOS Rosemont, IL, 2001.

34. Munjal S, Phillips MJ, Krackow KA. Revision total knee arthroplasty: planning, controversies, and management–infection. AAOS Inst Course Lect 2001; 50:367–377. AAOS Rosemont, IL, 2001.

35. Merkel KD, Brown ML, Dewange MK, Fitzgerald RH Jr. Comparison of Indium Labeled Leukocyte Imaging with Sequential Technetium-Gallium Scanning in the Diagnosis of Low Grade Musculoskeletal Infections. JBJS 1985; 67-A:465–476.

36. Potter HG, Sofka CM, Peters LE, Salvatti EA. Abstract: Evaluation of Total Hip Arthroplasty with Magnetic Resonance Imaging. Proceedings of the American Academy of Orthopaedic Surgeons 69th Annual Meeting, Dallas, TX. AAOS, Rosemont, IL, 2002, 692.

37. Wixson RL, Stulberg SD, Adams AD, Hendrix RW, Beanfield JB. Abstract: Monitoring Pelvic Osteolysis Following Total Hip Replacement Surgery: An Algorithm for Surveillance. Proceedings of the American Academy of Orthopaedic Surgeons 69th Annual Meeting, Dallas, TX. AAOS, Rosemont, IL: 2002, 734.

38. Sprangehl MJ, Masri BA, O'Connell JX, Duncan CP. Prospective Analysis of Preoperative and Intraoperative Investigations for the Diagnosis of Infection at

the Sites of Two-Hundred and Two Revision Total Hip Arthroplasties. JBJS 1999; 81-A:672–683.

39. Duff GP, Lachiewicz PF, Kelley SS. Aspiration before revision arthroplasty. CORR 1996; 331:132–139.

40. Barrack RL, Jennings RW, Wolfe MW, Bertot AJ. The Coventry Award: The Value of Preoperative Aspiration Before Total Knee Revision. CORR 1997; 345:8–16.

41. Mirra JM, Amstutz HC, Matos M, Gold R. The Pathology of the Joint Tissues and it's Relevance in Prosthesis Failure. CORR 1976; 117:221–240.

42. Lonner JH, Desai P, Dicesare PE, Steiner G, Zuckerman JD. The Reliability of Analysis of Intraoperative Frozen Sections for Identifying Active Infection During Revision Hip or Knee Arthroplasty. JBJS 1996; 78-A:1553–1558.

43. Engh GA, Koralewicz LM, Pereles TR. Clinical results of modular polyethylene insert exchange with retention of total knee arthroplasty components. JBJS 2000; 82-A:516–523.

44. Engh GA, Rao A, et al. Abstract: tibial baseplate wear: a major source of wear debris with contemporary modular knee implants. Proceedings of the American Academy of Orthopaedic Surgeons 67th Annual Meeting Orlando, FL. Rosemont, IL: AAOS, 2000, 283.

45. Tsahakis PJ, Beaver WB, Brick GW. Technique and results of allograft reconstruction in revision total knee arthroplasty. CORR 1994; 303:86–94.

46. Ghazavi MT, Stockley I, Yee G, Davis A, Gross AE. Reconstruction of Massive Bone Defects with Allograft in Revision Total Knee Arthroplasty. JBJS 1997; 79-A:17–25.

47. Engh GA, Herzwurm PJ, Parks NL. Treatment of Major Defects of Bone with Bulk Allografts and Stemmed Components During Total Knee Arthroplasty. JBJS 1997; 79-A:1030–1039.

48. Clatworthy MG, Ballance J, Brick GW, Chandler HP, Gross AE. The Use of Structural Allograft for Uncontained Defects in Revision Total Knee Arthroplasty. JBJS 2001; 83-A:404.

49. Rand JA, Chao EY, Stauffer RN. Kinematic Rotating-Hinge Total Knee Arthroplasty. JBJS 1987; 69-A:489–497.

50. Shaw JA, Balcom W, Greer RB. III, Total Knee Arthroplasty Using the Kinematic Rotating Hinge Prosthesis. Orthopedics 1989; 12:647–654.

51. Jones RE, Skedros JG, Chan AJ, Beauchamp DH, Harkins PC. Total Knee Arthroplasty Using the S-ROM Mobile-Bearing Hinge Prosthesis. J. ArthroplastyÔ 2001; 16(3):279–287.

52. Barrack RL, Lyons TR, Ingraham RQ, Johnson JC. The Use of a Modular Rotating Hinge Component in Salvage Revision Total Knee Arthroplasty. J Arthroplasty 2000; 15(7):858–866.

6

Histopathology of Periprosthetic Tissues

Stuart B. Goodman

Department of Orthopaedic Surgery, Stanford University Medical Center, Stanford, California, U.S.A.

Victor Fornasier

Department of Pathology, St. Michael's Hospital, University of Toronto, Toronto, Ontario, Canada

INTRODUCTION

Total joint replacements are generally highly successful operations with acceptable longevity. Whether the prosthesis is cemented or cementless, if the materials selected are biocompatible, and based on the component design and surgical technique are optimized, hip and knee arthroplasties have a survivorship of 15 years with over a 90% probability. The key to the success of joint replacement is the host's biological response to the implant. In this chapter, we will explore the histopathology of total joint replacements including the tissue response to well-functioning orthopaedic joint prostheses, and those undergoing failure due to loosening and osteolysis.

HISTOPATHOLOGY OF WELL-FIXED JOINT REPLACEMENTS

Cemented Implants

The cemented joint implant is still the gold standard by which all other forms of fixation are compared. Sir John Charnley (1,2) popularized the use of polymethylmethacrylate (PMMA) to grout implants within bone. Although technical advances have been made in the delivery of bone cement to the bone bed (such as using a cement gun, distal plugging of the femoral canal, using pulsatile lavage, centralization of the prosthesis within the cement mantle, etc.), the aim is still to intrude the cement into the cleaned and dried interstices of bone (3,4). This provides a mechanical interlock between the cement and bone, as PMMA has no adhesive properties.

The histological stages of cemented prosthetic interfaces are well described by Charnley (1,2) in his textbook and others employing retrieved specimens and different animal models. Charnley retrieved 23 human specimens between one month and seven years after cemented total hip replacement. All of the cases were clinically successful and not loose radiographically. In femoral retrievals harvested several weeks after implantation, cellular damage (loss of the definition of fat and hematopoietic cells) was seen in an area 500 μm from the cement interface. Charnley presumed that this layer was due to chemical, thermal, and mechanical trauma to the surrounding bone during the initial implantation. A fibrous tissue layer then developed at the interface, with embedded impressions of the circular PMMA beads. The fibrous layer then underwent metaplasia to fibrocartilage in areas subjected to "mechanical pressure." In other areas, the PMMA beads directly abutted bony trabeculae and cortical bone. In some areas, the original bone adjacent to the cement became necrotic and was slowly replaced by new bone, with an intervening layer of fibrous tissue or fibrocartilage. According to Charnley, the fibrocartilage might then mature to lamellar bone over many years. A foreign-body giant cell reaction was seen on the surface of fibrous tissue in areas that Charnley believed were subject to minimal load.

In human retrieval studies, Harris and associates (5–7) demonstrated trabecular bone intimately interdigitated with the cement surrounding well-fixed femoral stems two weeks to 17 years postoperatively. Fibrous tissue was apparently uncommon at the cement–bone interface. After many years, the bone surrounding prostheses had undergone a remodeling process in which a secondary, circumferential, trabecular "neocortex" was formed surrounding the cement. This neocortex was connected to the outer cortex via radial spicules of bone. Failure of fixation of cemented femoral components was found to be initiated at the cement–prosthesis interface by separation or "debonding" and fracture in the cement mantle. This thesis was novel, as previous descriptions of the failure of cemented femoral stems emphasized failure of the bone–cement interface, rather than the stem–cement interface. Furthermore, the above observations led to the controversial concept of precoating of the femoral stem ex vivo, in order to create a chemical bond between the precoated cement and the cement placed into the canal at surgery.

Fornasier et al. (8) reported a detailed histomorphometric study of 14 hip arthroplasties harvested at postmortem. The implants were all functioning successfully two weeks to 14 years postoperatively. The radiographs apparently did not demonstrate evidence of prosthetic migration or radiolucent lines at the cement–bone interface. Despite these clinical and radiographic findings, the cemented components were surrounded by a fibrohistiocytic membrane in most cases; macrophages and foreign body giant cells were observed surrounding and engulfing cement and polyethylene debris; chronic inflammatory cells were also seen. Fibrocartilage often covered thickened bony trabeculae. The underlying bone demonstrated active remodeling. The density of macrophages and foreign body giant cells correlated with the time after prosthetic implantation, the membrane thickness, and the density of polyethylene particles. These asymptomatic, retrieved, well-fixated, cemented implants suggested a process of "loosening in evolution" at the cement–bone interface.

Apparently well-fixed cemented acetabular components harvested at autopsy also showed a progressive, centripetal resorption of the bone supporting the prosthetic bed, due to the ingress of polyethylene debris and subsequent foreign body reaction (9). The foreign body and chronic inflammatory reaction to plastic wear debris continued to undermine the cement–prosthesis bony support until motion at the bone–cement interface led to clinical failure of the implant. These observations also underlined the importance of wear of the articulation, and the subsequent biological reaction to the debris generated.

Cement that is well interdigitated into the interstices of bone can act as a barrier to the entry of polyethylene debris into the surrounding bone. This important sealant effect of bone cement undoubtedly contributes to the low incidence of periprosthetic osteolysis seen in cemented implants, even in the presence of significant polyethylene wear.

Cementless Implants

Cementless components for joint replacement may be covered in whole or part with a porous coating or possess surface modifications to enhance the ingrowth/ongrowth of bone (10–15). The aim of these implants is to provide a pain-free, stable, durable, functional hip joint with minimal adverse bone remodeling. Irrespective of whether bone is ingrown into a porous surface or opposed to the prosthesis (bone ongrowth), load must be transmitted with minimal micromotion at the interface.

Bone ingrowth/ongrowth occurs by a series of events that are analogous to fracture healing. Three phases are generally noted: inflammation, repair, and remodeling. In the first few days after surgery, voids are filled by coagulated blood (hematoma formation). In the first few weeks that follow, the hematoma is invaded by mesenchymal cells which have osteoprogenitor potential. Newly formed osteoblasts produce woven fiber bone (stage of repair). Around four weeks after surgery, remodeling begins and is characterized by the formation of parallel, lamellar, fiber bone via intramembranous ossification. Interfacial motion, pore size and gap between the host bone and the porous surface, all influence bone ingrowth (13,15). Prerequisites for the occurrence of bone ingrowth include intimate contact between the porous surface and the surrounding bone and "rigid" fixation (10–17). Excessive motion of approximately 25–50 μm or more between the implant and the host bone leads to fibrous tissue rather than bone ingrowth. The optimum pore size for bone ingrowth is in the range of 100–400 μm, although fiber-mesh porous coatings with a more open cancellous-like structure and macroporous implants also facilitate ingrowth of bone (12,13).

Implant retrieval studies are critical in assessing the degree of bone ingrowth or apposition but must be interpreted with caution. Autopsy retrievals from clinically well-functioning components are best. Retrievals from revision cases reflect clinical failure due to reasons such as polyethylene wear, recurrent dislocation, intractable pain, etc. Because of possible abnormal biomechanics of prosthetic loading and other potential confounding variables, the findings from these studies may not accurately reflect the degree of bone ingrowth into implants from patients with well-functioning implants.

The amount of bone ingrowth into porous coated prostheses is a controversial subject and depends on many factors, including the patient, the local biological and mechanical environment, surgical and prosthetic variables, and the postoperative loading protocol (11). A study by Cook et al. (18) reported 90 porous-coated cementless total joints (62 total knee arthoplasty (TKA) components and 28 total hip arthoplasty (THA) components) retrieved from 58 patients. Spherical-bead and fiber-metal porous implants were included. The components were all revised for reasons other than aseptic loosening or infection. Histologically, in approximately one-third of all components, the porous coating contained only mature fibrous tissue, and no bone ingrowth or apposition was observed. In another one-third of implants, ingrowth or apposition of bone was limited to less than 2% of the available surface area of the porous coating. In the remaining one-third of the components, between 2% and 10% of the porous coating contained bone. In all cases, the majority of the porous coating contained mature, oriented fibrous tissue rather than bone. These findings were extremely disappointing and cast doubt on the concept of bone ingrowth as a sustaining method of long-term prosthetic fixation.

Bone ingrowth has been more successful in other series. In a study by Jacobs et al. (19), 14 consecutively retrieved porous-fiber metal femoral components that had been removed for reasons other than loosening and infection were examined. In 10 of the 14 cases retrieved from primary hip replacements with normal femoral geometry, the mean extent of bone ingrowth (bone along the surface to a depth of at least 1/2 bead diameter) was 44.9% (range, 19.6–92.6%). The mean volume fraction of bone ingrowth (i.e., the degree to which pores were filled with bone) was 17.2% (range 6.8–64.8%). This and other similar studies emphasize the necessity of defining terms relating to bone ingrowth very specifically. Only by using a common, well-defined nomenclature of bone ingrowth/ongrowth can different studies be compared and logical conclusions derived.

In general, bone ingrowth is more extensive in hip rather than knee prostheses, and increases with time that the implant is in situ. Bone ingrowth is also increased in areas of close prosthesis–bone apposition and around screws and screw holes; a gap of 1.5–2.0 mm usually is too wide for bone ingrowth to take place (20–24). If optimal conditions are not fulfilled, fibrous tissue and fibrocartilage as well as bone marrow fill the interstices. However, despite the low percentage of bone ingrowth/ongrowth that is associated with cementless prostheses, these implants are highly successful clinically and have longevities that are comparable those from cemented implants, especially in younger, more active patients.

Bone ingrowth into porous coatings can also function as an impediment to the migration of wear particles; however, debris can migrate along fibrous or cancellous interfaces with cyclic loading of the joint to more remote sites along the prosthetic interface. This may result in localized or more widespread osteolytic areas along the bone–implant interface.

Implants with Bioactive Coatings

Two main calcium phosphate ceramics, hydroxylapatite [$Ca_{10}(PO_4)_6(OH)_6(OH)_2$, HA] and tricalcium phosphate [$Ca_3(PO_4)_2$, TCP] have been used to coat implants and enhance bone apposition. Synthetic HA and TCP have similar chemical compositions as the calcium phosphate in bone. Both HA and TCP are osteoconductive, nontoxic substances that are capable of bonding directly to bone, enhancing osseointegration. TCP gradually dissolves whereas HA dissolves very minimally.

Coating an uncemented prosthesis with HA by methods such as plasma spraying, electrophoresis, dipping, sputtering, and mechanical techniques increases the deposition of new bone both on the surface of the implant and on the host bone bed (25–34). No intervening fibrous tissue is found. This enhances bone ingrowth/ongrowth, linking newly formed bone with the HA at the atomic level. As a result, strength of the bone–implant interface is increased, and the time required to achieve adequate fixation strength is decreased. The osteoconductive properties of HA coating also facilitates bone apposition by mitigating the adverse effects of gaps (up to 2 mm) and micromotion (31–34), which are commonly found after initial placement of a cementless implant. Numerous mechanical and histological studies in animals and humans have demonstrated the efficacy of HA coatings in enhancing the processes of bone ingrowth and osseointegration. In retrieval studies of hip implants up to five years postoperatively, growth of bone onto the HA coating varied from 10% to 20% of the surface after three weeks, 48% after 12 weeks, and 32–78% after 5–25 months (27).

Because of the osteoconductive properties of hydroxyapatite and the direct mineralization of the HA-coated implant surface with bone, no intervening fibrous tissue layer is found. Thus HA coating, like PMMA may impede the ingress of wear particles to the bone–prosthesis interface. This may curtail more widespread undermining of the surrounding bone by the foreign body and chronic inflammatory reaction associated with particulate wear debris, limiting the extent of periprosthetic osteolysis. However, mechanical loss of the HA coating during prosthetic insertion, or during the lifetime of the prosthesis with migration of the particles into the joint may potentially result in third body wear.

HISTOPATHOLOGY OF LOOSE JOINT REPLACEMENTS

Implants for total joint replacement (TJR) and internal fixation of fractures are similar situations that provide two alternatives: a biologically and mechanically favorable outcome with implant stability and enhanced function versus instability and poor function due to excessive interfacial motion with subsequent failure of the construct. Mechanically loose implants undergo excessive displacement with physiological loads. Motion at the interface of loose joint replacements leads to a reactive fibrosis. Furthermore, a synovial lining layer may subsequently develop between the moving surfaces. This is true for implants that are cemented, cementless, and those covered by bioactive coatings. Pressure necrosis of bone may occur when a loose implant subsides and/or abuts the cortex, and loading becomes excessive and concentrated over a small area. Debris from articulating and nonarticulating surfaces of the implants, the surrounding bone, and other structures accumulates locally; this debris incites a foreign body and chronic inflammatory reaction composed primarily of macrophages and foreign body giant cells in a fibrous stroma (35–42). These circumstances begin a cascade of events culminating in periprosthetic bone resorption which further undermines the prosthetic bed. With intermittent loading, waves of increased pressure within the joint distribute the wear particles and by-products, cellular constituents, and inflammatory mediators to more remote sites along the interface and beyond.

Failed loose cemented joint arthroplasties are typically surrounded by a thick, frond-like, tan-colored, rubbery tissue that is composed of mono- and multi-nucleated foreign body cells (macrophages) and chronic inflammatory cells in a fibrous stroma (Fig. 1) (35,36). A synovial-like lining layer is sometimes found on the membrane surface, adjacent to the cement layer (37,38). This one- to two-cell layer is composed of large polygonal cells with eccentric nuclei located away from the cement surface. This synovial-like layer is supported by a loose fibrovascular stroma containing macrophages and wear particles. A third layer of more dense fibrous tissue supports the second layer, and abuts the surrounding bone. Small particles of PMMA, polyethylene and metals, depending on the materials in the implant are intermixed with the above cellular reaction (Figs. 1–3). PMMA is dissolved during conventional processing of the tissue specimens but can be identified by the round vacant cement "ghosts" of PMMA and the presence of residual,

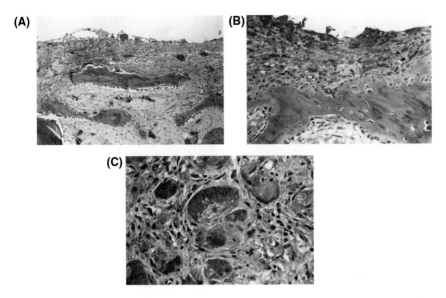

Figure 1 Interface membrane surrounding a revised loose cemented total hip replacement. (**A**) Cement has been dissolved during tissue processing producing the empty space at the top of the photomicrograph. The interface membrane is cellular with active osteoclastic resorption of the trabeculae of bone on the side facing the implant. Plump osteoblasts are seen on the side away from the implant. This is the typical pattern of remodeling occurring at the periprosthetic interface at revision for aseptic loosening. [Decalcified paraffin embedded World Health Organization (WHO) stained section, transmitted light, 100× magnification.] (**B**) This high power photomicrograph of the interface surrounding a revised loose cemented hip replacement demonstrates a highly cellular tissue adjacent to small granular cement remnants. Note both osteoclasts and osteoblasts lining the trabecular bone that is undergoing active remodeling. (Decalcified paraffin embedded WHO stained section, transmitted light, 250× magnification.) (**C**) This section from a revised loose cemented hip replacement demonstrates numerous multinucleated giant cells in a highly cellular stroma containing mononuclear phagocytes, scattered lymphocytes, and fibroblasts. Near the center of the photomicrograph is a large multinucleated giant cell containing an asteroid body (the star-shaped figure). (Decalcified paraffin embedded WHO stained section, transmitted light, 500× magnification.)

undissolved particles of barium sulfate or other radio-opaque device. Polyethylene debris can be identified with the use of polarized light or oil red O staining methods (39,40). The polyethylene debris is generally in the submicron range and found in macrophages; larger shards are surrounded by numerous multinucleated giant cells in a fibrous stroma (41).

Tissues from loose cementless implants are usually more fibrous in nature and do not contain PMMA debris (39). The interface tissues may also have a

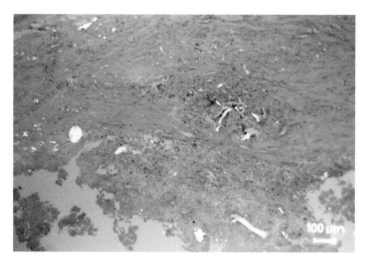

Figure 2 Tissue from a total hip replacement revised because of polyethylene wear. The fibrohistiocytic membrane contains areas of necrosis. Polarized light has been used to highlight the positively birefringent shards of polyethylene. (Decalcified paraffin embedded WHO stained section, partially-polarized light, 100× magnification.) *Abbreviation*: WHO, World Health Organization.

synovial-like lining layer. If polyethylene wear has been excessive, the synovium and capsular tissues can be exuberant, frond-like and necrotic in areas. Black wear particles of various metal alloys and their by-products (such as those from stainless steel, cobalt–chrome, or titanium alloy) are micron or submicron in size in diameter and located both intra- and extra-cellularly. When in small numbers, these particles are often intermixed within the fibrous tissue stroma. The tissues may have a black discoloration to gross examination if metallic wear has been excessive.

The cellular response to particulate debris has classically been designated a nonspecific foreign body type reaction. In some patients, however, there may be a type IV hypersensitivity immune reaction to the particle-protein complex (43). This type IV immune reaction may be specific to a small subset of patients with prostheses that contain either titanium alloy or cobalt–chrome alloy. Thus, one may see significant numbers of T lymphocytes in the tissues in some cases, sometimes with perivascular cuffing. A phenomenon labeled "aggressive granulomatous reaction" has been described in which progressive, locally expanding periprosthetic osteolytic lesions are seen (44). These cases are associated with activated fibroblasts and macrophages. It has been hypothesized that this phenomenon may be due to an uncoupling of the events encompassing the nonspecific foreign body response and reactive fibrosis.

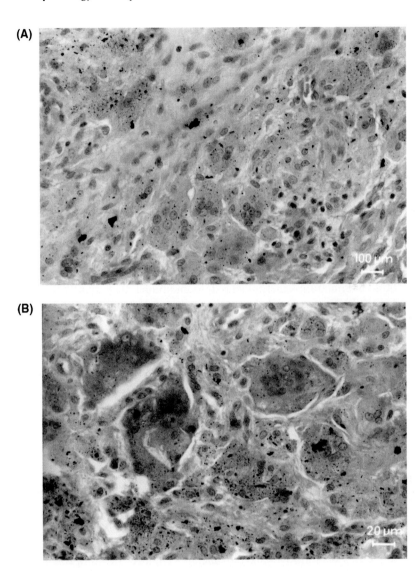

Figure 3 Low power (**A**) and high power (**B**) photomicrographs of tissues from a failed total hip replacement in which unwanted metal-on-metal articulation resulted from severe polyethylene liner wear. Numerous mono- and multi-nucleated macrophages are observed containing small black specks of metallic wear particles. [Decalcified paraffin embedded WHO stained section, transmitted light. (**A**) 200× magnification, (**B**) 400× magnification.] *Abbreviation*: WHO, World Health Organization.

Cell and organ culture studies have documented that the tissues surrounding loose cemented and cementless implants are biologically very active (37–39,47). These tissues produce high levels of prostaglandin E2, pro-inflammatory cytokines (such as interleukins 1 and 6 and tumor necrosis factor), chemokines, nitric oxide, and superoxide anions (see below). Tissues from both loose cemented and cementless implants are capable of producing these factors which have been linked to periprosthetic bone resorption (47).

Histochemistry, immunohistochemistry, in situ hybridization, and other cellular and molecular biological techniques have yielded important information on the biological processes of the periprosthetic tissues (45–54). Activated macrophages which stain positively for the proinflammatory cytokines interleukin-1, interleukin-6, and tumor necrosis factor alpha are found in high numbers in the tissues; these cytokines undoubtedly play a major role in the process of osteolysis (47,48). These activated macrophages are correlated with the presence of polyethylene particles (55,56). Granulocyte-macrophage colony stimulating factor (GM-CSF), a growth factor that regulates the transformation of immature macrophages into multinucleated giant cells and osteoclasts, is highly expressed by phagocytic macrophages (57). Interestingly, histomorphometric analysis has documented the prominence of markers of bone formation (heightened alkaline phosphatase activity) on the surrounding bony surface, indicating attempts at repair of bone (46). Furthermore, transforming growth factor beta, an anti-inflammatory cytokine was also strongly expressed by multinucleated giant cells of the pseudosynovium (58).

Chemokines are a family of proinflammatory cytokines that act primarily as chemoattractants for cells of the immune system (49–54). The C–C chemokine subfamily consists of monocyte chemoattractant proteins-1, 2, 3, 4 (MCP-1, 2, 3, 4), macrophage inflammatory proteins-1-α, 1-β, 3-α, 3-β (MIP-l-α, 1-β 3-α, 3-β) and regulated upon activation normal T expressed and secreted protein (RANTES). Immunohistochemical and other analyses of retrieved periprosthetic tissues have demonstrated MCP-1 and MIP-l-α expression but RANTES expression was not observed (53). Expression of macrophage migration inhibitory factor (MIF) has also been observed in retrieved tissues harvested from failed total joint arthroplasties using immunohistochemistry.

Numerous degradative enzymes including matrix metalloproteinases (MMPs) and their inhibitors tissue inhibitor of matrix metalloproteinase (TIMPs) are highly expressed in tissues harvested from loose prostheses. These proinflammatory molecules include collagenases MMP-1, MMP-2 and MMP-9 gelatinases, stromolysin MMP-3, extracellular matrix metalloproteinase inducer (EMMPRIN)—an MMP upregulator, cathepsin C, alpha 1-antichymotrypsin, tenascin, elastase, etc. (59–69). Proinflammatory factors such as the prostanoids and leukotrienes, especially prostaglandin E2 and nitric oxide metabolites are also highly expressed (37–39,69,70). These degradative enzymes and other factors are important in the cascade of events leading to undermining of the bony support of an implant.

Biomaterial particles not only stimulate macrophages but also activate T cells in the presence of a suitable antigen (a protein-coated particle) and co-stimulatory molecules such as CD80 and CD86. Immunochemical studies have recently confirmed the presence of this pathway, indicating the importance of T cells and immune processes in the periprosthetic tissues (71,72). However, the exact role of T cells and related immune processes in modulating the periprosthetic events is controversial.

The osteoclast is the final common pathway in effecting periprosthetic bone resorption. Osteoblasts and stromal cells, however are integral parts of this process by releasing Receptor Activate of NFKB Light (RANKL), which together with M-CSF are essential for osteoclast differentiation from monocytes/macrophages. Osteoprotegerin (OPG), the soluble receptor for RANKL inhibits the above pathways. Studies of macrophages isolated from loose arthroplasties have confirmed these principles and the importance of osteoblasts/stromal cells-macrophage interaction in osteolysis (73–77). These concepts are discussed in more detail in the chapter by Haynes and Crotti later in this book.

Information concerning novel bearing couples, such as ceramic on ceramic and metal on metal, is now being reported. These bearing couples have been introduced in the hope of decreasing wear and its biological consequences, and potentially allowing a more active lifestyle in younger patients, thus extending the longevity of joint replacements. Specifications and tolerances have been improved compared to similar, older prostheses. Thus, catastrophic breakage of a ceramic head is now a rare occurrence. Wear particles from ceramic prostheses are much smaller in size and less in number compared to polyethylene particles, and appear to be relatively benign. Particles from revised metal-on-metal articulations that have been introduced more recently have been reported by Willert et al. (77) to be associated with a diffuse and perivascular lymphocytic infiltration, and swelling and obliteration of blood vessel walls. Five to ten percent of the lymphocytes expressed the proliferation-associated antigen Ki-67. These findings are suggestive of a cell-mediated immune reaction. Interestingly, this reaction also appeared to be of a much higher intensity compared to older metal-on-metal prostheses retrieved during revision surgery. The clinical significance of these findings is unknown.

IMPROVING OSSEOINTEGRATION AND LONGEVITY OF JOINT REPLACEMENTS: THE FUTURE

The key to improving osseointegration of implants for joint replacement is to optimize all variables pertaining to patient selection, prosthetic design, surgical technique, and postoperative rehabilitation. While it is not the purpose of this chapter to discuss the salient points pertinent to all of the above factors, some general comments will be offered with reference to the bone–implant interface. Whether the implant is cemented, cementless or covered by a bioactive coating, the initial interface that develops will be a major determinant of the longevity of the implant. Implants should be made of the most biocompatible materials available in a cost-effective manner. Enhancement of the initial biological and mechanical characteristics of the interface by chemical, mechanical, immunological, or other methods should be explored. Wear debris and other by-products should be minimized and incite bland, minimally-reactive, nontoxic sequelae. Strategies for mitigating the effects of osteolysis and stress shielding that jeopardize the longevity of the implant and restoring lost bone stock should be aggressively pursued. Some success has already been realized with the advent of bioactive prosthetic coatings, new cross-linked polyethylenes that demonstrate enhanced wear characteristics, bisphosphonate use, etc. Articulations such as metal-on-metal, ceramic on polyethylene, and ceramic on ceramic, etc., require clinical and scientific validation in comparative prospective randomized studies with currently available implants. Surface treatments that may potentially decrease wear need further study. With further research, it is hoped that implants for joint replacement may someday provide optimal function for the patient's entire lifetime. This is a particularly challenging goal in light of the fact that our population as a whole is aging and becoming more active.

REFERENCES

1. Charnley J. Low Friction Arthroplasty of the Hip. New York: Springer, 1979.
2. Charnley J. The reaction of bone to self-curing acrylic cement. A long term histological study in man. J Bone Joint Surg 1986; 52-B:340–353.
3. Mulroy WF, Estok DM, Harris WH. Total hip arthroplasty with use of so-called second-generation cementing techniques. A fifteen-year-average follow-up study 1995; 77-A(12):1845–1852.
4. Pierson JL, Harris WH. Effect of improved cementing techniques on the longevity of fixation in revision cemented femoral arthroplasties. J Arthroplasty 1995; 10(5):581–591.
5. Jasty MJ, Goldring SR, Harris WH. Comparison of bone cement membrane around rigidly fixed versus loose total hip implants. Trans 30th Annu Meet Orthop Res Soc 1984; 9:125.
6. Maloney WJ, Jasty MJ, Burke DW, Harris WH. Biomechanical and histological investigation of cemented total hip arthroplasties: a study of autopsy retrieved femurs after in vivo cycling. Clin Orthop 1989; 249:129–140.
7. Maloney WJ, Sychterz C, Bragdon C, McGovern T, Jasty M, Engh CA. Skeletal response to well fixed femoral components inserted with and without cement. Clin Orthop 1996; 333:15–26.
8. Fornasier VL, Wright J, Seligman J. The histomorphologic and morphometric study of asymptotic hip arthroplasty—a postmortem study. Clin Orthop 1991; 271:272–282.

9. Schmalzried TP, Kwong LM, Jasty M, Sedlacek RC, Haire TC, O'Connor DO, Bragdon CR, Kabo JM, Malcolm AJ, Harris WH. The mechanism of loosening of cemented acetabular components in total hip arthroplasty. Analysis of specimens retrieved at autopsy. Clin Orthop 1992; 274:60–78.

10. Galante J, Rostoker W, Lueck R, Ray RD. Sintered fiber metal composites as a basis for attachment of implants to bone. J Bone Joint Surg 1971; 53-A(1): 101–114.

11. Albrektsson T, Albrektsson B. Osseointegration of bone implants. A review of an alternative mode of fixation. Acta Orthop Scand 1987; 58:567–577.

12. Galante J. Bone ingrowth in porous materials. In: Lewis JL, Galante JO, eds. The Bone Implant Interface, Workshop Report. Park Ridge: American Academy of Orthopaedic Surgeons, 1985:172–183.

13. Bobyn JD, Pilliar RM, Cameron HU, Weatherly GC. The optimum pore size for the fixation of porous-surfaced metal implants by the ingrowth of bone. Clin Orthop 1980; 150:263–270.

14. Spector M. Historical review of porous coated implants. J Arthroplasty 1987; 2:163–177.

15. Harris WH, Jasty M. Bone ingrowth into porous-coated canine acetabular replacements: the effect of pore size, apposition and dislocation. In: Fitzgerald RH ed. The Hip: Proceedings of the Thirteenth Open Scientific Meeting of the Hip Society. St Louis, C. V. Mosby, 1985:214–234.

16. Jasty M, McGann W, Rubash HE, Paiement G, Bragdon C, Harris WH. Comparison of bone ingrowth into cobalt–chrome spheres vs. titanium fiber mesh coatings on canine cementless acetabular components. Trans Orthop Res Soc 1987; 12:433.

17. Turner TM, Sumner DR, Urban RM, Rivero DP, Galante JO. A comparison study of porous coatings in a weight-bearing total hip arthroplasty model. J Bone Joint Surg 1986; 68-A(9):1396–1409.

18. Cook SD, Thomas KA, Haddad PJ Jr. Histological analysis of retrieved human porous-coated total joint components. Clin Orthop 1988; 234:90–101.

19. Jacobs JJ, Sumner DR, Caviglia HA, Turner TM, Urban RM, Galante JO. A quantitative study for bone ingrowth into titanium total hip femoral components removed for reasons other than loosening. Orthop Trans 1989; 13:524.

20. Engh CA, Bobyn JD, Glassman AH. Porous-coated hip replacement—The factors governing bone ingrowth, stress shielding, and clinical results. J Bone Joint Surg 1987; 69-B(1):45–55.

21. Engh CA, McGovern TF, Bobyn JD, Harris WH. A quantitative evaluation of periprosthetic bone-remodeling after cementless total hip arthroplasty. J Bone Joint Surg 1992; 74-A(7):1009–1020.

22. Engh C, Zettl-Schaffer KF, Kukita Y, Sweet D, Jasty M, Bragdon C. Histological and radiographic assessment of well functioning porous-coated acetabular components. A human postmortem retrieval study. J Bone Joint Surg 1993; 75-A(6): 814–824.

23. Sumner DR, Jasty M, Jacobs JJ, Urban RM, Bragdon CP, Harris WH, Galante JO. Histology of porous-coated acetabular components. 25 cementless cups retrieved after arthroplasty. Acta Orthop Scand 1993; 64(6):619–626.

24. Pidhorz LE, Urban RM, Jacobs JJ, Sumner DR, Galante JO. A quantitative study of bone and soft tissues in cementless porous-coated acetabular components retrieved at autopsy. J Arthroplasty 1993; 8(2):213–225.
25. Furlong RJ, Osborn JF. Fixation of hip prostheses by hydroxyapatite ceramic coatings. J Bone Joint Surg 1991; 73-B(5):741–745.
26. Hardy DC, Frayssinet P, Quilhem A, Lafontain MA, Delince PE. Bonding of hydroxyapatite-coated femoral prostheses. Histology of specimens from four cases. J Bone Joint Surg 1991; 73-B(5):732–740.
27. Bauer TW, Geesink RCT, Zimmerman R, McMahon JT. Hydroxyapatite-coated femoral stems. Histological analysis of components retrieved at autopsy. J Bone Joint Surg 1991; 73-A(10):1439–1452.
28. Rivero DP, Fox J, Skipor AK, Urban RM, Galante JO. Calcium phosphate-coated porous titanium implants for enhanced skeletal fixation. J Biomed Mater Res 1988; 22:191–201.
29. Oonishi H, Yamamoto M, Ishimaru H, Tsuji E, Kushitani S, Aono M, Ukon Y. The effect of hydroxyapatite coating on bone growth into porous titanium alloy implants. J Bone Joint Surg 1989; 71-B:213–216.
30. Cook SD, Thomas KA, Kay JF, Jarcho M. Hydroxyapatite-coated titanium for orthopedic implant applications. Clin Orthop 1988; 232:225–243.
31. Søballe K, Hansen ES, Brockstedt-Rasmussen H, Pedersen M, Bünger C. Hydroxyapatite coating enhances fixation of porous coated implants. A comparison in dogs between press fit and noninterference fit. Acta Orthop Scand 1990; 61(4):299–306.
32. Søballe K. Hydroxyapatite ceramic coating for bone implant fixation. Mechanical and histological studies in dogs. Acta Orthop Scan Suppl 1993; (255):1–58.
33. Clemens JAM, Klein APAT, Sakkers RJB, Dhert WJA, Groot KD, Rozing PM. Healing of gaps around calcium phosphate-coated implants in trabecular bone of the goat. J Biomed Mater Res 1997; 36:55–64.
34. Søballe K, Hansen ES, B-Rasmussen H, Jørgensen PH, Bünger C. Tissue ingrowth into titanium and hydroxyapatite-coated implants during stable and unstable mechanical conditions. J Orthop Res 1992; 10:285–299.
35. Mirra JM, Marder RA, Amstutz HC. The pathology of failed total joint arthroplasty. Clin Orthop 1982; 17:175–183.
36. Willert HG, Semlitsch M. Reactions of the articular capsule to wear products of artificial joint prostheses. J Biomed Mater Res 1977; 11:157–164.
37. Goldring SR, Jasty M, Roelke MS, Rourke CM, Bringhurst FR, Harris WH. Formation of a synovial-like membrane at the bone–cement interface. Arthritis Rheum 1986; 29:836–842.
38. Goldring SR, Schiller AL, Roelke M, Rourke CM, O'Neill DA, Harris WH. The synovial-like membrane at the bone cement interface in loose total hip replacements and its proposed role in bone lysis. J Bone Joint Surg 1983; 65A:575–584.
39. Goodman SB, Chin RC, Chiou SS, Schurman DJ, Woolson ST, Masada MT. A clinical–pathological–biochemical study of the membrane surrounding loosened and nonloosened joint arthroplasty. Clin Orthop 1989; 244:182–187.
40. Schmalzried TP, Jasty M, Rosenberg A, Harris WH. Histologic identification of polyethylene wear debris using oil red O stain. J Appl Biomater 1993; 4: 119–125.

41. Willert HG, Bertram H, Buchhorn GH. Osteolysis in alloarthropasty of the hip. The role of ultra-high molecular weight polyethylene wear particles. Clin Orthop 1990; 258:95–107.

42. Charosky CB, Bullough PG, Wilson PD Jr. Total hip replacement failures. A histological evaluation. J Bone Joint Surg 1973; 55-A:49–58.

43. Hicks DG, Judkins AR, Sickel JZ, Rosier RN, Puzas JE, O'Keefe RJ. Granular histiocytosis of pelvic lymph nodes following total hip arthroplasty. The presence of wear debris, cytokine production and immunologically activated macrophages. J Bone Joint Surg 1996; 78-A:482–496.

44. Santavirta S, Konttinen YT, Begroth V. Aggressive granulomatous lesions associated with hip arthroplasty. Immunopathological studies. J Bone Joint Surg 1990; 72-A:252–258.

45. Jiranek WA, Machado M, Jasty M, Jevsevar D, Wolfe HJ, Goldring SR, Goldberg MJ, Harris WH. Production of cytokines around loosened cemented acetabular components. Analysis with immunohistochemical techniques and in situ hybridization. J Bone Joint Surg 1993; 75A:863–879.

46. Kodaya Y, Revell PA, Al-Saffar N, Kobayashi A, Scott G, Freeman MAR. Bone formation and bone resorption in failed total joint replacements arthroplasties: histomorphometric analysis with histochemical and immunohistochemical technique. J Orthop Res 1996; 14:473–482.

47. Shanbhag AS, Jacobs JJ, Black J, Galante JO, Glant TT. Cellular mediators secreted by interfacial membranes obtained at revision total hip arthroplasty. J Arthroplasty 1995; 10:498–506.

48. Goodman SB, Huie P, Song Y, Schurman D, Maloney W, Woolson S, Sibley R. Cellular profile and cytokine production at prosthetic interfaces. J Bone Joint Surg 1998; 80-B:531–539.

49. Ishiguro N, Kojima T, Kurokouchi K, Iwase T, Iwata H. mRNA expression of chemokines in interface tissue around of loosening total hip arthroplasty components. Trans Orthop Res Soc 1997; 22:735.

50. Frokjar J, Deleuran B, Lind M, Overgaard S, Soballe K, Bunger C. Polyethylene particles stimulate monocyte chemotactic and activating factor production in synovial mononuclear cells in vivo. Acta Orthop Scand 1995; 66: 303–307.

51. Chiba J, Oyama M, Sugawara S, Inoue K, Rubash HE. The role of chemokine, adhesion molecules, and cytokine receptor in femoral osteolysis after cementless total hip arthroplasty. Trans Orthop Res Soc 1996; 21:514.

52. Rollins BJ. Chemokines. Blood 1997; 90:909–928.

53. Nakashima Y, Sun D-H, Chun LE, Trindade M, Song Y, Maloney WJ, Goodman SB, Schurman DJ, Smith RL. Induction of macrophage C–C chemokine expression by titanium alloy and bone cement particles. J Bone Joint Surg 1999; 81-B:155–162.

54. Lind M, Trindade M, Nakashima Y, Schurman DJ, Goodman SB, Smith RL. Chemotaxis and activation of particle challenged human monocytes in response to monocyte migration inhibiting factor and C–C chemokines. J Biomed Mater Res Appl Biomater 1999; 48(3):246–250.

55. Kobayashi A, Freeman MA, Bonfield W, Kadoya Y, Yamac T, Al-Saffar N, Scott G, Revell PA. Number of polyethylene particles and osteolysis in total

joint replacements. A quantitative study using a tissue-digestion method. J Bone Joint Surg 1997; 79-B:844–848.

56. Kadoya Y, Revell PA, Kobayashi A, Al-Saffar N, Scott G, Freeman MA. Wear particulate species and bone loss in failed total joint arthroplasties. Clin Orthop 1997; 340:118–129.

57. Al-Saffar N, Khwaja HA, Kadoya Y, Revell PA. Assessment of the role of GM-CSF in the cellular transformation and the development of erosive lesions around orthopaedic implants. Am J Clin Pathol 1996; 105(5):628–639.

58. Al-Saffar N, Revell PA. Differential expression of transforming growth factor-alpha and macrophage colony-stimulating factor/colony-stimulating factor-1R (c-fms) by multinucleated giant cells involved in pathological bone resorption at the site of orthopaedic implants. J Orthop Res 2000; 18(5):800–807.

59. Takagi M, Konttinen YT, Lindy O, Sorsa T, Kurvinen H, Suda A, Santavirta S. Gelatinase/type IV collagenases in the loosening of total hip replacement endo-prostheses. Clin Orthop 1994; 306:135–144.

60. Tagaki M, Konttinen YT, Kemppinen P, Sorsa T, Tschesche H, Blaser J, Suda A, Santavirta S. Tissue inhibitor of metalloproteinase 1, collagenolytic and gelatino-lytic activity in loose hip endoprostheses. J Rheumatol 1995; 22:2285–2290.

61. Takagi M. Neutral proteinases and their inhibitors in the loosening of total hip prostheses. Acta Orthop Scand 1996; 67(suppl 271):1–29.

62. Takagi M, Santavirta S, Ida H, Ishii M, Akimoto K, Saotome K, Konttinen YT. The membrane-type matrix metalloproteinase/matrix metalloproteinase-2/ tissue inhibitor of metalloproteinase-2 system in periprosthetic connective-tissue remodeling in loose total-hip prostheses. Lab Invest 1998; 78:735–742.

63. Takagi M, Santavirta S, Ida H, Ishii M, Mandelin J, Konttinen YT. Matrix metalloproteinases and tissue inhibitors of metalloproteinases in loose artificial hip joints. Clin Orthop 1998; 352:35–45.

64. Takei I, Takagi M, Santavirta S, Ida H, Hamasaki M, Ishii M, Fukushima S, Ogina T, Konttinen YT. Metalloproteinases and tissue inhibitors of metallo-proteinases in joint fluid of the patients with loose artificial joints. J Biomed Mater Res 1999; 45:175–183.

65. Takagi M, Konttinen YT, Santavirta S, Kangaspunta P, Suda A, Rokkanen P. Cathepsin G and alpha 1-antichymotrypsin in the local host reaction to loosen-ing of total hip prostheses. J Bone Joint Surg 1995; 77-A:16–25.

66. Takagi M, Konttinen YT, Santavirta S, Kangaspunta P, Sorsa T, Yamakawa M, Suda A. Elastase activity, uninhibited by alpha 1-antitrypsin, in the peripros-thetic connective matrix around loose total hip prostheses. J Orthop Res 1995; 13(2):296–304.

67. Li TF, Warris V, Ma J, Lassus J, Yoshida T, Santavirta S, Virtanen I, Konttinen YT. Distribution of tenascin-X in different synovial samples and synovial membrane-like interface tissue from aseptic loosening of total hip replacement. Rheumatol Int 2000; 19(5):177–183.

68. Li TF, Santavirta S, Virtanen I, Kononen M, Takagi M, Konttinen YT. Increased expression of EMMPRIN in the tissue around loosened hip pros-theses. Acta Orthop Scand 1999; 70(5):446–451.

69. Takagi M, Konttinen YT, Santavirta S, Sorsa T, Eisen AZ, Nordsletten L, Suda A. Extracellular matrix metalloproteinases around loose total hip prostheses. Acta Orthop Scand 1994; 65(4):281–286.

70. Hukkanen M, Corbett SA, Platts LA, Konttinen YT, Santavirta S, Hughes SP, Polak JM. Nitric oxide in the local host reaction to total hip replacement. Clin Orthop 1998; 352:53–65.

71. Farber A, Chin R, Song Y, Huie P, Goodman SB. Chronic antigen-specific immune system activation may potentially be involved in the loosening of cemented acetabular components. J Biomed Mater Res 2001; 55:433–441.

72. Bainbridge JA, Revell PA, Al-Saffar N. Co-stimulatory molecule expression following exposure to orthopaedic implants wear debris. J Biomed Mater Res 2001; 54(3):328–334.

73. Neale SD, Haynes DR, Howie DW, Murray DW, Athanasou NA. The effect of particle phagocytosis and metallic wear particles on osteoclast formation and bone resorption in vitro. J Arthroplasty 2000; 15(5):654–662.

74. Neale SD, Fujikawa Y, Sabokbar A, Gundle R, Murray DW, Graves SE, Howie DW, Athanasou NA. Human bone-derived cells support formation of human osteoclasts from arthroplasty-derived cells in vitro. J Bone Joint Surg 2000; 82(6):892–900.

75. Fujikawa Y, Sabokbar A, Neale SD, Itonaga I, Torisu T, Athanasou NA. The effect of macrophage-colony stimulating factor and other humoral factors (interleukin-1, -3, -6, and -11, tumor necrosis factor-alpha, and granulocyte macrophage-colony stimulating factor) on human osteoclast formation from circulating cells. Bone 2001; 28(3):261–267.

76. Itonaga I, Sabokbar A, Murray DW, Athanasou NA. Effect of osteoprotegerin and osteoprotegerin ligand on osteoclast formation by arthroplasty membrane derived macrophages. Ann Rheum Dis 2000; 59(1):26–31.

77. Willert H-G, Buchhorn GH, Fayyazi A, Lohmann CH. Signs of delayed hypersensitivity and histopathological changes around metal-on-metal hip joints. Trans Soc Biomater 2001; 24:338.

7

Properties of Biomaterials Used in Joint Replacements

Timothy M. Wright

Department of Biomedical Mechanics and Materials, Hospital for Special Surgery, and Department of Orthopaedics, Weill Medical College of Cornell University, New York, New York, U.S.A.

Robert F. Closkey Jr.

Department of Biomedical Mechanics and Materials, Hospital for Special Surgery, New York, New York, and Department of Orthopaedic Surgery, Community Medical Center, Toms River, New Jersey, U.S.A.

INTRODUCTION

Biomaterials for use in total joint replacement must meet several criteria to perform successfully. They must be biocompatible, functioning in vivo without eliciting a detrimental local or systemic response. They must be resistant to corrosion and chemical degradation so that the harsh in vivo environment does not adversely affect any of their properties. They must possess adequate mechanical strength, since they must withstand the large forces that are transmitted across all of the articular joints in the body. In addition, materials for use in bearing surfaces must be wear resistant over tens of millions of cycles of use with minimal release of particulate debris. Finally, biomaterials must be easy to fabricate at a relatively low cost.

The failure of biomaterials to meet these criteria can be directly related to clinical failures of joint replacement systems. In some cases, failures can be linked back to inherent design flaws that compromise material performance. In other cases, failures can result from inadequate consideration of performance limitations in preclinical testing. To insure the appropriate use of implant devices and minimize the potential for failure requires that the orthopaedic surgeon understands the properties of orthopaedic biomaterials and how those properties affect clinical performance.

METALLIC ALLOYS

Metallic alloys, composed of mixtures of metallic and nonmetallic elements, possess the combination of high strength, flexibility, ductility, corrosion resistance, and biocompatibility required for load-bearing applications as implant components for total joint arthroplasty. Three common alloys are used: stainless steel, cobalt–chromium alloy, and titanium alloy. In general, these alloys were not developed specifically for orthopaedic applications. Instead, their proven performance in the aerospace, marine, and chemical industries made them acceptable candidates for implant use.

Stainless Steel

Steels are alloys primarily of iron and carbon. The properties of steels can be altered by three different approaches. The first is by adding or removing additional elements such as chromium, nickel, manganese, or molybdenum. Chromium additions provide corrosion resistance, so steels with high chromium contents are termed stainless steels. The chromium forms a strongly adherent oxide film that provides a passive layer shielding the bulk material from the environment. Chromium also imparts strength to the steel and contributes to its ability to harden when deformed. The second method for improving properties is by heat treatment that realigns the atomic structure of the steel. Heat treatment can be used to strengthen the steel, though it can have detrimental effects on properties as well. Most stainless steels used for orthopaedic instruments, for example, are heat treated to increase their strength, but are not used for devices because the increased strength comes with an unacceptable reduction in corrosion resistance if implanted in the body. The third method for improving properties is by cold working the raw material. Stainless steel is typically cold worked by about 30% for orthopaedic applications, meaning that it is forced to change shape under high stress that realigns the structure of the material and improves the strength (Fig. 1).

The most common form of stainless steel used in orthopaedic applications is 316L. The chemical composition and properties are designated by the American society for testing and materials (ASTM) in specification F138. The "L" denotes low carbon concentration (typically below 0.03 wt%). The carbon level must be kept low in stainless steel to maintain corrosion resistance (1,2). The recommended size of the individual grains that comprise the material is small (about 100 μm in any dimension) to

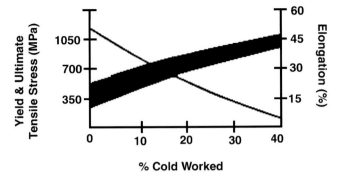

Figure 1 The mechanical properties of stainless steel can be altered by cold working. Deformation of the material beyond its yield stress can result in steel with improved strength. Though the remaining ductility is reduced with cold working, ample strain to failure exists for most common orthopaedic implant applications.

assure adequate strength for orthopaedic applications. Grain size can be controlled by the original solidification process used to make the steel and by postsolidification heat treatment and cold working. Grade 316L is commonly used for internal fracture fixation devices for its moderate strength, good machinability, good corrosion resistance, and relatively low cost.

When higher strength is required, a material with a different metallurgy can be used. One such alloy is 22Cr–13Ni–5Mn; the higher chromium, nickel, and manganese content increases static and fatigue strength and corrosion resistance over those of 316L (Table 1). Cost is higher due to higher material costs and increased difficulty in manufacturing. A recent introduction to the orthopaedic market is a steel that combines higher percentages of chromium,

Table 1 Mechanical Properties of Implant Materials for Total Joint Replacement

Material	Yield stress (MPa)	Ultimate stress (MPa)	Elastic modulus (GPa)	Fatigue strength (MPa)
Stainless steel (30% cold worked)	790	930	190	300–450
Cobalt alloy (as cast)	450–515	650–890	210	200–310
Cobalt alloy (forged)	900–1200	1400–1590	210	600–900
Titanium alloy (forged)	1000	1100	110	620
PMMA	–	35	3	10
UHMWPE (conventional)	14	27	1	–

cobalt, and molybdenum with an extremely low nickel content to increase further the material strength and decrease possible reactions in nickel-sensitive patients (compared to the 22Cr–13Ni–5Mn alloy). Again, difficulty in machining results in higher costs.

Cobalt–Chromium Alloys

Cobalt–chromium alloys include compositions intended to be manufactured by casting (ASTM F75 alloy) and by forging (ASTM F799 alloy), as well as alloy compositions that obtain excellent mechanical properties through cold working (ASTM F90 and F562). The base element of these alloys is cobalt with significant amounts of chromium added for corrosion resistance, again as an adherent passive layer of chromium oxide.

The ease of fabrication and the range of properties available for cobalt alloys make them ideal for a wide range of orthopaedic applications, including metallic components of all joint replacements. These alloys display superior resistance to crevice corrosion compared to stainless steel, though fretting and crevice corrosion at modular junctions have proven problematic (3). Long-term clinical use has proven that these alloys also have exceptional biocompatibility in bulk form, though particulate debris from bearing surfaces can contribute to osteolysis and the binding of metals to proteins contributes to systemic accumulation (4,5).

Care must be taken in casting implant components from F75 cobalt alloy. The ability to trap air and gases escaping from the solidification process can lead to porosity that in turn can serve as the initiation site for fatigue failure (Fig. 2). F75 alloy is used to fabricate porous coatings for biologic fixation of orthopaedic implants. The resulting properties of the porous-coated device will depend on the microstructures of the substrate metal and the porous beads, as well as the thermal sintering process used to connect the two. Sintering involves high temperatures, which can significantly decrease the fatigue strength of the substrate material. Together with the stress concentrations caused at the attachment points with the porous coating, the resulting fatigue strength is only about 200 MPa, even after additional thermal treatments are used to restore some of the strength (Table 1). This strength is well below that achieved for cobalt alloys that are not porous-coated.

Titanium and Its Alloys

Titanium is used in orthopaedic implants in both the commercially pure form and alloyed with other elements. Commercially pure titanium is typically used as a coating to enhance biological fixation of titanium alloy implants to the surrounding bone. Since titanium is highly osteoconductive, porous coatings with large titanium surface areas can facilitate bone ingrowth into the porous coatings and improve the bone–implant interface. Coatings are applied either through plasma spraying of titanium onto the implant to create a roughened,

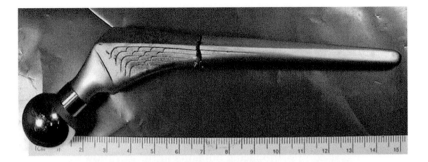

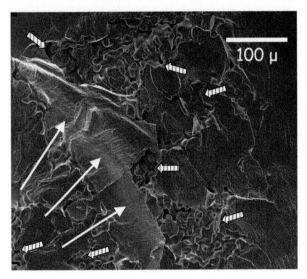

Figure 2 Total joint replacement components are susceptible to fatigue failure because of the large cyclic stresses they must withstand. This femoral component fabricated by casting cobalt alloy suffered a fatigue fracture. A close-up of the fracture surface shows clam shell markings (*solid arrows*) indicative of the direction that the fatigue crack propagated and evidence that porosity (*hatched arrows*), caused by the trapping of gases in the metal casting as it cooled, contributed to the failure.

porous surface or as a fiber metal coating that is pressed and sintered onto the underlying substrate to create a coating with interconnected porosity. The properties of commercially pure titanium depend in large part on the oxygen content; the higher the content, the greater the strength.

Titanium alloys are used in total joint replacement components because of their high strength, outstanding biocompatibility, and corrosion resistance. Unlike stainless steels and cobalt alloys, corrosion resistance is provided by an adherent passive layer of titanium oxide (TiO_2), which greatly reduces susceptibility to most corrosion conditions, even crevice and fretting corrosion. Long-term clinical use in humans confirms superior biocompatibility. Furthermore, the oxide surfaces of titanium alloys are well tolerated by bone tissue, leading to direct osseointegration between bone and implant with little evidence of a fibrous layer (6).

The most common alloy used in joint replacements is titanium–aluminum–vanadium alloy (ASTM F136). The alloy is often called Ti–6Al–4V or simply Ti–6–4 because the primary alloying elements, aluminum and vanadium, are limited to 5.5–6.5 and 3.5–4.5 wt%, respectively. Developed for the aerospace industry to possess a high strength-to-weight ratio, the alloy is used in orthopaedic implants in the extra low interstitials form, in which the oxygen concentration is kept very low to avoid embrittlement and to maximize strength and ductility.

The mechanical properties of Ti–6Al–4V are more than adequate for joint replacement applications (Table 1). The elastic modulus is about half that of stainless steels and cobalt alloys, making the alloy an ideal candidate for lowering the structural stiffness of an implant without changing its shape. The axial, bending, and torsion stiffnesses of a hip stem fabricated from titanium alloy will all be half that of a stem of the same size and shape made from either of the other two metallic alloys. Thus, the severity of stress shielding as the stem and the surrounding cortex share load should be less for the titanium alloy stem (7).

Titanium alloys have limitations, however. One disadvantage is notch sensitivity. A stress concentration, such as a deep scratch, on the surface of a titanium alloy implant significantly reduces the fatigue life of the part. Notch sensitivity can also arise at the junctions between the porous coating and the substrate of a titanium alloy component and even as a result of identification markings etched into the surface by the manufacturer (8).

Another limitation of titanium alloy is its lower hardness (in comparison, for example, to cobalt alloys). A somewhat ambiguous term, hardness encompasses a number of mechanical properties, but mostly measures the material's resistance to elastic and plastic deformation such as occurs during scratching of a bearing surface. Clinical performance of titanium alloy as a bearing material (for example, as a femoral head in a total hip replacement) has been poor, with significant scratching a common occurrence. Local and systemic measurements of the metal levels from around well-functioning hip replacements have confirmed the release of significant amounts of the alloying elements from the femoral head, though these levels increase markedly in the case of loosened implants (Fig. 3). Titanium alloys that have not undergone additional surface processing (for example, ion implantation) are no longer used as an articulating surface. Modular connections between cobalt alloy heads and titanium stems in total hip replacement also show elevated systemic levels of alloy constituents, consistent with susceptibility to fretting wear (5).

Long-term clinical evidence underscores the excellent biocompatibility of titanium 6–4 alloy. Nonetheless, the concern that the release of vanadium, a cytotoxic element, could cause local and systemic problems has led to

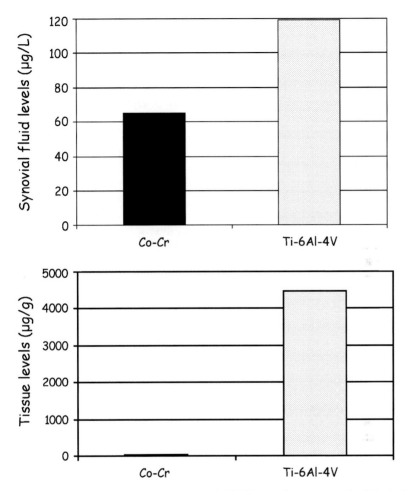

Figure 3 Total metal levels in the synovial fluids and tissues around solid cobalt alloy and solid Ti–6Al–4V total hip implants. The markedly higher titanium alloy levels than cobalt alloy levels are consistent with the poorer wear resistance of titanium alloy. *Source*: From Ref. 8a.

consideration of other titanium alloys in which the vanadium has been replaced by a more inert element such as niobium (9).

Tantalum

Tantalum (Ta: atomic number 73) is a pure metal in group VB of the periodic table. This metal was discovered in 1802 and has more than 50 years of clinical use with few reported side effects. It is chemically stable with excellent corrosion resistance and biocompatibility. The elastic modulus is

185 GPa, yield strength 165 MPa, elongation to failure 40%, tensile strength 205 MPa and the ASTM designation is F560-92 (10).

Recent orthopaedic applications of Ta are uses as a porous biomaterial in fracture and joint reconstruction. The Ta porous biomaterial is designed to mimic trabecular bone, in which the goal is to allow bone ingrowth into porous Ta stock. During manufacturing pure tantalum is deposited into a carbon skeleton using chemical vapor deposition/infiltration (CVD/CVI) which produces a porous metal construct. This produces a high volumetric porosity dodecahedron and highly interconnected network of consistent shaped pores (11). The structural biomaterial is 80% porous allowing 2–3 times greater bone ingrowth while doubling interference shear strength when compared to conventional porous coated materials. Osteointegration approaches 50% at four weeks (12). Limited adverse host responses include formation of fibrous capsules and membranes due to corrosion. No illness, immune responses or remote site effects have been reported. Limitations of tantalum uses are largely due to technical challenges in fabrication of clinically useful implants.

POLYMERS

Polymers are large molecules made from combinations of smaller molecules called "mers." The molecular weight of a polymer is determined by the number of monomer units used to make up the polymer. Some polymers, termed copolymers, contain more than one type of monomer. Bone cement, for example, is predominantly polymethylmethacrylate (PMMA), but in some cases also contains polystyrene or methacrylic acid to provide increased toughness. The properties of copolymers depend significantly on the distribution of the different monomers.

Bone Cement

PMMA has been used for implant fixation of joint replacement components since its introduction by Charnley in the 1970s. Typically, PMMA is supplied to the surgeon as a liquid in a sealed glass ampule and a powder in a bag. The liquid is methylmethacrylate monomer with small additions of hydroquinone to inhibit premature polymerization during storage and *N,N*,-dimethyl-*p*-toluidine to accelerate polymerization and offset the effect of the hydroquinone once the liquid is mixed with the powder and the polymerization reaction has begun.

The powder is composed of PMMA (or a copolymer blend) in the form of prepolymerized beads; bead size and the distribution of bead sizes can be altered to influence the viscosity of the doughy stage of the cement. The powder also contains an initiator, dibenzoyl peroxide, to insure polymerization begins, even in the presence of the hydroquinone inhibitor in the liquid. Finally, radiopaque powder particles, either barium sulfate

(BaSO$_4$) or zirconia (ZrO$_2$), are included in the powder so that the normally radiolucent cement can be visualized on radiographs.

Polymerization of PMMA generates considerable heat (about 130 calories/g of methylmethacrylate monomer). The accompanying temperature rise is controlled by several factors, including the bulk of the cement necessary for the intended fixation of the implant and the rate of heat transfer to adjacent implant components and biological structures. Though tissue necrosis caused by the temperature increase is often cited as a concern, the long-term success of cemented implants strongly suggests that thermal necrosis from cement polymerization and curing does not negatively impacted the overall performance of orthopaedic devices.

The cement interface that forms against a metallic implant can be influenced by the temperature of the metal itself. In vitro experiments, for example, showed that preheating the femoral stem portion markedly improved the shear strength and cement porosity of the interface (13), while not adversely affecting the mechanical properties of the bulk cement (14). Preheating causes increased polymerization temperatures at the cement–bone interface, but this has not had a detrimental effect in clinical use (15). In addition, preheating decreases polymerization time, reduces operative time, and decreases the risk of inadvertently moving the stem while the cement is curing.

Current common practice is to prepare lower viscosity cements using a vacuum mixing system to minimize the number of voids in the cement. Use of these techniques can reduce the porosity by greater than 50% over that of hand mixing. Removing the voids does not alter the material properties of the cement, but without voids the cement mantle has a greater cross-sectional area, adding structural strength (Fig. 4). The clinical relevance of improving the structural properties over that of hand-mixed cement is difficult to prove (16). Laboratory experiments show no significant improvement in the low cycle fatigue behavior of bone-implant systems with reduced porosity as compared to hand mixed cements (17).

Bone cement is also used to deliver antibiotics and osteoinductive agents. Cement properties can be altered by these additions, and the delivery of the agent to the surrounding tissue depends on the chemistry and surface area of the cement, as well as the manner in which the cement is prepared prior to delivery into the patient. This difference can be seen among commercial cements; diffusion of gentamycin from Simplex or CMW cements has been reported, for example, to be much less than that from Palacos (18). Although the mechanical properties of PMMA cement are reduced with the addition of large amounts of antibiotics, in general therapeutic levels of antibiotics can be added to the cement without any measurable reduction of properties (19). Interim placement of antibiotic-impregnated cement spacers as part of two-stage revision arthroplasty to treat infection has also proven effective (20). The recent approval by the FDA of antibiotic containing cements for commercial distribution

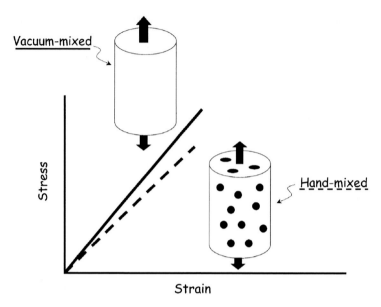

Figure 4 Porosity reduction in PMMA bone cement is advocated to increase strength. The strength increase comes about not by altering the material properties of the cement, but simply by providing more cement in a given cross-section. Stress is load divided by cross-sectional area; if the outer specimen diameter is used to calculate stress (ignoring the pores), the vacuum mixed specimen will appear stronger (i.e., a higher "stress"-strain curve. But if the appropriate area is used to calculate stress (i.e., if the porosity is accounted for in determining the area of the specimen on the right), the two "stress"-strain curves would overlap. *Abbreviation*: PMMA, polymethylmethacrylate.

provides the surgeon with a more controlled manner for delivering antibiotics in cement.

Polymeric Bearing Materials

Since the advent of total hip replacements, relatively few polymeric materials have actually been used in total joint replacements. In 1936, Judet introduced PMMA as the first synthetic polymeric material used as a replacement for the femoral head. However, the press-fit acrylic devices often loosened and wore and were not extensively used. Charnley, in developing his concept of low friction hip arthroplasty in the late 1950s, originally chose polytetrafluoroethylene (PTFE) as a bearing material based on its chemical inertness and low coefficient of friction. Rapid failure due to high wear rates and adverse reactions to PTFE debris caused him to search for alternative polymers, eventually deciding on ultra high molecular weight polyethylene (UHMWPE), the material that remains the most popular choice as a bearing surface in modern total joint replacements.

Three different methods are used to fabricate polyethylene joint replacement components. The first is to extrude UHMWPE resin particles under heat and pressure through a die to form a cylindrical bar; components are then machined from the bar into their final form. The second method is to compression mold the UHMWPE resin into a large sheet and then machine components from the sheet. The final method is to mold UHMWPE resin into the finished part (so-called net-shape or direct molding), though key features such as locking mechanisms are often subsequently machined into the part.

Polyethylene bearing surfaces have been used in joint arthroplasty for three decades with considerable success. Nonetheless, osteolysis secondary to the biological reaction to polyethylene wear debris particles is recognized as a significant problem that can limit the longevity of total joint replacements (21). Biomaterials research and development efforts to combat polyethylene wear have concentrated on improving the material's resistance to oxidative degradation and on making the material more resistant to the abrasive and adhesive wear mechanisms most responsible for the release of submicron wear particles.

The historical technique for sterilizing polyethylene implant components has been to expose them to gamma radiation above a dose of about 25 kGy in an ambient environment. This technique is now well recognized to cause oxidative degradation (22). The exposure to radiation energy causes chain scission, chain cross-linking, and the creation of free radicals in the material. The result is a decrease in molecular weight, an increase in density, and detrimental alterations in mechanical properties (an increase in elastic modulus and decreases in elongation to break and fracture toughness) that increase during shelf aging and that can add significantly to the wear problem (23).

Quality control problems have also been suggested to adversely affect the wear of polyethylene total joint components. Nonconsolidated polyethylene particles, perhaps left over from the extrusion or molding process, have been observed in components that also showed excessive wear (24). Most often, these defects formed in a band a millimeter or two below the component surface, the same location where oxidative degradation is maximum, suggesting that the defects and the degradation process combined to increase wear and wear-related damage to the bearing surface (25,26).

In response to the degradation problem, alternative sterilization techniques have been introduced that eliminate exposure to radiation altogether or that irradiate in inert environments. These methods are not equal, however, in terms of their effect on wear. Techniques that eliminate irradiation altogether, such as exposure to gas plasma and ethylene oxide, also eliminate the potential benefit of the additional cross-linking produced by irradiation. Indeed, wear rates in hip joint simulator studies are higher for both these techniques compared to gamma irradiation (27), and clinical wear rates for hip cups sterilized with ethylene oxide are nearly double that for conventional or reduced oxygen environment radiation (28,29). Little is known of the impact of irradiation-free sterilization techniques on the pitting and delamination surface damage that occurs in total knee polyethylene components. Studies of retrieved tibial components originally sterilized in ethylene oxide have, however, shown less evidence of cracking than conventionally sterilized components (30).

Sterilization techniques that employ irradiation in an inert or low oxygen environment are more beneficial in improving wear resistance as measured in laboratory hip simulator studies. The improved wear resistance is thought to be due to cross links that form between polyethylene chains. Unfortunately, free radicals produced at the ends of broken chains is a detrimental by-product of irradiation; postirradiation thermal treatments are performed to quench free radicals and prevent the degradation that could occur with subsequent exposure to an oxygen environment.

The fabrication technique also affects wear resistance of polyethylene components. Direct compression molding, for example, increases resistance to oxidative degradation. This resistance is combined with a lowering of the elastic modulus of the material. The resulting improvement in wear resistance has been established through studies of wear damage in retrieved components, laboratory wear tests, and most importantly clinical evidence (31,32). The lower elastic modulus that results from compression molding may be a key factor; under the same load conditions, a lower modulus polyethylene will have larger contacts areas and experience lower stresses than a higher modulus polyethylene under the same load conditions.

The most significant new fabrication technique for polyethylene joint replacement components is the incorporation of elevated levels of radiation to induce even higher levels of cross-linking than occur with the conventional (25 kGy) sterilization dose. Advantages of elevated cross-linking are significantly reduced wear as shown in hip and knee joint simulators (33,34), and in the case of knee joints, an increased resistance to pitting and delamination (35). Wear rates for elevated cross-linked polyethylenes approach zero, for example, in hip simulator tests (Fig. 5). Few well-controlled clinical studies exist to date in the peer-reviewed literature on the in vivo wear behavior of these materials, but short-term results suggest a marked improvement in wear (36–38).

The reduced wear resistance of elevated cross-linking polyethylene has also renewed interest in larger femoral heads for total hip replacement. The risk of dislocation is markedly reduced with a larger head size, but because sliding distance between the bearing surfaces and therefore the amount of wear increases with head size, conventional polyethylene metal bearings are typically small in diameter (32 mm or less). Larger head sizes are now commercially available with matching larger diameter elevated cross-linked polyethylene acetabular components. The wall thicknesses of the polyethylene liners in these components are less than 5 mm in some cases, however, making the strength and toughness of elevated cross-linked polyethylenes important considerations.

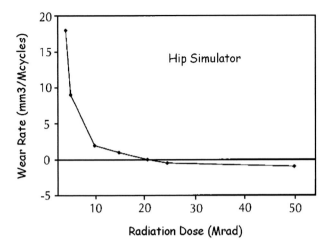

Figure 5 As ultra high molecular weight polyethylene is exposed to higher doses of radiation, the wear rate as measured in acetabular components tested in a hip simulator decreases, presumably due to the increased level of cross-linking. These data have been instrumental in the introduction of elevated cross-linked polyethylene into total joint components. *Source*: Data adapted from Ref. 30.

In fact, mechanical properties changes accompanying increased cross-linking may pose the biggest threat to the clinical efficacy of these materials. Reduced toughness and resistance to fatigue crack propagation have been shown in several laboratory studies using standardized specimens under controlled loading conditions (39,40). The clinical relevance of standardized fracture and fatigue test results is difficult to interpret, but reduced fracture properties could result in greater susceptibility to cracking as a form of wear damage (41), to gross component failure, and to dissociation of a polyethylene insert from its metal backing. Indeed, medical device reports to the Food and Drug Administration concerning elevated cross-linked polyethylene implant components include seven cases of gross fracture, four cases of component dissociation, and six cases of extensive wear.

Wear tests of knee-like geometries (with nonconforming bearing surfaces) and knee joint simulator studies show that elevated cross-linked materials perform quite well in comparison to conventional polyethylene (35). One possible explanation is the lowering of the elastic modulus that accompanies the post-cross-linking thermal treatment used to quench free radicals. As with compression molded polyethylene, the lower modulus creates larger contact areas, lower stresses, and better resistance to wear damage.

The recent findings of increased fatigue crack propagation rates in elevated cross-linked as compared to conventional polyethylenes might still prove problematic for in vivo wear behavior. These results suggest that if cracks were to form in vivo after a large number of cycles (larger than the number typically used in laboratory tests), failure might progress quickly. Thus, even if crack initiation is retarded because stresses are lower, the end results could still be worse.

CERAMICS

Ceramic materials are inorganic compounds, such as alumina (Al_2O_3), consisting of metallic and nonmetallic elements held together by ionic or covalent bonding. As with metals, ceramics have tightly packed atomic structures. Ceramic materials are very stiff and brittle. They are insoluble and chemically inert and, when processed to high purity, possess excellent biocompatibility and exceptional wear resistance with hard, hydrophilic surfaces. The brittle nature of ceramics limits their use in high load applications. In total joint replacement, ceramics have gained favor for two quite different applications. The first involves fully dense ceramics, such as alumina and zirconia, as bearing surfaces. The second involves the use of ceramics, such as hydroxyapatite, as less dense (even porous) coatings for metallic implants; these coatings are osteoconductive, providing surfaces to which bone will bond.

Alumina

Aluminum oxide (Al_2O_3), also known as alumina, has excellent abrasion resistance and when highly polished creates a very low coefficient of friction bearing surface against both UHMWPE and itself. Because of the excellent wettability of an alumina surface, better lubrication of the surface is possible. Wettability can be assessed through contact angle measurements, most commonly performed by placing a drop of liquid on the surface and measuring the angle between the plane of the surface and a line tangent to the edge of the liquid drop where it intersects the surface. The contact angle for alumina is about 45°, in comparison to those of polyethylene and metallic alloys, which are in the range of 70–85°.

Because of its excellent wear resistance, alumina has gained favor as a material for bearing surfaces in total hip replacement. Because of its brittle nature, however, it is used only for femoral heads and acetabular inserts and not for structural components such as femoral stems. Alumina femoral heads are attached to metallic stems through a taper connection. Early clinical experience showed fracture of alumina femoral heads to be a significant complication, with an incidence of more than 5% in some reported series. Improvements and standardization in alumina processing, including refinement of the grain size and hot isostatic pressing of the material after sintering to compact the material further, and in manufacturing taper connections have led to a dramatic improvement in performance (42). Grain sizes for alumina, for example, typically exceeded $4 \mu m$ in the 1970s with densities of about $4 g/mm^3$; grain sizes are now maintained at about $0.5 \mu m$ with densities of about $6 g/mm^3$, resulting in a 45% increase in strength. Even though alumina is considered biocompatible, recent reports of periprosthetic osteolysis secondary to alumina debris reinforce the concern that small particles ingested by cells can elicit an adverse biologic reaction regardless of their chemical nature (43).

Long-term experience with alumina-on-polyethylene bearings for hip replacement shows reduced wear rates over those typically seen with metal-on-polyethylene bearings, as well as an associated decrease in the presence of osteolysis, suggesting that these types of bearings are indeed beneficial in improving clinical performance (44). Alumina-on-polyethylene bearings in knee replacements have found much more limited use, and only mid-term results are available (45); the results are excellent but the absence of direct comparisons with conventional metal-on-polyethylene bearing surfaces of the same design and the lack of long-term results make it difficult to assess the clinical benefits.

Ceramic-on-ceramic bearings have been used extensively in total hip arthroplasty in Europe, though hip implants using this bearing combination have only recently received regulatory approval in the United States. In general, alumina-on-alumina joints have shown very low wear rates clinically, though the results are design-dependent, so that even these bearings can show excessive wear if incorporated into an inferior design (46). Recent reports also show excellent wear resistance in young patients with no measurable wear and no evidence of osteolysis even beyond a decade of follow-up (47). Furthermore, head fractures have not been observed even in this high demand patient population, lending further credence to the improved mechanical properties of alumina ceramic materials. Recent reports of stripe wear with metallic transfer have raised concern that edge loading of ceramic bearing surfaces could be problematic (Fig. 6).

Zirconia

Zirconium oxide (ZrO_2), also known as zirconia, is also used for femoral heads of total joint replacements, again because of its ability to create a low friction, wear resistant surface against UHMWPE. Unlike alumina, zirconia in pure form is unstable, changing phases between tetragonal, monoclinic, and cubic arrangements of molecules. The phase changes result in large volume changes that have a considerable effect on mechanical properties, often leading to internal cracks within the material. The tetragonal phase is the toughest of the three, and zirconia for joint replacements is stabilized with yttrium oxide to maintain this phase near room temperature. As another prevention of transformation to a less desirable phase, zirconia implants are often sterilized by exposure to ethylene oxide, a room temperature process. Intraoperative

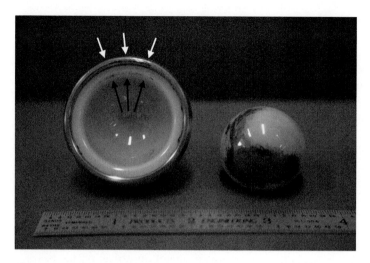

Figure 6   Impingement and dislocation remain problematic in total hip replacement. A retrieved ceramic-on-ceramic hip replacement shows considerable stripe wear on the femoral head and stripe wear on the rim of the ceramic acetabular insert (*black arrows*). Damage to the rim of the metallic acetabular shell (*white arrows*) is consistent with wear and transfer of metallic material to the ceramic surfaces.

steam resterilization of zirconia femoral head components can cause phase transformation and surface roughening and should never be performed.

Tougher than alumina with a much smaller grain size (less than half a micron), zirconia has found clinical use as an alternative bearing material to metallic alloys for articulating against UHMWPE. Zirconia does not, however, wear well against itself or against other ceramics such as alumina. Zirconia-on-polyethylene bearing surfaces have not proven as clinically successful as alumina-on-polyethylene bearings. High wear rates causing catastrophic failure as early as five years have been reported, though these failures might be due to the fact that a form of polyethylene (Hylamer), which has been prone to rapid oxidation and wear, was used in the acetabular component (48). More convincing data exist, however, from a direct comparison between alumina-, zirconia-, and metal-on-conventional polyethylene bearings in total hip patients that revealed the highest wear rate in the zirconia group, consistent with an increased monoclinic content on the surface of retrieved zirconia heads from the same series (49). Problems with manufacturing processes that led to a high incidence of fracture prompted a recent voluntary recall of nine batches of zirconia heads, further undermining confidence in this material.

More recently, an oxidized zirconium material has been introduced into both hip and knee replacement components for articulation against polyethylene, though few results are available and clinical experience with this material is short term (50).

Bioceramics

Certain ceramic materials are osteophilic, such that osteoblasts form bone with the mineral phase in direct contact with the ceramic surface. The chemical or physical bond that forms between the ceramic and the bone is not well understood, but results in sufficient interfacial strength that applications as ceramic coatings on joint replacement implants have been used in an attempt to improve implant fixation. Most coatings are variations on hydroxyapatite, a calcium phosphate, $Ca_{10}(PO_4)_6(OH)_2$, that forms the mineral phase of bone. The stability of calcium phosphate ceramics depends on the temperature and the environment and can be affected by substitution (for example, of a carbonate for a phosphate).

Hydroxyapatite coatings for fixation of load-bearing implants have been in clinical use for more than a decade, though the true composition of these coatings can be quite variable because of differences in manufacturing processes and alterations with time in vivo. Clinical results have shown hydroxyapatite coated implants perform well, even in young, high demand patients (51,52), though improvement in performance over noncoated implants has not always been found (53).

Studies of coatings on retrieved implants show that the coatings are often osteoconductive, but bonding with bone is inconsistent. The coatings themselves may not in fact be true hydroxyapatite, but a mixture of phases, including calcium oxide, tricalcium phosphate, and amorphous calcium phosphate. Coatings have been shown to dissolve and fracture from the implant substrate, as well as to be removed by an osteoclastic remodeling process (54).

SUMMARY

The biomaterials employed in total joint replacement have generally met all of the biocompatible, corrosion, mechanical, quality, and cost issues necessary for the rigorous environments within which they must perform. Despite problems such as osteolysis and ongoing concerns such as corrosion and systemic accumulation of metallic elements, the biomaterials in current use have performed well, most for more than 30 years.

Nonetheless, the search for biomaterials with increased performance (e.g., improved wear resistance) or with properties better suited for specific applications (e.g., small implants for implantation using less invasive surgical techniques) is continuing. Given the significant costs of developing new materials and the rigorous bench testing and clinical trials necessary to demonstrate safety and efficacy, this effort will probably concentrate more on altering the properties of existing materials than on developing new ones. Alteration in alloying elements in implant metals could improve properties and increase biocompatibility of released particulate debris. Biologically active coatings on metallic implants could be aimed at providing combination products that can improve fixation and treat infection and pain. Nanotechnology could be used to design surface shapes and chemistries more amenable to interactions with surrounding cells. The success of these developments in improving the performance of total joint replacements will depend not only on continued improvement in biomaterials science, but also on the ability to integrate new materials using appropriate engineering design principles and a keen understanding of the requirements of the orthopaedic surgeon.

REFERENCES

1. Cahoon JR, Holte RN. Corrosion fatigue of surgical stainless steel in synthetic physiological solution. J Biomed Mater Res 1981; 15:137–145.
2. Colangelo VJ, Greene ND. Corrosion and fracture of type 316 SMO orthopaedic implants. J Biomed Mater Res 1969; 3:247–265.
3. Goldberg JR, Gilbert JL, Jacobs JJ, Bauer TW, Paprosky W, Leurgans S. A multicenter retrieval study of the taper interfaces of modular hip prostheses. Clin Orthop 2002; 401:149–161.
4. Hallab NJ, Jacobs JJ, Skipor A, Black J, Mikecz K, Galante JO. Systemic metal-protein binding associated with total joint replacement arthroplasty. J Biomed Mater Res 2000; 49:353–361.
5. Jacobs JJ, Skipor AK, Patterson LM, Hallab NJ, Paprosky WG, Black J, Galante JO. Metal release in patients who have had a primary total hip arthroplasty. A prospective, controlled, longitudinal study. J Bone Joint Surg Am 1998; 80:1447–1458.
6. Jinno T, Goldberg VM, Davy D, Stevenson S. Osseointegration of surface-blasted implants made of titanium alloy and cobalt–chromium alloy in a rabbit intramedullary model. J Biomed Mater Res 1998; 42:20–29.
7. Wan Z, Dorr LD, Woodsome T, Ranawat A, Song M. Effect of stem stiffness and bone stiffness on bone remodeling in cemented total hip replacement. J Arthroplasty 1999; 14:149–158.
8. Woolson ST, Milbauer JP, Bobyn JD, Yue S, Maloney WJ. Fatigue fracture of a forged cobalt–chromium–molybdenum femoral component inserted with cement. A report of ten cases. J Bone Joint Surg Am 1997; 79:1842–1848.
8a. Brien WW, Salvati EA, Betts F, Bullough P, Wright T, Rimnac C, Buly R, Garvin K. Metal levels in cemented total hip arthroplasty. A comparison of well-fixed and loose implants. Clin Orthop Relat Res 1992; 276:66–74.
9. Eisenbarth E, Velten D, Muller M, Thull R, Breme J. Biocompatibility of beta-stabilizing elements of titanium alloys. Biomaterials 2004; 25:5705–5713.
10. Black J. Biological performance of tantalum. Clinical Materials 1994; 16: 167–173.
11. Bobyn JD, Stackpool GJ, Hacking SA, Tanzer M, Krygier JJ. Characteristics of bone ingrowth and interface mechanics of a new porous tantalum biomaterial. J Bone Joint Surg Br 1999; 81-B:907–914.
12. Hacking SA, Bobyn JD, Toh K, Tanzer M, Krygier JJ. Fibrous tissue ingrowth and attatchment to porous tantalum. J Biomed Mater Res 2000; 52:631–638.
13. Iesaka K, Jaffe WL, Kummer FJ. Effects of preheating of hip prostheses on the stem–cement interface. J Bone Joint Surg Am 2003; 85-A:421–427.

14. Parks ML, Walsh HA, Salvati EA, Li S. Effect of increasing temperature on the properties of four bone cements. Clin Orthop 1998; 355:238–248.

15. Salvati EA, Wright TM: Commentary and Perspective on "Effects of Preheating of Hip Prostheses on the Stem–Cement Interface" by K Iesaka, WL Jaffe, FJ Kummer, J Bone Joint Surg 2003; 85A:421–427, at http://www.jbjs.org/Comments/2003/cp_mar03_salvati.shtml

16. Ling RS, Lee AJ. Porosity reduction in acrylic cement is clinically irrelevant. Clin Orthop 1998; 355:249–253.

17. Chao EY, Chin HC, Stauffer RN. Roentgenographic and mechanical performance of centrifuged cement in a simulated total hip arthroplasty model. Clin Orthop 1992; 285:91–101.

18. Stevens CM, Tetsworth KD, Calhoun JH, Mader JT. An articulated antibiotic spacer used for infected total knee arthroplasty: a comparative in vitro elution study of Simplex and Palacos bone cements. J Orthop Res 2005; 23:27–33.

19. Wright TM, Sullivan DJ, Arnoczky SP. The effect of antibiotic additions on the fracture properties of bone cements. Acta Orthop Scand 1984; 55:414–418.

20. Masri BA, Duncan CP, Beauchamp CP. Long-term elution of antibiotics from bone-cement: an in vivo study using the prosthesis of antibiotic-loaded acrylic cement (PROSTALAC) system. J Arthroplasty 1998; 13:331–338.

21. Wright TM, Goodman SB. Implant Wear in Total Joint Replacement: Clinical and Biologic Issues, Materials and Design Considerations. Rosemont: American Academy of Orthopaedic Surgeons, 2001.

22. Rimnac CM, Klein RW, Betts F, Wright TM. Post-irradiation aging of ultra high molecular weight polyethylene. J Bone Joint Surg 1994; 76A:1052–1056.

23. Collier MB, Engh CA Jr, Engh GA. Shelf age of the polyethylene tibial component and outcome of unicondylar knee arthroplasty. J Bone Joint Surg Am 2004; 86-A:763–769.

24. Gomez-Barrena E, Li S, Furman BS, Masri BA, Wright TM, Salvati EA. Role of polyethylene oxidation and consolidation defects in cup performance. Clin Orthop 1998; 352:105–117.

25. Wrona M, Mayor MB, Collier JP, Jensen RE. The correlation between fusion defects and damage in tibial polyethylene bearings. Clin Orthop 1994; 299:92–103.

26. Sutula LC, Collier JP, Saum KA, et al. Impact of gamma sterilization on clinical performance of polyethylene in the hip. Clin Orthop 1995; 319:28–40.

27. Hopper RH Jr, Young AM, Orishimo KF, Engh CA Jr. Effect of terminal sterilization with gas plasma or gamma radiation on wear of polyethylene liners. J Bone Joint Surg Am 2003; 85-A:464–468.

28. Digas G, Thanner J, Nivbrant B, Rohrl S, Strom H, Karrholm J. Increase in early polyethylene wear after sterilization with ethylene oxide: radiostereometric analyses of 201 total hips. Acta Orthop Scand 2003; 74:531–541.

29. Orishimo KF, Hopper RH Jr, Engh CA. Long-term in vivo wear performance of porous-coated acetabular components sterilized with gamma irradiation in air or ethylene oxide. J Arthroplasty 2003; 18:546–552.

30. Williams IR, Mayor MB, Collier JP. The impact of sterilization method on wear in knee arthroplasty. Clin Orthop 1998; 356:170–180.

31. Berzins A, Jacobs JJ, Berger R, Ed C, Natarajan R, Andriacchi T, Galante JO. Surface damage in machined ram-extruded and net-shape molded retrieved

polyethylene tibial inserts of total knee replacements. J Bone Joint Surg Am 2002; 84-A:1534–1540.

32. Ritter MA. Direct compression molded polyethylene for total hip and knee replacements. Clin Orthop 2001; 393:94–100.

33. McKellop H, Shen FW, Lu B, Campbell P, Salovey R. Development of an extremely wear-resistant ultra high molecular weight polyethylene for total hip replacements. J Orthop Res 1999; 17:157–167.

34. Muratoglu OK, Bragdon CR, Jasty M, O'Connor DO, Von Knoch RS, Harris WH. Knee-simulator testing of conventional and cross-linked polyethylene tibial inserts. J Arthroplasty 2004; 19:887–897.

35. Maher SA, Furman BD, Wright TM. The reduced fracture toughness that accompanies elevated cross-linking of polyethylene is not associated with an increase in pitting and delamination type aear. In: Kurtz SM, Gsell R, Martell J, eds. Crosslinked and Ther-mally Treated Ultra-High Molecular Weight Polyethylene for Joint Replacements ASTM STP 1445. West Conshohocken: ASTM International 2004:137–150.

36. Digas G, Karrholm J, Thanner J, Malchau H, Herberts P. Highly cross-linked polyethylene in total hip arthroplasty: randomized evaluation of penetration rate in cemented and uncemented sockets using radiostereometric analysis. Clin Orthop 2004; 429:6–16.

37. Heisel C, Silva M, dela Rosa MA, Schmalzried TP. Short-term in vivo wear of cross-linked polyethylene. J Bone Joint Surg Am 2004; 86-A:748–751.

38. Martell JM, Verner JJ, Incavo SJ. Clinical performance of a highly cross-linked polyethylene at two years in total hip arthroplasty: a randomized prospective trial. J Arthroplasty 2003; 18:55–59.

39. Baker DA, Hastings RS, Pruitt L. Study of fatigue resistance of chemical and radiation crosslinked medical grade ultrahigh molecular weight polyethylene. J Biomed Mater Res 1999; 46(4):573–581.

40. Cole JC, Lemons JE, Eberhardt AW. Gamma irradiation alters fatigue-crack behavior and fracture toughness in 1900H and GUR 1050 UHMWPE. J Biomed Mater Res 2002; 63:559–566.

41. Bradford L, Baker DA, Graham J, Chawan A, Ries MD, Pruitt LA. Wear and surface cracking in early retrieved highly cross-linked polyethylene acetabular liners. J Bone Joint Surg Am 2004; 86-A:1271–1282.

42. Willmann G. Ceramics for total hip replacement—what a surgeon should know. Orthopaedics 1998; 21:173–177.

43. Yoon TR, Rowe SM, Jung ST, Seon KJ, Maloney WJ. Osteolysis in association with a total hip arthroplasty with ceramic bearing surfaces. J Bone Joint Surg Am 1998; 80:1459–1468.

44. Hamadouche M, Boutin P, Daussange J, Bolander ME, Sedel L. Alumina-on-alumina total hip arthroplasty: a minimum 18.5-year follow-up study. J Bone Joint Surg Am 2002; 84:69–77.

45. Akagi M, Nakamura T, Matsusue Y, Ueo T, Nishijyo K, Ohnishi E. The bisurface total knee replacement: a unique design for flexion. Four-to-nine-year follow-up study. J Bone Joint Surg Am 2000; 82-A:1626–1633.

46. Urban JA, Garvin KL, Boese CK, Bryson L, Pedersen DR, Callaghan JJ, Miller RK. Ceramic-on-polyethylene bearing surfaces in total hip arthroplasty.

Seventeen to twenty-one-year results. J Bone Joint Surg Am 2001; 83: 1688–1694.

47. Fenollosa J, Seminario P, Montijano C. Ceramic hip prostheses in young patients: a retrospective study of 74 patients. Clin Orthop 2000; 379:55–67.

48. Norton MR, Yarlagadda R, Anderson GH. Catastrophic failure of the Elite Plus total hip replacement, with a Hylamer acetabulum and Zirconia ceramic femoral head. J Bone Joint Surg Br 2002; 84:631–635.

49. Hernigou P, Bahrami T. Zirconia alumina ceramics in comparison with stainless-steel heads. Polyethylene wear after a minimum ten-year follow-up. J Bone Joint Surg Br 2003; 85:504–509.

50. Laskin RS. An oxidized Zr ceramic surfaced femoral component for total knee arthroplasty. Clin Orthop 2003; 416:191–196.

51. Dumbleton J, Manley MT. Hydroxyapatite-coated prostheses in total hip and knee arthroplasty. J Bone Joint Surg Am 2004; 86-A:2526–2540.

52. Singh S, Trikha SP, Edge AJ. Hydroxyapatite ceramic-coated femoral stems in young patients. A prospective ten-year study. J Bone Joint Surg Br 2004; 86:1118–1123.

53. Parvizi J, Sharkey PF, Hozack WJ, Orzoco F, Bissett GA, Rothman RH. Prospective matched-pair analysis of hydroxyapatite-coated and uncoated femoral stems in total hip arthroplasty. A concise follow-up of a previous report. J Bone Joint Surg Am 2004; 86-A:783–786.

54. Tonino A, Oosterbos C, Rahmy A, Therin M, Doyle C. Hydroxyapatite-coated acetabular components. Histological and histomorphometric analysis of six cups retrieved at autopsy between three and seven years after successful implantation. J Bone Joint Surg Am 2001; 83-A:817–825.

8

Wear of Joint Replacements

John Fisher

*Medical and Biological Engineering, School of Mechanical Engineering,
University of Leeds, Leeds, U.K.*

INTRODUCTION

The primary bearing couple that has been used in artificial joints over the last 40 years is a polished metallic convex femoral surface on a concave ultra high molecular weight polyethylene (UHMWPE) acetabular or tibial surface. This was first introduced in hip prostheses in the early 1960s, and since the early 1970s has also been used extensively in knee prostheses. An estimated number of over one million bearing couples are implanted in patients every year, and these remain one of the most successful surgical applications of any biomaterial. Over the majority of this 40-year period, wear of the UHMWPE bearing surfaces has not been considered to be a major clinical problem. The historical linear wear of polyethylene bearing surfaces has been between 0.1 and 0.2 mm/yr, and with UHMWPE bearing components having thickness of up to 10 mm, it could take 50–100 years to wear out an average bearing. This is well beyond the expected life time of the majority of patients. This perceived adequate tribological performance of UHMWPE bearing surfaces has meant that historically alternative bearing couples such as metal on metal or ceramic on ceramic had limited clinical application.

During the last 10 years, it has become recognized that, although UHMWPE bearing surfaces rarely wear out, adverse tissue reactions to small micrometer and submicrometer UHMWPE wear particles is a major cause of medium- to long-term failure of joint replacements. These were first identified in 1977 (1). However, the clinical impact of this wear debris-induced osteolysis was not recognized until the 1990s. It is a complex and interactive biomechanical and biological failure process (2), which remains one of the major challenges facing joint replacement surgery at the present time. This has prompted considerable research in recent years into new and improved bearing couples for joint replacements, which has, in parallel, allowed the research community to develop a deeper understanding of wear, wear debris generation and tribological processes in joint replacements.

In this chapter, the basic principles of wear will be introduced, the historical perspective of wear of UHMWPE described, and the current perspectives of recently introduced "improved" bearing couples presented. Finally, future perspectives on advanced bearing technologies that may further reduce wear and osteolysis are presented.

LUBRICATION, FRICTION, AND WEAR

Although wear properties of materials have been extensively described, it is extremely important to recognize that wear is not a fundamental property of a material, but is a functional performance criterion of an engineering or tribological system. The wear of a component in a tribological system is dependent on the properties of the opposing counterface material in the bearing couple, the lubrication regime and resulting frictional forces, as well as the loading regime and duty cycle. The dependency of the wear of a component on a range of other variables and conditions in the tribological system frequently leads to apparently contradictory results, both in vitro and in vivo.

The frictional force and the resulting wear of bearing couples are critically dependent on the lubrication regime (3). A schematic representation of variation in the coefficient of friction as a function of the lubrication regime is shown in Figure 1. The horizontal axis is the product of the sliding velocity and viscosity of the fluid divided by the load. For high values of viscosity and/or velocity and low values of load, the parameter has a large value and fluid film lubrication may be achieved. Fluid film lubrication occurs when the thickness of lubricating film produced by hydrodynamic or elastohydrodynamic lubrication action is greater than three times the combined surface roughness of the bearing surfaces. If fluid film lubrication is achieved, the bearing surfaces are separated by a fluid film and little or no wear will occur. Although smooth bearing surfaces are commonly used in joint replacements, (surface roughness R_a 0.01–0.1 μm), the relatively low sliding velocities, the variable viscosity of the pseudosynovial fluid, and the high loads during stance means that full fluid film lubrication is rarely achieved, and wear nearly always occurs in joint replacement. However, this does not mean that lubrication is not important in joint replacements. Under conditions of low viscosity fluid (or absence of fluid), very low sliding velocity and high load, boundary lubrication dominates, in (Figure 1), and

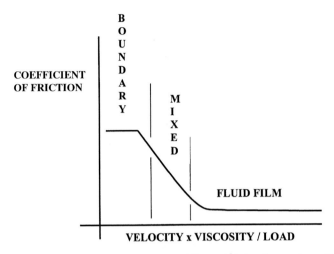

Figure 1 Friction coefficient for different lubrication regimes. The horizontal axis is the product of velocity and viscosity divided by load.

the solid asperities of the two bearing surfaces come into direct intimate contact, friction increases which increases wear. In practice, most joint replacements operate between the boundary and fluid film lubrication regimes. This is known as the mixed lubrication regime. In this regime, the coefficient of friction and hence wear is highly dependent on viscosity, velocity, and load, as the fluid has the ability to partially separate interacting solid asperities, sharing part of the load. Equally important in a biological fluid such as "pseudosynovial fluid" is the role of the larger protein and lipid molecules. These can attach to both wear surfaces acting as a solid phase boundary lubricant which can also reduce friction and wear. Additionally, and frequently overlooked in the orthopaedic literature, is the role of the wear debris itself, which can also act as a solid phase lubricant, as it becomes detached from the bearing surfaces and exits from the contact. This wear debris can act as a protective screen between the bearing surfaces, reducing friction and wear (4). This wear debris must be differentiated from the "foreign" third body particles arising from other sources, which may enter the contact and damage bearing surfaces and accelerate wear in joint replacements.

The prediction of the lubrication regime is extremely complex. Under conditions of continuous walking, which is most advantageous to film lubrication, the thickness of the lubricating film is critically dependent on the viscosity of the pseudosynovial fluid, elasticity of the bearing surfaces, head size, and geometrical clearances between the components (5). For a metal on UHMWPE bearing, a thicker fluid film may be achieved due to deformation of the polymer. However, the larger surface roughness of the polymer indicates these bearings operate towards the boundary end of the mixed lubrication regime with a coefficient of friction of 0.04–0.1. In the harder metal-on-metal and ceramic-on-ceramic bearings, film thickness may be less, but the surfaces, particularly in ceramic-on-ceramic bearings, are very smooth and these approach the fluid film end of the mixed regime. In the case of ceramic-on-ceramic, this can lead to friction coefficients as low as 0.01–0.02. However, patients walk for less than 5% of their lives and in other activities with lower velocities, the fluid film lubrication is depleted and the system moves towards the boundary end of the mixed regime. The maximum value for the coefficient of friction that bearings can reach in the boundary regimes is material dependent, with metal on UHMWPE being lowest 0.1–0.2 and metal-on-metal being highest 0.5–0.7. Under these boundary conditions, the larger molecular weight molecules in the fluid act as boundary lubricants to protect the bearing surface and reduce friction. Proteins appear to be particularly important in reducing friction in metal-on-metal bearing surfaces, under severe loading conditions, while in contrast proteins may slightly elevate friction in UHMWPE bearings (University of Leeds, Student Project Report). Under conditions of a constant load and low velocity, metal-on-polyethylene has the lowest coefficient of friction and metal on metal the highest.

Friction, of course, is not directly related to wear and some materials such as PTFE have very low friction and high wear. However, for a given bearing combination improving lubrication by increasing velocity, increasing viscosity, and reducing load in the mixed lubrication regime will reduce both friction and wear, as demonstrated in metal-on-metal bearings (6). While lubrication has an important role to play in reducing friction and wear, there are many other factors that influences wear and wear mechanisms in joint replacements.

BASIC MECHANISMS, TYPES OF WEAR AND DEBRIS GENERATION

Wear processes in tribological systems can be characterized by the basic mechanisms that generate the wear debris, which can be considered as the inputs to the system, and the types of wear or wear surfaces, which can be considered the outputs of the wear processes. Examples of wear mechanisms include adhesive, abrasive, corrosive, fatigue, while examples of types of wear include, burnishing, pitting, and delamination. Types of wear are often defined by simply observing the wear surfaces, and they do not require a knowledge or understanding of the wear process in the tribological system. In contrast, the definition of the wear mechanisms requires some knowledge of the wear process and tribological systems and conditions. Types of wear surfaces can be related to wear mechanisms, but this can only be done in specific conditions and systems, and no generic guidelines can be given to the relationships between wear mechanisms and types of wear in these complex tribological systems.

The most basic mechanisms of wear occur at a microscopic level due to interactions of the asperities of the rough surfaces. When two surfaces come into contact the asperities on the surfaces deform both elastically and plastically. When the surfaces slide over each other they have to shear the interface between the contacting asperities, which gives rise to adhesive friction and adhesive wear. Additionally, the sliding process produces further deformation of the asperities, which can give rise to deformation friction and abrasive wear. These two basic wear mechanisms are shown schematically in Figure 2. In dry contacts, adhesive forces are high, but in lubricated contacts particularly with biological fluids with large macromolecules that can act as boundary lubrication, the adhesive component of wear can be reduced (7). In a hard or soft bearing combination, such as metal on polyethylene, asperities of the metal surface plough or deform the softer polyethylene. If the metal asperities are large or sharp then abrasive wear is produced (8). By making the metal surface much smoother with smaller asperities with larger wavelengths, the abrasive wear is reduced (8,9) and the surface wear occurs due to deformation and adhesive forces. Single asperity interactions may not generate individual wear particles, and multiple asperity interactions are often required to generate a wear particle, and hence the mechanisms enter into a microscopic fatigue wear regime. This can result in a polished or burnished wear surface on the polymer. The above mechanisms occur at the lowest scale of interaction in which the level of the asperity on the metal surface typically has a height of a maximum of 0.1 μm (10). This gives rise to the smallest granular type wear particles generated in polyethylene-on-metal combinations (Fig. 3). Similarly, in highly polished metal-on-metal and ceramic-on-ceramic bearings, the microscopic asperity interactions and the micro fatigue wear will give rise to the smallest wear particles which are 5–30 nm in size.

However, materials are complex and have higher order structures and interactions that occur at larger dimensional scale, which can give rise to

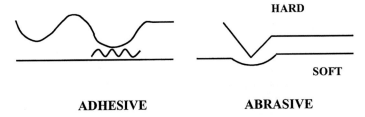

HARD

SOFT

ADHESIVE   **ABRASIVE**

Figure 2 Schematic diagram of adhesive and abrasive wear mechanisms in metal-on-polyethylene joints.

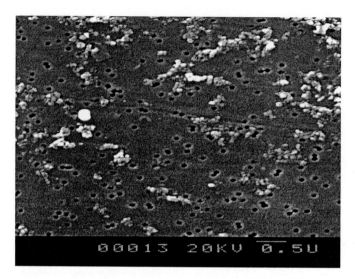

Figure 3 SEM of the smallest granular type UHMWPE wear debris isolated from periprosthetic tissues. *Abbreviation*: UHMWPE, ultra high molecular weight polyethylene.

different and larger wear particles (10). Metal-on-metal bearings for hip prostheses are made from cobalt–chrome alloys which have larger hard carbides in the surface. These hard carbides can cause large abrasive scratches and can also pull out of the surface producing larger debris in each case (11). In the ceramic-on-ceramic bearings the alumina ceramic has a grain structure of 1–2 μm, so in addition to microscopic asperity fatigue wear and relief polishing, in cases of very high stresses, such as with head–rim contact, intergranular fracture and grain pull out resulting in larger meter size debris can occur (12).

UHMWPE has by far the most complex wear mechanisms. In addition to the microscopic fatigue wear and burnishing by the smooth metal asperities, the UHMWPE can deform on a more macroscopic level. This gives rise to larger scale plastic deformation on the surface (13) and an increased surface roughness. This in turn can then lead to large flakes or fibers of wear debris being produced up to 10–100 μm in length (Fig. 4) (10). Most importantly, the UHMWPE also deforms and orientates at a molecular level which gives rise to an orthotropic surface, an orientation hardening in the principal direction of sliding and orientation softening in the transverse direction (14). The surface is frequently rippled transverse to the direction of sliding which can give rise to microfibrils of the order of 1–10 μm in length. The molecular orientation is very important and is dependent on the kinematic conditions. If the motion is primarily unidirectional, the polymer strain hardens in the direction of sliding and the wear resistance is high.

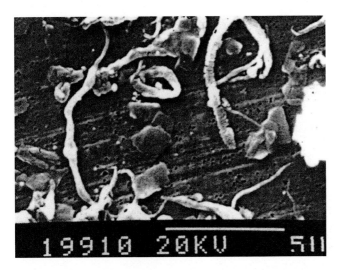

Figure 4 Examples of larger type UHMWPE wear debris from retrieved periprosthetic tissues. *Abbreviation*: UHMWPE, ultra high molecular weight polyethylene.

However, if the motion is multidirectional as in the case of the hip joint, the cross shearing by the friction force in the transverse direction accelerates wear due to the material being strain softened or weakened in this direction. It is this cross shearing that is claimed to break off the micro fibrils. The kinematic conditions can have a 10-fold effect on the wear rate (15).

These different scales of interactions give rise to a wide range of wear particles in polyethylene from 0.1 to 0.5 μm granules (Fig. 3) produced by micro asperity fatigue, micro fibrils produced by orientation and cross shearing and platelets, and larger fibres (Fig. 4) produced by macroscopic surface plastic deformation (16,17). Additionally, with highly stressed knees, even larger wear particles are produced by structural fatigue and cracking indicated at oxidized grain boundaries. These particles are in the range of 100 μm to 1 mm (10).

The types of wear surface produced are clearly dependent on the type of wear mechanisms and tribological conditions. Polishing or burnishing type wear surfaces due to microscopic asperity fatigue processes are found in UHMWPE, metal-on-metal and ceramic-on-ceramic bearings under mild wear conditions. On UHMWPE, rippling of the surface can also occur where there is a predominant direction of motion and high magnification SEM can detect fibril detachment from the rippled surface due to cross shear. In the presence of hard third body particles, abrasive wear tracks can be found on polyethylene surfaces, and discrete micrometer size scratches can also be found on the harder metallic surfaces (17) (Fig. 5). Larger scale plastic deformation can also be found on the UHMWPE

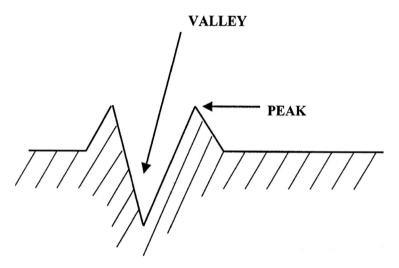

Figure 5 Example of a scratch profile to a metallic femoral head caused by third body particles. The raised lips of the scratch cause accelerated wear of the UHMWPE. *Abbreviation*: UHMWPE, ultra high molecular weight polyethylene.

surface, which gives the surface a waviness of height up to 1 µm and wavelength of the order of 100 µm. Plastic deformation on the surface due to cyclic strain accumulation can be detected by polarized light microscopy (13). UHMWPE is consolidated from grains up to 300 µm in size and pitting is also seen on wear surfaces due to grain pull out. Additionally, gross structural fatigue failure has been seen in highly stressed conditions and this has been termed delamination wear (Fig. 6). In metal-on-metal bearing surfaces, hard carbides can pull out of the surface and cause abrasive tracks and scratches to the opposing surface (11), which then get polished back with time. In ceramic-on-ceramic alumina bearings occasional partial grain pull out can occur which leaves a small hole or pit in the polished surface. However, the most common severe wear mode is a characteristic wear stripe on the femoral head associated with high stress contact with the rim of the cup, which cause intergranular fracture and roughening of the femoral head surface (Fig. 7) (12). The above provides examples of a few common types of wear surfaces, and their relationship to the wear processes and mechanisms that produce them. There are many types of wear surfaces. The frequency or incidence of wear surface features is not often reported and care has to be taken in interpretation of such data. Equally, observations of wear surfaces are frequently made only at one position on the surface, and this can mean that important features that may occur elsewhere are overlooked. Full quantitative mapping of wear surfaces is time consuming and is rarely undertaken.

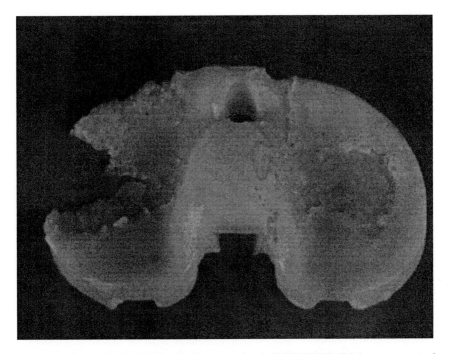

Figure 6 An example of delamination wear in the UHMWPE tibial component of the knee. *Abbreviation*: UHMWPE, ultra high molecular weight polyethylene.

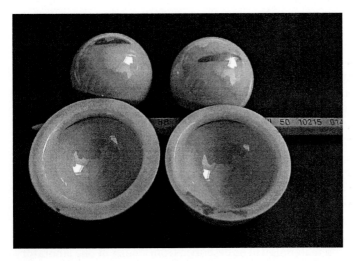

Figure 7 An example of intergranular fracture caused by head-on-rim contact of alumina ceramic on ceramic prosthesis.

BASIC LAWS OF WEAR AND FACTORS THAT INFLUENCE WEAR RATES

The simple experiments indicate that wear volume V is linearly proportional to sliding distance X. Additionally, wear volume has in certain conditions been shown to be proportional to load P. Caution has to be used in applying this proportionality which only extends over a limited range of contact stresses (19). A simple wear equation can be written as follows:

$$V = kPX$$

where k is an empirical constant (the wear factor) with units of mm^3/N m.

This simple wear equation and the wear function are used to compare wear of different materials and tribological conditions. The wear factor does not have a unique value for a single material, but is highly dependent on the tribological conditions under which the wear is being generated. For example, for a metal-on-polyethylene bearing combination the wear factor (or wear rate) is reduced if the counterface metal becomes smoother (20), if the protein lubricant has increased lipid concentration (21), or if the motion becomes less multidirectional and more unidirectional (22).

In contrast, the wear factor for metal on metal is reduced by more multidirectional motion (23), which produces a more effective polishing action, and is also reduced by increased protein concentration in the lubricant. The wear factor of metal on metal is reduced considerably in a hip joint simulator under cyclic loading due to squeeze film and elastohydrodynamic lubrication compared to a constant load wear test in which the lubricating film is depleted (24).

In ceramic-on-ceramic bearings the wear factor is less dependent on lubricant or loading conditions or motion (25), but does increase markedly under high contact stress or impact (12).

In general terms, it is predicted that the wear factor or wear rate is inversely proportional to the hardness of the bearing surface, which would indicate that UHMWPE would have the highest wear and ceramic (the hardest material) the lowest wear. The effect of the tribological conditions described above can change the relative wear rates. It is therefore important to compare materials under similar tribological conditions and that these conditions should replicate the conditions found in vivo. To this end sophisticated hip and knee joint simulators have been developed in a number of centers around the world. However, these are not all the same, and while it is acceptable to compare materials under the same conditions and simulators within one laboratory, it is not advisable to compare directly different materials studied by a variety of methods in different laboratories. In this review, comparison of the wear of different materials will be described from studies in one laboratory only. However for a given material, comparison will be made between different laboratories to highlight the influence of different conditions on wear.

WEAR OF POLYETHYLENE IN HIP PROSTHESES

UHMWPE acetabular cups articulating against polished metallic or ceramic femoral heads have been the most widely used bearing couple over the last 40 years. Metallic femoral heads have included stainless steel alloys and cobalt-chrome alloys. Additionally titanium has also been used, but this gave poor performance due to its poor abrasion resistance. Ceramic femoral heads have included zirconia ceramic and alumina ceramic. Head sizes have mainly been used in sizes 22, 28, and 32 mm diameters. The effect of head size on wear rates was comprehensively reported by Livermore et al. (26) who showed that as head size increased, the wear volume increased due to increased sliding distance as predicted by basic laws of wear. However, as the area being worn is proportional to the projected area of the head, (diameter squared) the actual linear wear penetration is reduced with head size. As the concern is osteolysis and volume of wear particles (not linear penetration), clinical advantages have been found with smaller diameter heads.

Several types of UHMWPE have been used during this period. One major difference has been molecular weight, with GUR1120 having a lower molecular weight of 2–4 million and GUR1150 having a higher molecular weight of 4–6 million. Wear studies have shown relatively little difference in their respective wear rates (27). There have also been different processing routes, including extrusion, compression molding, and in limited cases, direct compression molding. Little difference has been found in the wear resistance between extrusion and compression molding (28). Materials have also been made with and without calcium sterate additives. There is some indication that calcium sterate may lead to additional degradation following irradiation. Today, many UHMWPE materials are processed without calcium sterate.

The most important variable has been the method of sterilization of UHMWPE. The vast majority of historical polyethylene used during this period was gamma irradiated in the presence of oxygen. It has been shown in the last 10 years that this leads to the generation of free radicals, degradation of mechanical properties such as toughness and ductility, and an increase in wear rate (29).

The results of the wear of GUR 1120 UHMWPE gamma irradiated in air polyethylene in the Leeds Anatomical/Physiological hip joint simulators are shown in the following figures and compared to clinical data. The wear rate of 28 mm acetabular cups articulating against stainless steel, cobalt–chrome, and zirconia ceramic femoral heads is shown in Figure 8. A lower wear rate is achieved with the zirconia head due to its slightly better surface finish (30). Clinical wear rates for retrieved Charnley prostheses with undamaged femoral heads were similar but showed much greater variation (Fig. 9) (17). The Charnley hip had a smaller head size and therefore sliding distance which would reduce wear, but the UHMWPE was aged and that

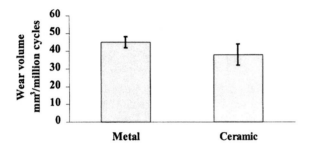

Volumetric Wear
γ-Irradiated in Air
Hip Joint Simulator
Femoral Heads

Figure 8 Simulator wear rate of UHMWPE acetabular cups articulating against different femoral heads. Wear against the zirconia ceramic femoral head is lowest. *Abbreviation*: UHMWPE, ultra high molecular weight polyethylene. *Source*: From Ref. 30.

would contribute to increased wear. Equally the activity of the patients in this study, who were mainly elderly, was not monitored. In prostheses with scratched or damaged metallic femoral heads the average wear rate was doubled (Fig. 9) (17). A laboratory model of deliberately scratching metallic femoral heads with discrete scratches has been shown to increase the wear rate by a factor of three (Fig. 10) (31). Although this was greater than the two-fold increase seen in vivo, it has to be recognised that the scratching in vivo occurred at some undetermined point in the prostheses lifetime, but the wear rate was averaged over its whole lifetime. Minakawa et al. (32) showed that ceramic femoral heads are much more damage resistant than metal femoral heads, retaining their surface finish for much longer. It is predicted that this will lead to lower long term wear rates of UHMWPE compared to metal heads that have been scratched or damaged.

Studies of the wear of gamma irradiated and aged UHMWPE can give an indication of the effect of oxidative degradation, firstly when aged in vitro, i.e., stored in the packaging prior to implantation and secondly, retrieved from patients after having little storage in vitro prior to implantation. The wear rate of GUR 1120 gamma irradiated in air increases with age on the shelf (33). The wear rate of GUR 1120 UHMWPE gamma irradiated in air and aged for five years in the packaging prior to implantation is compared to nonaged material in Figure 11. The oxidative ageing on the shelf produced a three-fold increase in wear rate. The wear rate of GUR 1120 gamma irradiated in air UHMWPE which had been implanted in patients for 15 years and tested in the hip joint simulator is compared to nonaged material in Figure 12 (34). Fifteen years in vivo produced a three-fold

Volumetric Wear
γ-Irradiated in Air In Vivo

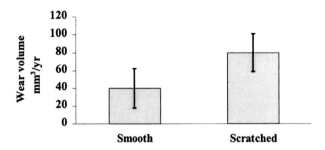

Figure 9 Clinical wear rates for retrieved Charnley prostheses with damaged and not damaged femoral heads. *Source*: From Ref. 17.

increase in wear. The available oxygen in vivo is less than outside the body in air, and this may indicate a lower rate of oxidative degradation in vivo. These and other studies have led to the recent development and clinical use of stabilized and crosslinked polyethylenes.

It is worth contrasting the wear rates found with different hip simulators in laboratories around the world for the historical gamma irradiated in air UHMWPE. For this comparison not aged material will be used. The University of Durham (35) used 25% (v/v) bovine serum as in the above studies and showed similar wear rates of 40 mm^3/million cycles under these standard conditions. Wang et al. (36) using an anatomical MTS biaxial

Volumetric Wear
γ-Irradiated in Air
Hip Joint Simulator

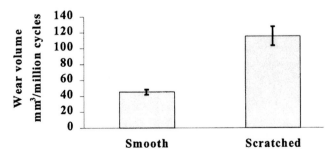

Figure 10 Simulator wear rates of UHMWPE against smooth and scratched femoral heads. *Abbreviation*: UHMWPE, ultra high molecular weight polyethylene. *Source*: From Ref. 31.

γ-Irradiated in Air UHMWPE, aged 5 yrs In Vitro
Tested in a Hip Joint Simulator,
Smooth Femoral Heads
Volumetric Wear Rates

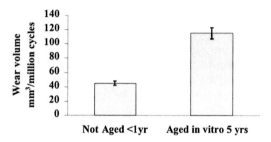

Figure 11 Hip joint simulator wear rates of aged for five years on the shelf and not aged GUR1120 gamma irradiated in air UHMWPE. *Abbreviation*: UHMWPE, ultra high molecular weight polyethylene.

rocking simulator showed similar, if not slightly higher, wear rates. The traditional inverted biaxial rocking simulators which have used higher serum concentrations (90–100%) have produced lower wear rates of 20–30 mm³/ million cycles (37,38). The Boston simulator which uses a high concentration serum lubricant also produced low wear rates for the traditional gamma irradiated UHMWPE (39). These differences are important when comparing data from different groups. There is growing evidence that high serum concentration and higher cycle rate reduce wear in in vitro simulators.

γ-Irradiated in Air, UHMWPE aged 15 yrs In Vivo
Tested in a Hip Joint Simulator, Smooth Femoral
Heads, Volumetric Wear Rates

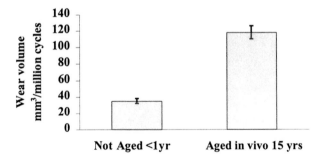

Figure 12 Hip joint simulator wear rates of 15 years old retrieved from patients GUR1120 UHMWPE compared to not aged gamma in air UHMWPE. *Abbreviation*: UHMWPE, ultra high molecular weight polyethylene.

WEAR OF STABILIZED AND CROSS-LINKED POLYETHYLENE IN HIP PROSTHESES

The introduction of stabilized and crosslinked UHMWPE for bearing surfaces in joint replacements which are highly resistant to oxidative degradation is one of the major advances in orthopaedic biomaterials in the last five years. Stabilized materials include UHMWPE sterilized with gas plasma (40,41) or ETO (42). Crosslinked materials include moderately crosslinked materials using 3–5 mrad in an inert atmosphere such as nitrogen or a vacuum (42), medium crosslinked 5 mrad irradiation in a vacuum followed by annealing at 150°C (43), or highly crosslinked UHMWPE 10 mrad gamma irradiation using an electron beam source followed by annealing (or melting) (44).

The use of nonirradiated material reduces the wear rate by a factor greater than 2 compared to the oxidized and aged materials (Fig. 13). Stabilized and crosslinked materials have the potential to reduce the wear further. The wear of moderately crosslinked 4 mrad GVF [gamma vacuum foil compared to ethylene oxide (ETO) sterilized GUR 1020 in the hip joint simulator (45)] showed a 30% reduction in wear rates (Fig. 14). However, against deliberately damaged femoral heads the wear rate of both materials increased markedly and the moderately crosslinked material showed a slightly higher wear rate (45) (Fig. 15). Analysis of the debris for the moderately crosslinked material showed it to be smaller and more biologically active (42,45,46).

Lower wear has been reported by McKellop et al. (43) for medium crosslinked UHMWPE (5 Mrad in a vacuum with 150°C annealing) with an 85% reduction compared to noncrosslinked UHMWPE, and by Muratoglo et al. (44) for highly crosslinked UHMWPE (10 Mrad E Beam and annealed) with a 100% reduction or zero wear compared to nonirradiated UHMWPE. Differences in the reduction in wear reported for various levels of crosslinking are related to conditions of the wear simulations. A recent study from our

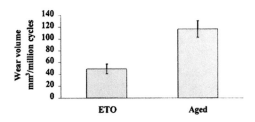

Figure 13 Hip joint simulator wear of ETO sterilized GUR 1020 UHMWPE compared to five years in vitro and 15 years in vivo aged UHMWPE. *Abbreviation*: UHMWPE, ultra high molecular weight polyethylene.

ETO and Cross-Linked UHMWPE
Hip Joint Simulator, Smooth Femoral Heads
Volumetric Wear Rate

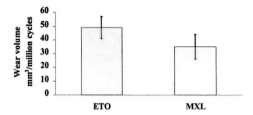

Figure 14 Simulator wear rates for moderately crosslinked and ETO sterilized GUR 1020 UHMWPE on smooth femoral heads. *Abbreviation*: UHMWPE, ultra high molecular weight polyethylene. *Source*: From Ref. 45.

group indicated that the wear reduction due to crosslinking was dependent on serum concentration, kinematics, and counterface conditions. A large reduction in wear was only found with the 10 Mrad highly crosslinked materials for high serum concentrations (90%) and high levels of cross shear in the motion which were similar conditions as those used in other studies (43,44). When serum protein concentrations were reduced to physiological levels as defined by the ISO standard, the reduction in wear found with highly crosslinked material was only 65% compared to the noncrosslinked value and this was lower still for rough counterfaces (<50%). No significant reduction was found when less multidirectional kinematics were used. These findings coupled with the understanding that the highly crosslinked material produced a greater percentage volume of smaller more biologically active particles raise questions about the osteolytic potential in young and active patients and also its application in knees.

ETO and Cross-Linked UHMWPE
Hip Joint Simulator, Scratched Femoral Heads
Volumetric Wear Rates

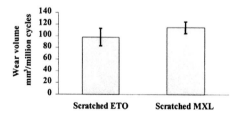

Figure 15 Simulator wear rates for moderately crosslinked and ETO sterilized GUR1020 UHMWPE on scratched femoral heads. *Abbreviation*: UHMWPE, ultra high molecular weight polyethylene. *Source*: From Ref. 45.

WEAR OF CERAMIC–CERAMIC HIPS

Alumina-on-alumina ceramic bearings for hip prostheses have been used in limited numbers for over 20 years and in some centers have shown excellent long-term results (47). During this period the grain size of the ceramic has been reduced, and the quality and fracture toughness of the alumina ceramic has been improved. Hip simulator studies of ceramic-on-ceramic bearings have shown very low wear (48,49) of the order of $0.1\,mm^3/yr$. This may be attributed to enhanced fluid film lubrication (5). Clinical retrieval specimens have low wear of the order of $1\,mm^3/yr$ (50) with a characteristic stripe wear pattern on the head and wear of the superior rim of the cup. It has recently been discovered that this is due to microseparation of the head and cup during the swing phase of walking which produces a small lateral displacement of the head (less than 0.5 mm), which on reapplication of the load at heel strike impacts on the superior rim of the cup before relocating fully in the socket. This microseparation has been simulated in vitro (51) and the wear rate of the alumina-on-alumina bearing has been shown to increase to approximately $1\,mm^3$/million cycles. The wear rates of alumina-on-alumina bearings under standard and microseparation conditions are shown in Figure 16. Even under microseparation conditions the wear rate of alumina on alumina is 40 times less than moderately crosslinked polyethylenes. The microseparation simulation produces clinically relevant wear rates, wear scars, mechanisms and wear debris, which is bimodal in distribution including both nanometer size particles and a smaller number of larger particles up to 1 μm in size associated with grain boundary fracture. The comparative osteolytic potential of crosslinked polyethylene and

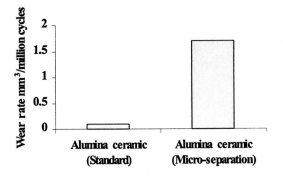

Figure 16 Simulator wear rates for Biolox Forte alumina ceramic-on-ceramic bearings under standard and microseparation conditions.

alumina debris has been determined through a novel model to predict functional biological activity, which integrates wear simulator studies, debris and in vitro cell culture cytokine assays (52). The lower volumes and lower specific biological activity of the ceramic debris combine to produce a 100-fold reduction in functional biological activity and osteolytic potential compared to moderately crosslinked polyethylene (53).

WEAR OF METAL–METAL HIPS

Cobalt–chrome metal-on-metal hips have also been used for over 30 years in limited numbers (54). The McKee Farrar hip reduced in popularity following problems with fixation and design and manufacturing variability which led to equatorial contact of the bearings, high friction and wear. The concerns about polyethylene wear debris-induced osteolysis led to the re-emergence of the metal-on-metal hip in the 1990s (55). Clinical wear rates of about $1 \, mm^3/yr$ have been recorded (57), but as with ceramic-on-ceramic bearings these have not always been replicated in vitro. It has been shown that wear is highly dependent on the serum concentration with high serum concentrations reducing wear to very low levels. Studies by Chan (58) also showed low wear rates ($0.1 \, mm^3/$million cycles) in high serum concentration. These studies also showed that fluid film lubrication had a role in reducing wear and that wear was increased by stop start motion. Wear has also been shown to be dependent on simulator kinematics (24) with more eccentric wear paths increasing wear. In terms of prosthesis design, increase in head size has also been shown to reduce wear (59), this reduction being attributed to improved lubrication. Similarly the use of high carbon on low carbon bearings reduced wear compared to low carbon alloy couples (60). The wear of cobalt–chrome metal on metal has been shown to be substantially less than moderately crosslinked polyethylene (Fig. 17). However, there remains some concern about the ion release from metal wear debris (61). The metal-on-metal wear debris is very small (30 nm) providing a large surface area for ion release (23,24,60). These very small particles have been shown to have a cytotoxic effect at high concentrations in vitro (62) and there remain some concerns about other adverse cellular reactions. However, large numbers of metal-on-metal hip prostheses, over 100,000, have been implanted in the last 10 years and at present they offer real potential as an osteolysis free bearing solution for young patients.

WEAR OF POLYETHYLENE IN KNEE PROSTHESES

In artificial knee prostheses, the primary bearing surface couple has been UHMWPE articulating on polished cobalt–chrome alloy metallic femoral components. The traditional wear and failure mode has been oxidative degradation followed by delamination fatigue failure (Fig. 6) (10). The

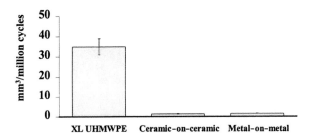

Metal-on-Metal Compared to Ceramic-on-Ceramic and XL UHMWPE Volumetric Wear Rate

Figure 17 Simulator wear rates of cobalt–chrome metal-on-metal hips compared to moderately crosslinked UHMWPE. *Abbreviation*: UHMWPE, ultra high molecular weight polyethylene.

introduction of stabilized (oxidation resistant) UHMWPE should reduce the incidence of this type of failure in currently manufactured and implanted devices. There is, of course, a clinical legacy of gamma irradiated in air bearings which have been historically implanted in patients, and will continue to oxidize and degrade in vivo.

The use of stabilized UHMWPE and the demand for knee prostheses in younger, more active patients means that attention is now focused on surface wear and the generation of micrometer and submicrometer size wear particles that can lead to osteolysis (63). Four key factors can influence the amount of surface wear of UHMWPE in the knee (64). Patient weight and activity (sliding distance) directly influence wear volume ("Basic Laws of Wear and Factors that Influence Wear Rates" Section) (19). Damage or scratching to the femoral counterface can also increase wear ("Basic Laws of Wear and Factors that Influence Wear Rates" Section). Both of these have a similar effect to that found in the hip. Additionally, in the knee the patient kinematics and motions at the knee prostheses markedly influence knee wear, as does the actual design of the knee itself.

It has been shown that an increase in the internal–external rotation from ± 2.5 to ± 5° and an increase in the anterior–posterior displacement from 4.5 to 9 mm can increase the volumetric wear of a fixed bearing knee by a factor of five. The increase in rotation and translation produces additional cross shear in strain orient UHMWPE increasing wear rate (14,65) (Fig. 18). A mobile bearing (rotating platform) design has the potential to address this by decoupling the rotation motion to a second tibial interface, producing more linear kinematics at the femoral articulation, hence reducing wear (Fig. 19) (66). These studies which have considerable impact for

Fixed Bearing Knee PFC Sigma
Gamma Irradiated in a Vacuum and Foil Packed
Low and High Kinematics

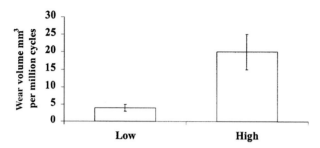

Figure 18   Simulator wear rates of cobalt–chrome metal-on-metal hips compared to moderately crosslinked UHMWPE. *Abbreviation*: UHMWPE, ultra high molecular weight polyethylene.

knee replacements in young active patients are described more fully in the literature (64–67).

FUTURE PERSPECTIVES—BEARING SURFACES AND REDUCTION IN WEAR

There is a continual need for further reduction in the wear and the biological responses to wear debris. This is being driven by the increase in joint replacements in younger patients, increased lifetimes, improved quality of life, and increase in the expectation of patients with prostheses. It is now recognized that the patient's response to wear debris is heterogenous, and the genetic predisposition of certain sections of the population can make them particularly susceptible to adverse biological reactions to different types of wear debris (2).

In the hip, the long-term osteolytic potential of highly crosslinked UHMWPE will be determined through clinical studies. For younger, more active patients, advances in ceramic-on-ceramic bearings with the introduction of zirconia toughened alumina (a ceramic matrix composite) which has improved toughness and wear resistance offer greater design flexibility and reduction in the incidence of fracture (67). Advances in metal-on-metal hips may also be achieved through the application of thick ceramic-like surface coatings which have the potential to reduce wear rates and metal ion release by a factor of 50 or more (68). These particular arc evaporated physical vapor deposition coatings have shown good durability to five million cycles. Longer term durability studies are underway.

In the knee, the introduction of the crosslinked UHMWPE may give a further reduction in wear, but care must be taken as there is potential for

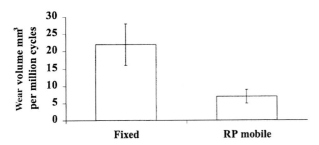

Figure 19 Comparison of the wear rate of a fixed bearing knee with a rotating platform mobile bearing knee in a knee joint simulator.

fracture and fatigue in less tough materials. The introduction of ceramic or ceramic-coated femoral components may lead to some reductions in UHMWPE wear particularly in the presence of third body damage. Understanding the relationships between design, kinematics, and wear may well give advantages both in terms of function and osteolytic potential in the knee.

Improvements may not only come from material and prosthetic design. Lubricants can reduce wear (21) and the potential for therapeutic lubrication has still to be investigated in joint replacements. Equally, understanding the patient-specific susceptibility to adverse reactions to wear debris could lead to further development of pharmaceutical therapies to address the osteolytic potential of different types of joint replacements.

All advances in wear reduction and bearing surface technologies have to be proven clinically. The predicted lifetimes of many of the new bearing surfaces are well beyond 20 years, and the time constants for clinical evaluations need to be extended to similar time periods. This will necessarily slow down the introduction of new biomaterial technologies for further reduction in wear. Considerations relating to other design variables, cost and individual patient specific requirements and responses are likely to play an increasing role in the selection of bearing surfaces in the future.

REFERENCES

1. Willert HG, Semlitsch M. Reactions of the articular capsule to wear products of artificial joint prostheses. J Med Mater Res 1977; 11:157–164.
2. Ingham E, Fisher J. Biological reactions to wear debris in total joint replacement. Proc Inst Mech Eng 1999; 214H:21–37.

3. Dowson D, Fisher J, Jin ZM, Auger DD, Jobbins B. Design considerations for cushion form bearings for artificial hip joints. Proc Inst Mech Eng 1991; 205H:59–68.

4. Godet M. Third bodies in tribology. Wear 1990; 136:29–45.

5. Jin ZM, Dowson D, Fisher J. Analysis of fluid film lubrication in artificial hip joint replacements with surfaces of high elastic modulus. Proc Inst Mech Eng 1997; 211H:247–256.

6. Chan FW, Bobyn JD, Medley JB. Engineering issues and wear performance of metal on metal hip implants. Clin Orthop 1996; 333:96–107.

7. Fisher J, Dowson D. Tribology of artificial joints. Proc Inst Mech Eng 1991; 205H:73–79.

8. Lancaster JG, Dowson D, Issac GH, Fisher J. The wear of UHMWPE sliding on metallic and ceramic counterfaces representative of current femoral surfaces in joint replacement. Proc Inst Mech Eng 1997; 211H:17–24.

9. McNie CM, Barton DC, Ingham E, Tipper JL, Fisher J, Stone MH. The prediction of polyethylene wear rate and debris morphology produced by microscopic asperities on femoral heads. Mater Sci Mater Med 2000; 11:163–174.

10. Fisher J. Wear of ultra high molecular weight polyethylene in total artificial joints. Cur Orthop 1994; 8:164–169.

11. Firkins PJ, Tipper JL, Saadatzadeh MR, Ingham E, Stone MH, Farrar R, Fisher J. Quantitative analysis of wear and wear debris from metal-on-metal hip prostheses tested in a physiological hip joint simulator. Bio-Med Mater Eng 2001; 11:143–157.

12. Nevelos J, Ingham E, Doyle C, Streicher R, Nevelos A, Walter W, Fisher J. Microseparation of the centers of alumina–alumna artificial hip joints during simulator testing produces clinically relevant wear and patterns. J Arthroplasty 2000; 15:793–795.

13. Cooper JR, Dowson D, Fisher J, Isaac GH, Wroblewski BM. Observations of residual sub-surface shear strain in ultra high molecular weight polyethylene acetabular cups. J Mater Sci Mater Med 1994; 5:52–57.

14. Wang A, Sun DC, Yau S-S, Edwards B, Stark C, Dumbleton JH. Orientation softening in the deformation and wear of UHMWPE. Wear 1997; 203:230–241.

15. Marrs H, Barton DC, Jones RA, Ward IM, Fisher J. Comparative wear under four different tribological conditions of acetylene enhanced crosslmked ultra high molecular weight polyethylene. J Mater Sci Mater Med 1999; 10:333–342.

16. Campbell P, Ma S, Yeom B, Schmalzried P, Amstutz HC. Isolation of predominantly submicron-sized UHMWPE wear particles from periprosthetic tissues. J Biomed Mater Res 1995; 29:127–131.

17. Tipper JL, Ingham E, Hailey JL, Besong AA, Fisher J, Wroblewski BM, Stone MH. Quantitative analysis of polyethylene wear debris, wear rate and head damage in retrieved Chamley hip prostheses. J Mater Sci Mater Med 2000; 11:117–124.

18. Jones SMG. Polyethylene wear in uncemented knee-placements. J Bone Joint Surg 1992; 74B:18–22.

19. Barbour PSM, Barton DC, Fisher J. The influence of contact stress on the wear of UHMWPE for total replacement hip prostheses. Wear 1995; 181:250–257.

20. Fisher J, Firkins P, Reeves EA, Hailey JL, Isaac GH. The influence of scratches to metallic counterfaces on the wear of ultra-high molecular weight polyethylene. Part H, Proc Inst Mech Eng 1995; 209H:263–264.

21. Bell J, Tipper JL, Ingham E, Stone MH, Fisher J. The influence of phospholipid concentration in protein-containing lubricants on the wear of ultra-high molecular weight polyethylene in artificial hip joints. Proc Inst Mech Eng 2001; 215H:259–263.

22. Besong AA, Tipper JL, Stone MH, Ingham E, Fisher J. The influence of joint kinematics on the number and morphology of polyethylene wear particles in models of hip and knee prostheses. Trans IMechE Conf Knee Replace 1999:70–73.

23. Tipper JL, Firkins PJ, Ingham E, Stone MH, Farrar R, Fisher J. Quantitative analysis of the wear and wear debris from low and high carbon content cobalt chrome alloys used in metal on metal total hip replacements. J Mater Sci Mater Med 1999; 10:355–362.

24. Firkins PJ, Tipper JL, Ingham E, Stone MH, Farrar R, Fisher J. Influence of simulator kinematics on the wear of metal-on-metal hip prostheses. Proc Inst Mech Eng 2001; 215H:119–121.

25. Nevelos JE, Ingham E, Doyle C, Nevelos AB, Fisher J. The influence of acetabular cup angle on the wear of "BIOLOX Forte" alumina ceramic bearing couples in a hip joint simulator. J Mater Sci Mater Med 2001; 12:141–144.

26. Livermore J, Duane I, Murray B. Effect of femoral head size on the wear of the polyethylene acetabular component. J Bone Joint Surg 1990; 72-A:518–528.

27. Endo MM, Barbour PSM, Barton DC, Wroblewslci BM, Fisher J, Tipper JL, Ingham E, Stone MH. A comparison of the wear and debris generation of GUR 1120 (compression moulded) and GUR 4150HP (ram extruded) ultra high molecular weight polyethylene. Bio-Med Mater Eng 1999; 9:113–124.

28. Barbour PSM, Stone MH, Fisher J. A study of the wear resistance of three types of clinically applied UHMWPE for total replacement hip prostheses. Biomaterials 1999; 20:2101–2106.

29. Fisher J, Chan KL, Hailey JL, Shaw D, Stone MH. Preliminary study of the effect of ageing following irradiation on the wear of ultrahigh-molecular-weight polyethylene. J Arthroplasty 1995; 10:689–692.

30. Barbour PSM, Stone MH, Fisher J. A hip joint simulator study using simplified loading and motion cycles generating physiological wear paths and rates. Proc Inst Mech Eng 1999; 214H:455–467.

31. Barbour PSM, Stone MH, Fisher J. A hip joint simulator study using new and physiologically scratched femoral heads with ultra-high molecular weight polyethylene acetabular cups. Proc Inst Mech Eng 2000; 214H:569–576.

32. Minakawa H, Stone MH, Wroblewski BM, Lancaster JG, Ingham E, Fisher J. Quantification of third-body damage and its effect on UHMWPE wear with different types of femoral head. J Bone Joint Surg 1998; 80-B:894–899.

33. Besong AA, Tipper JL, Ingham E, Stone MH, Wroblewski BM, Fisher J. Quantitative comparison of wear debris from UHMWPE that has and has not been sterilised by gamma irradiation. J Bone Joint Surg 1998; 80B:340–344.

34. Hardaker C., Isaac GH, Fisher J. Influence of in vivo and in vitro ageing on wear of polyethylene. Proc Eur Soc Biomater 2001.

35. Smith SL, Unsworth A. Wear of UHMWPE acetabular cups sliding against CoCr Mo femoral heads in a hip joint simulator. Proc Inst Mech Eng 1999; 213H:475–485.
36. Wang A, Stark C, Dumbleton JH. Mechanistic and morphological origins of UHMWPE wear. Proc Inst Mech Eng, 1996; 210H:141–155.
37. McKellop HA, Campbell P, Park SH. The origin of submicron wear in total hip arthroplasty. Clin Orthop 1995; 311:3–20.
38. Clarke IC, Gustafson A. Clinical and hip simulator comparisons of ceramic on polyethylene and metal on polyethylene wear. Clin Orthop 2000; 379:34–40.
39. Bragdon CR, O'Connor DO, Jasty M. The importance of multidirectional motion on wear of polyethylene. Proc Inst Mech Eng 1996; 210H:157–160.
40. Fisher J, Reeves EA, Issac GH. Comparison of the wear of aged and non-aged UHMWPE sterilised by gamma irradiation and gas plasma. J Mater Sci Mater Med 1997; 8:375–378.
41. Reeves EA, Barton DC, FitzPatrick D, Fisher J. Comparison of gas plasma and gamma irradiation in air sterilization on the delamination wear of the ultra-high molecular weight polyethylene used in knee replacements. Proc Inst Mech Eng 2000; 214H:249–255.
42. Endo MM, Barbour PSM, Barton DC, Fisher J, Tipper JL, Ingham E, Stone MH. Comparative wear and wear debris under three different counter-face conditions of crosslinked and non-crosslinked ultra high molecular weight polyethylene. Bio-Med Mater Eng 2001; 11:23–35.
43. McKellop H, Shen F, Lu B, Campbell P, Salovey R. Development of an extremely wear resistant UHMWPE. J Orthop Res 1997; 17:157–167.
44. Muratoglu OK, Bragdon CR, O'Connor DO, Jasty M, Harris WH. A novel method to crosslink UHMWPE to improve wear. J Arthroplasty 2001; 16:149–160.
45. Endo HM, Barton DC, Fisher J, Tipper JL, Ingham E, Stone MH. Wear of crosslinked and non-crosslinked polyethylene. Proc Inst Mech Eng Part H. 2002; 216:111–122.
46. Scott M, Widding KE, Ries M, Shanbhag A. Wear particle analysis of conventional and crosslinked UHMWPE. Trans 47th Orthop Res Soc 01, 2001.
47. Sedel L. Evolution of alumina alumina implants. Clin Orthop 2000; 379:48–54.
48. Clarke IC, Good V, Williams P, Schroeder H, Oonishi M. Ultra low wear rates with rigid on rigid bearings. Proc Inst Mech Eng 2000; 214H:221–347.
49. Nevelos JE, Ingham E, Doyle C, Nevelos AB, Fisher J. The influence of acetabular cup angle on the wear of "BIOLOX Forte" alumina ceramic bearing couples in a hip joint simulator. J Mater Sci Mater Med 2001; 12:141–144.
50. Nevelos JE, Ingham E, Doyle C, Nevelos AB, Fisher J. Analysis of retrieved alumina ceramic components for Mittelmeier total hip prostheses. Biomaterials 1999; 20:1833–1840.
51. Nevelos J, Ingham E, Doyle C, Streicher R, Nevelos A, Walter W, Fisher J. Microseparation of the centers of alumina-alumna artificial hip joints during simulator testing produces clinically relevant wear and patterns. J Arthroplasty 2000; 15:793–795.

52. Fisher J, Bell J, Barbour PSM, Tipper JL, Matthews JB, Besong AA, Stone MH, Ingham E. A novel method for the prediction of functional biological activity of polyethylene wear debris. Proc Inst Mech Eng 2001; 215H:127–132.
53. Fisher J. New bearing materials with improved functional biocompatibility. The way forward. Joint replacement—Once is forever? Proc Royal Acad Eng 2001.
54. Amstutz H, Grigoris P. Metal on metal bearings in hip arthroplasty. Clin Orthop 1996; 329:11–34.
55. Wagner M, Wagner H. Medium term results with modern metal on metal system. Clin Orthop 2000; 379:123–133.
56. Rieker C, Konrad R, Schon R. In vitro comparison of two hard on hard articulations. Proc Inst Mech Eng 2001; 215H:153–160.
57. Medley JB, Chan F, Kryger J, Bobyn JD. Comparison of alloys and designs of metal metal implants. Clin Orthop 1996; 3291:148–159.
58. Chan FW, Bobyn JD, Medley JB, Kryger J, Tanzer W. Wear and lubrication of metal on metal hips. Clin Orthop 1999; 369:10–24.
59. Smith SL, Dowson D, Goldsmith A. The effect of femoral head diameter upon lubrication and wear of metal on metal hip replacement. Proc Inst Mech Eng 2001; 215H:161–170.
60. Firkins PJ, Tipper JL, Saadatzadeh MR, Ingham E, Stone MH, Farrar R, Fisher J. Quantitative analysis of wear and wear debris from metal-on-metal hip prostheses tested in a physiological hip joint simulator. Bio-Med Mater Eng 2001; 11:143–157.
61. Hallab N, Merritt K, Jacobs J. Metal sensitivity in patients with orthopaedic implants. J Bone Joint Surg 2001; 83A:428–436.
62. Germain MA, Matthews JB, Stone MH, Fisher J, Ingham E. The effect of clinically relevant wear particles on viability of cells in vitro. Proc Eur Soc Biomater 2001; T76.
63. Howling GI, Barnett PI, Tipper JL, Stone MH, Fisher J, Ingham E. Quantitative characterisation of polyethylene debris isolated from periprosthetic tissue in early failure knee implants and early and late failure Charnley hip implants. J Biomed Mater Res Appl Biomater 2001; 58:415–420.
64. Fisher J. Wear of polyethylene in total knee replacements. Curr Orthop. 2001; 15:399–405.
65. Barnett PI, Auger DD, Ingham E, Stone MH, Fisher J. Influence of kinematics of wear of polyethylene. J Mater Sci Mater Med. 2001; 12:1039–1042.
66. McEwen H, Auger DD, Fisher J. Reduction in polyethylene wear by rotating platform mobile bearing knees. J Mater Sci Mater Med. 2001; 12:1049–1052.
67. Stewart TD, Streicher RM, Fisher J. Long term wear of alumina on alumina hip prostheses under microseparation conditions. J Mater Sci Mater Med. 2001; 12:1053–1056.
68. Fisher J. Wear of surface engineered metal-on-metal hip prostheses. J Mater Sci Mater, Med 2004; 15:225–235.

9

Human Motion and Its Relevance to Wear and Failure in Total Knee Arthroplasty

Markus A. Wimmer

Department of Orthopaedic Surgery, Rush University Medical Center, Chicago, Illinois, U.S.A.

Thomas P. Andriacchi

Department of Mechanical Engineering, Biomechanical Engineering, Stanford University, Palo Alto, California, U.S.A.

INTRODUCTION

The natural human knee is a complex and heavily loaded joint. The articulation must transmit large forces while allowing significant motion at the same time. Typically, the knee undergoes a six-degree-of-freedom movement including both rolling and sliding (1). For functional reasons, freedom of movement and stability are important characteristics for the artificial knee joint as well. Technically, the latter are demanding requirements because of mixed kinematics and the high stresses placed on the articulation (2). As a result, wear and fatigue of the tibial polyethylene bearing are common failure criteria.

Based on 30,000 artificial knees implanted between 1976 and 1992, the Swedish Knee Arthroplasty Register (3,4) reported a continuous improvement in prosthetic knee survival with a steady decline in complications. These promising observations have been reflected in the annual growth in the number of primary knee surgeries, which have already outnumbered the primary hip operations in the United States (5).[a] Nevertheless, revisions have been increasing at the same rate as primary surgeries, and demonstrate the problem of limited durability of total knee arthroplasty (TKA). While better patient selection and better surgical technique have helped to reduce early complications (3), the application of joint replacement to younger and more active people plus the general increase in life expectancy make wear and the consequences of wear the leading cause of failure in TKA (6). New material developments with higher wear resistance are therefore a priority research area. These new materials need to be accurately tested close to the physiological situation.

THE SYSTEM APPROACH OF TRIBOLOGY

While the mechanical properties of engineering materials can be described in terms of yield strength, Young's modulus, fracture toughness, etc., friction and wear are not intrinsic material properties but are characteristics of the system (7). The structure of such a tribological system consists of four principal elements: solid body, counterbody, interfacial medium, and environment (8). The "operating variables" are the input to the system, while the output can be defined as loss of energy and material (Fig. 1).

Because of the complex nature of friction and wear, the problems of tribology are difficult to assess by a simple model. In order to follow the system theory of Figure 1, it would be necessary to analyze the wear affected specimens under real conditions, i.e., implanted into the patient under defined operating conditions. Of course, for ethical reasons this is impossible and would be very time consuming and expensive. Therefore, a step-by-step analysis, where the models of wear approximate reality more and more, is probably the best approach one can take (9,10). Figure 2 describes different types of tribological testing.

A successful wear testing apparatus should reflect the structure of the tribosystem and the type of dynamic interaction between its elements. It should be considered that the proper modeling of the input parameters, e.g., loading and motion of the joint, may determine the acting wear mechanism. In fact, different material or design modifications may be appropriate depending on the acting wear mechanism (11). Fischer (12) stresses the importance of knowledge of the acting wear mechanisms,[b] since it is known

---

[a] Currently, 400,000 joint replacements are performed yearly in the United States alone, and this number is projected to increase to three-quarters of a million Americans a year by 2030. (Wright TM. Total joint replacement in the new millennium, 6th World Biomaterials Congress, Hawaii, 2000.)

[b] There are four basic mechanisms of wear: adhesion, abrasion, surface fatigue, and tribochemical reaction. See Appendix A for details. The wear mode is not a steady state condition and may transform from one to another.

Operating Variables

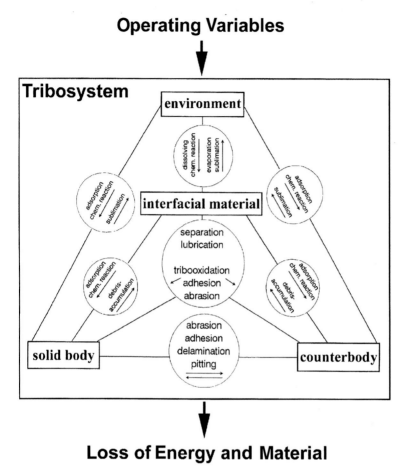

Loss of Energy and Material

Figure 1 General description of the tribosystem which consists of four principal elements: the two bodies in contact, the interfacial material, and the surrounding media. All these elements can affect each other and change the mechanism of inter-action. For example, interfacial material can scratch the counterbody in a way that the adhesive interaction between solid and counterbody is turned into abrasion. *Source*: Modified from Ref. 8.

that even for the same wear mode[c] different design or material modifications are appropriate. For example, the parameters of the wear mode "rolling abrasion" of a metal-on-metal bearing can be changed in such a way that either the mechanisms "adhesion" (mostly plastic interaction) or "surface fatigue" (mostly elastic interaction) apply. Thus, a successful plan to improve the bulk

---

[c] The general mechanical condition under which the system is functioning, when wear occurs. For example, a distinction can be made between sliding, rolling, impact, etc., wear.

Classification

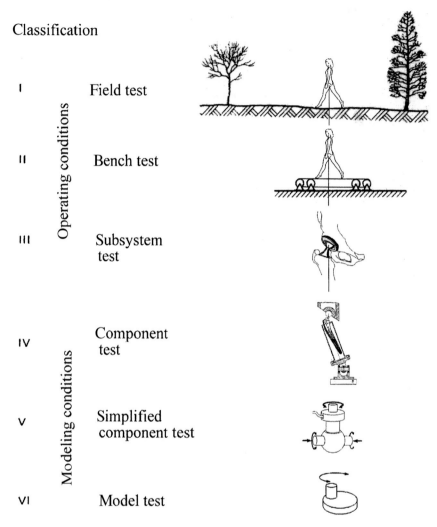

I	Field test	
II	Bench test	
III	Subsystem test	
IV	Component test	
V	Simplified component test	
VI	Model test	

Operating conditions (I–III)

Modeling conditions (IV–VI)

Figure 2 Classification of different types of tribological testing. *Source*: Adapted from Ref. 9.

characteristics of the materials in contact demands an exact understanding of the structure of the tribosystem, which requires information about the prostheses design, joint kinematics, and kinetics in the physiological situation.

EVOLUTION OF KNEE PROSTHESIS DESIGN

The original total knee arthroplasties were of hinged design and had a metal-on-metal articulation. They were used with reasonable clinical outcome for nearly two decades starting in 1960 (13). By then, experience indicated that such systems exhibited several problems, including implant loosening, stem breakage, progressive metal wear, and infection. Primarily, the difficulties occurring were associated with the uniaxial mechanics of the hinges, interfering with the multiaxial biomechanics of the joint, in other words, a rigidly hinged joint does not account for reasonable simulation of normal knee motion, in particular rotation. This causes inadequate stresses on all portions of the components, and fracture or loosening occurs with time.

When Gunston (14) described the first polycentric knee design to overcome these problems, efforts were also made to develop a prosthesis which relied purely on the natural, ligamentous constraints of the knee. In 1973, Coventry et al. (15) reported on the first two-component total knee arthroplasty, the "Geometric" prosthesis. It consisted of two metal femoral condyles and a tibial polyethylene plateau, attached directly to the bone by means of bone cement. Mechanical stability was provided by the ligaments (including the anterior cruciate ligament) and the surrounding soft tissue. Although the prosthesis was bicondylar, no attempt was made to duplicate the anatomy of the knee joint. A metal-on-polyethylene concept was chosen to tackle the problem of wear. While the early results were promising, poor instrumentation and failure to restore normal knee kinematics complicated the procedure leading to problems in the long term. Finally, in the mid-1970s the "Total Condylar" prosthesis became available (16). In contrast to the Geometric design the femoral condyles were shaped anatomically with different radii in the distal and posterior portion of the implant. The long term survivorship of this artificial joint was quite reasonable with a revision rate of less than 5% at 10 years (3).

Nowadays, many TKA designs consist of three components: a bicondylar metal part for the femoral surface, an ultra high molecular weight polyethylene (UHMWPE) insert for the tibial plateau, and again a polyethylene component to resurface the patella (Fig. 3). Many variations on this basic design have been developed, including the addition of metal backing and the modularity of polyethylene components. Parallel to the evolution of prosthetic design, an understanding of appropriate patient selection criteria, the importance of preoperative planning for surgery and operative technique have been developed (13). One of the key issues for further progress is to obey the rules of functional knee biomechanics.

FUNCTIONAL KNEE JOINT KINEMATICS AND KINETICS

Kinematics During Flexion and Extension of the Knee

The relative motion at the knee joint can be described by three translations and three rotations which constitute six degrees of freedom at the joint. The relative flexion–extension angle between the femur and tibia has been measured during human locomotion and found to be highly reproducible intraindividually (17). At heel strike the knee is almost fully extended.

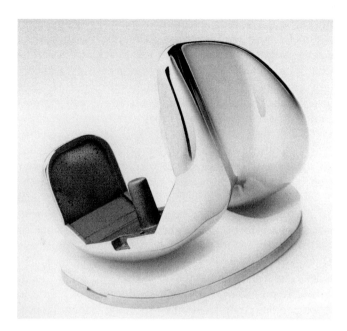

Figure 3 Total knee system showing the tibio-femoral bearing. The focus of this chapter is exclusively on this articulation.

It begins to flex, reaching a maximum of about 15–20° during midstance. At this point the direction of the angular progression reverses and the knee fully extends again (50% of gait cycle). The joint reverses direction once more to start the preswing phase until toe-off occurs at approximately 63% of the gait cycle (Fig. 4). Lafortune et al. (18) demonstrated that substantial angular and linear motions occur about all six degrees of freedom of the joint during walking. The complex motion pattern was studied using target markers that were fixed to the tibia and femur by means of intracortical traction pins.

Flexion of the knee progresses as a combination of rolling, sliding, and spin of the femoral condyles over the tibial plateau (1). Experiments demonstrating this mechanism were performed as early as 1836 by the Weber brothers (19). They evaluated the relative motion between the femoral condyles and the tibial surface by placing markers on the corresponding points of contact on both surfaces. Nearly a hundred years later it was demonstrated that the ratio of rolling to sliding varies during flexion and extension (20). One of the models to explain the mechanism is the crossed-four-bar linkage considered by Müller (21) and O'Connor (22,23). In this model, the insertions of both cruciate ligaments are rigidly attached to the femur and the tibia. They are represented by two crossed bars, which are not linked but held fixed firmly at their anatomical points of insertion (Fig. 5). During flexion and extension the linkage guides the motion of

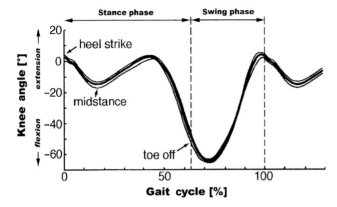

Figure 4 Flexion–extension angle at the knee during the gait cycle. The heavy line represents the mean of a single subject during several trials. The thin lines indicate the standard deviation.

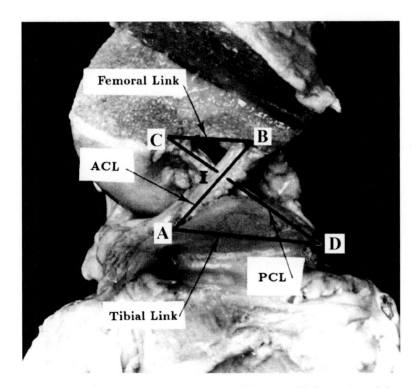

Figure 5 Section through a human knee with the medial femoral condyle removed exposing the cruciate ligaments and with the cruciate linkage ABCD superposed. *Source*: From Ref. 27a.

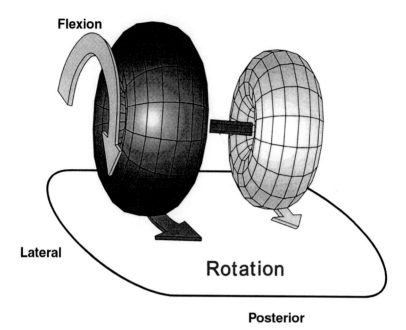

Figure 6   Knee flexion causes femoral rollback and rotation due to the bigger lateral condyle.

the knee and results in a slide-roll ratio of approximately 2:1 during the early stages of flexion, and 4:1 during late flexion (21).

Cadaver experiments have demonstrated that both the geometry of the joint surfaces and the soft tissue constraints determine the kinematic behavior of the knee (24). The rolling motion predominates early in flexion (0–20°), while sliding becomes dominant at flexion angles beyond 30°. As the knee is rolling on a larger curvature laterally than medially it moves a greater distance on the lateral plateau as compared to the medial plateau (25). As a result, during rollback, the femur not only moves posteriorly, but also rotates externally during flexion (Fig. 6). The so-called "screw-home" movement is the reverse situation and gives additional stability to the knee: "more, than would be possible if the tibiofemoral joint would be a simple hinge joint" (26).

More recent experiments, however, have shown that the particular kinematic behavior of the knee can be derived from observations during functional activity only. Using the so-called point cluster technique [a motion analysis method described in Ref. (27)], Andriacchi et al. (28,29) demonstrated that relative knee motion is dependent on activity rather than on knee flexion angle. As shown in Figure 7, the femur rotates externally during squatting but rotates internally during stair climbing with increasing knee flexion. This points to the fact that the natural knee cannot be regarded as

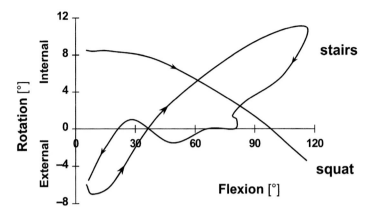

Figure 7   The femur rotates externally during squatting but rotates internally during stair climbing with increasing knee flexion.

a stiff mechanical linkage, but rather as a very flexible connection between femur and tibia, optimized for all the various activities of daily life.

The cruciate ligaments interact kinematically with the articulating surfaces (30,31). Along the orientation of their constituent fibers they are able to resist tensile forces in the anterior or posterior directions and play a role together with the collateral ligaments in restraining varus/valgus loading. The anterior cruciate ligament (ACL) usually has to be sacrificed in order to open the knee joint sufficiently and implant a total prosthesis. One of the controversies, however, is the retention or removal of the posterior cruciate ligament (PCL). An elevated cam or post, positioned between the medial and lateral bearing portion of the tibial component, restricts femoral glide off in the case of PCL removal. Moilanen and Freeman (32) argue that retention of the PCL makes the operation more complex because "balancing" the PCL often results in a PCL which is too slack or too tight, causing a decreased range of motion. If these altered movements are incompatible with the shape of the articular surfaces, constraint forces will be generated. On the other hand, a properly tightened PCL will guide the knee during femoral rollback (2). This femoral rollback has an important mechanical implication which will be discussed in more detail in the next section.

Dynamics of the Knee

As the femur moves posteriorly during femoral rollback, the distance from the points of contact of the femur on the tibia to the line of action of the quadriceps mechanism increases (25). This increase of the lever arm is substantial for the efficiency of the extensor muscles (Fig. 8A) and is reflected in TKA. It has been reported that patients from whom the PCL

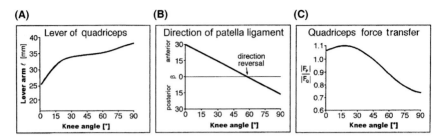

Figure 8 The three factors that influence the mechanical efficiency of the quadriceps with changing knee flexion: (**A**) Change of the lever-arm 1 of the quadriceps with knee flexion; (**B**) Change in the direction of the patellar ligament with knee flexion; (**C**) Change in the force transfer of quadriceps tendon F_Q and patellar ligament F_p. *Source*: From Refs. 25, 35, 37, 38.

was removed showed abnormal functional adaptations and had significantly more problems climbing stairs than those who had retained the PCL (33,34).

The orientation of the patellar ligament is another factor that influences the efficiency of the quadriceps mechanism. At full extension this ligament is angled between 22 and 30° anteriorly. As the knee flexes to about 60° the ligament is nearly vertical, and later in flexion it is angled posteriorly (Fig. 8B) (35,36). In addition to a third factor, namely, the transfer of quadriceps force from the quadriceps tendon over the patella to the patellar ligament (Fig. 8C) (37); those observations explain the varying efficiency of the extensor mechanism with flexion. It is greatest between 15 and 25° of knee flexion and declines rapidly beyond 30° (38). If the lever arm of this system is reduced, more quadriceps force will be needed to balance the external forces and moments at the knee joint. This may cause higher loading of the knee joint with potential functional problems during daily activity and increased risk of tibial component wear (39). Ground reaction forces, arising during human locomotion, impose external forces and external moments at the knee joint that must be balanced by a set of internal forces (Fig. 9). These internal forces consist of forces generated by muscles, bone-to-bone contact forces, and forces of soft tissues constraints. Of all these structures, the muscles are in the best position to resist the external moments, because they have sufficient lever arms, defined from their lines of action to the point of contact at the joint.

The external moment patterns during the stance and swing phases of gait are shown in Figure 10. Typically, at heel strike, there is an external flexion–extension moment tending to extend the knee joint. In order to balance this moment internally, the flexor muscles have to become active. As the knee moves into midstance, the external moment reverses direction, demanding the action of the extensor muscles. The external moment reverses

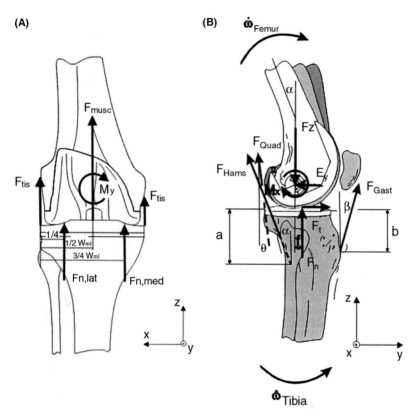

Figure 9 Frontal (**A**) and sagittal (**B**) view of the proximal portion of the tibia and the distal part of the femur with attached total knee prosthesis. Muscle groups (F_{Quad}, F_{Hams}, F_{Gast}), soft tissue structures (F_{Tis}), and contact forces (F_n, F_t) crossing the joint are represented by force vectors. Here, the external forces (F_z, F_y) and moments (M_x, M_y) are shown acting about the center of curvature of the femoral condyles. The internal (muscle, soft tissue, contact) forces balance the imposed external forces and moments.

direction again during late midstance, activating the flexor muscles. Finally, at toe-off the extensors have to become active once more (40).

The muscular activity pattern during normal gait can be obtained using electromyography (EMG). EMG signals, however, give no direct access to the muscle force generated or the moment produced (41–43). EMG can be used, however, to determine which muscle is active and to what extent. The electromyographic activity of the flexor and extensor group during level walking is shown above the flexion–extension moment graph (Fig. 10). The activity pattern follows complex rules: The extensor muscles are active although there is an external extending moment and the flexor muscles work despite the occurrence of an external flexing moment. This phenomenon is

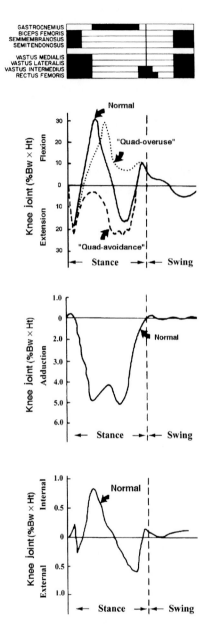

Figure 10 The moments at the knee joint during level walking along with myoelectric activity of various muscle groups. The flexion–extension moment, abduction–adduction moment, and internal–external moment act in the sagittal, frontal, and transverse plane, respectively. All moments are normalized to body weight × height. Note the occurrence of abnormal flexion–extension patterns, which are frequently observed in patients having a total knee replacement.

referred to as antagonistic muscle activity and increases the stability of the joint (44).

During walking the associated adduction moment (Fig. 10) produces an asymmetric load distribution in the frontal joint plane and forces the knee into varus. This can be related to the vector of the ground reaction force which typically passes the knee medially. The collateral ligaments help to balance the loads between the medial and lateral condyles of the knee. Proper tensioning of the lateral collateral ligament is therefore absolutely critical to prevent lift-off of the lateral condyle in TKA (45). Also the risk of leaving the knee in residual varus is evident: Residual varus results in increased adducting moments and, thus, higher medial compartment loads leading to subsequent failure of the implant (2).

The flexion–extension moments measured during gait can only be interpreted in terms of "net quadriceps" and "net flexor" demand (Fig. 11), while EMG is a valuable tool in defining whether the muscle is "on" or "off"; e.g., from the activity pattern of Figure 12 it can be deduced that at heel strike it is primarily the muscles of the hamstring group which are active to balance the extension moment, while during midstance the extension moment is accommodated by the medial and lateral gastrocnemius. The capability of muscles for synergistic activity (several muscles providing the same biomechanical function) and the presence of antagonistic muscle activity during human locomotion make the analysis of the effective load on the joint complex.

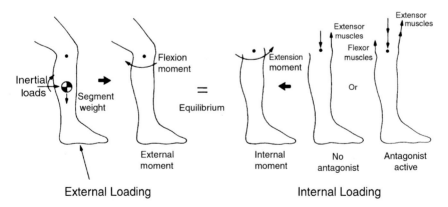

Figure 11 External loading of the knee has to be in equilibrium with internal loading. For example, the ground reaction force plus the inertia of the limb segments may produce a moment tending to flex the knee. In order to balance this external moment a moment of equal magnitude and opposite direction has to be produced by internal structures. This "net moment" can be generated either with or without antagonists. *Source*: From Ref. 47.

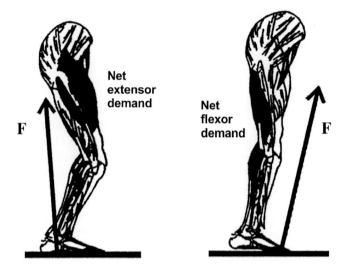

Figure 12   The line of action of the ground reaction force requires either "net extensor" or "net flexor" demand. The patient is capable to control the force direction with movement of the upper body.

Studies have shown that patients adapt to changes of the intrinsic mechanics of the system. Patients who no longer have an ACL usually adjust by avoiding the normal use of the quadriceps muscles (46,47). The patients achieve this by changing their upper body position in such a way that the vector of the ground reaction force passes the knee anteriorly, causing net flexor demand (Fig. 12). Due to this adaptation the patients protect their collateral ligaments and medial meniscus from stretching. The use of more quadriceps force would pull the tibia forward, since the ACL is missing. A similar gait pattern has been recognized in patients with total knee prostheses (and sacrificed ACL), although not to the same extent (50% vs. 75%) (34). Its influence on the contact mechanics of an artificial knee implant has been investigated by Wimmer and Andriacchi (48), and will be discussed in more detail later.

ESTIMATION OF CONTACT FORCES

Research has been performed to estimate the contact forces for different activities (e.g., walking, stair climbing and descending, rising from a chair, etc.). Most researchers have calculated the external forces and moments from measurement of the three-dimensional position of the limb segments [e.g., Refs. (49–52)]. It has been difficult to conduct direct contact force measurements at the knee prosthesis, whereas such measurements have been performed at the hip [e.g., Refs. (53,54)]. The surface replacement design and the more complex kinematics of knee implants make it difficult to build instrumented prostheses (although there have been recent successful attempts). In order to obtain insight into the kinetics of the joint, mathematical modeling is still the method of choice.

Mathematical Modeling of the Knee Joint—Principles of Approach

Basically, there are two options: the direct and the inverse dynamics approach. In the former, the forces are considered as causes and motions are treated as effects, whereas in the latter, inverse approach, the forces are recalculated from equilibrium positions. The inherent difficulty with the direct dynamic approach is that one has to deal with the exact mathematical description of the incorporated structures in order to determine the correct displacements. Hence, there are only a few examples in the literature [e.g., Refs. (55,56)] as most researchers have used the inverse dynamics approach.

Here, the external forces and moments are calculated from measurement of the three-dimensional position of the limb segments and the ground reaction force. The body segments are approximated as a system of rigid links connected by movable joints (40). It is then assumed that the external forces and moments must be balanced by a set of forces and moments acting internally, which are primarily generated by muscle contraction, other soft tissue tension, and articular reaction forces (Fig. 9). Due to the redundancy of the internal structures, this approach induces more unknowns than can be solved with the number of equations available. In general, two attempts have been made to solve this indeterminate problem. The first reduces the unknowns by grouping the muscles and other soft tissue structures into functional units. The second uses an optimization criterion to solve the supernumerary mechanical equations. The optimization criterion works based on either trying to maximize or minimize a physical parameter (e.g., muscle endurance) which is modeled as an objective function.

Compressive Contact Forces

Morrison (50,57,58) was the first to report a method to calculate contact loads at the tibio-femoral articulation. He grouped the muscles acting at the knee into the hamstrings, gastrocnemius, and quadriceps and divided the ligaments into the cruciate and collateral. Using this method he was able to turn the problem into a three-dimensional statically determinate one. The general characteristic of the calculated tibio-femoral contact force during the stance phase of level walking showed three peaks with a maximum as high as three times body weight (Fig. 13). Seireg and Arvikar (49) addressed the indeterminate nature of the problem using an optimization criterion. They modeled the lower extremities as a system of seven segments connected by 31 muscles. Together with the joint reaction components of each plane the model yielded 104 unkowns by 42 given equilibrium equations. In order to solve the problem they established a linear objective function which had

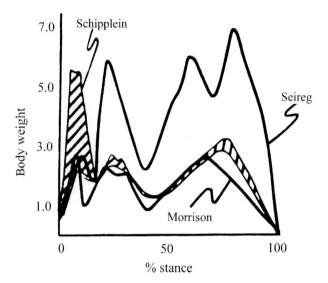

Figure 13 The resultant joint forces (bone-to-bone contact forces) at the normal knee joint from three different authors. The forces—normalized to body weight—are plotted against the stance phase of gait and have been calculated by solving the indeterminate problem by three different techniques. *Source*: Adapted from Refs. 45, 49, 58.

to be satisfied by all equations; the sum of the muscle forces plus a weighted sum of left-over joint moments (which were assumed to be taken by the ligaments) had to be minimized. The calculated tibio-femoral contact force showed a similar pattern to that found by Morrison (50), but with its maximum force exceeding seven times body weight (Fig. 13). This is certainly too high taking the measurements of Bergmann et al. (54) at the hip into account.

The difficulty with optimization methods has been to define the relevant physiological criterion. This problem has been discussed by several authors who tried to evaluate the most feasible criterion for human locomotion (59–61). The incomplete information about the physiological function and the role of the individual muscles, in addition to mathematical simplifications of the anatomy, make the calculation of the joint contact force disputable. The exact physiological function and role of synergistic and antagonistic muscles still remains unclear. Schipplein and Andriacchi (45), investigating the influence of antagonistic muscle activity on contact loads parametrically, reported forces between three and five times body weight during the stance phase of gait (Fig. 13). Unlike other studies, this relatively simple approach of Schipplein and Andriacchi points to the importance of antagonistic muscle activity for joint stabilization. In contrast, it is rather challenging to define an objective function considering muscle cocontraction. The problem then becomes even more complex when physiological and mechanical aspects are incorporated into the model. For example, the maximum force that can be physiologically generated by a muscle depends on its length and on the velocity of contraction, which makes the optimization process dependent on patient activity or pathological conditions.

Shear Contact Forces

All the models above have in common that they were applied to the normal knee. Because the coefficient of friction of cartilage on cartilage is extremely low, i.e., 0.0028–0.0054 (62,63), none of the models took surface friction (and hence shear contact forces) into account. In contrast, reported values of friction in artificial joints range from 0.04 to 0.2 (64–68) and can even rise to 0.35 if polymer transfer occurs (64). The increase in friction has important implications for the contact mechanics of a TKA. Friction introduces shear forces at the articulating surfaces, potentially damaging the polyethylene and stressing the underlying bone bed (69). These tangential shear forces can be generated not only during sliding but also during rolling motion. To exemplify such conditions of rolling movement, one might consider the wheels of a car which undergo driving and braking and as a result tangential load transfer during starting and stopping procedures on the road. Johnsen (71), therefore, suggested using the terms free rolling and tractive rolling to describe motions where the tangential surface loads are zero and nonzero, respectively.

Using a mathematical approach (48), it was shown that there was a substantial influence of gait characteristics and other patient factors on the shear contact forces generated during human motion. Briefly, the model was used to calculate the compressive (normal) and the tractive (shear) forces[d] at the knee from kinematic and kinetic measurements taken during the stance phase of gait of patients following TKA. The model of the artificial knee (Fig. 9) was based upon previously described models of the natural knee (45,71) with the following modifications: the kinematic linkage (pure rolling or sliding) between the femur and the tibia was determined by the static and dynamic coefficient of friction and the angle of knee flexion; the lines of action for each muscle group were approximated by force vectors that change direction as a function of knee flexion; and gait kinetics common to patients following TKA (34) were used.

Pure rolling between the femoral condyles and tibial plateau was simulated up to 18° of knee flexion (25). In addition, pure rolling was limited to the condition where the ratio F_t/F_n was less than the static coefficient of friction μ_s. The maximum static coefficient of friction used in the model

---

[d] Since most of these forces are generated during rolling motion they were called "tractive forces."

was twice the dynamic coefficient μ_d (72). Pure sliding with $\mu_d = 0.1$ (64,65) occurred beyond 18° (or anytime F_t/F_n was greater than μ_s). In addition to the knee flexion angle and EMG recordings, external moments and forces about the knee were entered into the model. Data were obtained from patients following total knee replacement during the stance phase of gait while level walking. Two characteristic gait patterns were analyzed (Fig. 14). The first pattern was characterized by a normal net flexion/extension moment ("Normal") while the second had a distinct reduction in the external flexion moment ("Quadriceps Avoidance"). The external forces obtained in the sagittal plane already included the effect of acceleration of the lower limb segments, and the external moments took the inertial moments into account. Both the external medio-lateral force component and the internal–external moment were neglected. The output of the model, F_n and F_t, was the sum of the respective forces acting on the medial and lateral plateau.

While the magnitude and pattern of the compression force F_n of Figure 15 was similar to previously published results (45,71), the variation of F_n and F_t along the tibial contact region (Fig. 16) was of significant interest. In the anterior region of the tibial plateau, F_t reached a peak, producing a posterior pull on tlie tibial surface. A second peak occurred in the posterior region as the femoral condyles rolled backwards. In contrast to sliding, the direction of the tangential force during tractive rolling is not necessarily in the direction of relative motion between the first and second body (Figs. 15 and 16) since accelerated and decelerated conditions

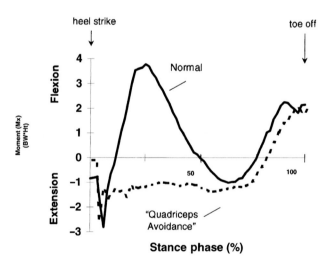

Figure 14 The two patterns of flexion/extension moment used for input to the model. The abnormal "quadriceps avoidance" pattern is common to patients following total knee replacement.

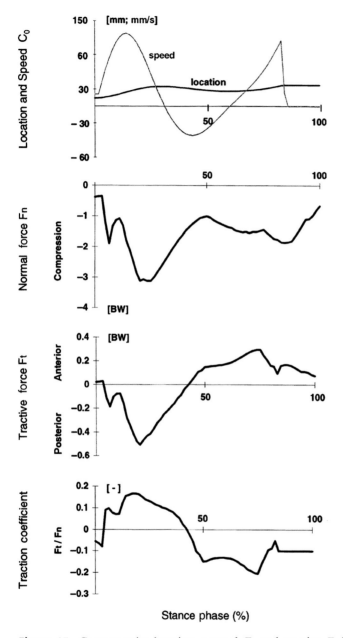

Figure 15 Contact point location, normal F_n and tractive F_t force for a normal walking pattern (0% antagonistic muscle activity). Note the biphasic shape of the traction force with its sign change around midstance. The latter is independent of the direction of relative motion. At about 85% of stance, rolling motion comes to an end and sliding takes place. The traction coefficient F_t/F_n between femoral condyle and tibial component remains between ±0.2 during normal walking.

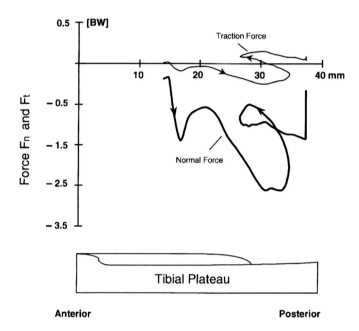

Figure 16 Sagittal view of the polyethylene component with loading history (normal gait pattern, no antagonistic muscle activity). The normal and traction force are shown with respect to their location on the articulating surface. Note that some tibial locations in the posterior region are overrun three times by the femoral condyles. Also the reversal in the direction of tractive force occurred in the posterior portion of the bearing.

are possible. A reversal of the tractive force occurred at the posterior end of the contact region. The knee rolled forward with knee extension following midstance flexion and F_t did not change its postero-anterior direction until the end of stance.

There was a substantial change in the characteristics of the traction force when the gait characteristics were changed to the "Quadriceps Avoidance" gait pattern. The posteriorly directed traction force in the posterior region of the tibial surface was reduced (Fig. 17). The reduction was primarily a result of the reduced quadriceps activity, diminishing the pull of the patellar ligament. The anteriorly directed traction force was not affected by the different gait characteristics, but it was dependent on the knee flexion angle at heel strike and antagonistic muscle activity. A detailed analysis of the influence of the antagonists can be found in Reference. 48.

The study suggests that there are conditions following TKA that can increase the magnitude of the tractive force acting at the knee. If the

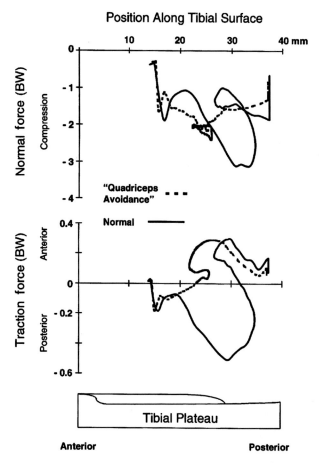

Figure 17 Sagittal view of the polyethylene component comparing the loading history of the normal (*solid*) with the "quadriceps avoidance" (*dashed*) gait pattern. Note that the antero-posterior pull in the posterior portion of the implant is missing for the quadriceps avoidance pattern. Also the normal force is reduced in that region.

coefficient of friction at the articulation increases beyond a certain value (approximately 0.1), the articulation becomes sensitive to factors such as gait mechanics, which then—in turn—can increase or decrease the tractive forces. Large variations in the tractive forces at the knee can result from different patterns of walking. For example, the quadriceps avoidance type of gait reduces the tractive forces of the joint. Also a more flexed position of the knee at heel strike would be beneficial for the articulation since it changes the slope of the patellar ligament to a more vertical direction, thus reducing the tractive pull during quadriceps activity (48). On the other hand, the tractive forces will increase if hyperextension occurs at heel strike and the magnitudes of the peak flexion and peak extension moments during the stance phase of gait are high. Interestingly, these theoretical considerations are in agreement with a clinical study reporting that gait affects the outcome of tibial component fixation (73). The patient group constituting the poor prognosis group had significantly ($p < 0.005$) larger peak flexion moments during level walking than the good prognosis group. Furthermore, the mean value of the peak extension moment at heel strike was significantly increased ($p < 0.01$). Both conditions suggest increased tractive forces (in antero-posterior direction) on the tibial plateau causing stress on the implant–bone anchorage and wear and fatigue at the polyethylene liner. Ultimately those conditions may result in aseptic loosening of the tibial plateau.

FATIGUE AND WEAR DUE TO TRACTIVE FORCES

Surface Fatigue

The repeated loading and unloading to which the polyethylene liner is exposed during antero-posterior motion of the knee may cause surface fatigue. In particular, the specific motion and force characteristics during tractive rolling will put increased stress on the articulation and have been analyzed using the method of finite elements (ADINA 7.0).

The two-dimensional model adopted for this study was originated and validated by Beard (74) and utilized for the analysis of residual stresses in polyethylene due to normal loading (75). Briefly, this model consists of a femoral component which is formed as a CoCr sphere (radius $= 55$ mm), and a tibial UHMWPE component approximated as plastic-multilinear material (dimensions: $40 \times 20 \times 10$ mm^3; Fig. 18). The elastic modulus $E = 572$ MPa, Poisson's ratio $v = 0.45$, and yield strength $\sigma = 12.7$ MPa were obtained from the experimental results of DeHeer (76) using ASTM D695 compression testing. The stress–strain curve found by DeHeer (77) was modeled as multilinear (Fig. 19). A von Mises yield criterion was included. Once plastified, the occurrence of residual stresses generated isotropic hardening of UHMWPE (74).

Rolling movement and tangential loading at the surface (as calculated in the previous model) were included to account for tractive forces generated on the tibial plateau. The normal load was applied to the bottom side of the tibial component as uniformly distributed pressure across the tibial length. The tractive forces were incorporated using a friction coefficient and a minimal displacement of the femoral condyle which was directed in the same direction as the tractive force. The friction coefficients were varied according to the ratio F_t/F_n as determined by the previous knee model. Rolling motion of the condyle on the tibia was included in a quasistatic manner and obtained by rotation and translation of the sphere nodes, assuming the same contact path as described in the previous section.

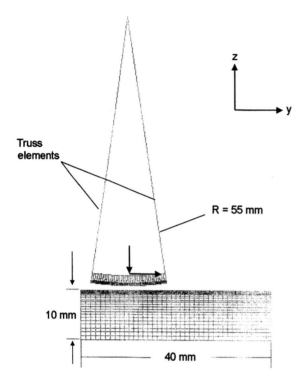

Figure 18 The two-dimensional finite element model. The bottom surface of the tibial component was constrained in all directions to prevent rigid body motion. *Source*: Adapted from Ref. 34.

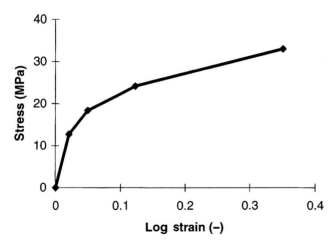

Figure 19 Stress–strain curve for UHMWPE in compression 76. A multilinear approximation was used to model the material properties of the tibial plateau.

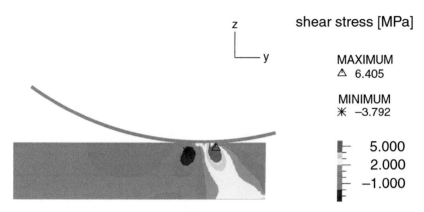

Figure 20 Shear–stress contours in the posterior region of the implant occurring at 21% of stance phase. Note the asymmetric character of the shear stress distribution.

As the femoral condyle rolled from anterior to posterior, the maximum shear stress moved from 1.3 to 0.6 mm towards the surface and became highest (6.4 MPa; Fig. 20) in the posterior region of the tibial plateau. The maximum of the von Mises stress stayed below the surface (0.6–2 mm) at all times, causing plastification and residual stresses in the posterior portion of the implant. Surface elements in the contact path of the femoral condyle became deformed and nondeformed undergoing tension and compression in tangential direction (Fig. 21). Hence, the moving contact between the articulating surfaces caused portions of the surface to be subjected to cyclic stress, providing necessary conditions leading to fatigue of the polyethylene.

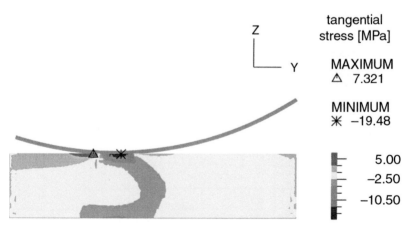

Figure 21 Tangential normal stress immediately after heel strike (at 8% of stance phase).

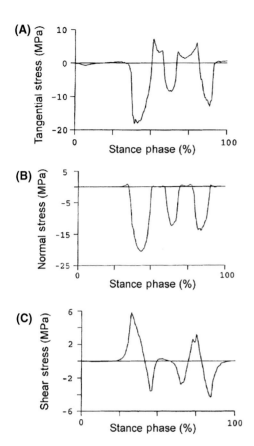

Figure 22 History of the tangential (**A**) and the normal (**B**) contact stress at one characteristic location (30.5 mm) during the stance phase of gait. Note the cyclic character of the stresses. Similar observations were made for the shear stress 0.75 mm below the surface (**C**).

Figure 22 visualizes the cyclic nature of the stress at certain locations of the implant. In a certain area of the posterior region (27–34 mm), the tangential contact stress (σ_{yy}) changed periodically three times between tension and compression during the stance phase of gait. In a similar, manner, the shear stress (σ_{yz}) underwent cyclic changes in direction, while the normal contact stress (σ_{zz}) exhibited a compressive-to-compressive cyclic characteristic. Assuming that a complete gait cycle lasts 1 second, a cyclic change of stresses at approximately 5 Hz (!) is generated in that particular region.

While surface fatigue cracks are usually associated with cyclic compressive–tensile stresses, Pruitt et al. (78) experimentally demonstrated that those cracks could also be initiated and propagated by fully compressive loading. The final length of the crack was dependent on the load ratio of the fatigue cycle: fatigue cracks propagated to greater lengths as the load ratio was increased. In this study it has been shown that both types of cyclic stresses—fully compressive and compressive–tensile—arise at the tibial plateau during normal walking. With increasing tractive force, the location of the maximum shear stress was found to come closer towards the surface. This may be a necessary condition for crack initiation, whereby it should be noted that the maximum shear stress did not rise above 0.6 mm below the surface. The coefficient of friction had to be increased to $\mu = 0.5$ to bring the maximum shear stress to the top of the material (79).

Although fatigue damage is associated with time, the loading history of only one gait cycle has been employed. As has been shown by Reeves et al. (80), the accumulation of stress residuals is dependent on the number of applied load cycles. The accumulated plastic deformation, caused by subsurface yielding of the polyethylene, leads to a region of compressive residual stress which is equilibrated by tensile residual stress at the surface. This tensile stress may combine with the tension generated by the femoral condyles at the edge of contact and may contribute to accelerated fatigue damage (81).

In summary, stress analysis confirmed that the fatigue life of tibial components may be shortened due to tractive rolling, especially when the same tibial contact spot is overrun several times during the stance phase of gait.

Surface Wear Due to Rolling Motion

Does pure rolling generate a wear scar? In the past, reciprocating sliding has been assumed to be the most relevant wear mode in total joint replacement and—as a result—has been simulated in wear studies using a variety of test set-ups [e.g., Refs. (65,82,83)]. The dominance of cyclic sliding versus rolling in wear production was demonstrated by Blunn et al. (84) who modified a pin-on-flat device to provide rolling and sliding under cyclic load. The femoral components were represented by cylinders with polished spherical ends of 25 and 75 mm radii which rolled or slid over a flat UHMWPE disc. Distilled water served as a lubricant. To produce rolling, the "tibial" disc was reciprocated and the "femoral" cylinder was rotated in synchrony. To achieve sliding the cylinder was blocked. Rolling resulted in the generation of shallow wear tracks without major damage, while sliding produced deeper impressions with evidence of subsurface cracking. Blunn et al. (84) attributed the reduced amount of wear during rolling to the lack of frictional shear forces across the surface. However, as shown above, shear forces do not only occur under sliding conditions but also under tractive rolling conditions.

In a separate study (85), the author and colleagues experimentally investigated the influence of increasing tractive forces on the kinematics

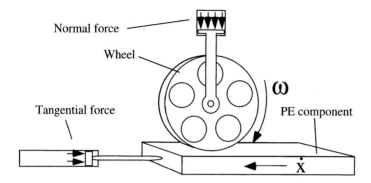

Figure 23 Mechanical concept of the "wheel-on-flat" apparatus: the sledge is driven by the wheel against a tangential force, actively produced by a pneumatic cylinder.

and early wear pattern of UHMWPE. For this reason, a special testing apparatus was designed to simulate increasing tractive force under conditions of pure rolling. The oscillating "wheel-on-flat" configuration consists of a driven cylindrical roller which is pressed against a flat polyethylene component under a constant normal load (Fig. 23). The polyethylene component is mounted on a slide block and, hence, driven by the roller until an increasing tangential force, generated by a pneumatic cylinder, causes a transition from rolling to sliding. Wheel and slide block are then separated from each other and set back to the starting position to begin a new cycle. The wear tests were conducted applying a constant normal force of 900N at the wheel. 900N reflect about half of the average normal load during the stance phase of gait (based on the results above) and were chosen because a single condyle was modeled in this wear test. After running in, a linearly increasing tractive force across the "tibial" plateau was simulated. The length of the wear track covered at least 70 mm. This approach, namely a defined linear increase of tangential force plus the stretched wear track, made it possible to determine the precise loading history for every specific location on the polyethylene component and wheel.

Repeated rolling of the wheel across the polyethylene surface generated a (macroscopically visible) deformed path, mostly from shakedown of the component, while the metal wheel showed only minor surface damage to the unaided eye. The severity of damage on the polyethylene surface changed with increasing tractive force (Fig. 24). Over the whole wear track, pitting was observed. The size of the pits was usually confined to a diameter of 10–20 μm. Longitudinal scratching also occurred, however, its appearance varied with location on the wear track. On the first 30 mm, random oriented scratches with 0–20° off-set from the direction of motion were visible. From 30 to 50 mm, these scratches were found to be deeper

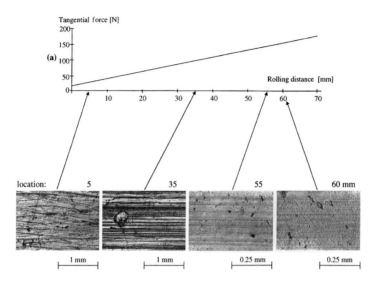

Figure 24 The appearance of wear on the tibial plateau changes with applied tractive force.

and more precisely oriented in the direction of the movement. In the last 20 mm of the wear track, the scratches disappeared and another mode of damage occurred. At that point, ridges perpendicular to the direction of motion came into view, pronounced in height and frequency on the last few millimeters of the wear track. In that area the ridges reached about 5–10 μm in length and seemed to be built up rather than separated from the surface. These perpendicular ridges have also been seen on retrieved tibial components (Fig. 25). They were found as a substructure occurring at the elevated islands of the so-called striated pattern (86). The latter comes about at locations that experience high tractive forces (87).

Overall, the damage of polyethylene was determined by the magnitude of the tractive force. While there were different damage modes present on the polyethylene samples, surface peeling and perpendicular ridges were only present at the end of the wear track where the highest tractive forces occurred. The kinetics of the rolling wheel on the polyethylene component induced cyclic compressive–tensile stresses located closer to the surface due to the higher tangential loads. If these stresses exceed the fatigue strength of the polymer, they may cause the release of near-surface polyethylene layers. Some of these released layers are then sheared into the direction of tractive force and appear as ridges perpendicular to the direction of movement. It should be noted that partially released surface layers and perpendicular ridges are capable of forming particulate debris and/or initiating progressive delamination. Both mechanisms are a potential problem in TKA.

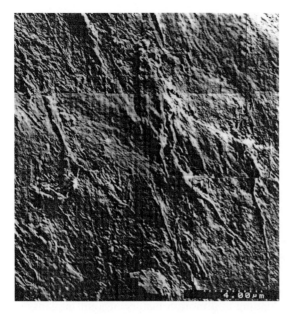

Figure 25 Polyethylene ridges seen on the summits of the striated pattern.

STATE-OF-THE-ART KNEE WEAR TESTING

Wear simulation is an important tool in the evaluation of the performance of the total knee implant under dynamic conditions. In the past, questions addressed have been mostly material or design related. According to Walker et al. (88) the existing wear testing machines can be divided into two basic groups: the first group of simulators model the complete foot–shank–thigh linkage. In this case, the "muscles" are wrapped around the knee and balance the ground reaction forces which are applied underneath the foot. These simulators have been in use since 30 years (89). An advanced example of such a knee simulator has been developed by MTS Systems Inc. in collaboration with researchers from the Mayo Clinic and Johns Hopkins University (90). The advantage of using this type of simulator is that the ground-to-foot reaction forces are well known and therefore highly accurate. However, the complexity of such a simulator limits the possibilities for long-term testing and, thus, for wear analysis.

The second group of simulators takes a more mechanistic approach towards testing, often by simplifying the true dynamics of the articulation of the joint. The reason for simplification is not only to reduce the costs and complexity of the testing device, but also to deal with the variability of joint forces, moments and motions. Early examples are the Stallforth (91) and Treharne (92) wear testing machines, which flex and extend the femoral condyle about a fixed axis. The "genuflector," developed by Paul et al. at the Massachusetts Institute of Technology [detailed description see (88)], uses a four-bar linkage to generate antero-posterior sliding during flexion and extension of the knee prosthesis. While these early simulators are all movement controlled, later models, including the Leeds knee simulator (93) and a simulator by Walker et al. (88), take a combination of motions and forces as input to achieve the desired kinematics.

Today, there are basically two testing options: the ap-motion controlled approach and the ap-force controlled approach. While the former approach allows exact reproduction of any observed in vivo wear scar, the latter more closely models reality (since the ap-motion of the artificial knee is force driven, not guided). Consequently, both approaches have their justification, whereby both have in common that they use a rather rough estimation of the wear relevant load spectrum. Currently, the complex tribological system of an implanted knee prosthesis is reduced to a model that typically consists of a sequence of gait cycles and is basically a copy of the standardized and simplified (but validated) hip wear testing protocol. Information about frequency (and duration) of activities in joint replacement patients is presently restricted to the number of walking steps per year (94,95). Hence, the annual loading and motion history of joint implants is reduced to one million gait cycles, continuously performed at 1–1.5 Hz (96). Human locomotion, however, is of an erratic nature due to the variety of activities during daily life. Recently, a study performed in the habitual environment of total knee patients found that walking only accounts for 10% of the total activity spectrum during the day (97).

The incorporation of different activities into knee wear testing protocols may be important, not only for an appropriate contact loading collective but also to simulate realistic knee motion. A study by Harman et al. (98) demonstrated an off-set in the wear scar dimensions between retrieved implants and the same type of implants tested on an ap-force controlled simulator. In general, the wear scar on the testing samples was well defined and by far shorter than on the retrieved components. This may be in part explained with the usage of an inappropriate loading and motion collective for knee wear testing. In fact, a gross validation of knee wear simulation with the clinical situation has never been performed. One of the inherent difficulties in this respect is the lack of radiographically based wear measurement techniques that are applicable during clinical follow-up. While the latter have been established and are well documented for the hip (99–101), clinically trustworthy wear data of the knee are only available from retrievals (86), These components, however, are mostly failures with a problematic—often incomplete—patient history. In addition, volumetric wear estimation on retrieved tibial liners is by far more challenging than for the hip cup because of the uncertainty of the starting condition (102). Contrary to the hip, where the tolerances of the cup half-sphere are well defined, the geometric and overall manufacturing tolerances of the tibial components are more loose. Hence, the threshold of volumetric wear determination of explants is in a region missing most of the moderately worn components (98).

As shown in the "functional biomechanics section" (Fig. 7), relative knee motion is dependent on the activity rather than on the knee flexion angle. Therefore, activities like chair rising, stair climbing and descending may be important. The wear and failure outcome of knee simulator studies will depend strongly on the input data, not only due to a changed wear path but also due to higher contact stresses generated (usually the posterior radius of the femoral condyle is smaller than the distal radius). In the aforementioned study (97) by one of the authors, it was shown that total knee patients are often in deep flexion ($\geq 60°$) with superimposed motion and load (e.g., sitting down, raising from a chair). These maneuvers are not modeled during simulation, whereas they should be of particular interest for new material developments, as for instance highly cross-linked polyethylene. The latter has proven its outstanding wear characteristics for total hip replacement, where abrasion and adhesion are the dominant wear mechanisms. In total knee replacement, however, fatigue related mechanisms (e.g., delamination) prevail as indicated by analysis of failed tibial components (103). Hence, one should be cautious using a material with decreased fracture mechanical properties [which may be the case for cross-linked UHMWPE (104)]. The benefit and the trade-off of new material developments need to be thoroughly analyzed before these materials are used clinically. Again, wear is a system property and, therefore, what seems good for the hip is not necessarily advantageous for the knee.

CONCLUSIONS

Improvements in the wear resistance of TKA will require an integrated view of the tribological system and the contact mechanics (kinematics and loading) at the knee joint. The structure of the tribological system and the contact mechanics of the knee joint are complex and interdependent. History has demonstrated that a single parameter (e.g., contact stress) will not address this problem and can produce results that do not represent in vivo wear conditions.

The kinematics of the knee joint is a critical factor influencing wear at the joint. Subtle variations in rolling, tractive rolling and sliding motion as well as the direction of the pathway of motion can have substantial affects on the production of wear debris or cyclic fatigue of the UHMWPE. Thus, a rigorous analysis of in vivo kinematics during various activities is crucial to establishing appropriate wear criteria for the bearing surfaces at the joint.

Clearly, the kinematics of the knee joint is activity dependent and is complicated by the fact that numerous parameters can influence the motion of the joint additionally. For example, there can be important variations in the kinematics within a single activity such as walking, since muscle activity will influence joint kinematics. Further, patients can adapt different walking characteristics that are dependent on the design of the implant. It has been shown that it is possible that some patients adapt gait characteristics that could potentially reduce wear relative to other patients with the same implant. The ability of patients to adapt different gait characteristics places additional burdens on in vivo testing protocols. Therefore, patient testing should be done with a minimal encumbrance to the natural movement of the patients, since the testing environment could cause a functional adaptation that does not reflect conditions during normal activities of daily living.

Finally, the basic science of human motion is critical to the solution of wear and failure in TKA. Information from in vivo patient testing is needed to establish design criteria as well as wear testing standards for TKA. In addition, joint kinematics is design specific and it might be possible that wear testing of different designs will require different loading and kinematic characteristics. The combination of an improved understanding of in vivo knee kinematics with the ability to modify the material characteristics of the UHMWPE should lead to substantial improvements in the wear characteristics of the knee joint.

APPENDIX

Wear is a direct result of the occurring mechanisms of friction at the interface which influence the physical and chemical reactions of the tribosystem. There are four basic mechanisms of wear, each of which obeys its own laws.

Adhesion

Adhesion occurs when two smooth bodies slide over each other and fragments of one surface are pulled out and adhere to the other. Later these fragments may come off the surface on to which they adhered and be transferred back to the original surface or they may form loose wear particles. The mechanism leads to the formation of local junctions between the surfaces which may be adhesive or cohesive. Some authors speak of cohesion, when similar materials are welded together.

Abrasion

Abrasive wear occurs when a rough hard surface, or a soft surface containing hard particles slides on a softer surface and ploughs or cuts grooves in it. The material removed from the grooves forms the particulate debris. "Microcutting" removes the material due to a single pass of one abrasive asperity or particle, "microploughing" displaces the material sideways. However, successive or simultaneous microploughing with many protuberances involved causes low cycle fatigue and eventually material break-off. In addition, microploughing and microcutting introduce large strains into the worn surface.

Surface Fatigue

Surface fatigue wear is observed during repeated rolling or sliding over a wear track. The repeated loading and unloading cycles to which the material is exposed may induce the formation of surface or subsurface cracks. Eventually this will result in the loss of large material fragments due to pitting and delamination. The cracks can originate from below or at the surface. Subsurface cracks are generated at locations of maximum shear stress, increased by internal voids or inclusion. The initiation of cracks, which propagate from the surface into the material, is caused due to oscillating, compressive and tensile stresses at the area of contact. Again, the cracks preferably start at "stress raisers," such as surface inclusions.

Tribochemical Reaction

The mechanism of tribochemical wear is usually discussed when materials are exposed to a corrosive environment. It results from the continual removal and new formation of chemical reaction products at the surfaces due to mechanical action. Although the knowledge of chemical or corrosive wear of polymers is even less well established than for metals, it still may play an important role in the process of surface break down.

It should be noted that the wear process itself can be very complex. On many occasions more than one mechanism is acting at a time. Then it becomes very difficult to disentangle the complex situation and find the primary reason for wear.

REFERENCES

1. Kapandji IA. The knee. In: The Physiology of the Joints. London, NY: Church Livingstone, 1970:72–106.
2. Andriacchi TP, Stanwick TS, Galante JO. Knee biomechanics and total knee replacement. J Arthroplasty 1986; 1:211–219.
3. Knutson K, Lewold S, Robertsson O, Lidgren L. The Swedish knee arthroplasty register: a nation wide study of 30,003 knees 1976–1992. Acta Orthop Scand 1994; 65:375–386.
4. Robertsson O, Knutson K, Lewold S, Goodman S, Lidgren L. Knee arthroplasty in rheumatoid arthritis. Acta Orthop Scand 1997; 6:545–553.
5. Hip and knee implant review. Orthop Network News 1995; 6:1–3.
6. Dorr LD, Serocki JH. Mechanisms of failure of total knee arthroplasty. In: Scott WN, ed. The Knee. St. Louis: Mosby, 1994:1239–1249.
7. Czichos H. Tribology—A systems approach to the science and technology of friction, lubrication and wear. Amsterdam: Elsevier, 1978.
8. Habig KH. Verschleißund Härte von Werkstoffen. München: Carl Hanser, 1980.
9. Uetz H, Sommer K, Khosrawi MA. Übertragbarkeit von Versuchs- und Prüfergebnissen bei abrasiver Verschleißbeanspruchung auf Bauteile. VDI-Berichte 1979; 354:107.

10. Fischer A. Einfluß der Temperatur auf das tribologische Verhalten metallischer Werkstoffe. Düsseldorf: VDI, 1994.
11. Uetz H, Wiedemeyer J. Tribologie der Polymere. München: Carl Hanser, 1984.
12. Fischer A. Well-founded selection of materials for improved wear resistance. Wear 1996; 194:238–245.
13. Rand JA. Introduction. In: Rand JA, ed. Total Knee Arthroplasty. New York: Raven Press, 1993.
14. Gunston FH. Polycentric knee arthroplasty. Prosthetic simulation of normal knee movement. Bone J Joint Surg 1971; 53-B:272–277.
15. Conventry MB, Jackson EU, Riley LH, Fimerman GAM, Turner RH. Geometric total knee arthroplasty. I. Conception, design, indications, and surgical technique. Clin Orthop 1973; 94:171–176.
16. Insall J, Ranawat CS, Scott WNS, Waler P. Total condylar knee replacement: preliminary report. Clin Orthop 1976; 120:149–154.
17. Andriacchi TP, Mikosz RP. Musculosceletal dynamics, locomotion and clinical applications. In: Mow VC, Hayes WC, eds. Basic Orthopaedic Biomechanics. New York: Raven Press, 1991:51–92.
18. Lafortune MA, Cavanagh PR, Sommer HJ, Kalenak A. Three-dimensional kinematics of the human knee during walking. Biomech J 1992; 25:347–357.
19. Weber W, Weber E. Mechanik der menschlichen. Gehwerkzeuge: Göttingen, 1836.
20. Strasser H. Lehrbuch der Muskel- und Gelenkmechanik. Berlin: Springer, 1917.
21. Müller W. The Knee: Form, Function, and Ligament Reconstruction. Berlin: Springer, 1983.
22. O'Connor JJ, Shercliff T, Fitzpatrick D. Geometry of the knee. In: Daniel DM, Akeson WH, O'Connor JJ, eds. Knee Ligaments: Structure, Function, Injury, and Repair. New York: Raven Press, 1990:163–199.
23. O'Connor JJ, Zavatsky A. Anterior cruciate ligament function in the normal knee. In: Jackson DW, ed. The Anterior Cruciate Ligament: Current and Future Concepts. New York: Raven Press, 1993:39–52.
24. Blankevoort L. Passive Motion Characteristics of the Human Knee Joint. Ph.D. dissertation, University of Nijmegen, The Netherlands, 1991.
25. Draganich LF, Andriacchi TP, Andersson GBJ. Interaction between intrinsic knee mechanics and the knee extensor mechanism. Orthop J Res 1987; 5: 539–547.
26. Rosenberg A, Mikosz RP, Mohler CG. Basic knee biomechanics. In: Scott WN, ed. The Knee. St. Louis: Mosby, 1994:75–94.
27. Andriacchi TP, Alexander EJ. Studies of human locomotion: past, present and future. Biomech J 2000; 33:1217–1224.
27a. O'Connor JJ, Zaratsky A. Kinematics and mechanics of the cruciate ligaments of the knee. In: Mow VC, Ratelitte A, Woo SX. Y, eds. Biomechanics of Diathrodial Joints. Vol. II. New York: Springer, 1990:197–241.
28. Dyrby CO, Andriacchi TP. Internal external knee rotation as a function of knee flexion for activities of daily living. Trans Am Soc Biomech 1997; 21:200–201.
29. Dyrby CO, Andriacchi TP. Deep knee flexion and tibio-femoral rotation during activities of daily living. Trans Orthop Res Soc 1998; 23:1110.

30. Blankevoort L, Huiskes R, de Lange A. Recruitment of knee-joint ligaments. Biomech J Eng 1991; 113:94–103.

31. Blankevoort L, Huiskes R, Kuiper JH, Grootenboer HJ. Articular contact in a three-dimesional model of the knee. Biomech J 1991; 24:1019–1031.

32. Moilanen T, Freeman MAR. Point–counterpoint of total knee arthroplasty: the case for resection of the posterior cruciate ligament. Arthroplasty J 1995; 10:564–568.

33. Dorr LD, Ochsner JL, Gronley J, Perry J. Functional comparison of posterior crucuiate-retained versus cruciate-sacrificed total knee arthroplasty. Clin Orthop 1988; 236:36–43.

34. Andriacchi TP, Galante JO, Fermier RW. The influence of total lcnee replacement design on function during walking and stair climbing. J Bone Joint Surg 1982; 64:1328–1335.

35. Matthews LS, Sonstegard DA, Henke JA. Load bearing characteristics of the patello-femoral joint. Acta Orthop Scand 1977; 48:511–516.

36. van Eijden TM, De Boer W, Weijs WA. The orientation of the distal part of the quadriceps femoris muscle as a function of the knee flexion–extension angle. Biomech J 1985; 18:803–809.

37. Ahmed AM, Burke DL, Hyder A. Force analysis of the patellar mechanism. Orthop J Res 1987; 5:69–85.

38. Andriacchi TP, Galante JO, Draganich LF. Relationship between knee extensor mechanics and function following total knee replacement. In: Dorr LD, ed. The Knee. Baltimore: University Park Press, 1985:83–94.

39. Li E, Ritter MA. Point – counterpoint of total knee arthroplasty: The case for retention of the posterior cruciate ligament. Arthroplasty J 1995; 10:560–564.

40. Andriacchi TP, Strickland AB. Gait analysis as a tool to assess joint kinetics. In: Berme N, Engin AE, Correia da Silva KM, eds. Biomechanics of Normal and Pathological Human Articulating Joints. NATO ASI Series # 93, 1985:83–102.

41. Olney SJ, Winter DA. Predictions of knee and ankle moments of force in walking from EMG and kinematic data. Biomech J 1985; 18:9–20.

42. Sepulveda F, Wells DM, Vaughan CL. A neural network presentation of electromyography and joint dynamics in human gait. J Biomech 1993; 26:101–109.

43. Cholewicki J, McGill SM. EMG assisted optimization: a hybrid approach for estimating muscle forces in an indeterminate biomechanical model. J Biomech 1994; 27:1287–1289.

44. Perry J. The mechanics of gait. In: Wright V, Radin EL, eds. Mechanics of Human Joints: Physiology, Pathophysiology, and Treatment. New York: Marcel Dekker, 1998:83–107.

45. Schipplein OD, Andriacchi TP. Interaction between active and passive knee stabilizers during level walking. Orthop J Res 1991; 9:113–119.

46. Berchuck M, Andriacchi TP, Bach BR, Reider B. Gait adaptions by patients who have a deficient anterior cruciate ligament. J Bone Joint Surg 1990; 72-A:871–877.

47. Andriacchi TP. Dynamics of pathological motion: applied to the anterior cruciate deficient knee. J Biomech 1990; 23:99–105.

48. Wimmer MA, Andriacchi TP. Tractive forces during rolling motion of the knee: implications for wear in total knee replacement. J Biomech 1997; 30:131–137.

49. Seireg A, Arvikar RJ. The prediction of muscular load sharing and joint forces in the lower extremities during walking. J Biomech 1975; 8:89–102.
50. Morrison JB. Function of the knee joint in various activities. Biomed Mater Eng 1969; 4:573–580.
51. Komistek RD, Stiehl JB, Dennis DA, Paxson RD, Soutas-Little RW. Mathematical model of the lower extremity joint reaction forces using Kane's method of dynamics. J Biomech 1998; 31:185–189.
52. Kuster MS, Wood GA, Stachowiak GW, Gächter A. Joint load considerations in total knee replacement. J Bone Joint Surg 1997; B-79:109–113.
53. Davy DT, Kotzar GM, Brown RH, Heiple KG, Goldberg VM, Berilla J, Bursteing AH. Telemetric force measurements across the hip after total hip arthroplasty. Bone J Joint Surg 1988; 70-A:45–50.
54. Bergmann G, Graichen F, Rohlmann A. Hip joint loading during walking and running measured in two patients. J Biomech 1993; 26:969–990.
55. Wismans J, Veldpaus F, Janssen J. A three-dimensional mathematical model of the knee-joint. J Biomech 1980; 13:677–685.
56. Andriacchi TP, Mikosz RP, Hampton SJ. Model studies of the stiffness characteristics of the human Knee joint. J Biomech 1983; 16:23–29.
57. Morrison JB. Bioengineering analysis of force actions transmitted by the knee joint. Biomed Mater Eng 1968; 3:164–170.
58. Morrison JB. The mechanics of the knee joint in relation to normal walking. J Biomech 1970; 3:51–61.
59. Crowninshield RD, Brand RA. A physiologically based criteria of muscle force prediction in locomotion. J Biomech 1981; 14:793–801.
60. Patriarco AG, Mann RW, Simon SR, Mansour JM. An evaluation of the approaches of optimization models in the prediction of muscle forces during human gait. J Biomech 1981; 14:513–525.
61. Kaufman KR, An KN, Litchy WJ, Chao EY. Physiological prediction of muscle forces—application to isokinetic exercises. Neuroscience 1991; 40:793–804.
62. Linn FC, Radin EL. Lubrication in animal joints—III. The effect of certain chemical alteration of the cartilage and lubricant. Arthritis Rheum 1968; 11: 674–680.
63. Unsworth A. Lubrication of human joints. In: Wright V, Radin EL, eds. Mechanics of Human Joints: Physiology, Pathophysiology, and Treatment. New York: Marcel Dekker, 1993:137–162.
64. McKellop H, Clarke IC, Markolf KL, Amstutz HC. Wear characteristics of UHMW polyethylene: a method for accurately measuring extremely low wear rates. J Biomed Mater Res 1978; 12:895–927.
65. Davidson JA, Mishra AK, Poggie RA, Wert JJ. Sliding friction and UHMWPE wear comparison between cobalt alloy and zirconia surfaces. Trans Orthop Res Soc 1992; 38:404.
66. Soudry M, Walker PS, Reilly DT, Kurosawa H, Sledge CB. Effects of total knee replacement design on femoral–tibial contact conditions. J Arthroplasty 1986; 1:35–45.
67. Fisher J, Dowson D, Hamdzah H, Lee HL. The effect of sliding velocity on the friction and wear of UHMWPE for use in total artificial joints. Wear 1994; 175:219–225.

68. Dumbleton JH. Tribology of Natural and Artificial Joints—Tribology Series 3, Amsterdam: Elsevier 1981.
69. Rullkoetter PJ, Hillberry BM. Tibio-femoral contact under dynamic loading. Trans Orthop Res Soc 1993; 39:425.
70. Johnsen KL. Contact Mechanics. 2nd. Cambridge: Cambridge University Press, 1985.
71. Morrison JB. The mechanics of the knee joint in relation to normal walking. J Biomech 1970; 3:51–61.
72. Lloyd AI, Noël RE. The effect of counterface surface roughness on the wear of UHMWPE in water and oil-in-water emulsion. Tribol Int 1988; 301:83–88.
73. Hilding MB, Lanshammer H, Ryd L. Knee joint loading and tibial component loosening. J Bone Joint Surg 1996; 78-B:66–73.
74. Beard BJ. Origins of wear in the polyethylene component of total knee replacements based on finite element analysis, M.S. Thesis, University of Illinois at Chicago, Chicago, 1996.
75. Beard BJ, Natarajan RN, Andriacchi TP, Amirouche FML. The stress origins of a new striated wear pattern in total knee replacements. Trans Orthop Res Soc 1996; 21:465.
76. DeHeer DC. Stresses in polyethylene components for total knee arthroplasty, M.S. thesis, Purdue University, West Lafayette, IN, 1992.
77. DeHeer DC, Hillberry BM. The effect of thickness and nonlinear material behavior on contact stresses in polyethylene tibial components. Trans Orthop Res Soc 1992; 38:327.
78. Pruitt L, Koo J, Rimnac CM, Suresh S, Wright TM. Cyclic compressive loading results in fatigue cracks in ultra high molecular weight polyethylene. J Orthop Res 1995; 13:143–146.
79. Schroeder U, Natarajan RN, Andriacchi TP, Wimmer MA. The influence of tractive force on the shear stresses in UHMWPE of a TKR component. Trans Orthop Res Soc 1997; 22:794.
80. Reeves EA, Barton DC, Fitzpatrick DP, Fisher J. A time dependent analysis of cyclic strain accumulation in UHMWPE knee replacements. Trans Orthop Res Soc 1997; 22:792.
81. Estupiñán JA, Bartel DL, Wright TM. Residual stresses in ultra-high molecular weight polyethylene loaded cyclically by a rigid moving indenter in nonconforming geometries. J Orthop Res 1998; 16:80–88.
82. White SE, Whiteside LA, McCarthy DS, Anthony M, Poggie RA. Simulated knee wear with cobalt chromium and oxidized zirconium knee femoral components. Clin Orthop 1994; 309:176–184.
83. Walker PS, Ben-Dov M, Askew MJ, Pugh J. The deformation and wear of plastic components in artificial knee joints—an experimental study. Eng Med 1981; 10:33–38.
84. Blunn GW, Walker PS, Joshi A, Hardinge K. The dominance of cyclic sliding in producing wear in total knee replacements. Clin Orthop 1991; 273: 253–260.
85. Wimmer MA, Birken LMO, Schimansky T, Morlock MM, Andriacchi TP, Schneider E. Simulated wear of the tibial components by tractive rolling, Trans EORS 1998; 8:15.

86. Wimmer MA. Wear of the Polyethylene Component Created by Rolling Motion of the Artificial Knee Joint. Aachen: Shaker 1999:78–112.

87. Wimmer MA, Andriacchi TP, Natarajan RN, Loos J, Karlhuber M, Petermann J, Schneider E, Rosenberg AG. A striated pattern of wear in ultra-high-molecular-weight polyethylene components of Miller–Galante Total Knee Arthroplasty. J Arthroplasty 1998; 13:8–16.

88. Walker PS, Blunn GW, Broome DR, Perry J, Watkins A, Sathasivam S, Dewar ME, Paul JP. A knee simulating machine for performance evaluation of total knee replacements. J Biomech 1997; 30:83–89.

89. Shaw JA, Murray DG. Knee joint simulator. Clin Orthop 1973; 94:15–23.

90. Mejia LC. Mechanical Testing Systems for Biomaterials/Biomechanics Research. Eden Prairie: MTS Systems Corporation, 1994.

91. Stallforth H, Ungethüm M. Die tribologische Testung von Knieendoprothesen. Biomed Techn 1978; 23:295–304.

92. Treharne RW, Young RW, Young SR. Wear of artificial joint materials III: Simulation of the knee joint using a computer-controlled system. Eng Med 1981; 10:137–142.

93. Dowson D, Gillis BJ, Atkinson JR. Penetration of metallic femoral components into polymeric tibial components observed in a knee joint simulator. In: Lee L-H, ed. Polymer Wear and Its Control. Washington DC: American Chemical Society 1985:215–228.

94. Schmalzried TP, Szuszczewicz ES, Northfield MR, Akizuki KH, Frankel RE, Belcher G, Amstutz HC. Quantitative assessment of walking activity after total hip or knee replacement. J Bone Joint Surg 1998; A-80:54–59.

95. Zahiri CA, Schmalzried TP, Szuszczewicz ES, Amstutz HC. Assessing activity in joint replacement patients. J Arthroplasty 1998; 13:890–895.

96. Ungethuem M, Winkler-Gniewek W. Tribologie in der Medizin. Tribol und Schmierungstechn 1990; 37:268–277.

97. Hänni M, DeWilde P, Morlock MM, Schneider E, Kehl T, Wimmer MA. Activity profile of total knee patients during the day. Proceedings of the Biomechanica IV, Davos. J Biomech 2001; 34(suppl l):50.

98. Harman M, DesJardins J, Banks S, Benson L, LaBerge M, Hodge W. Damage patterns on polyethylene inserts after retrieval and after wear simulation. Trans Orthop Res Soc 2001; 26:1003.

99. Bould M, Barnard S, Learmonth ID, Cunningham JL, Hardy JR. Digital image analysis: improving accuracy and reproducibility of radiographic measurement. Clin Biomech 1999; 14:434–437.

100. Martell JM, Berdia S. Determination of polyethylene wear in total hip replacements with use of digital radiographs. J Bone Joint Surg 1997; A-79:1635–1641.

101. Gölzhäuser G, Wimmer MA, Berzins A, Sumner DR, Scheuvens BJ, Schneider E. Aufbau und Validierung einer Methode zur Verschleißmessung von Polyethylen-Hüftpfannen mit Metallschale mit Hilfe von Röntgenbildern, Biomed. Technik 1998; 43(suppl l):66–67.

102. Seebeck J, Schneider E, Natarajan RN, Wimmer MA. Volumetric deformation of retrieved polyethylene tibial inserts with consideration of the initial

manufacturing variation. Proceedings of the International Society of Biomechanics XVIIIth Congress, Zurich, 2001, #O356.
103. Wright TM, Bartel DL. The Problem of surface damage in polyethylene total knee components. Clin Orthop 1986; 205:67–74.
104. Baker DA, Hastings RS, Pruitt L. Study of fatigue resistance of chemical and radiation cross-linked medical grade ultrahigh molecular weight polyethylene. J Biomed Mater Res 1999; 46:573–581.

10

Corrosion of Metallic Implants

Nadim James Hallab and Joshua J. Jacobs

Department of Orthopaedic Surgery, Rush University Medical Center, Chicago, Illinois, U.S.A.

Jeremy L. Gilbert

Department of Bioengineering and Neuroscience, Syracuse University, Syracuse, New York, U.S.A.

INTRODUCTION

Electrochemical corrosion occurs to some extent on all metallic implants. This is primarily undesirable for two main reasons: (i) the process of degradation may reduce the structural integrity of the implant, and (ii) the release of degradation products may react unfavorably with the host. Metallic implant degradation may result from either electrochemical dissolution or wear, but most commonly occurs through a synergistic combination of the two (1,2). Corrosion processes include both generalized degradation uniformly affecting an entire surface, and localized corrosion affecting either areas of a device relatively shielded from the environment (e.g., crevice corrosion), or seemingly random sites on the surface (e.g., pitting corrosion). Although generally phenomena of the past, these electrochemical and other mechanical processes can and have interacted to cause premature structural failure and accelerated metal release (e.g., stress corrosion cracking, corrosion fatigue, and fretting corrosion). What remains problematic is the prevalence of elevated local and systemic metal concentrations and particulate corrosion products in peri-implant tissues associated with the corrosion of both past and contemporary metallic implant devices.

This chapter will overview electrochemical corrosion of implant alloys (focusing on orthopaedic alloys) and how this impacts us all from a more clinical perspective. A summary of implant corrosion basic science, in vitro corrosion testing techniques, and corrosion properties of orthopaedic alloy will be followed by more clinical reviews of metal release, local tissue response to implant corrosion products, and implications for potential systemic effects.

GENERAL CORROSION CONCEPT

There are two essential features associated with how and why metal implants corrode. These features have to do with (i) the extent of the thermodynamic driving forces, which cause corrosion (oxidation/reduction reactions), and (ii) physical barriers which limit the kinetics of corrosion. Of course, in practice, corrosion of orthopaedic biomaterials is complex, and is dependent on a number of variables: geometric variables (e.g., taper geometry in modular component hip prostheses), metallurgical variables (e.g., surface microstructure, oxide structure, and composition), mechanical variables (e.g., stress and/or relative motion), and solution variables (e.g., pH, solution proteins, and enzymes).

Thermodynamic Considerations

The basic underlying reaction which occurs during corrosion is the increasing of the valence state (i.e., loss of electrons) of the metal atom.

$$M \rightarrow M^{z+} + ze^- \ (\text{oxidation})$$

This oxidation event (loss of electrons and increase in valence) may result in the release of free ions from the metal surface into solution (which then can migrate away from the metal surface), or may result in other reactions such as the formation of metal oxides, metal chlorides, organo-metallic compounds, or other species. These "end" products may also be soluble in solution or may precipitate to form solid phases. Solid oxidation products may be subdivided into either those which form adherent compact oxide films or those which form nonadherent oxide (or other) particles which can migrate away from the metal surface.

For corrosion to occur at all there must be a thermodynamic driving force for the oxidation of metal atoms. This driving force can be quantified thermodynamically using "Gibbs function" or free energy (Gibbs function incorporates both the entropy and enthalpy changes of the above chemical reaction, or the total work to reach equilibrium).

$$\Delta G_{red} = \Delta G^0 + RT \ \ln \frac{[M]}{[M^{z+}][e^-]^z}$$

where

ΔG_{red} is the free energy change for the reduction reaction (i.e., the reverse reaction from above),

ΔG^0 is the free energy of the reaction in some quantifiable standard state (typically where the ions are at unit activity or fully saturated), [M], [M^{z+}], and [e^-]^z are approximate activities (or concentrations) of the species involved in the reaction. This assumption is only really true in infinitely dilute solutions where released ion do not interact and molality equals activity, but it remains a good approximation for dilute solutions as well.

By convention, if $\Delta G > 0$ then the process requires energy or, if $\Delta G < 0$, the oxidation process releases energy and corrosion will spontaneously occur.

Categorically, there are two sources of energy to be considered in corrosion processes; (i) chemical and (ii) electrical (charge separation). The chemical driving force (ΔG) determines whether or not corrosion will take place under the conditions of interest. When the free energy for oxidation is less than zero then oxidation is energetically favorable and will take place spontaneously. The second energy force relates to the positive and negative charges (metal ions and electrons, respectively) separated from one another during corrosion. The ions are released into the solution or go to form an oxide or other compound and the electrons are left behind in the metal (or undergo other electrochemical reactions like the reduction of oxygen or hydrolysis of water). This charge separation contributes to what is known as the electrical double layer and creates an electrical potential across the metal–solution interface (similar to that of a capacitor) which can be quantified by the expression:

$$\Delta G = -zF\Delta E$$

where

ΔG is the free energy change,
z is the valence of the ion,
F is known as the Faraday constant (i.e., 96,500 C/mole electrons) and
ΔE is the voltage across the metal–solution interface.

This potential is also a measure of the reactivity of the metals or the driving force for metal oxidation. It shows that the more negative the potential of a metal in solution, the more reactive it will tend to be (i.e., the greater is ΔG for reduction).

At equilibrium, the chemical energy balances with the electrical energy yielding the Nernst equation, which defines the electrical potential across an ideal metal–solution interface when in a solution.

$$\Delta E = \Delta E^{o} + \frac{RT}{zF} \ln \frac{[M^{z+}]}{[M]}$$

where

> ΔE is the potential of the metal,
> ΔE° is the standard electrode potential of the metal,
> R is the gas constant (8.314 J/mole),
> T is temperature in Kelvin (25°C is 298 K),
> z is the valency, and
> F is the Faraday constant (96,490 C/mole).

From this equation, a theoretical scale of metal reactivity can be established, known as the electrochemical series, which is a ranking of the equilibrium potential from most positive (i.e., least reactive or most Noble) to most negative (most reactive, most Base). Be aware that this ranking is based only on thermodynamic equilibrium. That is, it is only true if we assume that there are no barriers (i.e., no surface oxide formation) to the oxidation (loss of electrons/corrosion) of the metal, these potentials would be the ones that would exist across the metal–solution interface. Table 1 shows some selected reactions and their electrochemical potential (using a standard hydrogen electrode). Certain metals owe their corrosion resistance to the fact that their equilibrium potentials are very positive. Gold and platinum are examples of metals, which have little or no driving force for oxidation in aqueous solutions and thus they tend to corrode very little in the human body. However, other metals which are commonly used in orthopaedics have more negative potentials indicating that, from a chemical driving force perspective, they are much more likely to corrode. For example, titanium has a very large negative potential, -1.6 V (SHE), indicating that there is a large chemical driving force for corrosion (oxidation). If something like surface oxide formation (or passivation) did not intervene, pure titanium would violently corrode with its surroundings (typically oxygen, water, or other oxidizing species). For example, unoxidized pure titanium powder sprayed into an oxygen containing atmosphere will react exothermically and burn violently.

Kinetic Barriers to Corrosion

The second factor which governs the corrosion process of metallic biomaterials is the formation of stable surface barriers or limitations to the kinetics of corrosion. These barriers prevent corrosion by physically limiting the rate at which oxidation or reduction processes can take place. The formation of

Table 1 Standard Electrochemical Series for Selected Metals

		Reaction	Potential (V)
(corrosion resistant)			
Noble	$Au^{3+} + 3e^-$	$\Leftrightarrow Au$	1.42
↑	$Pt^{2+} + 2e^-$	$\Leftrightarrow Pt$	1.20
	$Ag^+ + e^-$	$\Leftrightarrow Ag$	0.80
	$O_2 + 2H_2O + 4e^-$	$\Leftrightarrow OH^-$	0.40
	$Ti(OH)^{3+} + H^+ + e^-$	$\Leftrightarrow Ti^{3+} + H_2O$	0.06
	$H^+ + e^-$	$\Leftrightarrow 1/2\ H_2$	0.00
	$Fe^{3+} + 3e^-$	$\Leftrightarrow Fe$	−0.04
	$Co^{2+} + 2e^-$	$\Leftrightarrow Co$	−0.28
	$Fe^{2+} + 2e^-$	$\Leftrightarrow Fe$	−0.41
	$Cr^{2+} + 2e^-$	$\Leftrightarrow Cr$	−0.56
	$Cr^{3+} + 3e^-$	$\Leftrightarrow Cr$	−0.74
	$2H_2O + 2e^-$	$\Leftrightarrow 2OH^-$	−0.83
	$TiO_2 + 4H^+ + 4e^-$	$\Leftrightarrow Ti + 2H_2O$	−0.86
	$Ti^{2+} + 2e^-$	$\Leftrightarrow Ti$	−1.60
↓	$Mg^+ + e^-$	$\Leftrightarrow Mg$	−2.37
Active	$Na^+ + e^-$	$\Leftrightarrow Na$	−2.71
(corrosion prone)			

Note: These values are based on the standard hydrogen electrode scale. The more noble metals at the top of the list are less reactive, while the more active metals (towards the bottom) are more reactive and have a higher driving force for oxidation (corrosion). Note that titanium and chromium (particularly the trivalent form) are both very reactive and have a high driving force for oxidation.

a metal-oxide passive film on a metal surface is one example of a kinetic limitation to corrosion. The general reaction which governs this formation is as follows.

$$M^{z+} + \frac{z}{2}H_2O \rightarrow \frac{z}{2}MO + zH + ze^-$$

In general, kinetic barriers to corrosion prevent either the migration of metallic ions from the metal to the solution, the migration of anions from solution to metal, or the migration of electrons across the metal–solution interface. Passive oxide films are the most well-known forms of kinetic barriers in corrosion, but other kinetic barriers exist including polymeric coatings.

Most orthopaedic alloys rely entirely on the formation of passive films to prevent significant oxidation (corrosion) from taking place. These films consist of metal oxides (ceramic films) which form spontaneously on the surface of the metal in such a way that they prevent further transport of metallic ions and/or electrons across the film. Passive films must have certain characteristics to be effective barriers. The films must be compact and fully cover the metal surface, they must have an atomic structure which limits the migration of ions and/or electrons across the metal-oxide–solution interface, and they must be able to remain on the surface of these alloys even with mechanical stressing or abrasion, expected with orthopaedic devices.

Passivating oxide films spontaneously grow on the surface of metals. These oxide films may be amorphous or crystalline and are very thin, (on the order of 5 to 70 Å[1]) which depends on the potential across the interface[1] as well as solution variables like pH (3,4). Since the potentials across the metal–solution interface for these reactive metals is typically 1–2 V and the distances are so small, the electric field across the oxide is very high, on the order of 10^6–10^7 V/cm. One of the more widely accepted models of oxide film growth at low temperatures is based on the theory of Cabrera and Mott (5) which states that oxide film growth depends on the electric field across the oxide. If the potential across the metal-oxide–solution interface is decreased (i.e., made closer to the electrochemical series potential) then the film thickness will decrease by reductive dissolution processes at the oxide to make the electric field strength constant. Increasing the voltage will correspondingly increase the thickness of the film. In fact, oxide thickness is often determined by the anodization rate which is given as oxide thickness per volt (4). The film will change its thickness by growth or dissolution until the rates of both are equal, giving rise to a film thickness which is dependent on metal-oxide–solution potential. If the interfacial potential is made sufficiently negative or the pH of the solution is made low enough, then these oxide films will no longer be thermodynamically stable and will undergo reductive dissolution, or, there will be no driving force for the formation of the oxide and the metal surface will become open to corrosion.

Oxide films are not flat smooth continuous sheets of adherent oxide covering the metal. Transmission electron microscopy (TEM) and atomic force microscopy (AFM) techniques have shown that oxides of titanium, for instance, consist of needle (6) or dome (7) shapes.

Mechanical factors such as fretting, micromotion, or applied stresses may be such that the oxide films are abraded or fractured. When an oxide film is ruptured from the metal substrate, unoxidized metal is exposed to solution. These films will tend to reform or repassivate and the magnitude of the repassivation currents may be large. This is due to the normally large driving forces that are present for the oxidation process and when the kinetic barrier is removed these large driving forces can operate to cause oxidation. However, the extent and duration of the oxidation currents will depend on the repassivation kinetics for oxide film formation. Hence, the mechanical stability of the oxide films as well as the driving force associated with their formation is central to the performance of oxide films in orthopaedic applications.

The Nature of the Solution/Metal Interface

The interface between a passivating metal and body environment can then be summed up with the following description (Fig. 1). The metal surface spontaneously reacts with its surroundings to form a passive metal-oxide film which may be nonuniform in cross section (domed or needle shaped) and, at least initially, amorphous. An oxide film nucleates and grows on a metal surface and contains within it defects which allow for electronic and ionic transport of charged species across the film. There are species such as oxygen, phosphates (8), hydroxides or proteins (9) adsorbed from solution onto the surface of the oxide film which may change the properties of the film. There also exists a large electric field which is the driving force

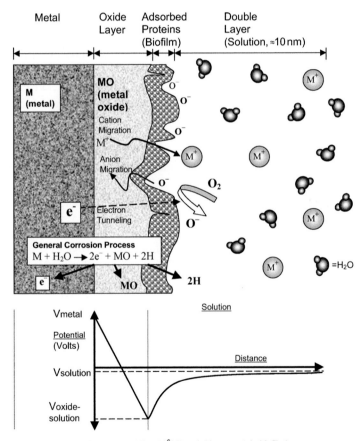

Figure 1 A schematic showing the interface of a metal surface in contact with a biological environment. The metal is covered by an oxide layer followed by the adsorbed proteins (biofilm) through which metal ions can pass into the solution as shown.

for the movement of these ions across the film. If the electric field strength is changed (by changing the applied potential, for instance) then the oxide film will grow or shrink to maintain a constant field strength (at least at low temperatures). Also, depending on conditions, the oxide film will change crystal structure, size, and thickness. Several treatments have been investigated to see if improvements in the barrier effect of the oxide films can be achieved. These treatments include a hot, concentrated nitric acid bath treatment, boiling in distilled water (10), and anodization. However, detailed investigations into the changes in oxide film structure with these treatments are incomplete.

Oxidation and reduction reactions upon metal surfaces are typically separated spatially from each other (i.e., the rate of oxidation of a species may be heterogeneously distributed about a metal surface), i.e., regions where oxidation is occurring may be well-separated spatially from where the corresponding reduction process is operating. These variations can be due to local microstructural heterogeneities or differences between grain boundaries and grain interiors in the alloy, differences in strain energy, or due to geometry as occurs in crevice corrosion or pitting corrosion. During crevice corrosion the region inside the crevice develops into a deaerated environment and may have a lower pH than the bulk solution. This may accelerate the release of metal ions in the crevice, while away from the crevice the reduction reactions involving oxygen can take place. In this case, oxidation will be localized inside the crevice and reduction will take place outside of the crevice.

IN VITRO CORROSION TESTING METHODS

There are a wide variety of corrosion test methodologies used to assess the corrosion properties of orthopaedic alloys. These include immersion tests such as anodic polarization, linear polarization, and other specialized tests such as impedance spectroscopy (11), stripping analysis, and newer techniques such as scanning electrochemical microscopy (12). All these tests are used to investigate the rate of ion release, the electrochemical conditions which cause oxidation and reduction processes, and the electrical nature of the interface. Additionally, there are several test methods related to combined mechanical–electrochemical processes such as fretting corrosion, stress corrosion, and corrosion fatigue. These tests typically evaluate how an alloy resists corrosion during physiologically relevant loading.

Open Circuit Potential

There are several electrochemical tests which are used to assess the corrosion properties of orthopaedic alloys. These tests typically investigate the electrical currents (A) and potentials (V) of the metal–solution interface. Metal–solution interfaces have an associated potential which is determined by the concentration of species present at the interface, i.e., the oxide films and other species which may adsorb to the surface (Fig. 1). In the more complicated environment of the human body and the presence of multiple metals in an alloy, the potential of the interface (known as the open circuit potential, OCP) will represent the sum of all reactions that are ongoing at the interface. At equilibrium for this "multi-electrode system," the net external current which flows is zero. This means that any and all oxidation processes ongoing at the surface must be balanced by reduction processes which are also occurring at the same surface.

Polarization Testing—Current Potential Response

The standard electrochemical test used to evaluate the corrosion resistance of metals and alloys is the polarization test. This test assesses the current-potential characteristics of the metal–solution interface by varying the potential of the interface and measuring the resulting current. This test forces the potential across the metal-oxide–solution interface to vary in a controlled fashion and forces the oxidation and reduction reactions, which are at a dynamic equilibrium at the OCP to deviate from equilibrium. For metals which do not form passivating films (none of the implant alloys), the current potential relationship is given by the Butler–Volmer equation (13):

$$i_{corr} = i_o \left[\exp^{\frac{\eta}{b_c}} - \exp^{\frac{\eta}{b_a}} \right]$$

where

i_{corr} is the corrosion current at the applied potential,
η is the overpotential (the potential difference between open circuit and the applied potential),
b_a and b_c are the Tafel constants, and
i_o is the exchange current density.

From these polarization tests, information concerning the corrosion current at the open circuit potential can be obtained as well as the nature of the electrochemical behavior when the potential of the interface is different from the resting OCP.

Polarization tests are performed by applying a potential (voltage) to a metal sample (working electrode) relative to a standardized reference electrode. The typical instrumentation used for this purpose is a potentiostat. A counter electrode is used to complete the circuit and to provide a current sink or source so that the reference electrode is not affected by the current which flows. A typical curve for a polarization test of a passivating metal is shown schematically in Figure 2. Here there are several features worthy of note.

Polarization of Passive Metals

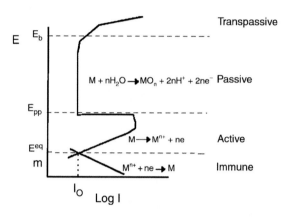

Figure 2 A schematic for a polarization test of an idealized metal with no other electrochemical reactions taking place. The y-axis represents the voltage of the metal surface relative to a standard electrode of some sort and the x-axis represents the log of the current produced by the corrosion. The areas of different corrosion behavior are indicated by the dotted lines. Below the equilibrium potential (E_m), metal ions tend to come out of solution onto the metal surface. Between the equilibrium potential and the passivation potential (E_{pp}) metal ion release from the surface is thermodynamically favorable, without inhibition by surface oxide formation. However, between the passivation potential and the breakdown potential (E_b) the surface of the metal is protected by the formation of an oxide layer (i.e., passive region). Above E_b the driving force for ionization overcomes the protective surface oxide resulting in corrosion within the transpassive region.

There are four regions of this plot which are the result of different behavior of the electrode surface. At sufficiently negative potentials (i.e., below the equilibrium potential of the metal in question), there is no driving force for oxidation of the metal to form either ions in solution or oxide on the metal surface. At this potential the metal is said to be immune. At potentials positive of the equilibrium potential, the metal has a thermodynamic driving force for oxidation. At these potentials the metal is in the active region. In this range of potentials the metal surface is actively corroding and releasing ions into the solution. A passive film has not formed to the extent that it can limit the rate of corrosion, although incomplete oxide film formation may be occurring. As the potential is increased in the active range, a greater current flows and more of the metal is oxidized. At a sufficiently more positive potential (or less negative), the metal will spontaneously begin to form an oxide film on its surface. When this film fully covers the metal substrate, the metal is said to become passive and the potential at which this occurs is known as the passivating potential, E_{pp}.

Because there is now a kinetic barrier to further oxidation, the current which flows drops dramatically and the electrode enters into the passive range of behavior. As long as the oxide layer remains intact on the surface, further increases in electrode potential will not significantly increase the current which flows through the metal–solution interface. However, as the potential is increased in the passive range there is an increase in the thickness of the oxide film. This process is known as anodization and can be used to thicken the oxide film. For titanium, the anodization rate has been reported to be in the range of 20 Å/V (4).

If the potential is increased to a value where there is a change in the oxide layer which reduces its ability to kinetically limit further oxidation, the corrosion currents can increase and the electrode is said to enter transpassive behavior. This potential is referred to as the breakdown potential, E_b. Any changes in the barrier effect of the oxide film may be the result of changes in the oxide structure or composition, valence of the metal ions in the oxide, or fracture of the oxide layer. For titanium, the breakdown potential is several tens of volts, well outside of any potential developed in the body. However, Co–Cr and stainless steel alloys have a breakdown potential of about +550 mV. This breakdown potential is most likely due to the Cr_2O_3 undergoing a reaction to a chromate ion which is soluble, as is predicted by the equilibrium potential–pH diagram termed a Pourbaix diagram (14).

Please note that Figure 2 is an idealized plot of passive behavior and does not show any other oxidation or reduction reactions which may be ongoing concurrently (i.e., no oxide layer formation, precipitates, and/or ion interactions in solution). If a second electrode reaction, typically the reduction of oxygen, is present, the resultant polarization curve will be the sum of the two reactions. The summation effect can be seen in Figure 3. In this case, the overall polarization curve will be the sum of the two curves shown. In this case, the corrosion potential (or OCP) for the combined reactions will be where the O_2 reduction reaction curve intersects with the oxidation reaction of the metal. Also, the active to passive loop for the metal may be significantly suppressed on the combined curve because the reduction reaction will generate so much current as to overwhelm the currents associated with active to passive behavior. This more complex graph more accurately represents what happens when performing this type of testing on implant alloys using physiologically relevant solutions where there are hundreds to thousands of reactions occurring.

Electrochemical Impedance Spectroscopy

This technique is based on the fact that metal-oxide interfaces have characteristics which are related to electrical circuits. For instance, the transfer of metal ions across the interface can be thought of as a current whose driving force is the potential drop across the interface and the resistance is due to

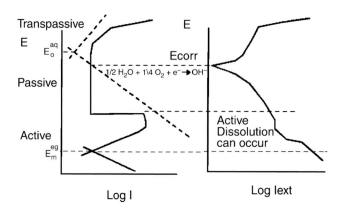

Figure 3 A schematic showing a polarization test in which there are two electrode reactions. One is a passivating metal and the other a reduction reaction (i.e., oxygen reduction). This more realistic schematic of an actual metal implant surface demonstrates the difficulty in ascertaining distinct electrochemical characteristics from real world samples (e.g., Ti-based alloy in bovine serum electrolyte).

the kinetic barriers to the movement of these ions. Also, at the interface there are positive and negative charges separated from one another known as the electrical double layer which creates an equivalent capacitor at the interface. Thus, the interface can be analogous to a resistor in parallel with a capacitor. Impedance spectroscopy uses alternating current techniques to determine the resistive and capacitive nature of the interface. From these experiments one can determine how difficult or easy it is to transport charge across the interface and also to determine the nature of the electrical double layer. With passivating metals, there is additional information which can be obtained about the growth and structure of the oxide layer as well (11). One of the results of these types of experiments is the determination of the polarization resistance. This is a term which describes the ease of ion transport across the interface. Higher polarization resistance implies lower corrosion rates. This technique has been used to assess the polarization resistance of Ti–6Al–4V in Ringers solution, Ringers with serum, and Ringers at pH = 1 (15). It was found that the polarization resistance of this alloy decreased (implying that the corrosion rate increased) with the addition of bovine serum and with a decrease in pH.

Metal Release Immersion Testing

During one type of immersion testing, samples are placed in a representative electrolyte solution for various periods of time and the concentration of ionic species released into solution is measured using atomic absorption spectroscopy (AAS) and inductively coupled plasma atomic emission spectroscopy to quantify the concentration of ions released. These techniques work by heating small volumes of solution containing the ions of interest until they are vaporized and further ionized. These ions form a plasma which will absorb or emit photons, respectively, at specific energies characteristic of the species and in proportion to the concentration of the species present. The above spectroscopic analysis techniques have high sensitivity (in parts per billion with proper experimental technique) but they cannot provide information about the valence state of the ions released. Valence state may be important to understand how these ions interact with proteins and ultimately influence the surrounding tissues.

Scanning Electrochemical Microscopy

This is a new technique which can be used to analyze and image the local microscopic heterogeneous corrosion behavior of metal–solution interfaces (12). This technique uses a solid microelectrode probe to investigate the release of ions from a metal surface on the microscopic scale. It has the ability to obtain images of the corrosion reactions at a metallic surface under a wide variety of conditions. These include assessment of the ease and distribution of oxidation and reduction processes on metal surfaces. While this technique is relatively new to orthopaedic biomaterials analysis, it may have significant application to the study of electrochemical processes at implant surfaces.

Surface Analytical Techniques

These techniques are used to evaluate the surface of metal alloys after they have been exposed to body simulating environments. Surface sensitive techniques include X-ray photoelectron spectroscopy (XPS), Auger electron spectroscopy (AES), secondary ion mass spectroscopy (SIMS), and others. These techniques are very sensitive and are used to evaluate the outermost surfaces of alloys. These techniques rely on photon-surface interactions and electron surface interactions to provide chemical information about the oxide layer. They are surface sensitive because the signal generated comes only from the outer 5 nm or so of the surface. Detailed description of these techniques is out of the scope of this chapter. One limitation with these techniques include the use of instruments which require very high vacuums and may alter or affect the nature of the surface.

CORROSION OF ORTHOPAEDIC ALLOYS

Metals provide the appropriate material properties such as high strength, ductility, fracture toughness, hardness, corrosion resistance, formability, and biocompatibility necessary for use in load bearing roles required in fracture fixation and total joint arthroplasty (TJA). There are three principal metal alloys used in orthopaedics and particularly in total joint replacement: (i) titanium based alloys, (ii) cobalt based alloys, and (iii) stainless steel alloys. The elemental composition of these three alloys is shown in Table 2. Alloy specific differences in strength, ductility, and hardness generally determine which of these three alloys is used for a particular application or implant component. However, it is primarily the high corrosion resistance of all metal alloys which has lead to their widespread use as implant materials. Implant alloys were originally developed for maritime and aviation uses where mechanical properties such as corrosion resistance and high strength are paramount.

It is important to understand that corrosion of orthopaedic biomaterials is not just an exercise in physics and chemistry. There are significant problems relating to corrosion of implant alloys in the current state-of-the-art implants which will likely continue to be a potential hazard for the near future. One of the current issues is the corrosion event observed in the taper connections of retrieved modular joint replacement components. With the large and growing number of total joint designs which use modular connections (i.e., metal-on-metal press-fit conical tapered connections), the effects of crevices, stress and motion take on increasing importance. Retrieval studies (16,17) have shown that severe corrosion attack can take place in the crevices formed by these tapers in vivo (Fig. 4). This attack was observed in components which consisted of Ti–6Al–4V alloy stems and Co–Cr heads as well as Co–Cr stems on Co–Cr heads. It has been postulated that this corrosion process is the result of a combination of stress and motion at the taper connection and the crevice geometry of the taper. The stresses resulting from use cause fracturing and abrasion of the oxide film covering these passive metal surfaces. This, in turn, causes significant changes in the metal surface potential (makes it more negative) and in the crevice solution chemistry as the oxides continuously fracture and repassivate. These changes may result in deaeration (loss of O_2) of the crevice solution and a lowering of the pH in the crevice (18) as is expected in crevice corrosion attack. The ultimate result of this process is a loss of the oxide film and its kinetic barrier effect and an increase in the rate of corrosive attack in the taper region.

Severe corrosion attack has been associated with Co–Cr alloy modular taper connections. While less common, corrosion attack of titanium alloy stems can also occur. In general, Co–Cr alloys undergo intergranular corrosion, etching, selective dissolution of cobalt, and the formation of Cr rich particles which are most likely oxides or oxychlorides. The corrosion products generated at the taper connections can migrate into periprosthetic tissues and in-between articulating polymeric surfaces. In the past there have been instances where retrieved implants have corroded to such an extent that intergranular corrosion resulted in fatigue failure in the neck of Co–Cr stems. These observations point to the important effect of combined

Table 2 Approximate Weight Percent of Different Metals Within Major Orthopaedic Alloys

Alloy	Ni	N	Co	Cr	Ti	Mo	Al	Fe	Mn	Cu	W	C	Si	V
Stainless steel (ASTM F138)	10–15.5	<0.5	–	17–19	–	2–4	–	61–68	–	<0.5	<2.0	<0.06	<1.0	–
CoCrMo alloys (ASTM F75)	<2.0	–	61–66	27–30	–	4.5–7.0	–	<1.5	<1.0	–	–	<0.35	<1.0	–
(ASTM F90)	9–11	–	46–51	19–20	–	–	–	<3.0	<2.5	–	14–16	<0.15	<1.0	–
(ASTM F562)	33–37	–	35	19–21	<1	9.0–11	–	<1	<0.15	–	–	–	<0.15	–
Ti alloys CPTi (ASTM F67)	–	–	–	–	99	–	–	0.2–0.5	–	–	–	<0.1	–	–
Ti–6Al–4V (ASTM F136)	–	–	–	–	89–91	–	5.5–6.5	–	–	–	–	<0.08	–	3.5–4.5
45TiNi	55	–	–	–	45	–	–	–	–	–	–	–	–	–

Note: Alloy composition are standardized by the American Society for Testing and Materials (ASTM vol. 13.01).
– Indicates less than 0.05%.

(A)   **(B)**

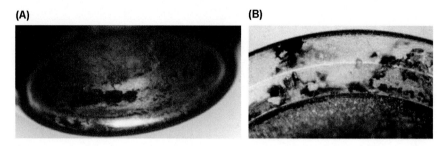

Figure 4 Retrieved joint replacement components showing corrosion around the rims of metal conical taper connections. **(A)** Cobalt-base alloy head showing evidence of corrosion precipitates. **(B)** Macrograph of deposits of $CrPO_4$ corrosion products on the rim of a modular cobalt–chrome femoral component. Both fretting and crevice corrosion are responsible for generating this type of implant degradation.

stresses and motion, and the electrochemical processes present at metal-oxide–solution interfaces. It cannot be stressed enough that it is the mechanical integrity of the oxide films which form on these alloys that determine long-term stability and performance of metallic components. Very little is known about the mechanical stability of oxide films and the electrochemical reactions, which occur when an oxide film is fractured. What is known is that when the oxide films of these orthopaedic alloys are abraded or removed from the surface by rubbing, that the open circuit potential can decrease to values as low as −500 mV (vs. SCE) (19).

These potential excursions may be significant enough and prolonged enough to cause changes in the oxide structure and stability by bringing the interface potential into the active range of the alloy, thereby dramatically accelerating the corrosion rate. Known corrosion properties of popular implant alloys are listed in Table 3 and discussed in the following sections.

Stainless Steel Alloys

Stainless steels were the first metals to be widely used for orthopaedic applications in 1926. However, it was 1943 before ASTM 304 was developed as a standard implant material. All steels are comprised of iron and carbon and commonly contain chromium, nickel, and molybdenum. Trace elements such as manganese, phosphorous, sulfur, and silicon are also present. Carbon and the other alloying elements affect the mechanical properties of steel through alteration of its microstructure.

The form of stainless steel most commonly used in orthopaedic practice is designated 316LV (American Society for Testing and Materials F138, ASTM F138). The number "316" classifies the material as austenitic, the "L" denotes the low carbon content and "V" the vacuum under which it is formed. The carbon content must be kept at a low level to prevent carbide

Table 3 Electrochemical Properties of Implant Metals (Corrosion Resistance) in 0.1 M NaCl at pH = 7

Alloy	ASTM Designation	Density (g/cm³)	Corrosion Potential (vs. Calomel) (mV)	Passive Current Density (mA/cm²)	Breakdown Potential (mV)
Stainless steel	ASTM F138	8.0	−400	0.56	200–770
Co–Cr–Mo alloys	ASTM F75	8.3	−390	1.36	420
Ti alloys CPTi	ASTM F67	4.5	−90 to −630	0.72–9.0	>2000
Ti-6Al-4V	ASTM 136	4.43	−180 to −510	0.9–2.0	>1500
Ti5Al2.5Fe	⁻	4.45	−530	0.68	>1500
Ni45Ti	⁻	6.4–6.5	−430	0.44	890

Note: The corrosion potential represents the open circuit potential (OCP) between the metal and a calomel electrode. The more negative the OCP, the more chemically reactive and thus the less corrosion resistance. Generally low current density indicates greater corrosion resistance. The higher the breakdown potential the better (i.e., the more elevated the breakdown potential, the more stable the protective layer).
⁻ Indicates no current ASTM standard.

(chromium–carbon) accumulation at the grain boundaries. This carbide formation weakens the material by allowing a combination of corrosion and stress to degrade the material at its grain boundaries. In the past, elevated levels of carbon have been associated with the fracture of some orthopaedic implants in vivo. Molybdenum is added to enhance the corrosion resistance of the grain boundaries, while chromium dissipated evenly within the microstructure allows the formation of chromium oxide (Cr_2O_3) on the surface of the metal. The ionic bonds associated with this coating protect the surface from electrochemical degradation. Stainless steels are surface treated (e.g., in nitric acid) to promote the growth and thickening of this passive oxide layer (2,20–22).

Cobalt–Chromium Alloys

Cobalt-based alloys were developed in 1926. In 1929 they were used in dentistry but were not used in orthopaedics until 1937 Co–Cr–Mo alloys were first used in orthopaedics (under the trade name Vitallium). The two basic constituents of all Co–Cr alloys are Co (approximately 65%) and Cr (approximately 35%). Co and Cr form a solid solution of large FCC grains.

Molybdenum is added to decrease the grain size and thus improve the mechanical properties. This homogeneous solid solution of Co, Cr, and Mo is comprised of a face centered cubic (austenitic) crystal, which is only retained if the metal is worked when it is still hot ($>650°C$, hot forging). However, when the metal is worked at room temperature (cold worked) an hexagonal close packed (HCP) phase is introduced which acts to harden and strengthen the metal, but which also reduces properties such as fatigue strength and ductility (Table 4). Cobalt–chromium implant alloys fall into one of two categories, those with nickel and other alloying elements and those without. Of the many Co–Cr alloys available, there are two most commonly used as implant alloys (Table 2): (i) cobalt–chromium–molybdenum (CoCrMo), which is designated ASTM F-75 and F-76, and (ii) cobalt–nickel–chromium–molybdenum (CoNiCrMo) designated as ASTM F-562. Others approved for implant use include one which incorporates tungsten (W) (CoCrNiW, ASTM F-90) and another with iron (CoNiCrMoWFe, ASTM F-563). Co–Ni–Cr–Mo alloys which contain large percentages of Ni (25–37%) promise increased corrosion resistance, yet raise concerns of possible toxicity and/or immunogenic reactivity (discussed later) from released Ni. The biologic reactivity of released Ni from Co–Ni–Cr alloys is cause for concern under static conditions. Due to their poor frictional (wear) properties, Co–Ni–Cr alloys are also inappropriate for use in articulating components. Therefore, the dominant implant alloy used for total joint components remains CoCrMo (ASTM F-75).

Titanium Alloys

Titanium alloys were developed in the mid-1940s for the aviation industry and were first used in orthopaedics around the same time. Two post-World War II alloys, commercially pure titanium (CpTi) and Ti–6Al–4V, remain the two dominant titanium alloys used in implants. Commercially pure titanium (CpTi, ASTM F67) is 98–99.6% pure titanium. The crystal structure of CpTi is HCP yet it can be cold worked for further improvement in the mechanical properties. The addition of other elements within a CpTi alloy drastically affects the mechanical properties. For example, the difference between 0.18% and 0.4% oxygen increases the yield strength three-fold (from 170 to 450 MPa). While CpTi is most commonly used in dental applications, the stability of the oxide layer formed on CpTi (and consequently its high corrosion resistance) and its relatively higher ductility (i.e., the ability to be cold worked) compared to Ti–6Al–4V has led to its use in porous coatings (e.g., fiber metal) of TJA components. Generally, Ti–6Al–4V (ASTM F-136) is used for joint replacement components because of its superior mechanical properties in comparison to CpTi (Table 4). The Ti–6Al–4V alloy (also known as Ti-6-4) is composed of grains of two phases: an HCP phase and a BCC phase referred to as the alpha and beta phases,

Table 4 Mechanical Properties of Implant Alloys

Implant Alloy	ASTM Designation	Trade Name and Company (Examples)	Elastic Modulus (GPa)	Yield Strength (MPa)	Ultimate Strength (MPa)	Fatigue Strength (Endurance Limit) (MPa)	Hardness, HVN	Elongation at Fracture (%)
Stainless Steel								
	ASTM F138	Protusul S30-Sulzer	190	792	930	241–820	130–180	43–45
CoCrMo alloys								
	ASTM F75	Alivium-Biomet CoCrMo-Biomet Endocast SIL-Krupp Francobal-Benoist Girard Orthochrome-DePuy Protosul 2-Sultzer Vinertia-Deloro Vitallium C-Howmedica Vitallium FHS-Howmedica Zimaloy-Zimmer Zimalloy Micrograin-Zimmer	210–253	448–841	655–1277	207–950	300–400	4–14
	ASTM F90	Vitallium W-Howdmedica	210	448–1606	1896	586–1220	300–400	10–22
	ASTM F562	HS251-Haynes Stellite	200–230	300–2000	800–2068	340–520	8–50 (RC)	10–40
		MP35N-Std Pressed Steel Corp.						

(*Continued*)

Table 4 Mechanical Properties of Implant Alloys (*Continued*)

Implant Alloy	ASTM Designation	Trade Name and Company (Examples)	Elastic Modulus (GPa)	Yield Strength (MPa)	Ultimate Strength (MPa)	Fatigue Strength (Endurance Limit) (MPa)	Hardness, HVN	Elongation at Fracture (%)
	ASTM 1537	TJA 1537-Allevac Metasul-Sulzer	200–300	960	1,300	200–300	41 (RC)	20
Ti alloys CPTi	ASTM F67	CSTi-Sulzer	110	485	760	300	120–200	14–18
Ti-6Al-4V	ASTM 136	Isotan-Aesculap Werke Protosul 64WF-Sulzer Tilastan-Waldemar Link Tivaloy 12-Biomet Tivanium-Zimmer	116	897–1034	965–1103	620–689	310	8
Ti5Al2.5Fe	—		100–110	780	860	300–725	310	7–13
Ni45Ti	—	Nitinol-Nitinol Medical Technologies	28–110	621–793	827–1172	<200	40–62 (RC)	1–60

— Indicates no current ASTM standard.
Abbreviations: RC, rockwell hardness scale; HVN, vickers hardness number (kg/mm).

respectively. Aluminum (Al, 5.5–6.5% by weight) stabilizes the HCP phase and vanadium (V, 3.5–4.5% by weight) stabilizes the BCC phase. The microstructure and mechanical properties of this alloy are highly dependent on the thermomechanical processing treatments. The Ti–6Al–4V alloy microstructure is generally composed of a fine-grained HCP phase with a sparse distribution of the BCC phase. If the material is cooled too slowly the BCC phase becomes more prominent and lowers the strength and corrosion resistance of the alloy.

Titanium alloys are particularly good implant materials because of their high corrosion resistance compared with stainless steel and Co–Cr–Mo alloys. A passive oxide film (primarily of TiO_2) protects both Ti–6Al–4V and CpTi. This stable and adherent passive oxide film protects Ti alloys from pitting corrosion, intergranular corrosion, and crevice corrosion attack and in large part is responsible for the excellent biocompatibility of Ti alloys. Generally, the strength of Ti–6Al–4V exceeds that of stainless steel, with a flexural rigidity roughly half of stainless steel and Co–Cr–Mo alloys. The torsional and the axial stiffness of Ti alloys are therefore closer to bone and theoretically provide less stress shielding than do Co alloys and stainless steel. This attribute, along with excellent biocompatibility and corrosion resistance, is primarily responsible for the popularity of titanium alloys in fracture fixation devices (plates, screws), spinal fixation devices, and total hip replacement femoral components. Ti–6Al–4V alloy is an example of a material which can be approximately 15% softer than Co–Cr–Mo alloys, yet when used in bearing applications results in significantly more than 15% greater wear than Co–Cr–Mo when used in orthopaedic applications, e.g., TKA or THA femoral heads. Thus, Ti alloys are seldom used as materials where resistance to wear is the primary concern (1,21–25).

New Alloys and Surface Coatings

The quest for new metal alloys with improved corrosion resistance, biocompatibility, and mechanical properties is ongoing. The use of Ti alloys, Co–Cr–Mo alloys, or stainless steels in a specific application generally involves trade-offs of one desirable property for another. New alloys seek improved material properties to overcome or minimize necessary trade-offs. "New" alloys are usually slight variations of alloys within the three categories of implant metals previously described which are already approved for use as implant materials.

New Titanium Alloys

One new group of Ti alloys proposed for orthopaedic applications are the so-called beta-titanium alloys which contain metal alloying elements that stabilize the beta (BCC) phase. One such alloy contains >10% Mo, a known beta stabilizer. These beta Ti alloys promise an increased fatigue strength and 20% reduction in the elastic modulus, which is closer to bone, minimizing the potential for stress shielding.

Other attempts at improving traditional Ti–6Al–4V alloys seek to improve biocompatibility and mechanical properties by the substitution of V (a relatively toxic metal) with other less toxic metals. Two such Ti alloys include Ti5Al2.5Fe and Ti6Al17Nb. These alloys have higher fatigue strength and a lower modulus, compared to Ti-6-4, thus enhancing bone to implant load transfer (Table 4).

Other Ti alloys are being developed for specific applications, such as TiTa30 which has been found to possess the same thermal coefficient of expansion as alumina (a ceramic currently used as femoral and head components), and can be bonded to the ceramic without induction of cracks within the metal. The combination of metal bonded to ceramic has the advantages of high fatigue resistance and high wear resistance. This couple is currently used in dental applications.

"Nitinol" is a nickel–titanium alloy which has "shape memory" properties and appears promising for orthopaedic applications. After these alloys are preformed into specific shapes, they can be manipulated into new shapes at temperatures below their transition temperature (T_s). Then when heated to temperatures above their transition temperature (15–75°C) they revert to their original shape. Biocompatibility concerns regarding Nitinols are centered on the Ni composition (55%) of these alloys. Despite this high amount of a relatively toxic metal, these "memory alloys" may allow implant shape changes in situ thereby expanding the capabilities of current implants.

New Stainless Steels

The relatively poor corrosion resistance and biocompatibility of stainless steels when compared to Ti and Co–Cr–Mo alloys provides incentive for development of improved stainless steels. New alloys such as BioDur 108 (Carpenter Technology Corp, Redington, Pensylvania U.S.A.) attempt to solve the problem of corrosion with an essentially nickel-free austenitic stainless alloy. This steel contains a high nitrogen content to maintain its austenitic structure and boasts improved levels of tensile yield strength, fatigue strength, and improved resistance to pitting corrosion and crevice corrosion as compared to nickel-containing alloys such as Type 316L (ASTM F138).

New Zirconium and Tantalum Alloys

Zirconium (Zr) and tantalum (Ta) are characterized as refractory metals (others include molybdenum and tungsten) because of their relative chemical stability (passive oxide layer) and high melting points. Zr and Ta alloys are currently in use and may be gaining popularity as orthopaedic metals. Because of the surface layer stability Zr and Ta (like Ti) are highly corrosion resistant. Corrosion resistance generally correlates with biocompatibility (although not always) because more stable metal alloys tend to be less chemically active and less participatory in biologic reactions. While elemental tantalum unites strength and corrosion resistance and has been used for more than 50 years in applications such nonload bearing applications as cranioplasty plates and pacemaker leads. Newer vapor deposition manufacturing techniques for Ta have enabled new orthopaedic applications such as the fabrication of metallic strut configurations similar in morphology to trabecular bone. This tantalum trabecular metal consists of interconnecting struts forming pores, results in a structural biomaterial and is 80% porous, which theoretically allows approximately two to three times greater bone ingrowth compared to conventional porous coatings. This new application promises double the interface shear strengths where the crystalline microtexture of a trabecular Ta strut is conductive to direct bone apposition.

Refractory metals such as Zr generally possess high levels of hardness (12 GPa) and wear resistance (approximately 10-fold that of Co and Ti alloys, using abrasion testing), which makes them well suited for bearing surface applications. The thickness of the surface oxide layer (approximately 5 μm) and ability to extend ceramic-like material properties (i.e., hardness) into the material through techniques such as oxygen enrichment has resulted in the production of TJA components using these alloys (e.g. oxidized zirconium TKA femoral components, Smith and Nephew). As difficulties associated with forming and machining these metals are overcome, the use of these materials is expected to grow (2,21,23–25).

METAL RELEASE

The issue of metal released from implants can be broken down into four basic questions: (i) How much metal is released from the implant? (ii) Where is the metal transported and in what quantity? (iii) What is the chemical form of the released metal (e.g., inorganic precipitate vs. soluble organometallic complex) and (iv) What are the pathophysiological consequences of such metal release? With regard to the first two questions, there is a growing body of literature addressing these issues. What little is currently known with regard to the latter two questions is discussed later.

There is a considerable body of literature concerning serum and urine chromium, cobalt, and nickel levels following total joint replacement, but relatively fewer studies examining titanium, aluminum, and vanadium levels. Many investigations have been hampered by technical limitations of the analytical instrumentation, inadequate contamination precautions, and/or suboptimal study designs. Furthermore, it is difficult to compare the results from different laboratories since different techniques and protocols produce different results.

Normal human serum levels of prominent implant metals are approximately 1–10 ng/mL aluminum, 0.15 ng/mL chromium, <0.01 ng/mL vanadium, 0.1–0.2 ng/mL cobalt, and <4.1 ng/mL titanium. Following total joint arthroplasty levels of circulating metal (Co, Cr, Ni, Al, and V) have been shown to increase (Table 5).

Multiple studies have demonstrated chronic elevations in serum and urine cobalt and chromium following total primary total joint replacement. Chronic elevations in serum titanium concentrations in subjects with well-functioning THR with titanium-containing components have also been reported without measurable differences in urine titanium concentrations, serum aluminum concentrations, or urine aluminum concentrations. Vanadium concentrations have not been found to be elevated in patients with TJA partially due to the technical difficulty associated with measuring the small concentrations present in serum.

Metal ion levels within serum and urine of TJA patients can be affected by a variety of factors. For example, patients with total knee

Table 5 Approximate Concentrations of Metal in Human Body Fluids and in Human Tissue with and Without Total Joint Replacements (34,126)

		Ti	Al	V	Co	Cr	Mo	Ni
Human body fluids ($\times 10^{-3}$ mM)								
Serum	Normal	0.06	0.08	<0.02	0.003	0.001	–	0.007
	TJA	0.09	0.09	0.03	0.007	0.006	–	<0.16
Urine	Normal	<0.04	0.24	0.01	–	0.001	–	–
	TJA	0.07	0.24	<0.01	–	0.009	–	–
Whole blood	Normal	0.35	0.48	0.12	0.002	0.058	0.009	0.078
	TJA	1.4	8.1	0.45	0.33	2.1	0.104	0.50
Human tissue (µg/g) (roughly equivalent to 0.1–0.01 mM)								
Skeletal muscle	Normal	–	–	–	<12	<12	–	–
	TJA	–	–	–	160	570	–	–
Liver	Normal	100	890	14	120	<14	–	–
	TJA	560	680	22	15200	1130	–	–
Lung	Normal	710	9830	26	–	–	–	–
	TJA	980	8740	23	–	–	–	–
Spleen	Normal	70	800	<9	30	10	–	–
	TJA	1280	1070	12	1600	180	–	–
Kidney	Normal	–	–	–	30	<40	–	–
	TJA	–	–	–	60	<40	–	–
Lymphatic Tissue	Normal	–	–	–	10	690	–	–
	TJA	–	–	–	390	690	–	–
Heart	Normal	–	–	–	30	30	–	–
	TJA	–	–	–	280	90	–	–

Note: Normal, Subjects without any metallic prosthesis (not including dental); TJA, Subjects with well functioning total joint arthroplasty.
– Data Not Available (33,87,127,128).

replacement components containing titanium-base alloy and carbon fiber reinforced polyethylene wear couples demonstrated 10-fold elevations in serum titanium concentration at an average of four years after implantation. Substantial serum titanium elevations have also been reported in patients with failed metal-backed patellar components where unintended metal/metal articulation was possible. These individuals contained serum titanium levels up to a hundred times higher than normal. However, even among these THA patients, there was no elevation in serum or urine aluminum, serum or urine vanadium levels, or urine titanium levels.

Mechanically-assisted crevice corrosion of modular total hip arthroplasty components has been associated with elevations in serum cobalt and urine chromium. It has been previously assumed that extensively porous coated cementless stems would give rise to higher serum and urine chromium concentrations due to the larger surface area available for passive dissolution. However, some studies suggest that a predominant source of disseminated chromium degradation products is most likely the fretting corrosion modular junctions.

The form(s) of released metal in vivo remain relatively uncharacterized. What metal bioreactivity has been characterized in vitro using metal ions in culture medium with 10% serum (as is the case with most in vitro investigations) may differ from in vivo conditions of essentially 100% serum, where relatively inert compounds (e.g., metal oxides) and complexes (e.g., metal–albumin) may more readily form and abrogate (or exaggerate) the toxic effects of metals. Metal ions released in vivo (26) and in vitro (27) are bound by specific serum proteins. Where two molecular weight ranges of human serum proteins were determined to be associated with the binding of Cr from Co–Cr–Mo (ASTM F-75) implant alloy degradation (at approximately 68 and 180 kDa), only one range of serum protein(s) (at approximately 68 kDa) is associated with the binding of Ti released from Ti–6Al–4V implant alloy. The role of serum or tissue proteins in the mediation of metal-induced effects remains largely unknown.

While it has been repeatedly demonstrated that chronic elevations in serum and urine metal content are associated with total joint replacement components, the toxicological importance of these findings are not known. Currently, there is quite limited information in the literature which describes the chemical form of the degradation products of metallic joint replacement prostheses. Ultimately, specific toxicological experiments of relevant chemical species identified by bioavailability studies will be used in animal models and cell cultures to define specific toxicities of the degradation products. However, at the present time this information is not available.

Postmortem studies: Homogenates of remote organs and tissue obtained postmortem from subjects with cobalt base alloy total joint replacement components have indicated that significant increases in cobalt and chromium concentrations occur in the heart, liver, kidney, spleen, and lymphatic tissue (Table 5). Similarly, patients with titanium-base alloy implants demonstrated elevated titanium, aluminum, and vanadium levels around their metal implants (with up to 200 ppm of titanium, six orders of magnitude greater than that of controls, 880 ppb of aluminum, and 250 ppb of vanadium). Spleen aluminum levels and liver titanium concentrations can also be markedly elevated in patients with failed titanium-alloy implants. It has been found that even in the absence of significant elevations in serum metal concentrations, deposition of metal can occur locally and in remote organ stores in association with a well-functioning device (28–30).

Particle Release and Distribution

Particulate debris comprises the large portion of degradation products generated by joint replacement prostheses. Although polyethylene particles are generally recognized as the most prevalent particles in the periprosthetic milieu, metallic and ceramic particulate species are also present in variable amounts and may have important sequelae. When present in sufficient amounts, particulates generated by wear, corrosion, or a combination of processes which then induce the formation of an inflammatory, foreign-body granulation tissue with the ability to invade the bone-implant interface. This may result in progressive, periprosthetic bone loss that threatens the fixation of both cemented and cementless devices, limiting the survivorship of total joint replacement prosthesis.

Consequently, particulate wear debris of polymers, ceramic material, and metal alloys used in prosthetic components have been the subject of intense study concerning their role in bone resorption and aseptic loosening. There have been numerous reports indicating that modular femoral total hip replacement components can undergo severe corrosion at the tapered interface between their head and neck. The clinical significance of corrosion at the modular head/neck junction lies, in part, in the effects that solid corrosion products increase the particulate burden within the joint and migrate along bone-implant interface membranes to sites remote from their origin. They can also migrate to the prosthetic bearing surface where they may result in three-body wear, thereby increasing the production of polyethylene debris. All of these factors can contribute to periprosthetic bone loss and aseptic loosening.

Generally, metal particles found disseminated beyond the periprosthetic tissue are submicron in size. Although variables influencing accumulation of wear debris in remote organs are not clearly identified, numerous case reports document the presence of metallic, ceramic, or polymeric wear debris from hip and knee prostheses in regional and pelvic lymph nodes. Postmortem studies have demonstrated that dissemination of wear particles to the liver, spleen, or abdominal lymph nodes is a common occurrence in patients who have a total hip or knee replacement (31–33). These studies also revealed both metallic and polyethylene wear particles in the para-aortic lymph nodes of approximately 90% of patients with a joint replacement prosthesis. Whereas metallic wear particles alone were present in the para-aortic lymph nodes of approximately 70% of patients with a hip or knee. Of these approximately 40% of TJA patients were reported to have particles disseminated to the liver or spleen. Most disseminated metallic particles have been reported to be less than 1 μm in size, but the range of particle sizes is material dependant. Particles of commercially pure titanium and titanium–aluminum–vanadium alloy may range from 0.1 μm to as large as 50 μm in the lymph nodes and as large as 10 μm in the liver and spleen. In contrast, particles of cobalt–chromium and stainless steel alloys rarely exceed 3 μm. The response to metallic (and polymeric) debris in lymph nodes includes immune activation of macrophages and associated production of inflammatory cytokines. Metallic and polyethylene wear particles in the liver or spleen are more prevalent in patients who have had a previously failed reconstruction when compared to patients with primary hip or knee arthroplasties (34). While there have been numerous investigations concerning particulate debris of the periprosthetic tissues, particularly with regard to the phenomenon of particle-induced, macrophage-mediated osteolysis, relatively little is known about the dissemination of wear debris beyond the local tissues. Identification of orthopaedic wear debris can be difficult, even in regional lymph nodes, due to the coexistence of particles from other sources.

The clinical significance of orthopaedic wear debris accumulation at remote sites has been understood based largely on examination of lymph nodes biopsied at revision surgery or for cancer staging in patients who also happened to have a total joint replacement. Numerous case reports document the presence of metallic, ceramic, or polymeric wear debris from hip and knee prostheses in regional and pelvic lymph nodes (along with the findings of lymphadenopathy, gross pigmentation due to metallic debris, fibrosis, lymph node necrosis, and histiocytosis, including complete effacement of nodal architecture). The inflammatory response to metallic and polymeric debris in lymph nodes has been demonstrated to include immune activation of macrophages and associated production of cytokines. Accumulation of debris in remote organs and lymph nodes may explain, in part, past observations suggest that circulating peripheral blood monocytes from patients with joint replacements are more reactive to particulate wear debris stimulation than monocytes from individuals without implants (35–40).

LOCAL TISSUE EFFECTS

The tissues surrounding modern implants may include areas of bone ingrowth (osseointegration), fibrous encapsulation, and a variable presence of the foreign-body responses. There are no generalized types of metal release known to occur with all metallic implants. However, accelerated corrosion and a tissue response that can be directly related to identifiable corrosion products have been demonstrated in the tissues surrounding multipart devices.

Histological sections of the tissues surrounding stainless steel internal fixation devices generally show encapsulation by a fibrous membrane with little or no inflammation over most of the device. However, at screw-plate junctions, surrounding tissue membranes often contain cells such as macrophage, foreign-body giant cells, and lymphocytes. These cells are present in reaction to two types of particulate debris, (i) predominantly iron contain granules and microplates, and (ii) larger particles of predominantly chromium compounds, e.g. chromium phosphate.

Chromium microplates are of variable morphology and are found within the tissues as closely packed, plate-like particle aggregates ranging in size from 0.5 to 5.0 μm. They are often found free within acellular collagen or within frankly necrotic tissue. Several multinucleated foreign-body giant cells are usually present within or bordering collections of these particles. In hematoxylin and eosin preparations, the majority of microplates are yellow or "apple-green." Many microplates, however, stain darkly with hematoxylin and these microplates also react strongly to staining for iron. Electron microprobe energy-dispersive X-ray analyses indicate that microplates are a chromium compound containing iron and a substantial amount of phosphorous.

Iron granules are often seen surrounding chromium microplates, but the granules are found alone as well. Iron granules are yellow-brown, mainly spherical, and 0.1–3 μm in diameter. They are predominantly intracellular, most often in macrophages, but may also be found in fibrocytes. X-ray diffraction indicates that the granules consist of a mixture of two or more of the iron oxides, αFe_2O_3 and σFe_2O_3, and the hydrated iron oxides, $\alpha Fe_2O_3 \cdot H_2O$ and $\sigma Fe_2O_3 \cdot H_2O$.

The nature of the corrosion products were similar whether the modular heads had been mated with cobalt–chromium alloy or Ti–6Al–4V alloy femoral stems. The principal corrosion product was identified by electron microprobe energy-dispersive X-ray analysis and Fourier-transform infrared microprobe spectroscopy as a chromium orthophosphate hydrate rich material. This corrosion product was present at the modular head–neck junction and as particles within the joint pseudocapsules, the bone–implant interface membranes, and at sites of femoral osteolytic lesions.

Particles of the chromium–phosphate hydrate rich material can be found at the bearing surface of the UHMWPE acetabular liners, suggesting they may participate in articular surface three-body wear resulting in an increased production of polyethylene debris. Particles of the chromium-phosphate hydrate rich corrosion product found in tissues range in size from submicron to aggregates of particles up to 500 μm. These particles are similar in appearance to the chromium containing microplates observed in association with corroded stainless steel implants when viewed through a light microscope. Larger particles are often found within areas of marked fibrosis or necrosis or associated with foreign-body giant cells, although most of these particles are less than 5 μm in size and are found within macrophages.

The degradation products that can be observed in histologic sections of tissues adjacent to titanium base alloys are of a different nature than the precipitates associated with stainless steel and cobalt base alloys that have undergone accelerated corrosion. Titanium base alloys, although very corrosion resistant, typically discolor darkly stain adjacent tissue due to metallic debris. Examination has found the ratios of titanium, aluminum, and vanadium concentrations in the periprosthetic tissues are similar to those of the bulk alloy. This suggests that the metallic debris represented wear particles from the head or stem rather than precipitated corrosion products. This wear debris presents enormous surface areas for electrochemical dissolution. This additional metal available for dissolution is likely a major factor contributing to observed systemic elevations in titanium (Table 5).

REMOTE AND SYSTEMIC EFFECTS

General Considerations

As previously noted above, there is a long clinical experience with permanent and temporary metallic implants. The biocompatibility of such implants has always been of concern with regard to the local tissue reaction. The use of porous metallic coatings for cementless fixation of total joint replacement components with surface areas an order of magnitude higher than solid implants of comparable dimensions has intensified this concern, particularly because these prostheses are intended for use in younger, more active patient populations. The implants, or wear debris generated from the implant, may release chemically active metal ions into the surrounding tissues. While these ions may stay bound to local tissues, there is an increasing recognition that metal ions may also bind to protein moieties that are transported in the bloodstream and/or lymphatics and hence to remote organs (41). As previously stated the problem of "metal ion release" can be broken down into four basic questions: (i) How much metal is released from the implant? (ii) Where is the metal transported and in what quantity? (iii) What is the chemical form of the released metal (e.g., inorganic precipitate vs. soluble organometallic complex), and (iv) What are the pathophysiological consequences of such metal release? The little that is currently known about the latter two questions will be discussed in the following section.

The concern about the release and distribution of metallic degradation products is justified by the known potential toxicities of the elements used in modern orthopaedic implant alloys—titanium, aluminum, vanadium, cobalt, chromium, and nickel. Broad reviews of the toxicology of these elements are available (42,43) and are summarized below. In general terms, metal toxicity may be by virtue of (i) metabolic alterations, (ii) alterations in host/parasite interactions, (iii) immunologic interactions of metal moieties by virtue of their ability to act as haptens (specific immunological activation) or anti-chemotactic agents (nonspecific immunological suppression) (44,45), and (iv) by chemical carcinogenesis (46).

Cobalt, chromium, nickel, and vanadium are all essential trace metals in that they are required for certain enzymatic reactions (47). In excessive amounts however, these elements are also toxic. Excessive cobalt may lead to polycythemia (48), hypothyroidism (48), cardiomyopathy and carcinogenesis (49,50). Chromium can lead to nephropathy, hypersensitivity, and carcinogenesis (51,52). Nickel can lead to eczematous dermatitis, hypersensitivity, and carcinogenesis (53). Vanadium can lead to cardiac and renal dysfunction, and has been associated with hypertension (54) and depressive psychosis (55). The nonessential metallic elements also possess specific toxicities. Titanium, although generally regarded as inert, has been associated with pulmonary disease in patients with occupational exposure (56) and in animal models (57). Aluminum toxicity is well documented in the setting of renal failure and can lead to anemia (58), osteomalacia (59), and neurological dysfunction possibly including Alzheimer's disease (60). However, considering the litany of documented toxicities of these elements, it is important to remember that the toxicities generally apply to soluble forms of these elements and may not apply to the chemical species that are the degradation products of prosthetic implants.

The carcinogenic potential of the metallic elements used in THA is obviously an area of concern, particularly because the high surface area of cementless porous coated devices is intended for implantation in younger more active patient population that may have implant life expectancies exceeding 30 years. Animal studies have documented the carcinogenic potential of these implant materials. For example, Memoli et al. (61) reported a small increase in sarcoma in rats with implants which had high cobalt, chromium, or nickel contents. Furthermore, lymphomas with bone involvement were found to be more common in rats with metallic implants.

There are a significant number of reports of implant site tumors in dogs and cats—primarily osteosarcoma and fibrosarcoma associated with stainless steel internal fixation devices (1). There are relatively few case reports of malignant tumors associated with human total joint replacements (62) but the number of case reports is increasing. Concerted efforts are under way to accumulate cases of implant site malignant neoplasm associated with total joint replacements to better define the prospective risks (63).

Large-scale epidemiological studies are even fewer in number. One such recent epidemiological investigation documented increased incidence of implant site tumors and leukemia/lymphoma in patients with cobalt-base alloy THA (44), while another study reaffirmed the increased incidence of leukemia/lymphoma (64). Interestingly, both of these studies demonstrated a decreased incidence of breast carcinoma.

At this point in time, the association of metal release from orthopaedic implants with any metabolic, bacteriologic, immunologic, or carcinogenic toxicity is conjectural since cause and effect have not been established in human subjects. However, this is due in large part to the difficulty of observation in that most symptoms attributable to systemic and remote toxicity can be expected to occur in a finite frequency in any population of orthopaedic patients. Thus, the identification of implant referable disease processes at sites remote from the implant depends upon the availability of comparative epidemiology or the ability to perform tests upon the patient before and after device removal. There is insufficient epidemiological follow-up data on joint replacement procedures, except for a few selected aspects such as pain, joint mobilization, and device survivorship which relates only to the implant procedure itself and not to any remote or systemic effects.

Effects of Metal on Cells

In vitro investigations indicate that specific metals in ionic form can affect the functionality of a variety of peri-implant cells such as fibroblasts, osteoblasts, macrophages, and lymphocytes within the ranges of metal concentrations reported to exist in periprosthetic tissue. Generally, the most toxic metal ions have been found to be Ni, Fe, Cu, Mn, and V while others such as Na, Cr, Mg, Mo, Al, Ta, and Co demonstrate relatively less cellular reactivity in vitro. Different metals act through different cellular mechanisms to induce distinct responses. There is mounting evidence that adverse local and remote tissue responses that in the past have been entirely associated with metal particles, to some extent may be due to soluble forms of specific metal degradation products (26,65). However, the effects of soluble metals on periprosthetic cells is a complex function of cell type, composition, and concentration of metal. In vitro investigation has determined the stimulatory effect of some metals (e.g., Al and V) on cells such as lymphocytes and fibroblasts, while the same metals (and concentrations) can suppress the viability and proliferation of other cell types (e.g., osteoblast-like cells). This differential impact of metal ions on some cell types and not others (particularly fibroblasts and osteoblasts) may potentially explain how fibrous membranes so readily form around implants initially placed in intimate contact with bone (i.e., osteoblasts). This contention is supported by past investigations (66,67) where metal ions such as Al, V, and Ti have been shown to inhibit apatite formation in vitro by blinding and blocking potential crystal growth sites. This poisoning of crystal growth sites by metal ions may thus act to interfere with normal in vivo osteoid mineralization and remodeling process of bone (66,67). Adverse local and remote tissue responses purportedly associated with particulate debris may be due in part to specific soluble metals resulting from implant degradation.

High concentrations of metals negatively impact all types of cells at some level (68–79). For certain cell types, such as human osteoblasts, these effects have been somewhat characterized. One of the main functions of osteoblasts (if not the main function) is to produce organic bone matrix, 90% of which is Type I collagen. Type I collagen is comprised of three helical chains. Two of the three helical protein chains are $\alpha1(I)$. The third chain, $\alpha2(I)$, is similar in structure yet genetically distinct from $\alpha1(I)$. Metal particles and ions have been found to decrease gene expression of procollagen $\alpha1(I)$ before decreases could be observed in other more osteoblast-specific markers of bone deposition such as gene expression of osteocalcin, and osteonectin and alkaline phosphatase (80–82). Other metal-induced effects on osteoblasts have been noted such as the production of cytokines which recruit and prime activate inflammatory cells. Interleukin-6 is secreted by osteoblasts in response to Al, Fe, Mn, Na, Ni, and V chloride solutions (more toxic metals). The concentrations of metal ions associated with toxic osteoblast responses can be detected within some ranges of metal concentrations reported to exist in periprosthetic tissue (Table 4) (75). The comparison of the effects of metal ions on osteoblasts to the effects of particles previously reported (82) demonstrates the potential of specific metal ions released from implants or particulate implant debris to play a role clinically in the pathogenesis of osteolysis. Whether through indirect osteoclast activation (i.e., IL-6 release via osteoblasts) or direct inhibitory effects on osteoblasts, it is apparent that metal ions released from implants have the potential to diminish bone formation, which previously has been largely attributed to particulate implant debris alone.

Important to the assessment of metal-induced osteolysis is the role of other peri-implant cells such as fibroblasts, osteoclasts, macrophages, and lymphocytes, which, after exposure to metal ions, may affect osteoblast function through paracrine mediators (69). Although osteoclast activity has been reportedly impaired by exposure to metal ions at sublethal concentrations (72) these effects may be overridden by metal-induced autocrine and paracrine induction of IL-6, which can act to directly stimulate osteoclast activity. Thus, further study using mixed cell populations is required to more comprehensively assess released implant metal effects within the peri-implant milieu.

Immunogenicity of Metallic Implants

Some adverse responses to orthopaedic biomaterials are subtle and continue to foster debate and investigation. One of these responses is "metal allergy" or hypersensitivity to metallic biomaterials. Dermal hypersensitivity to metal is common, affecting about 10–15% of the population (83–86). Dermal contact and ingestion of metals have been reported to cause immune reactions which most typically manifest as skin hives, eczema, redness and itching (83,87,88). As previously stated, all metals in contact with biological systems corrode (89,90) and the released ions, while not sensitizers on their own, can activate the immune system by forming complexes with native proteins (85,91,92). These metal–protein complexes are considered to be candidate antigens (or more loosely termed, allergens) for eliciting hypersensitivity responses. Metals known as sensitizers include beryllium (93), nickel (86–88,93), cobalt (93), and chromium (93), while occasional responses have been reported to tantalum (94), titanium (95,96), and vanadium (94). Nickel is the most common metal sensitizer in humans followed by cobalt and chromium (83,86–88). The prevalence of metal sensitivity among the general population is approximately 10–15%, with nickel sensitivity the highest (approximately 14%) (83). Cross reactivity between nickel and cobalt is most common (83,85). The amounts of these metals found in medical grade alloys were shown in Table 2.

Hypersensitivity can be either an immediate (within minutes) humoral response (initiated by antibody or formation of antibody–antigen complexes of types I, II and III reactions), or a delayed (hours to days) cell-mediated response (97,98). It is the latter response with which implant related hypersensitivity reactions are generally associated, in particular Type IV Delayed Type Hypersensitivity (DTH).

Cell mediated delayed type hypersensitivity is characterized by antigen activation of sensitized T_{DTH} lymphocytes releasing various cytokines which result in the recruitment and activation of macrophages. T_{DTH} lymphocytes are subset populations of T helper (T_H) lymphocytes purported to be of the CD4+ T_{H-1} subtype (and in rare instances CD8+, cytotoxic T cells, T_C). This T_{H-1} subpopulation of T cells is characterized by their cytokine release profile, e.g., interferon-γ (IFN-γ), tumor necrosis factor-α (TNF-α), interleukin-1 (IL-1), and interleukin-2 (IL-2). T_{H-1} cells are generally associated with responses to intracellular pathogens and autoimmune diseases. Although T_{DTH} cells mediate a DTH reaction, only 5% of the participating cells are antigen specific T_{DTH} cells within a fully developed DTH response. The majority of DTH participating cells are macrophages.

Metals from implant corrosion have been shown in case studies to be temporally associated with specific responses such as severe dermatitis, urticaria, vasculitis (99–104), and/or nonspecific immune suppression (44,45 105–107).

Generally, there are more case reports of hypersensitivity reactions associated with stainless steel and cobalt alloy implants than with titanium alloy components (1,84,85,99,100,102,108–111). One such case report implicated cobalt hypersensitivity in the poor performance of cobalt alloy plates and screws used in the fracture fixation of 45-year-old woman's left radius and ulna. In this case, the patient presented with periprosthetic fibrosis, patchy muscular necrosis and chronic inflammatory changes peripherally, seven years after implantation. After removal of all metal hardware, the swelling (48) isappeared and eventually the patient became complaint free. However, there remained a hypersensitivity to cobalt as evaluated by patch testing (104).

This and similar case reports prompted a number of larger patient cohort studies in the late 1970s and 1980s investigating the possible correlation between metal sensitivity and implant failure (84,111–123). Data (from these different investigations) regarding the prevalence of metal sensitivity are compiled in Figure 5. Unfortunately, these studies include heterogeneous patient populations and testing methodologies and consequently reach a variety of conclusions. However, all patient populations included in Figure 5

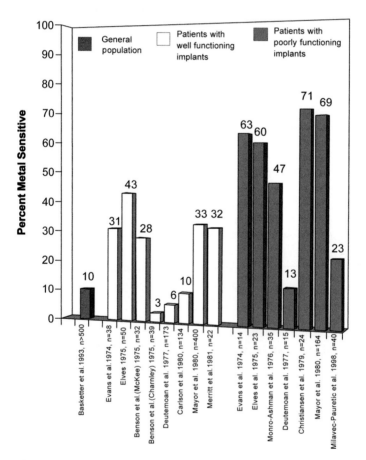

Figure 5 The bars indicate the average percentages of metal sensitivity (for nickel, cobalt, or chromium) among the general population and total arthroplasty patients with poorly and well-functioning implants based on a number of published reports. Note that the average incidence of metal sensitivity is 10, 25, and 60% for the population at large, patients with well-functioning total joint prosthesis and patients with poorly functioning implants, respectively.

were metal allergy tested to one or a combination of metals including nickel, cobalt, and/or chromium after receiving an implant. The prevalence of metal sensitivity among patients with well functioning implants is approximately 25%, roughly twice as high as that of the general population (108,111 114,116,118,121,122,124,125). Overall, the prevalence of metal sensitivity in patients with failed or failing implants is approximately six times that of the general population and approximately two to three times that of all patients with metal implants. Unfortunately, this association does not ascertain what is the cause of this effect; i.e., are these patients sensitive because the device has failed or has the device failed because the patient had a pre-existing metal sensitivity or are alternate dominating mechanisms (e.g., genetic auto-immunity) responsible for both?

Specific types of implants with greater propensity to corrosde and/or release metal in vivo may be more prone to induce metal sensitivity. Failures of total hip prostheses with metal-on-metal bearing surfaces have been associated with greater prevalence of metal sensitivity than similar designs with metal-on-ultrahigh molecular weight polyethylene bearing surfaces (112,125).

It is unclear whether hypersensitivity responses to metallic biomaterials affect implant performance in other than a few highly predisposed people (85,97,126). It is clear that some patients experience excessive eczemic immune reactions directly associated with implanted metallic materials (84,99,101). Metal sensitivity may exist as an extreme complication in only a few highly susceptible patients (i.e., less than 1% of joint replacement recipients), or it may be a more common subtle contributor to implant failure. Continuing improvements in immunologic testing methods will likely enhance future assessment of patients susceptible to hypersensitivity responses. The importance of this line of investigation is growing, as the use of metallic implants is increasing and as expectations of implant durability and performance increase (25,127,128).

Carcinogenesis

The carcinogenic potential of the metals used in TJA and other implants (e.g., nickel–titanium alloy arterial stents) remains an area of concern. Animal studies have documented the carcinogenic potential of orthopaedic implant materials. Small increases in rat sarcomas were noted to correlate with high serum cobalt, chromium, or nickel content from metal implants. Furthermore, lymphomas with bone involvement were also more common in rats with metallic implants. Implant site tumors in dogs and cats—primarily osteosarcoma and fibrosarcoma have been associated with stainless steel internal fixation devices.

Initially, epidemiological studies implicated cancer incidence in the first and second decades following total hip replacement. However, larger, more recent studies have found no significant increase in leukemia or lymphoma, although these studies did not include as large a proportion of subjects with a metal-on-metal prostheses. There are constitutive differences in the populations with and without implants that are independent of the implant itself, which confound the interpretation of epidemiological investigations.

The association of metal release from orthopaedic implants with carcinogenesis remains conjectural since causality has not been definitely established in human subjects. The identification of such an association depends both on the availability of comparative epidemiology and on the ability to perform tests on the patient before and after device removal. Due to a number of factors such as patient age, the actual number of reported cases of tumors associated with orthopaedic implants is likely under-reported. However, with respect to the number of devices implanted on a yearly basis the incidence of cancer at the site of implantation is relatively rare. Continued surveillance and longer term epidemiological studies are required to fully address these issues.

FUTURE DIRECTIONS AND CONCLUSIONS

Corrosion of orthopaedic implants remains a significant clinical concern. Even though past implant alloys have been replaced with modern corrosion resistant "super alloys," deleterious corrosion processes have been observed in certain clinical settings. There is reason to believe that attention to (i) metallurgical processing variables, (ii) tolerances of modular connections, (iii) surface processing modalities, and (iv) appropriate material selection all can diminish corrosion and minimize the potential for adverse clinical outcome. The potential exists for future surface treatments (e.g., nitriding, ion implantation, etc.) to significantly reduce the magnitude of fretting corrosion of titanium alloy and other metal implant devices.

There remains a need to further investigate the mechanical–electrochemical interactions of metal surfaces. Characterization of the stresses and motion needed to fracture passivating oxide films as well as the effects of repeated oxide abrasion on the electrochemical behavior of the interface and ultimately the implant continue to be actively investigated. Evaluating the role of particulate corrosion products in adverse local tissue reactions also requires continuing investigation. Thus, further clinical retrieval studies and in vitro cell culture experiments are needed to more fully characterize this relationship. Finally, the clinical significance of metal release and elevated metal content in body fluids and remote organs of patients with metallic implants needs to be elucidated. Considerable work will be required in discerning the chemical form(s) of released metal and the nature of its ligands to ultimately resolve questions of potential toxicity.

This chapter has focused on what is known of both the corrosion of implant metals and the local and systemic biologic effects over the long term. It is important to note that when evaluating the biocompatibility of a particular metal component, the results do not necessarily apply to all implants made of the same material. The definition of "biocompatibility" remains the ability of a material to demonstrate host and material response appropriate to its intended application. Reasons for poor implant performance can be attributed to many factors, which include manufacturing errors, mechanical design errors, surgical errors, and inappropriate choice of material for a given application. Wise material selection cannot compensate for poor implant design or surgical error. It must be emphasized that currently there is no universal "best" metal for all implant applications. Ultimately, the most prudent choice of a corrosion resistant metal for a particular application depends on careful evaluation of which specific mechanical properties of available materials (in addition to corrosion resistance) best satisfy the in situ demands and design characteristics of a particular implant component.

REFERENCES

1. Black J. Orthopaedic Biomaterials in Research and Practice. New York: Churchill Livingstone, 1988.
2. Jacobs JJ, Gilbert JL, Urban RM. Corrosion of metal orthopaedic implants. J Bone Joint Surg Am 1998; 80:268–282.
3. Lacombe P. Corrosion and oxidation of Ti and Ti alloys. In: Ti, Ti Alloys, Williams JC, Belor AF, eds. New York: Plenum Press, 1982:847–880.
4. Aladjem A. Review: Anodic oxidation of titanium and its alloys. J Mater Sci 1973; 8:688–704.
5. Cabrera N, Mott NF. Physics 1948; 12:163–164
6. Fraker A, Ruff AW, Yeager M. Studies of oxide film formation on titanium alloys in physiological solutions. Corros Sci 1973; 11:763–765.
7. Brown GM, Thundat T, Allison DA, Warmack RJ. Electrochemical and in-situ atomic force microscopy investigation of tiatnium in oxalic acid. J Vac Sci Technol 1992; 10:3001–3006.
8. Healy KE, Ducheyne P. The mechanisms of passive dissolution of titanium in model physiologic environment. J Biomed Mater Res 1992; 26:181–186.
9. Williams RL, Brown SA, Merritt K. Electrochemical studies on the influence of proteins on the corrosion of implant alloys. Biomaterials 1988; 9:181–186.
10. Wishey A, Gregson PJ, Peter LM. Effect of surface treatment on the dissolution of titanium based implant materials. Biomaterials 1991; 12:470–473.
11. MacDonald JR. Impedance Spectroscopy New York: Wiley Interscience, 1987.
12. Gilbert JL, Smith SM, Lautenschlager EP. Scanning electrochemical microscopy of metallic biomaterials: reaction rate and ion release imaging modes. J Biomed Mater Res 1993; 27:1357–1366.
13. Bard AJ, Faulkner LR. Electrochemical Methods. New York: Wiley, 1980.
14. Pourbaix M. Electrochemical corrosion of metallic biomaterials. Biomaterials 1984; 5:122–134.

15. Lewis G, Daigle K. Electrochemical behavior of T–6A1–4V alloy in static bio-simulationg solutions. J Biomed Mater Res Appl Biomater 1993; 4:47–54.
16. Gilbert JL, Buckley CA, Jacobs JJ, Bertin KC, Zernich MR. Intergranular corrosion-fatigue failure of cobalt-alloy femoral stems. A failure analysis of two implants. J Bone Joint Surg Am 1994; 76:110–115.
17. Collier JP, Suprenant VA, Jensen RE, Mayor MB, Suprenant HP. Corrosion between the components of modular femoral hip prosthesis. J Bone Joint Surg 1992; 74B:511–517.
18. Gilbert JL, Buckley CA, Jacobs JJ. In vivo corrosion of modular hip prosthesis components in mixed and similar metal combinations. The effect of crevice, stress, motion, and alloy coupling. J Biomed Mater Res 1993; 27:1533–1544.
19. Gilbert JL, Jacobs J. The mechanical and electrochemical processes associated with taper frettg crevice corrosion: a review. In: ASTM STP 1301 Modularity of Orthopaedic Implants. Philidelphia: ASTM, 1997:45–59.
20. Bundy K. Bone prosthesis and implant materials. In: Cowin SC, ed. Bone Mechanics. Boca Raton: CRC Press, 1989:160–184.
21. Park JB. Biomaterials Science and Engineering. New York: Plenum Press, 1984.
22. Silver FH, Christiansen DL. Biomaterials Science and Biocompatibility. New York: Springer, 1999.
23. Breme J, Biehl V. Metallic biomaterials. In: Black J, Hastings G, eds. Handbook of Biomaterial Properties. London: Chapman & Hall, 2001.
24. Black J. Biomaterials. New York: Marcel Dekker, 1992.
25. Black J. Prosthetic Materials. New York: VCH Publishers, 1996.
26. Hallab NJ, Jacobs JJ, Skipor A, Black J, Mikecz K, Galante JO. Systemic metal–protein binding associated with total joint replacement arthroplasty. J Biomed Mater Res 2000; 49:353–361.
27. Hallab NJ, Mikecz K, Akrami J, Jacobs J. Differential metal release and protein binding associated with titanium and cobalt–chromium implant alloys. Trans 46th Orthop Res Soc Orlando, Fl, 2000.
28. Michel R, Nolte M, Reich M, Loer F. Systemic effects of implanted prostheses made of cobalt–chromium alloys. Arch Orthop Trauma Surg 1991; 110:61–74.
29. Jacobs JJ, Silverton C, Hallab NJ, Skipor AK, Patterson L, Black J, Galante JO. Metal release and excretion from cementless titanium alloy total knee replacements. Clin Orthop 1999; 358:173–180.
30. Jacobs JJ, Skipor AK, Patterson LM, Hallab NJ, Paprosky WG, Black J, Galante JO. Metal release in patients who have had a primary total hip arthroplasty. A prospective, controlled, longitudinal study. J Bone Joint Surg Am 1998; 80:1447–1458.
31. Urban RM, Jacobs J, Gilbert JL, Rice SB, Jasty M, Bragdon CR, Galante GO. Characterization of solid products of corrosion generated by modular-head femoral stems of different designs and materials. In: Marlowe DE, Parr JE, Mayor MB, eds. STP 1301 Modularity of Orthopaedic Implants. Philadelphia: ASTM, 1997:33–44.
32. Urban RM, Jacobs JJ, Tomlinson MJ, Gavrilovic J, Black J, Peoc'h M. Dissemination of wear particles to the liver, spleen, and abdominal lymph nodes of patients with hip or knee replacement. J Bone Joint Surg Am 2000; 82:457–476.

33. Urban RM, Jacobs JJ, Gilbert JL, Galante JO. Migration of corrosion products from modular hip prostheses. Particle microanalysis and histopathological findings. J Bone Joint Surg Am 1994; 76:1345–1359.
34. Jasty M, Goetz DD, Bragdon CR, Lee KR, Hanson AE, Elder JR, Harris WH. Wear of polyethylene acetabular components in total hip arthroplasty. An analysis of one hundred and twenty-eight components retrieved at autopsy or revision operations. J Bone Joint Surg Am 1997; 79:349–358.
35. Jacobs JJ, Urban RM, Gilbert JL, Skipor AK, Black J, Jasty M, Galante JO. Local and distant products from modularity. Clin Orthop 1995; 319:94–105.
36. Jacobs JJ, Skipor AK, Urban RM, Black J, Manion LM, Starr A, Talbert LF, Galante JO. Systemic distribution of metal degradation products from titanium alloy total hip replacements an autopsy study. Trans Orthop Res Soc 1994:838.
37. Stulberg BN, Merritt K, Bauer T. Metallic wear debris in metal-backed patellar failure. J Biomed Mater Res Appl Biomater 1994; 5:9–16.
38. Jacobs JJ, Shanbhag A, Glant JJ, Black J, Galante JO. Wear debris in total joints. J Am Acad Orthop Surg 1994; 2:212–220.
39. Jacabs JJ. NIH Consensus Conference. Total hip replacement. JAMA 1995; 273:1950–1956.
40. Glant TT, Jacobs JJ, Molnar G, Shanbagh AS, Valyon M, Galante JO. Bone resorption activity of particulate-stimulated macrophages. J Bone and Mineral Res 1993; 8:1071–1079.
41. Woodman JL, Jacobs JJ, Galante JO, Urban RM. Metal ion release from titanium-based prosthetic segmental replacements of long bones in baboons: a long-term study. J Orthop Res 1984; 1:421–430.
42. Gitelman H. Aluminum and Health, a Critical Review. New York: Dekker, 1989.
43. Williams DF. Biological effects of titanium. In: Williams DF, ed. Systemic Aspects of Biocompatibility. Boca Ratan: CRC Press, 1981:169–177.
44. Gillespie WJ, Frampton CM, Henderson RJ, Ryan PM. The incidence of cancer following total hip replacement. J Bone Joint Surg Br 1988; 70:539–542.
45. Bravo I, Carvalho GS, Barbosa MA, de Sousa M. Differential effects of eight metal ions on lymphocyte differentiation antigens in vitro. J Biomed Mater Res 1990; 24:1059–1068.
46. Sinibaldi K, Rosen H, Liu SK, DeAngelis M. Tumors associated with metallic implants in animals. Clin Orthop 1976:257–266.
47. Luckey TD, Venugopal B. Metal Toxicity in Mammals. New York: Plenum, 1979.
48. Sederholm T, Kouvalainen K, Lamberg BA. Cobalt–induced hypothyroidism and polycythemia in lipoid nephrosis. Acta Med Scand 1968; 184:301–306.
49. Hartwig A. Carcinogenicity of metal compounds: possible role of DNA repair inhibition. Toxicol Lett 1998; 102-103:235–239.
50. Hayes RB. The carcinogenicity of metals in humans. Cancer Causes Control 1997; 8:371–385.
51. Costa M. Toxicity and carcinogenicity of Cr(VI) in animal models and humans. Crit Rev Toxicol 1997; 27:431–442.
52. Beyersmann D. Interactions in metal carcinogenicity. Toxicol Lett 1994; 72: 333–338.

53. Sunderman FW. Carcinogenicity of metal alloys in orthopaedic prosthesis: Clinical and experimental studies. Fundam Appl Toxicol 1989; 13:205–216.
54. Jandhyala BS, Hom GJ. Minireview. Physiological and pharmacological properties of vanadium. Life Sci 1983; 33:1325–1340.
55. Naylor GJ, Smith AH, Bryce-Smith D, Ward NI. Tissue vanadium levels in manic-depressive psychosis. Psychol Med 1984; 14:767–772.
56. Garabrant DH, Fine LJ, Oliver C, Bernstein L, Peters JM. Abnormalities of pulmonary function and pleural disease among titanium metal production workers. Scand J Work Environ Health 1987; 13:47–51.
57. Lee KP, Henry NW III, Trochimowicz HJ, Reinhardt CF. Pulmonary response to impaired lung clearance in rats following excessive TiO_2 dust deposition. Environ Res 1986; 41:144–167.
58. Altmann P, Plowman D, Marsh F, Cunningham J. Aluminium chelation therapy in dialysis patients: evidence for inhibition of haemoglobin synthesis by low levels of aluminium. Lancet 1988; 1:1012–1015.
59. Coburn JW, Norris KC, Nebeker HG. Osteomalacia and bone disease arising from aluminum. Semin Nephrol 1986; 6:68–89.
60. Good PF, Perl DP. Aluminium in Alzheimer's. Nature 1993; 362:418.
61. Memoli VA, Urban RM, Alroy J, Galante JO. Malignant neoplasms associated with orthopaedic implant materials in rats. J Orthop Res 1986; 4:346–355.
62. Jacobs JJ, Rosenbaum DH, Hay RM, Gitelis S, Black J. Early sarcomatous degeneration near a cementless hip replacement. A case report and review. J Bone Joint Surg Br 1992; 74:740–744.
63. Goodfellow J. Malignancy and joint replacement. J Bone Joint Surg Br 1992; 74:645.
64. Visuri T, Koskenvuo M. Cancer risk after Mckee–Farrar total hip replacement. Orthopaedics 1991; 14:137–142.
65. Sunderman FW, Hopfer SM, Swift T, Rezuke WN, Ziebka L, Highman P, Edwards B, Folcik M, Gossling HR. Cobalt, chromium, and nickel concentrations in body fluids of patients with porous-coated knee or hip prostheses. J Orthop Res 1989; 7:307–315.
66. Blumenthal NC, Cosma V. Inhibition of apatite formation by titanium and vanadium ions. J Biomed Mater Res 1989; 23:13–22.
67. Blumenthal NC, Cosma V. The effect of aluminum and gallium ions on the mineralization process. Bull Hosp Joint Dis Orthop Inst 1989; 49:192–204.
68. Sun ZL, Wataha JC, Hanks CT. Effects of metal ions on osteoblast-like cell metabolism and differentiation. J Biomed Mater Res 1997; 34:29–37.
69. Wataha JC, Hanks CT, Sun Z. Effect of cell line on in vitro metal ion cytotoxicity. Dent Mater 1994; 10:156–161.
70. Wataha JC, Hanks CT, Craig RG. In vitro effects of metal ions on cellular metabolism and the correlation between these effects and the uptake of the ions. J Biomed Mater Res 1994; 28:427–433.
71. Wataha JC, Hanks CT, Craig RG. The effect of cell monolayer density on the cytotoxicity of metal ions which are released from dental alloys. Dent Mater 1993; 9:172–176.
72. Nichols KG, Puleo DA. Effect of metal ions on the formation and function of osteoclastic cells in vitro. J Biomed Mater Res 1997; 35:265–271.

73. Thompson GJ, Puleo DA. Ti–6Al–4V ion solution inhibition of osteogenic cell phenotype as a function of differentiation timecourse in vitro. Biomaterials 1996; 17:1949–1954.

74. Thompson GJ, Puleo DA. Effects of sublethal metal ion concentrations on osteogenic cells derived from bone marrow stromal cells. J Appl Biomater 1995; 6:249–258.

75. Puleo DA, Huh WW. Acute toxicity of metal ions in cultures of osteogenic cells derived from bone marrow stromal cells. J Appl Biomater 1995; 6: 109–116.

76. Morais S, Dias N, Sousa JP, Fernandes MH, Carvalho GS. In vitro osteoblastic differentiation of human bone marrow cells in the presence of metal ions. J Biomed Mater Res 1999; 44:176–190.

77. Morais S, Sousa JP, Fernandes MH, Carvalho GS, de Bruijn JD, van Blitterswijk CA. Effects of AISI 316L corrosion products in invitro bone formation. Biomaterials 1998; 19:999–1007.

78. Morais S, Sousa JP, Fernandes MH, Carvalho GS. In vitro biomineralization by osteoblast-like cells. I. Retardation of tissue mineralization by metal salts. Biomaterials 1998; 19:13–21.

79. Wagner M, Klein CL, van Kooten TG, Kirkpatrick CJ. Mechanisms of cell activation by heavy metal ions. J Biomed Mater Res 1998; 42:443–452.

80. Roebuck KA, Vermes C, Carpenter LR, Fritz EA, Narayanan R, Glant TT. Down-regulation of procollagen alpha1(I) messenger RNA by titanium particles correlates with nuclear factor kappaB (NF-kappaB) activation and increased rel A and NF-kappaB1 binding to the collagen promoter. J Bone Miner Res 2001; 16:501–510.

81. Vermes C, Chandrasekaran R, Jacobs JJ, Galante JO, Roebuck KA, Glant TT. The effects of particulate wear debris, cytokines, and growth factors on the functions of MG-63 osteoblasts. J Bone Joint Surg Am 2001; 83:201–211.

82. Vermes C, Roebuck KA, Chandrasekaran R, Dobai JG, Jacobs JJ, Glant TT. Particulate wear debris activates protein tyrosine kinases and nuclear factor kappaB, which down-regulates type I collagen synthesis in human osteoblasts. J Bone Miner Res 2000; 15:1756–1765.

83. Basketter DA, Briatico-Vangosa G, Kaestner W, Lally C, Bontinck WJ. Nickel, cobalt and chromium in consumer products: a role in allergic contact dermatitis? Contact Dermat 1993; 28:15–25

84. Cramers M, Lucht U. Metal sensitivity in patients treated for tibial fractures with plates of stainless steel. Acta Orthop Scand 1977; 48:245–249.

85. Merritt K, Rodrigo JJ. Immune response to synthetic materials, Sensitization of patients receiving orthopaedic implants. Clin Orthop Rel Res 1996; 326:71–79.

86. Gawkrodger DJ. Nickel sensitivity and the implantation of orthopaedic prostheses. Contact Dermat 1993; 28:257–259.

87. Kanerva L, Sipilainen-Malm T, Estlander T, Zitting A, Jolanki R, Tarvainen K. Nickel release from metals, and a case of allergic contact dermatitis from stainless steel. Contact Dermat 1994; 31:299–303.

88. Haudrechy P, Foussereau J, Mantout B, Baroux B. Nickel release from nickel-plated metals and stainless steels. Contact Dermat 1994; 31:249–255.

89. Black J. Systemic effects of biomaterials. Biomaterials 1984; 5:12–17.

90. Jacobs JJ, Gilbert JL, Urban RM. Corrosion of metallic implants. In: Stauffer RN, ed. Advances in Orthopaedic Surgery. Vol. 2. St. Louis: Mosby, 1994:279–319.
91. Yang J, Black J. Competitive binding of chromium cobalt and nickel to serum proteins. Biomaterials 1994; 15:262–268.
92. Yang J, Merritt K. Production of monoclonal antibodies to study corrosion of Co–Cr biomaterials. J Biomed Mater Res 1996; 31:71–80.
93. Liden C, Wahlberg JE, Maibach HI. Skin. New York: Academic Press, 1995: 447–464.
94. Angle C. Organ-Specific Therapeutic Intervention. New York: Academic Press, 1995:71–110.
95. Lalor PA, Revell PA, Gray AB, Wright S, Railton GT, Freeman MA. Sensitivity to titanium. A cause of implant failure. J Bone Joint Surg 1991; 73-B:25–28.
96. Parker AW, Drez D Jr, Jacobs JJ. Titanium dermatitis after failure of a metal-backed patellas. Am J Knee Surg 1993; 6:129–131.
97. Hensten-Pettersen A. Allergy and hypersensitivity. In: Morrey BF, ed. Biological, Material and Mechanical Considerations of Joint Replacements. New York: Raven Press, 1993:353–360.
98. Kuby J. Immunology. New York: W.H. Freeman and Company, 1991.
99. Merle C, Vigan M, Devred D, Girardin P, Adessi B, Laurent R. Generalized eczema from vitallium osteosynthesis material. Contact Dermat 1992; 27: 257–258.
100. King J, Fransway A, Adkins RB. Chronic urticaria due to surgical clips. N Engl J Med 1993; 329:1583–1584.
101. Barranco VP, Solloman H. Eczematous dermatitis from nickel. J Am Med Assoc 1972; 220:1244.
102. Thomas RH, Rademaker M, Goddard NJ, Munro DD. Severe eczema of the hands due to an orthopaedic plate made of vitallium. Br Med J 1987; 294: 106–107.
103. Abdallah HI, Balsara RK, O'Riordan AC. Pacemaker contact sensitivity: Clinical recognition and management. Ann Thora Surg 1994; 57:1017–1018.
104. Halpin DS. An unusual reaction in muscle in association with a vitallium plate: a report of possible metal hypersensitivity. J Bone Joint Surg 1975; 57-B:451–453.
105. Merritt K, Brown SA. Biological Effects of Corrosion Products from Metal. Philadelphia: American Society for Testing and Materials, 1985:195–207.
106. Poss R, Thornhill TS, Ewald FC, Thomas WH, Batte NJ, Sledge CB. Factors influencing the incidence and outcome of infection following total joint arthoplasty. Clin Orthop 1984:182.
107. Wang JY, Wicklund BH, Gustilo RB, Tsukayama DT. Prosthetic metals interfere with the functions of human osteoblast cells in vitro. Clin Orthop 1997: 216–226.
108. Elves MW, Wilson JN, Scales JT, Kemp HB. Incidence of metal sensitivity in patients with total joint replacements. Br Med J 1975; 4:376–378.
109. Gordon PM, White MI, Scotland TR. Generalized sensitivity from an implanted orthopaedic antibiotic minichain containing nickel. Contact Dermat 1994; 30: 181–182.

110. Peters MS, Schroeter AL, Hale HM, Broadbent JC. Pacemaker contact sensitivity. Contact Dermat 1984; 11:214–218.
111. Rostoker G, Robin J, Binet O, Blamutier J, Paupe J, Lessana-Liebowitch M, Bedouelle J, Sonneck JM, Garrel JB, Millet P. Dermatitis due to orthopaedic implants. A review of the literature and report of three cases. J Bone Joint Surg 1987; 69-A:1408–1412.
112. Benson MK, Goodwin PG, Brostoff J. Metal sensitivity in patients with joint replacement arthroplasties. Br Med J 1975; 4:374–375.
113. Brown GC, Lockshin MD, Salvati EA, Bullough PG. Sensitivity to metal as a possible cause of sterile loosening after cobalt–chromium total hip-replacement arthroplasty. J Bone Joint Surg Am 1977; 59-A:164–168.
114. Deutman R, Mulder TH, Brian R, Nater JP. Metal sensitivity before and after total hip arthroplasty. J Bone Joint Surg Am 1977; 59-A:862–865.
115. Kubba R, Taylor JS, Marks KE. Cutaneous complications of orthopaedic implants. A two-year prospective study. Arch Dermatol 1981; 117:554–560.
116. Mayor MB, Merritt K, Brown SA. Metal allergy and the surgical patient. Am J Surg 1980; 139:477–479.
117. Merritt K, Brown S. Tissue reaction and metal sensitivity. Acta Orthop Scand 1980; 51:403–411.
118. Merritt K, Brown S. Metal sensitivity reactions to orthopaedic implants. Int J Dermatol 1981; 20:89–94.
119. Merritt K. Role of medical materials, both in implant and surface applications, in immune response and in resistance to infection. Biomaterials 1984; 5:53–57.
120. Pinkston JA, Finch SC. A method for the differentiation of T and B lymphocytes and monocytes migrating under agarose. Stain Technol 1979; 54: 233–239.
121. Rooker GD, Wilkinson JD. Metal sensitivity in patients undergoing hip replacement. A prospective study. J Bone Joint Surg 1980; 62-B:502–505.
122. Carlsson AS, Macnusson B, Moller H. Metal sensitivity in patients with metal-to-plastic total hip arthroplasties. Acta Orthop Scand 1980; 51:57–62.
123. Fischer T, Rystedt I, Safwenberg J, Egle I. HLA -A, -B, -C and -DR antigens in individuals with sensitivity to cobalt. Acta Derm Venereol Stockh 1984; 64:121–124.
124. Munro-Ashman D, Miller AJ. Rejection of metal to metal prosthesis and skin sensitivity to cobalt. Contact Dermat 1976; 2:65.
125. Evans EM, Freeman MA, Miller AJ, Vernon–Roberts B. Metal sensitivity as a cause of bone necrosis and loosening of the prosthesis in total joint replacement. J Bone Joint Surg 1974; 56-B:626–642.
126. Boyan BD. Discussion of Toxicity and Allergy. New York: Raven Press, 1993.
127. Jacobs JJ, Skipor AK, Patterson LM, Black J, Galante JO. Serum titanium concentration in patients with cementless TKR: a 5-year prospective study. Trans ORS 1997; 22:235.
128. Jacobs JJ, Skipor AK, Patterson LM, Paprosky WG, Black J, Galante JO. A prospective, controlled, longitidunal study of metal release in patients undergoing primary total hip arthroplasty. J Bone Joint Surg 2001.

11

Inflammation and the Role of Macrophages in the Foreign Body Reaction

James M. Anderson

Institute of Pathology and Departments of Macromolecular Science and Biomedical Engineering, Case Western Reserve University, Cleveland, Ohio, U.S.A.

INTRODUCTION

The aim of this chapter is to provide practicing orthopaedic surgeons, scientists involved in joint replacement research and development, fellows, residents, and biomedical engineering students with an overview and an appreciation of the fundamental aspects of tissue/material interactions with emphasis on the inflammatory response and the foreign body reaction. In this overview, tissue/material interactions and the foreign body reaction are viewed from the classical medical perspective of the pathologist. Tissue/material interactions are commonly referred to as the tissue response continuum which is the series of responses that are initiated by the implantation procedure, as well as by the presence of the biomaterial, medical device, or prosthesis. In this chapter, we divide the series of tissue/material responses into the early, transient tissue responses and the late, persistent tissue responses. Early, transient tissue/material responses include injury, blood/material interactions, provisional matrix formation, temporal sequence of inflammation and wound healing, acute inflammation, chronic inflammation, and granulation tissue development. These responses are usually of short duration, occurring over the first 2–3 weeks following implantation of a medical device or prosthesis.

Late, persistent tissue responses include macrophage interactions, foreign body giant cell (FBGC) formation and interactions, and fibrosis and fibrous encapsulation of the medical device or prosthesis. The early, transient tissue responses form the basis for safety or biocompatibility considerations of the medical device or prosthesis. Late, persistent tissue/material responses, while important to the safety and biocompatibility considerations, may be more important in modulating the performance characteristics of the medical device or prosthesis as well as providing a biological basis for device or prosthesis failure such as osteolysis or loosening with total joint prostheses.

EARLY, TRANSIENT TISSUE/MATERIAL RESPONSES

Injury

The process of implantation of a biomaterial, prosthesis, or medical device results in injury to tissues or organs (1–3). It is this injury and the subsequent perturbation of homeostatic mechanisms which lead to the inflammatory responses, foreign body reaction, and wound healing. In regard to total joint replacement, both soft and hard tissues are injured in the process of implantation. The response to injury is dependent on multiple factors which include the extent of injury, the loss of basement membrane structures, blood–material interactions, provisional matrix formation, the extent or degree of cellular necrosis, and the extent of the inflammatory response. These events, in turn, may affect the extent or degree of granulation tissue formation, foreign body reaction, and fibrosis or fibrous capsule development. These events are summarized in Table 1, the sequence of host reactions following implantation of medical devices. The host reactions are considered to be tissue dependent, organ dependent, and species dependent. In addition, it is important to recognize that these reactions occur or are initiated early, i.e., within 2–3 weeks of the time of implantation.

In considering these host reactions following injury, it is important to consider whether tissue resolution or organization occurs within the injured

Table 1 Sequence of Host Reactions Following Implantation of Medical Devices

Injury
Blood–material interactions
Provisional matrix formation
Acute inflammation
Chronic inflammation
Granulation tissue
Foreign body reaction
Fibrosis/fibrous capsule development

tissue. In situations where injury has occurred and exudative inflammation is present, but no cellular necrosis or loss of basement membrane structures has occurred, the process of resolution occurs. Resolution is the restitution of the pre-existing architecture of the tissue. On the other hand, with necrosis (cell death), granulation tissue grows into the inflammatory exudate and the process of organization with development of fibrous (scar) tissue occurs. With implants, the process of organization with development of fibrous tissue leads to the well-known fibrous capsule formation at the tissue/material interface. The proliferative capacity of cells within the tissue also plays a role in determining whether resolution or organization occurs. In general, the process of implantation in vascularized tissues leads to organization with fibrous tissue development and fibrous encapsulation. As is well known, the development of fibrotic tissue at the prosthesis/tissue interface leads to total joint prosthesis loosening, a common failure mechanism.

With total joint prostheses, implantation first involves soft tissue injury followed by injury to bone as the surgeon prepares the implant site. Thus, initiation of the inflammatory response occurs just prior to the implantation of the prosthesis and blood–material interactions and provisional matrix formation occur at the time of prosthesis implantation.

Blood–Material Interactions and Initiation of the Inflammatory Response

Blood–material interactions and the inflammatory response are intimately linked, and in fact, early responses to injury involve mainly blood and the vasculature (1–5). Regardless of the tissue into which a biomaterial is implanted, the initial inflammatory response is activated by injury to vascularized connective tissue (Table 2). Because blood and its components are involved in the initial inflammatory responses, thrombus and/or blood clot also forms. Thrombus formation involves activation of the extrinsic and intrinsic coagulation systems, the complement system, the fibrinolytic system, the kinin-generating system, and platelets. Thrombus or blood clot formation on the surface of a biomaterial is related to the well-known Vroman effect of protein adsorption. From a wound healing perspective, blood protein deposition on a biomaterial surface is described as provisional matrix formation.

Immediately following injury, i.e., the initiation of surgery, changes occur in vascular flow, caliber, and permeability. Fluid, proteins, and blood cells escape from the vascular system into the injured tissue in a process called exudation. Following changes in the vascular system, which also include changes induced in blood and its components, cellular events occur and characterize the inflammatory response (4–7). The effect of the injury and/or biomaterial in situ on plasma or cells can produce chemical factors that mediate many of the vascular and cellular responses of inflammation.

Table 2 Cells and Components of Vascularized Connective Tissue

Intravascular (blood) cells
   Erythryocytes (BBC)
   Neutrophils
   Monocytes
   Eosinophils
   Lymphocytes
   Basophils
   Platelets
Connective tissue cells
   Mast cells
   Fibroblasts
   Macrophages
   Lymphocytes
Extracellular matrix components
   Collagens
   Elastin
   Proteoglycans
   Fibronectin
   Laminin

Although injury initiates the inflammatory response, released chemicals from plasma, cells, and injured tissue mediate the response. Important classes of chemical mediators of inflammation are presented in Table 3. Several important points must be noted in order to understand the inflammatory response and how it relates to biomaterials. First, although chemical mediators are classified on a structural or functional basis, different mediator systems interact and provide a system of checks and balances regarding their respective activities and functions. Second, chemical mediators are quickly inactivated or destroyed, suggesting that their action is predominantly local (i.e., at the implant site). Third, generally acid, lysosomal proteases and oxygen-derived free radicals produce the most significant damage or injury. These chemical mediators are also important in the degradation of biomaterials.

The predominant cell type present in the inflammatory response varies with the age of the injury. In general, neutrophils, commonly called polymorphonuclear leukocytes or polys, predominate during the first several days following injury and then are replaced by monocytes as the predominant cell type. Three factors account for this change in cell type: (i) Neutrophils are short lived and disintegrate and disappear after 24–48 hour; neutrophil emigration is of short duration because chemotactic factors for neutrophil migration are activated early in the inflammatory response. (ii) Following emigration from the vasculature, monocytes differentiate into

Table 3 Important Chemical Mediators of Inflammation Derived from Plasma, Cells, or Injured

Mediators	Examples
Vasoactive agents	Histamines, serotonin, adenosine, endothelial derived relaxing factor (EDRF), prostacyclin, endothelin, thromboxane a_2
Plasma proteases	
Kinin system	Bradykinin, kallikrein
Complement system	C3a, C5a, C3b, C5b-C9
Coagulation/fibrinolytic system	Fibrin degradation products, activated Hageman factor (FXIIA), tissue plasminogen activator (tPA)
Leukotrienes	Leukotriene B4 (LTB_4), hydroxyeicosa-tetraenoic acid (HETE)
Lysosomal proteases	Collagenase, elastase
Oxygen-derived free radicals	H_2O_2, superoxide anion, nitric oxide
Platelet activating factors	Cell membrane lipids
Cytokines	Interleukin 1 (IL-1), tumor necrosis factor (TNF)
Growth factors	Platelet derived growth factor (PDGF), fibroblast growth factor (FGF), transforming growth factor (TGF-α or TGF-β), epithelial growth factor (EGF)

macrophages, and these cells are very long lived (up to months). (iii) Monocyte emigration may continue for days to weeks, depending on the injury and implanted biomaterial, and chemotactic factors for monocytes are activated over longer periods of time.

Provisional Matrix Formation

Injury to vascularized tissue in the implantation procedure leads to immediate development of the provisional matrix at the implant site. This provisional matrix consists of fibrin, produced by activation of the coagulative and thrombosis systems, and inflammatory products released by the complement system, activated platelets, inflammatory cells, and endothelial cells (8–10). These events occur early, within minutes to hours following implantation of a medical device. Components within or released from the provisional matrix, i.e., fibrin network (thrombosis or clot), initiate the resolution, reorganization, and repair processes such as inflammatory cell and fibroblast recruitment. Platelets, activated during the fibrin network formation, release platelet factor 4, platelet-derived growth factor (PDGF), and transforming growth factor β (TGF-β), which contribute to fibroblast recruitment (11,12). Monocytes and lymphocytes, upon activation, generate additional chemotactic factors including LTB$_4$, PDGF, and TGF-β to recruit fibroblasts.

Fibrin, the major component of the provisional matrix, has been shown to play a major role in the development of neovascularization, i.e., angiogenesis. Implanted porous surfaces filled with fibrin exhibit new vessel growth within four days. The intensity of this angiogenic response is enhanced when zymosan-activated serum or PDGF is incorporated in the fibrin matrix (13).

The provisional matrix is composed of adhesive molecules such as fibronectin and thrombospondin bound to fibrin as well as platelet granule components released during platelet aggregation. Platelet granule components include thrombospondin, released from the platelet α-granule, and cytokines including TGF-α, TGF-β, PDGF, platelet factor 4, and platelet-derived endothelial cell growth factor. The provisional matrix is stabilized by the cross-linking of fibrin by factor XIIIa.

The provisional matrix appears to provide both structural and biochemical components to the process of wound healing. The complex three-dimensional structure of the fibrin network with attached adhesive proteins provides a substrate for cell adhesion and migration. The presence of mitogens, chemoattractants, cytokines, and growth factors within the provisional matrix provide for a rich milieu of activating and inhibiting substances for various cellular proliferative and synthetic processes.

The provisional matrix may be viewed as a naturally derived, biodegradable, sustained release system in which mitogens, chemoattractants, cytokines, and growth factors are released to control subsequent wound healing processes (14–19). In spite of the rapid increase in our knowledge of the provisional matrix and its capabilities, our knowledge of the control of the formation of the provisional matrix and its effect on subsequent wound healing events is poor. In part, this lack of knowledge is due to the fact that much of our knowledge regarding the provisional matrix has been derived from in vitro studies, and there is a paucity of in vivo studies which provide for a more complex perspective. Little is known regarding the provisional matrix which forms at biomaterial and medical device interfaces in vivo. Attractive hypotheses have been presented regarding the presumed ability of materials and protein adsorbed materials to modulate cellular interactions through their interactions with adhesive molecules and cells.

Temporal Sequence of Inflammation and Wound Healing

Inflammation is generally defined as the reaction of vascularized living tissue to local injury. Inflammation serves to contain, neutralize, dilute, or wall off the injurious agent or process. In addition, it sets into motion a series of events that may heal and reconstitute the implant site through replacement

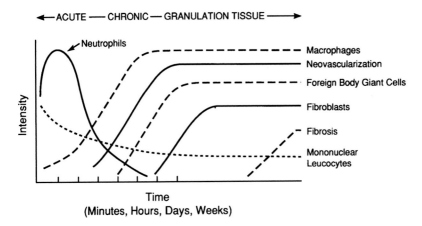

Figure 1 The temporal variation in the acute inflammatory response, chronic inflammatory response, granulation tissue development, and foreign body reaction to implanted biomaterials. The intensity and time variables are dependent upon the extent of injury created in the implantation and the size, shape, topography, and chemical and physical properties of the biomaterial.

of the injured tissue by regeneration of native parenchymal cells, formation of fibroblastic scar tissue, or a combination of these two processes (4,5).

The sequence of events following implantation of a biomaterial is illustrated in Figure 1. The size, shape, and chemical and physical properties of the biomaterial and the physical dimensions and properties of the prosthesis or device may be responsible for variations in the intensity and time duration of the inflammatory and wound healing processes. Thus, intensity and/or time duration of inflammatory reaction may characterize the biocompatibility of a biomaterial, prosthesis, or device.

In general, the biocompatibility of a material with tissue has been described in terms of the acute and chronic inflammatory responses and of the fibrous capsule formation that is seen over various time periods following implantation. Histologic evaluation of tissue adjacent to implanted materials as a function of implant time has been the most commonly used method of evaluating the biocompatibility. Classically, the biocompatibility of an implanted material has been described in terms of the morphological appearance of the inflammatory reaction to the material; however, the inflammatory response is a series of complex reactions involving various types of cells the densities, activities, and functions of which are controlled by various endogenous and autocoid mediators. The simplistic view of the acute inflammatory response progressing to the chronic inflammatory response may be misleading with respect to biocompatibility studies and the inflammatory response to implants. Studies using the cage implant system show that monocytes and macrophages are present in highest concentrations when neutrophils are also at their highest concentrations, i.e., the acute inflammatory response (20,21). Neutrophils have short lifetimes—hours to days—and disappear from the exudate more rapidly than do macrophages, which have lifetimes of days to weeks to months. Eventually macrophages become the predominant cell type in the exudate, resulting in a chronic inflammatory response. Monocytes rapidly differentiate into macrophages, the cells principally responsible for normal wound healing in the foreign body reaction. Classically, the development of granulation tissue has been considered to be a part of chronic inflammation, but because of unique tissue–material interactions, it is preferable to differentiate the foreign body reaction—with its varying degree of granulation tissue development, including macrophages, fibroblasts, and capillary formation—from chronic inflammation.

Acute Inflammation

Acute inflammation is of relatively short duration, lasting from minutes to days, depending on the extent of injury. The main characteristics of acute inflammation are the exudation of fluid and plasma proteins (edema) and the emigration of leukocytes (predominantly neutrophils). Neutrophils and other motile white cells emigrate or move from the blood vessels to the perivascular tissues and the injury (implant) site (22–24).

The accumulation of leukocytes, in particular neutrophils and monocytes, is the most important feature of the inflammatory reaction. Leukocytes accumulate through a series of processes including margination, adhesion, emigration, phagocytosis, and extracellular release of leukocyte products (25). Increased leukocytic adhesion in inflammation involves specific interactions between complementary "adhesion molecules" present on the leukocyte and endothelial surfaces (26,27). The surface expression of these adhesion molecules is modulated by inflammatory agents; mechanisms of interaction include stimulation of leukocyte adhesion molecules (C5a, LTB_4), stimulation of endothelial adhesion molecules (IL-1), or both effects (TNF-α). Integrins comprise a family of transmembrane glycoproteins that modulate cell–matrix and cell–cell relationships by acting as receptors to extracellular protein ligands and also as direct adhesion molecules (28). An important group of integrins (adhesion molecules) on leukocytes include the CD11/CD18 family of adhesion molecules. Inflammatory mediators, i.e., cytokines, stimulate a rapid increase in these adhesion molecules on the leukocyte surface as well as increased leukocyte adhesion to endothelium. Leukocyte–endothelial cell interactions are also controlled by endothelial–leukocyte adhesion molecules (ELAMs, E-selectins) or intracellular adhesion molecules (ICAM-1, ICAM-2, and VCAMs) on endothelial cells (29).

White cell emigration is controlled in part by chemotaxis, which is the unidirectional migration of cells along a chemical gradient. A wide variety of exogenous and endogenous substances have been identified as chemotactic agents (6,22–33). Important to the emigration or movement of leukocytes is the presence of specific receptors for chemotactic agents on the cell membranes of leukocytes. These and other receptors may also play a role in the activation of leukocytes. Following localization of leukocytes at the injury (implant) site, phagocytosis and the release of enzymes occur following activation of neutrophils and macrophages. The major role of the neutrophils in acute inflammation is to phagocytose microorganisms and foreign materials. Phagocytosis is seen as a three-step process in which the injurious agent undergoes recognition and neutrophil attachment, engulfment, and killing or degradation. With regard to biomaterials, engulfment and degradation may or may not occur depending on the properties of the biomaterial.

Although biomaterials are not generally phagocytosed by neutrophils or macrophages because of the size disparity (i.e., the surface of the biomaterial is greater than the size of the cell), certain events in phagocytosis may occur. The process of recognition and attachment is expedited when the injurious agent is coated by naturally occurring serum factors called opsonins. The two major opsonins are IgG and the complement-activated fragment, C3b. Both of these plasma-derived proteins are known to adsorb to biomaterials, and neutrophils and macrophages have corresponding cell membrane receptors for these opsonization proteins. These receptors may also play a role in the activation of the attached neutrophil or macrophage. Because of the size disparity between the biomaterial surface and the attached cell, "frustrated phagocytosis" may occur (30,31). This process does not involve engulfment of the biomaterial but does cause the extracellular release of leukocyte products in an attempt to degrade the biomaterial. Neutrophils adherent to complement-coated and immunoglobulin-coated nonphagocytosable surfaces may release enzymes by direct extrusion or exocytosis from the cell (30,31). The amount of enzyme released during this process depends on the size of the polymer particle, with larger particles inducing greater amounts of enzyme release. This suggests that the specific mode of cell activation in the inflammatory response in tissue is dependent upon the size of the implant and that a material in a phagocytosable form (e.g., powder or particulate) may provoke a degree of inflammatory response different from that of the same material in a nonphagocytosable form (e.g., film).

Chronic Inflammation

Chronic inflammation is less uniform histologically than is acute inflammation. In general, chronic inflammation is characterized by the presence of monocytes, and lymphocytes with the early proliferation of blood vessels and connective tissue (4,5,34,35). It must be noted that many factors modify the course and histologic appearance of chronic inflammation.

Persistent inflammatory stimuli lead to chronic inflammation. Although the chemical and physical properties of the biomaterial may lead to chronic inflammation, motion in the implant site by the biomaterial may also produce chronic inflammation. The chronic inflammatory response to biomaterials is confined to the implant site. Inflammation with the presence of mononuclear cells, including lymphocytes and plasma cells, is given the designation chronic inflammation, whereas the foreign body reaction with granulation tissue development is considered the normal wound healing response to implanted biomaterials (i.e., the normal foreign body reaction). Chronic inflammation with biocompatible materials is usually of very short duration, i.e., a few days.

Lymphocytes and plasma cells are involved principally in immune reactions and are key mediators of antibody production and delayed hypersensitivity responses. Their roles in nonimmunologic injuries and inflammation are largely unknown. Little is known regarding humoral immune responses and cell-mediated immunity to synthetic biomaterials. The role of macrophages must be considered in the possible development of immune responses to synthetic biomaterials. Macrophages process and present the antigen to immunocompetent cells and thus are key mediators in the development of immune reactions.

The macrophage is probably the most important cell in chronic inflammation because of the great number of biologically active products it produces (34). Important classes of products produced and secreted by macrophages include neutral proteases, chemotactic factors, arachidonic acid metabolites, reactive oxygen metabolites, complement components, coagulation factors, growth-promoting factors, and cytokines.

Growth factors such as PDGF, FGF, TFG-β, TGF-α/EGF, and IL-1 or TNF are important to the growth of fibroblasts and blood vessels and the regeneration of epithelial cells. Growth factors, released by activated cells, stimulate production of a wide variety of cells; initiate cell migration, differentiation, and tissue remodeling; and may be involved in various stages of wound healing (36–41). It is clear that there is a lack of information regarding interaction and synergy among various cytokines and growth factors and their abilities to exhibit chemotactic, mitogenic, and angiogenic properties.

Granulation Tissue

Within one day following implantation of a biomaterial (i.e., injury), the healing response is initiated by the action of monocytes and macrophages, followed by proliferation of fibroblasts and vascular endothelial cells at the implant site, leading to the formation of granulation tissue, the hallmark of healing inflammation. Granulation tissue derives its name from the pink, soft granular appearance on the surface of healing wounds, and its characteristic histologic features include the proliferation of new small blood vessels and fibroblasts. Depending on the extent of injury, granulation tissue may be seen as early as 3–5 days following implantation of a biomaterial.

The new small blood vessels are formed by budding or sprouting of pre-existing vessels in a process known as neovascularization or angiogenesis (42–44). This process involves proliferation, maturation, and organization of endothelial cells into capillary tubes. Fibroblasts also proliferate in developing granulation tissue and are active in synthesizing collagen and proteoglycans. In the early stages of granulation tissue development, proteoglycans predominate; later, however, collagen—especially type I collagen—predominates and forms the fibrous capsule. Some fibroblasts in developing granulation tissue may have features of smooth muscle cells. These cells are called myofibroblasts and are considered to be responsible for the wound contraction seen during the development of granulation tissue.

LATE, PERSISTENT TISSUE RESPONSES

Macrophage Interactions

Two factors which play a role in monocyte/macrophage adhesion and activation and foreign body giant cell formation are the surface chemistry of the substrate onto which the cells adhere and the protein adsorption which occurs before cell adhesion. These two factors have been hypothesized to play significant roles in the inflammatory and wound healing responses to biomaterials and medical devices in vivo.

Macrophage interactions with biomaterials are initiated when blood borne monocytes in the early, transient responses migrate to the implant site and adhere to the blood protein adsorbed biomaterial through monocyte integrin interactions. Following adhesion, adherent monocytes differentiate into macrophages which may then fuse to form FBGCs. Figure 2 demonstrates the progression from circulating blood monocyte to tissue macrophage to FBGC development that is most commonly observed. Because of the progression of monocytes to macrophages to FBGCs (Fig. 2), the following discussion of macrophage interactions also includes perspectives on how macrophages are formed, i.e., monocyte adhesion, and what happens to macrophages on biomaterial surfaces, i.e., FBGC formation.

Material surface property-dependent blood protein adsorption occurs immediately upon surgical implantation of a biomaterial and it is the protein-modified biomaterial that inflammatory cells subsequently encounter. Monocytes express receptors for various blood components, but they recognize naturally occurring foreign surfaces by receptors for opsonins such as fragments of complement component C3. Because complement activation

MONOCYTE   MACROPHAGE   FOREIGN BODY GIANT CELL

BLOOD   *TISSUE*   *TISSUE/BIOMATERIAL*   *BIOMATERIAL*

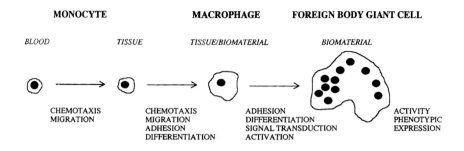

CHEMOTAXIS   CHEMOTAXIS   ADHESION   ACTIVITY
MIGRATION   MIGRATION   DIFFERENTIATION   PHENOTYPIC
                  ADHESION   SIGNAL TRANSDUCTION   EXPRESSION
                  DIFFERENTIATION   ACTIVATION

Figure 2 In vivo transition from blood-borne monocyte to biomaterial adherent monocyte/macrophage to foreign body giant cell at the tissue/biomaterial interface. Little is known regarding the indicated biological responses which are considered to play important roles in the transition to FBGC development.

by biomaterials has been well documented, we have investigated monocyte interactions with foreign surfaces. Exposure to blood during biomaterial implantation may permit extensive opsonization with the labile fragment C3b and the rapid conversion of C3b to its hemolytically inactive but nevertheless opsonic and more stable form, C3bi. C3b is bound by the CD35 receptor, but C3bi is recognized by distinct receptors, CDllb/CD18 and CDllc/CD18 on monocytes. Fibrinogen, a major plasma protein that adsorbs to biomaterials, is another ligand for these receptors which together with CDlla/CD18 constitutes a subfamily of integrins that is restricted to leukocytes. Studies with monoclonal antibodies to their common β_2 subunit (CD 18) and distinct α chains have implicated CDllb/CD18 and CDllc/CD18 in monocyte/macrophage responses. Other potential adhesion-mediating proteins that adsorb to biomaterials include IgG, which may interact with monocytes via various receptors and fibronectin, for which monocytes also express multiple types of receptors.

In our studies to explore the role of surface chemistry in monocyte adhesion, macrophage phenotypic expression and FBGC formation (45,46), we initially utilized chemically modified polystyrene surfaces. We have utilized only human monocytes in our studies because of their clinical relevance. Human monocyte in vitro adhesion with fluorinated, siliconized, nitrogenated, and oxygenated surfaces were reduced by 50–100% when complement component C3-depleted serum was used for adsorption. The fluorinated surfaces exhibited the greatest inhibition of monocyte adhesion with C3-depleted serum. Monocyte adhesion was restored on all surfaces when C3-depleted serum was replenished with purified C3. Monocyte adhesion to serum-adsorbed surfaces was inhibited by monoclonal antibodies to the leukocyte integrin beta subunit, CD18, and partially inhibited by a monoclonal antibody to the alpha subunit, CD11b. These findings suggest adhesive interactions between adsorbed C3bi, the hemolytically inactive form of the C3b fragment, and the leukocyte integrin, CDllb/CD18.

Additional studies demonstrated that adsorbed fibrinogen reduced the effectiveness of these inhibiting monoclonal antibodies, indicating that alternative adhesion mechanisms may operate depending on the critical adhesion-mediating blood protein components adsorbed onto the different surfaces.

Following adhesion to biomaterial surfaces, monocytes/macrophages may become activated with release of cytokines such as interleukin-1-β (IL-1-β), interleukin-6, and tumor necrosis factor-α (TNF-α) (47–53). These cytokines as well as other cytokines and growth factors released by activated macrophages on biomaterial surfaces can influence the subsequent inflammatory and wound healing responses (Fig. 3). In vitro studies of macrophages on biomaterial surfaces have indicated that polyethylene is similar to other biomedical polymers such as polydimethylsiloxane, expanded polytetrafluoroethylene, and Dacron® in its ability to produce cytokines following adherent macrophage activation. Cytokines and growth factors released from adherent macrophages may function in a paracrine fashion to activate other cells in the wound healing response as shown in Figure 3.

We have extensively investigated the effect of substrate surface chemistry on monocyte/macrophage adhesion, macrophage fusion, and FBGC development (54–63). The overall goal of these studies was to identify

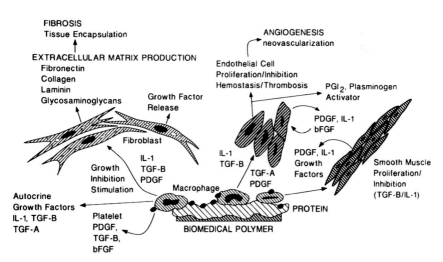

Figure 3 Polymer/protein/macrophage interfacial interactions leading to cellular activation, proliferation, and synthesis. Cytokines and growth factors control cellular processes important in biocompatibility, the foreign body reaction, and the wound healing response.

surfaces which do not permit monocyte/macrophage adhesion and/or macrophage fusion to form FBGC. Long-chain hydrocarbon groups on glass surfaces markedly reduce monocyte/macrophage adhesion and nearly eliminate IL-4-induced FBGCs (61). In contrast, polyethylene oxide (PEO) chains on glass surfaces do permit monocyte/macrophage adhesion but the level of IL-4-induced FBGC formation is markedly reduced (59). In the case of clean glass surfaces, adherent monocyte/macrophage densities are high enough to allow maximal levels of FBGC formation, however, negligible FBGC formation is observed. A comparison of these three different types of surfaces support the hypothesis that the composition and conformation of proteins adsorbed on surfaces provide signals or ligands for the adhesion of monocytes/macrophages as well as the macrophage fusion process itself. Thus, long-term macrophage adhesion and IL-4- or IL-13-induced FBGC formation are surface-dependent phenomena.

Cytoskeletal and adhesive structure studies of in vitro macrophages and FBGCs have demonstrated that podosomal structures, and not focal contacts, are the major adhesive structures present within macrophages and FBGC on surfaces (64,65). The podosomal structures are present at the ventral periphery of the FBGC and contain vinculin, talin, and paxillin in a ring-like structure surrounding a F-actin core (Fig. 4) These podosomal adhesion structures are similar to those identified for osteoclast adhesion. The podosomal structure present at the ventral and peripheral macrophage and FBGC surface implies a functional polarization and suggests the presence of frustrated phagocytosis via the formation of a closed compartment between the macrophage or FBGC and the underlying substrate where acid, degradative enzymes, reactive oxygen intermediates, and/or other products are secreted.

Macrophage interactions play a major role in total joint prosthesis failure through wear mechanisms. Polymethylmethacrylate (PMMA) bone cement particulate at the bone/bone cement interface may elicit inflammatory bone resorption, i.e., osteolysis, through macrophage and FBGC frustrated phagocytosis of the particulate. Macrophage interactions with PMMA particulate lead to macrophage activation with cytokine release and interleukin-1 stimulation of fibroblast proliferation and extracellular matrix synthesis (Fig. 3). PMMA bone cement particulate is commonly generated at the bone/bone cement interface by a mismatch in mechanical properties leading to fracture of the PMMA bone cement and production of particulate. The over-exuberant use of bone cement may lead to the generation of PMMA bone cement particulate with migration into the joint space where the PMMA particulate virtually functions as a grit to wear both the metallic and polyethylene articular surfaces. Migration of metal and polyethylene particulate then occurs from the synovial fluid in the joint space through the synovium and into the underlying tissue where focal granulomas composed of macrophages and FBGCs surrounding the particulate are

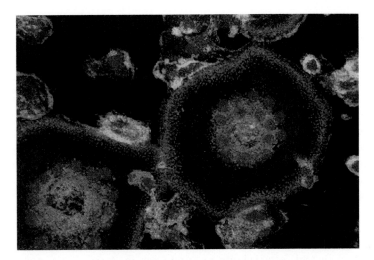

Figure 4 Macrophage fusion and foreign body giant cell formation in vitro. Human monocytes were cultured for three days to promote macrophage development. Monocyte-derived macrophages were then treated with interleukin-4 to induce macrophage fusion leading to multinucleated foreign body giant cell formation after four additional days of culture. Fluorescence confocal scanning laser microscopy was used to evaluate immunofluorescent staining of fusing macrophages and giant cells for beta2 integrins (*green*), filamentous actin (*red*), and nuclei (*blue*). The yellow fluorescence represents co-localization of beta2 integrins with actin. Punctate actin structures at the cell periphery indicate podosomal adhesion to the underlying substrate. (*See color insert.*)

present. Metal particulate generally does not form granulomas as its size is such that macrophages phagocytose these smaller particles, less than 1 μm in largest dimension. Sheets of macrophages containing metal particulate then form within the subsynovial tissue.

Foreign Body Giant Cell Formation and Interactions

The foreign body reaction is composed of FBGCs and the components of granulation tissue, which consist of macrophages, fibroblasts, and capillaries in varying amounts, depending upon the form and topography of the implanted material. Relatively flat and smooth surfaces, such as those found on breast prostheses, have a foreign body reaction that is composed of a layer of macrophages one to two cells in thickness. Relatively rough surfaces, such as those found on the outer surfaces of expanded poly(tetrafluoroethylene) (eTPFE) vascular prostheses or PMMA bone cement, have a foreign body reaction composed of several layers of macrophages and FBGCs at the surface. Fabric materials generally have a surface response composed of macrophages and FBGCs with varying degrees of granulation tissue subjacent to the surface response.

As previously discussed, the form and topography of the surface of the biomaterial determines the composition of the foreign body reaction. With biocompatible materials, the composition of the foreign body reaction in the implant site may be controlled by the surface properties of the biomaterial, the form of the implant, and the relationship between the surface area of the biomaterial and the volume of the implant. For example, high surface-to-volume implants such as fabrics or porous materials will have higher ratios of macrophages and FBGCs in the implant site than will smooth-surface implants, which will have fibrosis as a significant component of the implant site.

The foreign body reaction consisting mainly of macrophages and/or FBGCs may persist at the tissue–implant interface for the lifetime of the implant (1–3,66–69). Generally, fibrosis (i.e., fibrous encapsulation) surrounds the biomaterial or implant with its interfacial foreign body reaction, isolating the implant and foreign body reaction from the local tissue environment. Early in the inflammatory and wound healing response, the macrophages are activated upon adherence to the material surface. Although it is generally considered that the chemical and physical properties of the biomaterial are responsible for macrophage activation, the nature of the subsequent events regarding the activity of macrophages at the surface is not clear. Tissue macrophages, derived from circulating blood monocytes, may coalesce to form multinucleated FBGCs. FBGCs containing large numbers of nuclei are typically present on the surface of biomaterials. Although these FBGCs may persist for the lifetime of the implant, it is not known if they remain activated, releasing their lysosomal constituents, or become quiescent.

Efforts in our laboratory have focused on differential lymphokine regulation of macrophage fusion which leads to morphological variants of multinucleated giant cells, and the role played by the surface chemistry and other properties of the foreign material in facilitating monocyte adhesion, macrophage development, and giant cell formation. FBGCs are observed at the tissue–material interface of medical devices implanted in soft and hard tissue and remain at the implant–tissue interface for the lifetime of the device in vivo, which in some cases may extend beyond 20 years. In addition, FBGC have been implicated in the biodegradation of polymeric medical devices (70–72). FBGC and macrophages constituting the foreign body reaction at the tissue/device interface are surface area dependent. For these and other reasons, we have sought to identify the mechanism of induction of FBGC on biomaterials and the physiological and material bases for their formation.

Early studies utilizing lymphokines in the induction of FBGC formation utilized a wide variety of experimental conditions and resulted in both positive and negative modulation of FBGC formation (69). A number of these studies utilized conditioned media or supernatants. To provide a clearer identification of cell-derived agents which produce FBGC, we utilized recombinant human lymphokines with freshly isolated human monocytes in our culture systems. We believe that these conditions provide greater insight into FBGC formation and obviate unidentified problems that may result from the use of transformed cell lines and conditioned media and supernatants.

In our studies, human interleukin-4 (IL-4) induced the formation of FBGC from human monocyte-derived macrophages, an effect that was optimized with either GM-CSF or IL-3, dependent on the concentration of IL-4, and specifically prevented by anti-IL-4 (46,54). Very large FBGC with randomly arranged nuclei and extensive cytoplasmic spreading (285 ± 121 nuclei and 1.151 ± 0.303 mm^2/FBGC) were consistently obtained (Fig. 4). Rates of macrophage fusion in this system were high: $72 \pm 5\%$.

Most et al. (73) have shown that the fusion rates of monocytes/macrophages decrease with advancing differentiation and almost no giant cell formation was observed with 8-day-old macrophages which were derived from freshly isolated monocytes stimulated with cytokine-containing supernatants. A distinct difference in adhesion was seen in our studies when IL-4 was added to freshly adherent (2 hour) monocytes (46). IL-4 under these conditions resulted in a detachment of adherent cells and an inhibition of initial monocyte adhesion by IL-4. To accelerate the development of macrophage morphology, we added GM-CSF initially and at three days added IL-4 to induce macrophage fusion and FBGC formation. While positive effects may result from the use of conditioned media or inflammatory cell-derived supernatants, it must also be considered that negative autocrine or paracrine effects with downregulation of biological interactions important to macrophage differentiation and FBGC development may occur. It is obvious that the utilization of human cells together with appropriate recombinant human cytokines and antibodies provide for cleaner and more relevant systems in mechanistic studies of macrophage differentiation and fusion with FBGC formation.

Figure 5 demonstrates the sequence of events involved in inflammation and wound healing when medical devices are implanted. In general, the PMN predominant acute inflammatory response and the lymphocyte/monocyte predominant chronic inflammatory response resolve quickly, i.e., within two weeks depending on the type and location of implant. Studies utilizing IL-4 by ourselves and others demonstrate the role for Th2 helper lymphocytes in the development of the foreign body reaction at the tissue/material interface. Th2 helper lymphocytes have been described as "anti-inflammatory" based on their cytokine profile of which IL-4 is a significant component. Th2 helper lymphocytes also produce IL-13 and we have utilized this to demonstrate its similar effect to IL-4 on FBGC formation (55). In this regard, it is noteworthy that anti-IL-4 antibody does not

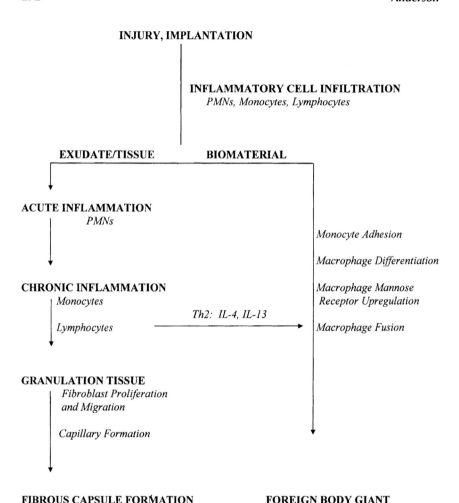

Figure 5 Sequence of events involved in inflammatory and wound healing responses leading to foreign body giant cell formation. This shows the importance of Th2 lymphocytes in the transient chronic inflammatory phase with the production of IL-4 and IL-3 which can induce monocyte/macrophage fusion to form foreign body giant cells.

inhibit IL-13 induced FBGC formation nor does anti-IL-13 antibody inhibit IL-4 induced FBGC formation. In our IL-4 and IL-13 FBGC culture systems, the macrophage mannose receptor (MMR) has been identified as critical to the fusion of macrophages in the formation of FBGC (55,56). FBGC formation can be prevented by competitive inhibitors of MMR activity, i.e., α-mannan, or inhibitors of glycoprotein processing that restrict MMR surface expression.

The lifetime of FBGCs at tissue/material interfaces is still unknown. Early publications had suggested that they were relatively short lived, lasting for several days. This is probably not true as clinical specimens show the presence of FBGCs for years and, in some cases, decades. Honma and Hamasaki (74) have reported on the ultrastructure of multinucleated giant cell apoptosis in a collagen sponge granuloma. They noted the disappearance of giant cells coincident with the resorption of the collagen sponge. This is most probably correct as once the inciting agent for giant cell formation is no longer present, the presence of giant cells is no longer necessary.

The osteoclast, the multinucleated giant cell responsible for bone resorption, is the most widely studied of all types of giant cells. Unlike the other types of giant cells which are found with pathological conditions, the osteoclast is found at bone surfaces where it participates in the constant process of bone remodelling. Excessive osteoclast activity in bone resorption has been implicated in pathological processes such as the advanced stages of multiple myeloma with lytic lesions in bone, postmenopausal osteoporosis, and osteolysis leading to total joint prosthesis failure. The majority of studies suggest that the CFU-GM, the granulocyte–macrophage progenitor, a cell in the monocyte–macrophage lineage, is the earliest osteoclast precursor. While the osteoclast, like the Langhans giant cell and the FBGC may have a hematopoietic precursor, molecular and cell biology studies have shown that the osteoclast has distinctly different functional and phenotypic characteristics (75,76). Table 4 demonstrates the functional

Table 4 Phenotypic and Functional Differences Between Osteoclasts and Monocyte–Macrophage-Derived Giant Cells[a]

	Osteoclasts	Monocyte–macrophage-derived giant cells
Podosomal adhesion structures to substrates	+	+
Resorption lacunae formation	+	−
Ruffled cell border	+	±
Vitronectin receptor expression	+	±
Calcitonin receptor expression	+	−
Calcitonin response	+	−
Tartrate-resistance acid phosphatase in vitro expression	+	−
Fc receptor expression	−	+
Nonspecific esterase expression	−	+

[a]The presence of phenotypic markers on the cell is denoted by the *plus sign* (+); the absence of phenotypic markers is denoted by the *minus sign* (−). Low abundance of phenotypic markers is denoted by the *plus-or-minus* sign (±).

and phenotypic differences between osteoclasts and monocyte/macrophage-derived giant cells.

The calcitonin receptor is the best marker for distinguishing mammalian osteoclasts as this receptor is not expressed on monocyte/macrophage-derived giant cells. A wide variety of factors can influence osteoclast formation and function. These include systemic hormones, cytokines, and growth factors. It is noteworthy that neither IL-4 (FBGC formation) or γ-Interferon (Langhans giant cell formation) is described as a significant factor in the formation or activation of osteoclasts. These findings suggest that although the CFU-GM progenitor is of monocytic lineage, its differentiation does not include expression of IL-4 or IFN-γ receptors or perhaps even a common signal transduction pathway. This is somewhat surprising as both FEGC and osteoclasts adhere to substrates through podosomal structures.

Recent studies demonstrate the ability of IL-1 and TNF-α to induce osteoclast formation and the bone-resorbing activity of osteoclasts (77–79). These studies suggest that activated macrophages may facilitate bone resorption by participating in osteoclast formation and activation. The role of TNF-α in regulating osteoclastic bone resorption continues to be elucidated with studies demonstrating that osteoblasts/stromal cells express a new member of the TNF-ligand family "osteoclast differentiation factor (ODF)/osteoprotegerin (OPGL)/TNF-related activation-induced cytokine (TRANCE)/receptor activation of NF-kB ligand (RANKL)" as a membrane associated factor (79–81).

Fibrosis and Fibrous Encapsulation

The end-stage healing response to biomaterials is generally fibrosis or fibrous encapsulation. However, there may be exceptions to this general statement (e.g., porous materials inoculated with parenchymal cells or porous materials implanted into bone).

Repair of implant sites involves two distinct processes: regeneration, which is the replacement of injured tissue by parenchymal cells of the same type, or replacement by connective tissue that constitutes the fibrous capsule. These processes are generally controlled by either (i) the proliferative capacity of the cells in the tissue receiving the implant and the extent of injury as it relates to the destruction, or (ii) persistence of the tissue framework of the implant site. The regenerative capacity of cells permits classification into three groups: labile, stable (or expanding), and permanent (or static) cells. Labile cells continue to proliferate throughout life, stable cells retain this capacity but do not normally replicate, and permanent cells cannot reproduce themselves after birth. Perfect repair with restitution of normal structure theoretically occurs only in tissues consisting of stable and labile cells, whereas all injuries to tissues composed of permanent cells may give rise to fibrosis and fibrous capsule formation with very little restitution of the normal tissue or organ structure. Tissues composed of permanent cells (e.g., nerve cells, skeletal muscle cells, and cardiac muscle cells) most commonly undergo an organization of the inflammatory exudate, leading to fibrosis. Tissues composed of stable cells (e.g., parenchymal cells of the liver, kidney, and pancreas), mesenchymal cells (e.g., fibroblasts, smooth muscle cells, osteoblasts, and chrondroblasts), and vascular endothelial and labile cells (e.g., epithelial cells and lymphoid and hematopoietic cells) may also follow this pathway to fibrosis or may undergo resolution of the inflammatory exudate, leading to restitution of the normal tissue structure. The condition of the underlying framework or supporting stroma of the parenchymal cells following an injury plays an important role in the restoration of normal tissue structure. Retention of the framework may lead to restitution of the normal tissue structure, whereas destruction of the framework most commonly leads to fibrosis. It is important to consider the species-dependent nature of the regenerative capacity of cells. For example, cells from the same organ or tissue but from different species may exhibit different regenerative capacities and/or connective tissue repair.

With total joint prostheses, the important interfaces are those involved in fixation of the components, i.e., metal, ceramic, or bone cement, with bone. It is these interfaces where inflammatory responses, provisional matrix formation, and/or healing responses may compromise the ultimate function of the total joint prosthesis. The extent of provisional matrix formation is an important factor as it is related to wound healing by first or second intention. First intention (primary union) wound healing occurs when there is minimal to no space between the bone and device whereas second intention (secondary union) wound healing occurs when a large space, providing for extensive provisional matrix formation, is present. Obviously, inappropriate or inadequate preparation of the implant site leading to extensive provisional matrix formation predisposes the total joint prosthesis to failure through mechanisms related to fibrous capsule formation.

FUTURE PERSPECTIVES

The concept of regenerative medicine and the development of biomaterials, prostheses, and medical devices which play a distinct functional role in the efficacy of implants requires an enhanced knowledge base and a molecular and cellular biology approach to inflammation and the role of macrophages and FBGCs in the foreign body reaction. It is clear that the foreign body reaction and fibrous encapsulation, commonly seen with so-called passive implants over the past four decades, may lead to functional impairment with a loss of efficacy of new types of devices based on tissue engineering and other approaches. Current and future technologies for investigating the cell and molecular biology of the foreign body reaction and fibrous encapsulation must be used to identify mechanisms such that the foreign body reaction and fibrous encapsulation are negated or inhibited with new functional devices. In particular, efforts must be undertaken to better understand protein adsorption on surfaces, monocyte/macrophage/FBGC adhesion, activation, and signal transduction and the role played by bioactive molecules generated through these processes must be better understood. New biomaterials, prostheses, and medical devices must be developed using biological criteria in addition to chemical, physical, mechanical, and other types of criteria traditionally used in the past.

The development and utilization of biological criteria for the development of new prostheses and devices requires, in part, a better understanding of gene induction and upregulation or downregulation when monocytes/macrophages/FBGCs, osteoblasts, osteoclasts, fibroblasts, and other cells present at implant/tissue interfaces adhere and are activated. Only recently have these approaches been initiated to understand the role of genes in modulating cytokine and growth factor participation by the aforementioned cell types. The identification of genes which may modulate cytokine and growth factor participation in the foreign body reaction and fibrous encapsulation is a research area currently in its infancy and in need of further growth and expansion. Modulation and control of cell function at material interfaces, the identification of gene induction by cell/material interactions, and the subsequent autocrine, paracrine, and endocrine effects generated by cell activation products offer broad as well as in-depth areas of research in cell–cell interactions and cell–material interactions for the future.

REFERENCES

1. Anderson JM. Mechanisms of inflammation and infection with implanted devices. Cardiovasc Pathol 1993; 2:199S–208S.
2. Anderson JM. Inflammation and the foreign body response. Prob Gen Surg 1994; 11:147–160.
3. Anderson JM. Inflammatory response to implants. ASAIO 1988; 11:101–107.
4. Acute and chronic inflammation, tissue repair: cellular growth, fibrosis and wound healing. In: Cotran RZ, Kumar V, Robbins SL, eds. Pathologic Basis of Disease, 6th ed. Philadelphia: W.B. Saunders, 1999:50–112.
5. Gallin JI, Synderman R, eds. Inflammation: Basic Principles and Clinical Correlates. 2nd ed. New York: Raven Press; 1999.
6. Weissman G, Smolen JE, Korchak HM. Release of inflammatory mediators from stimulated neutrophils. N Engl J Med 1980; 303:27–34.
7. Salthouse TN. Cellular enzyme activity at the polymer–tissue interface: a review. J Biomed Mater Res 1976; 10:197–229.
8. Clark RA, Lanigan JM, DellePelle P, Manseau E, Dvorak HF, Colvin RB. Fibronectin and fibrin provide a provisional matrix for epidermal cell migration during wound reepithelialization. J Invest Dermatol 1982; 79:264.
9. Tang L, Eaton JW. Fibrin(ogen) mediates acute inflammatory responses to biomaterials. J Exp Med 1993; 178:2147–2156.

10. Tang L. Mechanism of pro-inflammatory fibrinogen:biomaterial interactions. J biomater Sci Polym Ed 1998; 9:1257–1266.
11. Riches DWF. Macrophage involvement in wound repair, remodeling, and fibrosis. In: Clark RAP, Henson PM, eds. The Molecular and Cellular Biology of Wound Repair. New York: Plenum Press, 1998:213.
12. Wahl SM, Wong H, McCartney FN. Role of growth factors in inflammation and repair. J Cell Biochem 1989; 40:193.
13. Dvorak HF, Harvey VS, Estrella P, Brown LF, McDonagh J, Dvorak AM. Fibrin containing gels induce angiogenesis. Implications for tumor stroma generation and wound healing. Lab Invest 1987; 57:673.
14. Broadley KN, Aquino AM, Woodward SC, A Buckley-Sturrock, Sato Y, Rifkin DB, Davidson JM. Monospecific antibodies implicate basic fibroblast growth factor in normal wound repair. Lab Invest 1989; 61:571.
15. Sporn MB, Roberts AB. Peptide growth factors are multifunctional. Nature 1988; 332:217.
16. Muller G, Behrens J, Nussbaumer U, Böhlen P, Birchmeier W. Inhibitor action of transforming growth factor beta on endothelial cells. Proc Natl Acad Sci USA 1987; 84:5600.
17. Madri JA, Pratt BM, Tucker AM. Phenotypic modulation of endothelial cells by transforming growth factor-beta depends upon the composition and organization of the extracellular matrix. J Cell Biol 1988; 106:1375.
18. Wahl SM, Hunt DA, Wakefield LM, Roberts AB, Sporn MB. Transforming growth factor-beta (TGF-β) induces monocyte chemotaxis and growth factor production. Proc Natl Acad Sci USA 1987; 84:5788.
19. Ignotz R, Endo T, Massague J. Regulation of fibronectin and type I collagen mRNA levels by transforming growth factor-beta. J Biol Chem 1987; 262:6443.
20. Marchant R, Hiltner A, Hamlin C, Rabinovitch A, Slobodkin R, Anderson JM. In vivo biocompatibility studies: I. The cage implant system and a biodegradable hydrogel. J Biomed Mater Res 1983; 17:301–325.
21. Spilizewski KL, Marchant RE, Hamlin CR, Anderson JM, Tice TR, Dappert TO, Meyers WE. The effect of hydrocortisone acetate loaded poly(DL-lactide) films on the inflammatory response. J Contr Res 1985; 2:197–203.
22. Ganz T. Nentrophil receptors. In: Lehrer RI (moderator). Neutrophils and Host Defense. Ann Intern Med 1988; 109:127–142.
23. Henson PM, Johnston RB Jr. Tissue injury in inflammation: oxidants, proteinases, and cationic proteins. J Clin Invest 1987; 79:669–674.
24. Malech HL, Gallin JI. Current concepts: immunology. Neutrophils in human diseases. N Engl J Med 1987; 317:687–694.
25. Jutila MA. Leukocyte traffic to sites of inflammation. APMIS 1992; 100:191–201.
26. Pober JS, Cotran RS. The role of endothelial cells in inflammation. Transplantation 1990; 50:537–544.
27. Cotran RS, Pober JS. Cytokine–endothelial interactions in inflammation, immunity, and vascular injury. J Am Soc Nephrol 1990; 1:225–235.
28. Hynes RO. Integrins: versatility, modulation, and signaling in cell adhesion. Cell 1992; 69:11–25.
29. Butcher EC. Leukocyte-endothelial cell recognition: three (or more) steps to specificity and diversity. Cell 1991; 67:1033–1036.

30. Henson PM. The immunologic release of constituents from neutrophil leuko-cytes. II. Mechanisms of release during phagocytosis, and adherence to nonpha-gocytosable surfaces. J Immunol 1971; 107:1547–1557.
31. Henson PM. Mechanisms of exocytosis in phagocytic inflammatory cells. Am J Pathol 1980; 101:494–511.
32. Weiss SJ. Tissue destruction by neutrophils. N Engl J Med 1989; 320:365–376.
33. Paty PB, Graeff RW, Mathes SJ, Hunt TK. Superoxide production by wound neutrophils: evidence for increased activity of the NADPH oxidase. Arch Surg 1990; 125:65–69.
34. Johnston RB Jr. Monocytes and macrophages. N Engl J Med 1988; 318:747–752.
35. Williams GT, Williams WJ. Granulomatous inflammation—a review. J Clin Pathol 1983; 36:723–733.
36. Wahl SM, Wong H, McCartney-Francis N. Role of growth factors in inflam-mation and repair. J Cell Biochem 1989; 40:193–199.
37. Sporn MB, Roberts AB, eds. Peptide Growth Factors and Their Receptors I. New York: Springer, 1990.
38. Fong Y, Moldawer LL, Shires GT, Lowry SF. The biologic characteristics of cytokines and their implication in surgical injury. Surg Gynecol Obstet 1990; 170:363–378.
39. Kovacs EJ. Fibrogenic cytokines: the role of immune mediators in the develop-ment of scar tissue. Immunol Today 1991; 12:17–23.
40. Golden MA, Au YP, Kirkman TR, Wilcox JN, Raines EW, Ross R, Clowes AW. Platelet-derived growth factor activity and RNA expression in healing vas-cular grafts in baboons. J Clin Invest 1991; 87:406–414.
41. Mustoe TA, Pierce GF, Thomason A, Gramats P, Sporn MB, Deuel TF. Accel-erated healing of incisional wounds in rats induced by transforming growth factor. Science 1987; 237:1333–1336.
42. Maciag T. Molecular and cellular mechanisms of angiogenesis. In: VT DeVita, Hellman S, Rosenberg S, eds. Important Advances in Oncology. Philadelphia: Lippincott 1990:85.
43. Thompson JA, Anderson KD, DiPetro JM, Zweibel JA, Zmaetta M, Anderson WF, Maciag T. Site-directed neovessel formation in vivo. Science 1988; 241; 1349–1352.
44. Ziats NP, Miller KM, Anderson JM. In vitro and in vivo interactions of cells with biomaterials. Biomaterials 1985; 9:5–13.
45. McNally AK, Anderson JM. Complement C3 participation in monocyte adhe-sion to different surfaces. Proc Natl Acad Sci USA 1994; 91:10119–10123.
46. McNally AK, Anderson JM. Interleukin-4 induces foreign body giant cells from human monocytes/macrophages. Differential lymphokine regulation of macrophage fusion leads to morphological variants of multinucleated giant cells. Amer J Pathol 1995; 147:1487–1499.
47. Miller KM, Anderson JM. Human monocyte/macrophage activation and interleukin 1 generation by biomedical polymers. J Biomed Mater Res 1988; 22:713–731.
48. Miller KM, Hnskey RA, Bigby LF, Anderson JM. Characterization of bio-medical polymer-adherent macrophages: interleukin 1 generation and scanning electron microscopy studies. Biomaterials 1989; 10:187–196.

49. Bonfield TL, Colton E, Anderson JM. Plasma protein adsorbed biomedical polymers: activation of human monocytes and inductin of interleukin 1. J Biomed Mater Res 1989; 23:535–548.
50. Miller KM, Anderson JM. In vitro stimulation of fibroblast activity by factors generated from human monocytes activated by biomedical polymers. J Biomed Mater Res 1989; 23:911–930.
51. Miller KM, Rose-Caprara V, Anderson JM. Generation of IL-like activity in response to biomedical polymer implants: a comparison of in vitro and in vivo models. J Biomed Mater Res 1989; 23:1007–1026.
52. Bonfield TL, Colton E, Marchant RE, Anderson JM. Cytokine and growth factor production by monocytes/macrophages on protein preadsorbed polymers. J Biomed Mater Res 1992; 26:837–850.
53. Bonfield TL, Anderson JM. Functional versus quantitative comparison of IL-1β from monocytes/macrophages on biomedical polymers. J Biomed Mater Res 1993; 27:1195–1199.
54. Kao WJ, McNally AK, Hiltner A, Anderson JM. Role for interleukin-4 in foreign-body giant cell formation on a poly(etherurethane urea) in vivo. J Biomed Mater Res 1995; 29:1267–1276.
55. DeFife KM, McNally AK, Colton E, Anderson JM. Interleukin-13 induces human monocyte/macrophage fusion and macrophage mannose receptor expression. J Immunol 1997; 158:319–328.
56. McNally AK, DeFife KM, Anderson JM. Interleukin-4-induced macrophage fusion is prevented by inhibitors of mannose receptor activity. Am J Pathol 1996; 149:975–985.
57. Jenney CR, DeFife KM, Colton E, Anderson JM. Human monocyte/ macrophage adhesion, macrophage motility, and IL-4-induced foreign body giant cell formation on silane-modified surfaces in vitro. J Biomed Mater Res 1998; 41:171–184.
58. DeFife KM, Shive MS, Hagen KM, Clapper DL, Anderson JM. Effects of photochemically immobilized polymer coatings on protein adsorption, cell adhesion and the foreign body reaction to silicone rubber. J Biomed Mater Res 1999; 44:298–307.
59. Jenney CR, Anderson JM. Effects of surface-coupled polyethylene oxide on human macrophage adhesion and foreign body giant cell formation in vitro. J Biomed Mater Res 1998; 44:206–216.
60. DeFife KM, Colton E, Nakayama Y, Matsuda T, Anderson JM. Spatial regulation and surface chemistry control of monocyte/macrophage adhesion and foreign body giant cell formation by photochemically micropatterned surfaces. J Biomed Mater Res 1999; 45:148–154.
61. Jenney CR, Anderson JM. Alkylsilane-modified surfaces: inhibition of human macrophage adhesion and foreign body giant cell formation. J Biomed Mater Res 1999; 46:11–21.
62. Jenney CR, Anderson JM. Adsorbed serum proteins responsible for surface dependent human macrophage behavior. J Biomed Mater Res 2000; 49: 435–447.
63. Jenney CR, Anderson JM. Adsorbed IgG: a potent adhesive substrate for human macrophages. J Biomed Mater Res 2000; 50:281–290.

64. DeFife KM, Jenney CR, Colton E, Anderson JM. Cytoskeletal and adhesive structural polarizations accompany IL-13-induced human macrophage fusion. J Histochem Cytochem 1999; 47:65–74.

65. DeFife KM, Jenney CR, Colton E, Anderson JM. Disruption of filamentous actin inhibits human macrophage fusion. FASEB J 1999; 13:823–832.

66. Rae T. The macrophage response to implant materials. Crit Rev Biocompatibility 1986; 2:97–126.

67. Greisler H. Macrophage–biomaterial interactions with bioresorbable vascular prostheses. Trans Am Soc Artif Intern Organs 1988; 34:1051–1057.

68. Chambers TJ, Spector WG. Inflammatory giant cells. Immunobiology 1982; 161:283–289.

69. Anderson JM. Multinucleated giant cells. Curr Opin Hematol 2000; 7:40–47.

70. Zhao Q, Agger MP, Fitzpatrick M, Anderson JM, Hiltner A, Stokes K, Urbanski P. Cellular interactions with biomaterials: in vivo cracking of prestressed Pellethane 2363–80A. J Biomed Mater Res 1990; 24:621–637.

71. Zhao Q, Topham N, Anderson JM, Hiltner A, Lodoen G, Payet CR. Foreign-body giant cells and polyurethane biostability: *in vivo* correlation of cell adhesion and surface cracking. J Bio med Mater Res 1991; 25:177–183.

72. Wiggins MJ, Wilkoff B, Anderson JM, Hiltner A. Biodegradation of polyether polyurethane inner insulation in bipolar pacemaker leads. J Biomed Mater Res (Appl Biomater) 2001; 58:302–307, 2001.

73. Möst J, Spotl L, Mayr G, Gasser A, Sarti A, Dierich MP. Formation of multinucleated giant cells in vitro is dependent on the stage of monocyte to macrophage maturation. Blood 1997; 89(2):662–671.

74. Honma T, Hamasaki T. Ultrastructure of multinucleated giant cell apoptosis in foreign-body granulomas. Virchows Arch 1996; 428:165–176.

75. Roodman GD. Advances in bone biology: the osteoclast. Endocr Rev 1996; 17: 308–332.

76. Greenfield EM, Bi Y, Miyauchi A. Regulation of osteoclast activity. Life Sci 1999; 65:1087–1102.

77. Merkel KD, Erdmann JM, McHugh KP, Abu-Amer Y, Ross FP, Teitelbaum SL. Tumor necrosis factor-α mediates orthopedic implant osteolysis. Am J Pathol 1999; 154:203–210.

78. Jimi E, Nakamura I, Duong LT, Ikebe T, Takahashi N, Rodan GA, Suda T. Interleukin 1 induces multinucleation and bone-resorbing activity of osteoclasts in the absence of osteoblasts/stromal cells. Exp Cell Res 1999; 247:84–93.

79. Takahashi N, Udagawa N, Suda T. A new member of tumor necrosis factor ligand family, ODF/OPGL/TRANCE/RANKL, regulates osteoclast differentiation and function. Biochem Biophys Res Commun 1999; 256:449–455.

80. Burgess TL, Qian Y, Kaufman S, Ring BD, Van G, Capparelli C, Kelley M, Asu H, Boyle WJ, Dunstan CR, Hu S, Lacey DL. The ligand for osteoprotegerin (OPGL) directly activates mature osteoclasts. J Cell Biol 1999; 145:527–538.

81. Lum L, Wong BR, Josien R, Becherer JD, Erdjument-Bromage H, Schlondorff J, Tempst P, Choi Y, CP. Evidence for a role of a tumor necrosis factor-alpha (TNA-alpha)-converting enzyme-like protease in shedding of TRANCE, a TNF family member involved in osteoclastogenesis and dendritic cell survival. J Biol Chem 1999; 75:783–790.

12

Cytokines and Mediators in Physiologic and Pathologic Bone Resorption

David R. Haynes

Department of Pathology, Adelaide University, South Australia, Australia

Tania N. Crotti

New England Baptist Bone and Joint Institute, Beth Israel Deaconess Medical Center, Harvard Medical School, Boston, Massachusetts, U.S.A.

INTRODUCTION

Peri-implant Bone Remodeling

Maintaining healthy bone at the surface of prosthetic implants is vital for the longterm stability of artificial joints. Healthy bone is in a dynamic state continually being lost and replaced through the process of remodeling. Remodeling of bone relies on the integrated activity of the osteoblast (bone forming) and osteoclast (bone resorbing) cells to maintain the balance of bone metabolism (1). An imbalance in bone metabolism due to either excessive resorption or decreased bone formation can result in bone loss. While we have known for well over a decade about the factors, such as the bone morphogenic proteins, which regulate bone formation by osteoblasts, it is only relatively recently that we understand how osteoclasts form and resorb bone. While this review of peri-implant osteolysis will focus on the mediators that regulate osteoclasts it is important to recognize that bone formation by osteoblasts may also be disrupted in this pathology.

Localized bone loss is seen in several pathological states, such as adjacent to prosthetic joints, in periodontal disease and in rheumatoid arthritis

(RA). These three diseases are similar in that the bone loss is associated with a chronic inflammatory response in the surrounding soft tissues. This appears to be initiated in response to foreign material such as wear debris, in the case of peri-implant loosening, bacteria in the case of periodontitis, or an auto-immune response as suggested in the case of RA.

Osteolysis in bone loss pathologies is carried out by osteoclasts that form and then resorb bone under the control of cytokines and other mediators. Factors that regulate physiologic bone resorption may also regulate pathologic bone loss. We will explore the possibility that excessive peri-implant bone lysis is caused by an abnormal expression of factors that regulate osteoclast formation and activity. In this chapter, we will endeavor to not only describe these factors but also to elucidate a possible mechanism by which osteolytic mediators induce peri-implant bone lysis.

Osteoclast Activity and Peri-implant Bone Loss

Osteoclasts are defined as being multinucleated giant cells with the ability to resorb mineralized tissue (2). It is generally believed that they arise from hematopoietic stem cells of the monocyte–macrophage lineage that, in the process of osteoclast differentiation, lose macrophage markers (such as CD11a, CD11b, CD14, HLA-DR, and CD68) and acquire markers specific to osteoclasts (3–5). Osteoclasts are negative for these markers, but possess tartrate-resistant acid phosphatase (TRAP) with calcitonin receptors (CTR) (2,6), and express the cell surface integrin CD51, the alpha chain of the vitronectin receptor (VNR) (2,7), the ability to produce acids and the ability to resorb pits on mineralized tissue (6).

Additional osteoclast markers include carbonic anhydrase II (CAII), cathepsin K (cath K), matrix metalloproteinase MMP9, osteopontin (OPN), and β3 Integrin (4,8). The receptor for macrophage colony stimulating factor (M-CSF) on peripheral blood monocytes and macrophages, which is encoded by the proto-oncogene, *c-fms* (9–11) is also present on pre-osteoclasts and mature osteoclasts (12–14). More recently, the receptor activator of necrosis factor κB (RANK) has been identified as a differential marker of pre-osteoclasts and osteoclasts (15–20). The changes in expression of the various cell surface markers are summarized in Figure 1.

There is strong evidence for the presence of osteoclastic cells in the peri-implant tissues. Immunohistochemical studies using monoclonal antibodies have demonstrated macrophages and foreign body giant cells in the pseudomembrane surrounding loose prostheses express cytokine receptors found on osteoclastic cells (21). In addition, macrophages and foreign body giant cells, which are seen in the pseudomembrane surrounding loose prostheses, express similar markers to that found on mature osteoclasts (21,22). It is also likely that there are cells present in the peri-implant tissues that are in the process of differentiating from macrophages to mature osteoclasts (23).

The large numbers of macrophages present in the peri-implant tissues have the ability to become osteoclasts. Furthermore, large numbers of cells

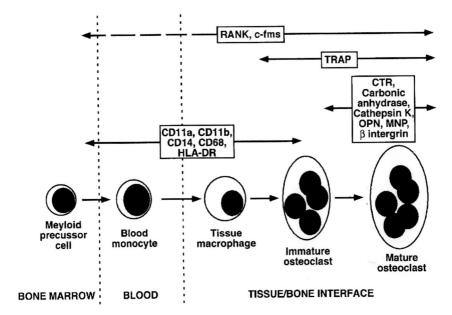

Figure 1 Schematic of the changes in the expression of cell markers expressed by cells of the monocyte/macrophage lineage as they mature to become osteoclasts. The abbreviations are described in the text and the broken line indicates that studies are yet to be carried out to determine when monocyte/macrophages first express RANK.

of the macrophage–monocyte lineage in the peri-implant tissues may be associated with the extent of osteolysis. Kadoya et al. (22) found interface tissue obtained during revision surgery adjacent to areas with osteolysis contained significantly more cells expressing the macrophage marker, CD llb, than areas without lysis. This concept is supported by similar studies in patients with RA where the degree of joint erosion significantly correlated with the number of synovial macrophages (24).

Osteoclast formation from macrophages and monocytes in the peri-implant tissues is considered to significantly contribute to peri-implant osteolysis. Several studies show that mononuclear cells from the peri-implant tissues of patients with implant loosening are capable of differentiating into bone resorbing osteoclasts when cultured under appropriate conditions (25–28,48). Similar studies have also shown that osteoclasts can form from cells isolated from the joints of patients with RA (29–33).

Macrophages from the inflammatory cell infiltrates in the pseudocapsules and pseudomembranes around failed joints that form osteoclasts ex vivo usually require co-culture with osteoblastic cells (25,26,34). Support for osteoclast formation can be provided by culture with either rat UMR 106 cells, murine ST2 cells (25,34,35), or human bone-derived cells (26,28,36). In

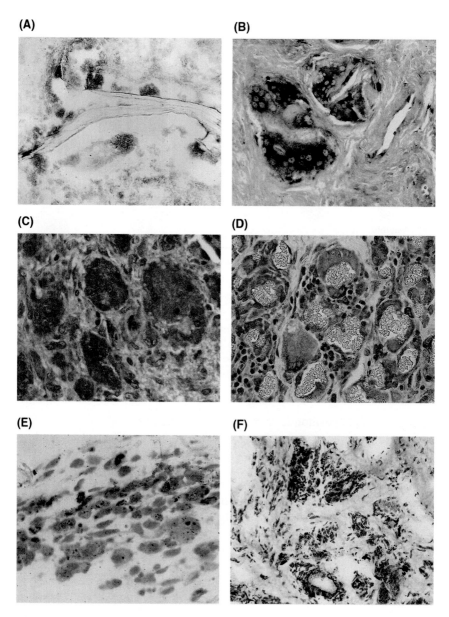

Figure 2 (*Caption on facing page*)

addition, vitamin D_3 $(1,25(OH)_2D_3)$ and M-CSF are required for up to three weeks before precursor cells differentiate into osteoclasts that resorb bone (37).

Our recent studies have shown that the cells isolated from peri-implant tissues of certain patients with failed implants may not require additional stromal or osteoblastic cell support to form bone resorbing cells (28). This indicates that, at least in some cases, cells with ability to provide stromal support for osteoclast differentiation are present in the peri-implant tissues. These cells provide important osteoclastogenic factors that are discussed later in this chapter. It is also important to note that mature osteoclasts may form within several days of culture (28). This indicates that the cells of the osteoclast lineage that are present in the peri-implant tissues may be almost, or have already, fully differentiated into mature osteoclasts.

Numerous studies of osteoclast activity have used the expression of TRAP to identify individual osteoclasts. The presence of cells expressing TRAP in the peri-implant tissues is strong evidence that osteoclasts are present in the tissues surrounding loose implants (Figure 2A). However,

---

Figure 2 (*Facing page*) TRAP, in situ and immunostaining of peri-implant tissues obtained at revision of patients with peri-implant osteolysis. Panel **A** shows a group of multinucleated giant cells, staining red (shown here in gray scale) for the presence of TRAP, surrounding a large polyethylene particle (approximately $300\times$ magnification). TRAP staining of a frozen tissue section was carried out using a staining kit from Sigma Chem. Co. (Castle Hills, Australia) and counter stained with methyl green (shown here in gray scale). Panel **B** shows two large multinucleated giant cells containing particles of polyethylene (approximately $500\times$ magnification). The purple stain (shown here in gray scale) indicates the presence of RANK mRNA. In situ hybridization was carried out using a digoxigenin (DIG)-labeled riboprobe constructed from primers described previously (28,33). Panel **C** and **D** show cells in revision tissue staining brown (shown here in gray scale) indicating TNF-α and IL-1β, respectively (approximately 300 and $150\times$ magnification). Staining was carried out using the methods described previously (247). Panel **E** shows cells have engulfed particles of polyethylene (only seen under polarized light). Panel **F** shows cells engulfing particles of silicone in peri-implant tissue from patient with failed silastic implant described previously (28). The red cytoplasmic staining in panel **E** (shown here in gray scale) indicates the presence of RANKL protein (approximately $300\times$ magnification). Many of these positive cells contain particles of metal. In panel **F**, the endothelial cells and lining blood vessels are stained red (shown here in gray scale) indicating the presence of OPG protein (approximately $300\times$ magnification). The immunostaining shown in the panels **E** and **F** was carried out using the monoclonal RANKL antibody (MAB 626) or OPG antibody (MAB 805), respectively, which were obtained from R&D Systems Inc. (Minneapolis, Minnesota, U.S.A.). Double enhancement-AEC immunohistochemistry was used to stain for RANKL and OPG as previously described (248). The authors wish to acknowledge the assistance of Dr. M. Smith and Mrs. H. Weedon in carrying out the immunostaining. *Abbreviations*: TRAP, tartrate-resistant acid phosphatase; OPG, oseoprotegerin; RANK, receptor activator of necrosis factor-κB.

caution needs to be taken when using TRAP as the sole marker for mature osteoclasts as positive staining has not always been a reliable marker for osteoclast phenotype in bone (38). It is important to note that TRAP is also expressed by human alveolar macrophages (39) and develops in macrophages activated in vivo (40). TRAP has been detected on foreign body giant cells in peri-implant tissues (22), although because the ability to resorb bone was not assessed these cells may actually have been functional osteoclasts. Chun et al. (41) suggested that the TRAP positive, VNR positive cells within the peri-implant tissue away from the bone be referred to as "osteoclast-like cells" or "osteoclast precursors" because they were not located in Howship's lacunae and therefore were not fully differentiated osteoclasts. The observations that many cells isolated from the peri-implant tissues express TRAP but usually require additional support in culture to become active osteoclasts is evidence that pre-osteoclasts that have not yet acquired the ability to resorb bone may express TRAP. More than one marker may be needed to conclusively identify mature osteoclasts (33,42).

CTR expression may better identify mature osteoclasts in tissues near pathological bone resorption. Studies have shown that this receptor is present on differentiated osteoclasts capable of resorbing bone (5,30,43–46). CTR is considered the most reliable marker of osteoclast differentiation as it is thought to distinguish osteoclasts from macrophage polykaryons (3,42,46). Takeshita (8) proposed three stages of osteoclast differentiation: the pro-osteoclast (spindle shaped macrophage cells), the pre-osteoclast (small rounded TRAP-positive cells), and the mature osteoclast (multinucleated TRAP-positive cells) stage. In this model, TRAP was expressed from the pro-osteoclast stage while CTR was strongly expressed in the multinucleated mature osteoclast stage.

Many of the large multinucleated cells that resemble mature osteoclasts (Figure 2B) often contain particles of prosthetic material. These cells are very similar to giant cells seen in granulomatous tissue during the immune reaction to foreign bodies and it is possible that these are mature osteoclasts which have phagocytosed particles during differentiation (23). Previously it was believed that osteoclasts do not phagocytose wear particles at the bone–implant interface (2). However, in vitro studies have shown that human osteoclasts derived from giant-cell tumors have the ability to phagocytose small particles of latex, poly methylmethacrylate (PMMA), and titanium in culture and retain the ability to resorb bone (47). Murine macrophages that have phagocytosed PMMA, Polyethylene (PE), titanium, or cobalt chromium particles are also able to differentiate into TRAP positive cells that resorb bone when cultured with UMR 106 cells and VD3 (48). It is therefore possible that the multinucleated cells in the granulomatous tissues that form in response to foreign bodies, such as prosthetic wear particles, share many features in common with mature osteoclasts.

Osteoclast Formation

Recent research has made major advances in our understanding of the process of osteoclast formation. Most of this has been based on studies made using human and animal physiologic models of osteoclast formation in vitro and relatively few studies have been carried out in human pathologies thus far.

Models of osteoclast formation have been based on simple co-cultures of cells from the monocyte lineage and osteoblastic cells. It appears cells of the macrophage/monocyte lineage at all stages of differentiation may have the potential to become osteoclasts and that only relatively immature hemopoietic cells, derived from the bone marrow itself, are capable of resorbing bone on bone slices in the absence of added bone stromal cells (49).

When mouse or rat monocytes or spleen cells are cultured with $1,25(OH)_2D_3$ and murine osteoblasts, TRAP +ve cells form within eight days of culture (43,50). In studies with human monocytes isolated from the peripheral blood (positive for CD11a, CD11b, CD14, and HLA-DR) expressed TRAP, vitronectin and calcitonin receptors when incubated with UMR 106 cells in the presence of M-CSF, VD3, were able to resorb bone by day 14 (49).

More mature monocytes from the peripheral blood can also become osteoclasts (5,49,51). Even cells that may be considered to be terminally differentiated, such as murine alveolar macrophages, can develop into active osteoclasts (52). The precursors of osteoclasts can be derived from a variety of tissues. Quinn et al. (49) demonstrated that human monocytes, peritoneal macrophages, and bone marrow cells (expressing monocyte/macrophage specific antigens), are capable of differentiating into mature osteoclasts when cultured with a stromal element (UMR 106 cells), M-CSF and dexamethasone. These studies show that cells of the monocyte/macrophage lineage, at various stages of differentiation, present at various sites throughout the body, are capable of becoming osteoclasts. Osteoclasts may, therefore, arise from several sources near orthopaedic implants. These can include immature cells present in the bone marrow, recruited monocytes from the peripheral blood, and mature tissue macrophages (5,28–32,43,49).

Rodan and Martin (53) were the first to hypothesize that osteoblasts played a significant role in the regulation of osteolysis. The early work of Martin and Ng (54) supported this hypothesis and took it further by proposing the mechanism by which cells of the osteoblast lineage controlled osteoclast formation and activity. Multiple studies have now established the requirement for co-culture with a stromal element in order for osteoclast differentiation to occur.

Not only is the presence of a stromal element required to stimulate osteoclast differentiation and activation but actual cell–cell contact between osteoclast precursors and stromal cells in the microenvironment of the bone must occur (5,28–32,43,49). Separation of monocytes from stromal cells via a membrane filter prevents osteoclasts from forming (5,43,55). In addition, replacing stromal cells with conditioned media from stromal cell cultures fails to support osteoclast formation (5,35,49). It is, therefore, likely that the signals needed for osteoclast formation act via membrane bound receptors and ligands on both the stromal and osteoclast cells rather than soluble factors (54). These factors are important regulators of osteoclast formation in the peri-implant tissues and will be discussed in detail later in this chapter.

FACTORS REGULATING PERI-IMPLANT OSTEOCLAST FORMATION

Recruitment of Osteoclasts to the Peri-implant Tissues

Aggressive granulomatous lesions are often associated with the ingrowth of a synovial-like membrane at the bone–cement interface in loose total hip implants [Santavirta, 1990 #50] (56). The accumulation of large numbers of cells of the macrophage/monocyte lineage, resulting in granuloma formation, is a characteristic of several other pathologies. This is significant as cells of this lineage differentiate into osteoclasts. The accumulation of the macrophage/monocytes is thought to be due to locally produced chemokines that recruit peripheral blood monocytes into the tissues. In peri-implant bone lysis, large numbers of macrophages containing wear particles are seen in the surrounding tissues (57,58). Since these cells may differentiate into mature osteoclasts, the accumulation of macrophages in the peri-implant tissues is likely to be a significant initial event in the pathology of aseptic joint loosening.

Over the past decade we have begun to understand the role chemokines play in the recruitment of macrophages in the formation of granulomas such as that seen in peri-implant loosening. There have been numerous chemokines identified over the past decade and recent studies have shown that a number of chemokines are likely to be involved in peri-implant recruitment of macrophages and other cells that form granulomas. These chemotactic molecules have been classified into four distinct groups according to the arrangement of cystine amino acid groups in their structure and several recent papers review the classification of both chemokines and their receptors (59–61).

Chemokines can be involved in the recruitment of many types of cells but it is those that are involved in the recruitment of monocytes/macrophages and, probably to a lesser extent, lymphocytes that are likely to be most important in peri-implant osteolysis. Chemokines belong to a family of molecules that are different from the more classical chemoattractants such as fragments C3a and C5a of complement, platelet activating factor, other metabolites of arachidonic acid, and bacterial products. It is those that belong to the group of chemokines known as the CC chemokines that are most likely to be involved in granuloma formation in the peri-implant tissues. Three important CC chemokines are chemoattractant protein (MCP)-l, macrophage inflammatory protein (MIP)-lα, and RANTES, as these are chemotactic for monocytes (60).

There is strong evidence that MCP-1 is important in granulomatous formation as abnormalities in monocyte recruitment and granuloma formation are seen in MCP-1 deficient mice (62) as well as in mice with knockout of the chemokine receptor (CCR)2 gene, the cell surface receptor for MCP-1 (63–65). Several other chemotactic molecules have been implicated in studies on experimental and human granulomatous diseases showing strong expression of MIP-1α (66) and RANTES (67–69) as well as MCP-1 (66,70–73). MCP-1 and MIP-1α are also implicated in the recruitment of osteoclasts (74–76) and MIP-1α may also mediate osteoclast differentiation (77).

There are reports that chemokines are present in the interface tissue around loosening implants (78), and that prosthetic particles stimulate production of molecules chemotactic for monocytes (78–80). The release of MCP-1, MIP-1α, and RANTES is reported to be stimulated by prosthetic particles in vitro (80). The in vitro studies also indicate that different types of prosthetic particles may induce different patterns of chemokines.

Interleukin (IL)-8 is a chemokine that functions as a mediator in diverse inflammatory disorders by promoting the recruitment, proliferation, and activation of vascular and immune cells. The IL-8 has also been linked to aseptic loosening (81,82). In a recent study, synovial-like interface membrane and pseudocapsular tissues from revision samples obtained at total hip replacement were found to have significantly higher levels of IL-8 compared to normal knee synovium (81). Histological assessment of the interfacial membrane between prosthesis and host showed IL-8 present in the peri-implant tissues. Using a dual immunostaining technique, fibroblastic cells were identified as the type of cell producing IL-8 in the peri-implant tissue (82).

Human osteoclasts isolated from osteoporotic femoral heads have also been shown to synthesize mRNA for IL-8 and release IL-8 protein in culture (83). Inflammatory stimuli such as lipopolysaccharide (LPS), IL-1α, and tumor necrosis factor (TNF)-α significantly increase mRNA expression and the levels of IL-8 protein released from osteoclasts. In contrast noninflammatory cytokines and systemic hormones such as IL-6, transforming growth factor (TGF)-β1 and TGF-β3 did not stimulate IL-8 release. IL-8 is also elevated in other similar bone loss pathologies such as RA (83). Rothe suggested human osteoclast derived IL-8 may be an important autocrine/paracrine mediator of bone cell physiology and immunoregulation involved in normal or pathological bone remodeling.

It is likely that a variety of chemokines play a key role in the bone loss seen in implant loosening and other similar pathologies. As yet we do not know which particular chemokines are the most important in the formation of osteoclasts in peri-implant osteolysis. This information may be important as it could identify targets for therapy in the future as new drugs become available which inhibit the activity of specific chemokines.

Inflammatory Mediators Regulating Osteoclasts

Osteoclast formation occurs in an environment driven by positive and negative influences. Normal bone metabolism is regulated by a plethora of cytokines whose negative and positive influences are in balance. In pathological conditions, where there is excessive bone loss, there is likely to be an excess of factors that stimulate bone resorption relative to the levels in those factors that inhibit bone resorption. Macrophages, foreign body giant cells, and osteoclasts isolated from peri-implant tissues express a variety of receptors including IL-1β, IL-4, TNF-α, IL-6, M-CSF, GM-CSF, and SCF (21). It is, therefore, possible that osteoclast formation may be mediated by many factors. The contention that these receptor ligand interactions are important for osteoclast formation in the peri-implant tissues of patients with loose implants is supported by the observation that ligands for several of these receptors are also found in these tissues (84).

Of the large number of inflammatory cytokines, IL-1β and TNF-α are considered to be the most important inflammatory mediators. Figure 2C and D show that macrophages containing wear particles in the peri-implant tissues express IL-1β and TNF-α protein. This is consistent with several other reports (84–87). Besides having a multitude of inflammatory effects on cells and tissues, these molecules also have an important role in regulating osteoclast formation. The ability of IL-1β to stimulate bone loss in disease is well recognized (88). IL-β acts directly on pre-osteoclasts and osteoclasts via functional IL-1R and appears to be important in the coordinated signaling between pre-osteoclasts and osteoblastic cells during osteoclast formation (51). Addition of IL-1β to mononuclear osteoclast like cells in vitro prolongs the survival of these cells and induces multinucleation (89). IL-1β may act by inducing actin ring formation by multinucleated cells in cultures of osteoclast like cells, in the absence of stromal cells, as well as bone resorption on dentine. In addition, IL-1β may also extend the life of osteoclasts by preventing apoptosis (89).

Like IL-1β, TNFα has long been recognized as a molecule that stimulates bone resorption (90). It is also reported to suppress osteoblast activation involved in bone formation (91,92). Both IL-1β and TNF-α are released by activated macrophages and there are numerous reports of how many types of prosthetic wear particles stimulate their release in vitro (93,94). As well as having a direct effect on osteoclast formation, these molecules also act indirectly to induce factors expressed by osteoblasts that promote osteoclast formation (95).

IL-6 is thought to have a regulatory role in maintaining the inflammatory response within the bone–implant interface as well as having an adverse effect on the process of bone remodeling (96). The importance of IL-6 in osteoclast formation is demonstrated by experiments using an IL-6 receptor antagonist (Sant 5) in human marrow cultures. Sant 5 blocks

IL-6, as well as IL-1 and TNF induced osteoclast formation, whereas addition of recombinant IL-6 stimulates osteoclast formation (96). This also indicates that IL-6 mediates the effects of IL-1 and TNF during human osteoclast formation, further highlighting its role in bone metabolism (96). This is further supported by in vitro experiments where osteoclasts are formed from cells present in the peri-implant tissues. Not only is IL-6 produced by cells present in the peri-implant tissues during osteoclast formation (97) but blocking IL-6 with antibodies markedly reduces the numbers of osteoclast which form ex vivo. Furthermore, IL-6 receptor is present on the macrophages and giant cells, possible precursors of osteoclasts, that are present in these peri-implant tissues (21). Together these findings show that IL-6 produced near the interface of bone and implant may regulate differentiation of osteoclast precursors and the activity of osteoclasts at the interface.

Prostaglandins affect both osteoblastic cells and cells of the mononuclear phagocyte lineage. A recent study has demonstrated that arthroplasty-derived bone cells cultured with human bone cells form bone resorbing osteoclasts after 14 days incubation (26). In this cell culture system, the addition of exogenous PGE_2 caused a dose-dependent increase in lacunar bone resorption of two to three times greater than untreated controls after 14 days incubation (26). While it appears to be a requirement for normal osteoclast formation, excessive PGEs may inhibit osteoclast formation (98,99). It appears that PGEs may have different effects on osteoclast development at different stages of osteoclast differentiation. Other arachidonate metabolites may also be involved in osteoclast formation in the peri-implant tissues. Anderson et al. (100) have developed a culture system that uses particles to stimulate osteoclast formation. Using this model they showed inhibition of osteoclast formation by specific inhibitors of leukotriene synthesis. While prostaglandins and leukotrienes are important mediators of osteoclast formation, it is not known if they have a direct effect on the process or if their effects are mediated via regulation of other important factors involved in osteoclastogenesis.

Parathyroid hormone is a hormone involved in bone remodeling that has a critical role in calcium metabolism. Its effects are usually systemic and its role in local bone loss pathologies, such as in prosthetic loosening, is yet to be demonstrated. In parathyroidectomized rats, continuous infusion of PTH results in a dose-dependent increase in serum-ionized calcium and a corresponding dose-dependent increase in osteoclast number (101). Conversely, when delivered in low doses intermittently, PTH causes an increase in bone mass (102) that is thought to be due to its ability to increase the number of osteoblasts in bone (103). The main stimulus of PTH is a fall in serum ionized calcium levels. The levels of PTH are also affected by the serum levels of magnesium, vitamin D metabolites, prostaglandins, and hormones (103).

M-CSF has been known for some time to be an important, if not essential, cytokine regulating bone metabolism. The action of M-CSF is mediated by a receptor encoded by the *c-fms* proto-oncogene (9). M-CSF can be produced by a variety of cell types that are present in the peri-implant tissues, such as fibroblasts, bone marrow stromal cells, osteoblast cells, and activated macrophages. M-CSF is believed to be an essential factor for both proliferation of osteoclast progenitors, and their differentiation into mature osteoclasts, in mouse and human in vitro and in vivo models (30,35,37,104–107).

M-CSF is known to enhance osteoclast formation at two different stages. M-CSF is important during the early stages of in vitro osteoclast formation, possibly inducing proliferation of pre-osteoclasts and, secondly, during the final differentiation phase of osteoclast formation. M-CSF may also prolong the survival of mature osteoclasts, as well as modulate their osteoclastic activity in vitro (108).

As M-CSF is considered to be an essential mediator of physiologic osteoclast formation, the release of M-CSF by activated cells in the peri-implant region is likely to be an important factor in peri-implant bone loss. M-CSF is present in the synovial fhuid (109) and in the synovial-like membrane of peri-implant tissues taken from patients with aseptic loosening (110). Higher levels of M-CSF were found in the tissue at the interface of implant and bone and pseudocapsular tissues in these patients than in the synovial membrane of patients undergoing primary hip replacement (110).

The localization of M-CSF to macrophages containing debris indicates that the macrophage response to wear particles resulted in the release of high levels of M-CSF. The ability of prosthetic wear particles to stimulate M-CSF mRNA expression in monocytes in vitro supports the contention that macrophages are a major source of M-CSF in the peri-implant tissues (28).

Granulocyte-macrophage colony stimulating factor (GM-CSF), a growth factor closely related to M-CSF, is also present in the bone–implant interface tissues (111). Like M-CSF it regulates the growth and maturation of cells of the macrophage–monocyte lineage and is reported to stimulate osteoclast formation in much the same way as M-CSF. Generally, it has been shown that GM-CSF is not a strong stimulator of osteoclast formation when compared to M-CSF and, therefore, it may not be as important as M-CSF in mediating peri-implant osteolysis.

It is significant that M-CSF receptor is present on the surface of macrophages and foreign body giant cells in the peri-implant tissues (97). Studies of osteoclast formation from these cells isolated from the peri-implant tissues illustrate the importance of M-CSF and its receptor in peri-implant osteolysis. High levels of M-CSF are produced during osteoclast formation in vitro in co-cultures of arthroplasty derived mononuclear cells and rat osteoblastic cells (97). The addition of antibodies to block endogenous human M-CSF binding to its receptor markedly reduced the numbers of osteoclasts that formed in these co-cultures. Antibodies blocking IL-6 also markedly reduced osteoclast formation but antibodies blocking IL-1β and TNFα had little effect. The addition of exogenous M-CSF or IL-6 to these cultures only slightly increased the numbers of osteoclasts that formed. It is significant to note that additional M-CSF was not required for osteoclast formation from these cells as additional M-CSF is normally required for osteoclast formation in vitro. This suggests that there are cells present in the peri-implant tissue which are releasing levels of M-CSF required to mediate osteoclast formation (97).

IL-11 is a multifunctional cytokine, closely related to IL-6 that has been implicated in the regulation of bone metabolism in normal physiology and disease (112). It can act by inducing osteoclastogenesis (113) and osteoblast-mediated osteoid degradation (114). IL-11 is not produced by T cells or monocytes but is probably produced by cells of the mesenchymal lineage (115). Cells of the murine osteoblast cell line, ST-2, express mRNA encoding IL-11 in vitro (116).

Immunohistochemical staining has identified IL-11 in the interface and pseudocapsular tissues obtained during total hip replacement (THR) for aseptic loosening (117). Cells expressing IL-11 are more numerous at the bone–implant interface and pseudocapsular tissues from patients with aseptic loosening than in control synovial tissues from patients undergoing primary hip replacement. The presence of IL-11 in revision tissue suggests it may be another factor involved in stimulating peri-implant osteolysis.

IL-17 is a factor reported to stimulate osteoclast activity but its involvement in peri-implant osteolysis is yet to be demonstrated. For example, IL-17 is associated with bone lysis in RA (118,119). However, as IL-17 is a T-cell derived mflammatory cytokine (87) its role in peri-implant osteolysis may not be as important as the factors men tioned above that are produced by other types of cells such as macrophages and fibroblastic cells because T cells are in low numbers in this tissue (57,84,120).

Other factors involved in tissue degradation may not directly be involved in osteoclast formation but could contribute to peri-implant osteolysis. Matrix metalloproteinases (MMP) that cause extracellular matrix degradation associated with osteolysis are reported near loose artificial hip joints (121). More recently it has been disputed that the acid- and cathepsin-K-driven pathological mechanism of bone resorption in aseptic loosening of total hip replacements is mediated by macrophages rather than by osteoclasts in the subosteoclastic space (122). The proposed mechanism is based on acidification and bone mineral dissolution. However, the localization of the enzyme in the interface tissue macrophage/giant cells, pseudosynovial fluid, and tissue extracts indicates that this occurs in the peri-prosthetic soft tissue–bone interface rather than the subosteoclastic space (122).

Receptor Activator NFκB Ligand Regulation of Peri-implant Osteolysis

Although the factors described above were thought to influence osteoclast formation, it had been suggested that there was a previously unidentified factor essential for the differentiation of osteoclasts from their precursors. It is established that M-CSF and vitamin D_3 are usually required for osteoclastogenesis in vitro but there was at least one additional factor, provided by osteoblastic cells, that was needed for osteoclast formation. The requirement for cell-to-cell contact between osteoclast precursors, such as monocytes, and osteoblastic cells led to the concept that an essential signal promoting osteoclast differentiation was mediated via ligands or receptors expressed by stromal or osteoblast cells (54).

The membrane bound factor regulating osteoclast differentiation on the surface of stromal and/or osteoblast cells was the focus of much investigation (1). This factor was eventually cloned simultaneously by two groups, Snow Brand Milk Co. in Japan (123) and AMGEN Inc. in the United States (124), and named osteoclast differentiating factor and Osteoprotegerin (OPG)-ligand, respectively. Using an expression library of the murine myelomonocytic cell line 32D, a ligand for OPG, the soluble inhibitor of osteoclastogenesis, was cloned and found to be identical to osteoclast differentiation factor (ODF) (OPG is discussed in detail below). Osteoprotegerin-ligand (OPGL) was also found to be identical to TRANCE (TNF-related activation induced cytokine) (125) and RANKL (receptor activator of nuclear factor (NF)-κB ligand) (126), previously identified by independent groups as a novel member of the TNF ligand family. TRANCE was identified in murine T-cell hybridomas (127) while RANKL was cloned from a cDNA library of murine thymoma EL4-5 cells (126). Soon, after identifying the elusive osteoclast differentiating factor (identical to TRANCE, RANKL, and OPGL) many studies demonstrated that it is an essential factor in human osteoclastogenesis (37,123,128).

The nomenclature of this molecule has recently been resolved. It has been decided that RANKL (or RANK ligand) will be the term used for the molecule known as OPGL/TRANCE/ODF (107) and we will use this term in our discussion.

RANKL plays a key role in several bone pathologies. In RA (129,130) and periodontal disease (131) T cells have been suggested as the major source of RANKL. In culture, human peripheral blood mononuclear cells (PBMC) derived T cells express RANKL when activated (132). Production of RANKL by activated T cells may enhance dendritic cell survival by interacting with high levels of its receptor present on dendritic cells (125).

While the production of RANKL by T cells may stimulate osteoclast formation particularly RA and periodontal disease this is yet to be proven in peri-implant osteolysis. The relatively low numbers of T cells present near peri-implant osteolysis make it unlikely that T cells are the major source of RANKL in peri-implant osteolysis (57,84,120).

Fibroblasts have also been suggested as a major source of RANKL in RA and peri-implant tissue (130,133,134). Murine fibroblastic cells from various tissues express RANKL mRNA and are able to support osteoclast formation from spleen cells in culture in the presence of dexamethasone (133). RA synovial fibroblasts from peri-implant granulomatous tissues have also been shown to be able to support osteoclast formation directly via RANKL expression (134). Immunohistochemical studies have shown RANKL protein to be associated with subintimal fibroblast-like cells in RA synovium (135) and granulomatous tissue from the pseudocapsule of revision arthroplasties (134). These data indicate it is likely that fibroblasts present near peri-implant bone loss can stimulate osteoclast formation by presenting RANKL to monocyte/macrophages in these tissues.

It is suggested that RANKL is not expressed by cells of the osteoclast lineage (136) but is bound to the membrane of osteoblastic cells (123). However, our recent report shows that human monocytes can express RANKL mRNA and RANKL is stimulated by prosthetic particles (28). In addition, staining for RANKL in the tissues has shown that cells having phagocytosed wear particles can express RANKL (Fig. 2E). Although the protein appeared to be in the cytoplasm further studies need to be carried out to prove that this is not membrane bound RANKL produced by other cells. If the large numbers of macrophages in peri-implant tissues are a major source of RANKL it is possible that autocrine stimulation of osteoclast formation may be involved in bone lysis in this region.

RANK is thought to be the sole cell surface receptor for RANKL (20) and is present on pre-osteoclasts (15) as well as mature osteoclasts (137). RANKL affects mature osteoclasts by signaling through RANK to induce rearrangement of the actin cytoskeleton into actin rings and formation of the specialized extracellular bone resorbing compartments (17,138). Activation of the mature osteoclasts can occur in the absence of M-CSF (17). Although RANKL does not increase the number of multinucleate osteoclasts, it increases the surface area of bone resorbed by each cell, causing multiple, spatially associated cycles of resorption in vitro (102). RANKL administration causes an immediate rise in serum calcium levels in mice indicating that it has a rapid and direct effect on osteoclast activity. OPG was able to block the effects of RANKL on both actin ring formation and bone resorption in these animals (17).

In the absence of stromal cells, soluble forms of RANKL can stimulate osteoclast formation when added to mouse or human monocytes (124). While the presence of soluble RANKL has not yet been reported in the synovial fluid of patients with joint loosening, it has been identified in the synovial fluid from patients with RA (135). Interestingly, elevated levels were also associated with active osteolysis in this disease (135). While it is likely the levels of soluble RANKL in the joint fluids of patients with peri-implant osteolysis are raised the significance is yet to be determined, as membrane-bound RANKL is reported to work much more efficiently than soluble RANKL (139).

There are claims that RANKL alone is sufficient for osteoclast formation from precursor cells (37), however, these need to be further investigated. It appears that RANKL is only active in the presence of M-CSF (124) a cytokine likely to act as a survival factor for both mature osteoclasts and their precursors. Other studies have shown that, under certain conditions, RANKL may not be an essential factor for osteoclast formation.

TNF-α and IL-1β stimulation, independent of RANKL, has been reported to induce osteoclast formation in vitro (89,140,141). This is quite important in the light of new data that IL-1 may act as a cofactor for and may be synergistic with RANKL, or induce osteoclast formation without a stromal population (141,142). In addition to having a direct effect on osteoclast formation, TNF can act indirectly to induce factors expressed by osteoblasts that promote osteoclast formation (95). TNF is also reported to suppress osteoblast activation involved in bone formation (91,92). It is important to note that recent studies have suggested that TNF-α may stimulate osteoclastogenesis directly, in the absence of RANKL (140). However, this may be dependent on exposure of macrophages to permissive levels of RANK ligand (143).

TNF-α and IL-1β are present in the tissues near loose implants, so it is possible that osteoclasts could form in the absence of RANKL if these levels of these cytokines were high enough.

RANK Expression

If RANKL is a significant (if not essential) mediator of osteoclast formation in the peri-implant tissues, then expression of its sole cell surface receptor RANK (20) is also important. RANK is a new member of the TNF receptor family that was first cloned by Anderson et al. (126) from a cDNA library of human dendritic cells. Northern blot analysis on mRNA from human tissues found ubiquitous expression of RANK with highest levels in skeletal muscles and the thymus. RANKL acts by direct binding to the receptor activator of RANK (NFκB) on the cell surface of osteoclast precursor cells (126). It is present on pre-osteoclasts (15) as well as mature osteoclasts (137).

Addition of genetically engineered soluble RANK blocks the binding of RANKL to RANK and inhibits osteoclastogenesis, indicating that RANK is essential for signal transduction in RANKL-mediated osteoclastogenesis (15,124,144). This is supported by the lack of osteoclasts and bone resorption in RANK$-/-$ mice (19,20) that is restored on transfer of RANK cDNA back into hematopoietic precursors (20). RANK interacts with tumor necrosis factor receptor associated factors (TRAF) 1, 2, 3, 5, and 6 in vitro. There are multiple TRAP binding sites clustered in two domains in the RANK cytoplasmic tail. These sites have selective binding for different TRAP proteins and are important for RANK dependent induction of NFκB and cJun NH2 terminal kinase activities (145). Cytoskeletal rearrangement and integrin engagement after osteoclast attachment to substrate is enhanced by the stimulation of RANK (17).

Little is known about RANK expression in pathologic bone resorption. However, we have reported that RANK mRNA is expressed in tissues near loose implants (28) similar to that seen in the synovial tissues from patients with active RA (33). While there is some speculation that the presence of mRNA may not necessarily prove the expression of RANK protein it may be significant to note that the high levels of RANK mRNA was found in tissues from which large numbers of osteoclast formed ex vivo (28). In the absence of commercially available antibodies for immunostaining we have carried out in situ hybridization on revision tissues using a riboprobe specific for RANK (Figure 2B). We found that many of the cells that expressed RANK mRNA also contained particles. This is consistent with observations that osteoclasts that form in the peri-implant tissues may contain wear particles (146).

Osteoprotegerin and Other Inhibitors of Osteolysis

While we tend to focus on the activity of factors stimulating osteolysis, those factors that inhibit osteolysis are just as important. Bone levels may be maintained by the balance of factors stimulating and inhibiting osteolysis. Elevated osteolysis by osteoclasts in bone pathologies might be due to a reduction in the levels of factors that inhibit osteoclast activity. Numerous inhibitors of osteoclast formation and activity have been identified. The relevance of each individual factor to peri-implant osteolysis is yet to be determined, however, the identification of the major factors stimulating osteolysis discussed above gives us some insight into those inhibitory factors that are likely to be most important in peri-implant osteolysis.

There is increasing evidence that the interaction of RANK and RANKL is fundamental to the formation of osteoclasts in health and disease. The natural inhibitor of RANKL, OPG, is therefore an important factor to consider in peri-implant osteolysis. The identification of an osteoclastogenesis-inhibitory factor, OPG, preceded the discovery of RANKL (147). Within the same year an independent group isolated osteoclastogenesis inhibitory factor (OCIF) from human fibroblast cultures and found its cDNA sequence to be identical to OPG (148).

OPG is expressed in various human osteoblast lineage cells including marrow stromal cells, normal trabecular osteoblasts, and immortalized fetal osteoblasts with expression possibly related to the stage of differentiation (149). OPG is a member of the TNF receptor family, however unlike other members of this family, it lacks a transmembrane domain. It was, therefore, predicted to be membrane bound and a secreted protein similar to other members of the soluble TNF receptor family (147). The OPG molecule is a heparin binding basic glycoprotein (148) that acts as a decoy receptor, specifically inhibiting osteoclastogenesis both in vivo and in vitro, and possibly regulates the function of mature osteoclasts.

The osteoclastogenic inhibitory action of OPG can be blocked by TNF-related apoptosis-inducing ligand (TRAIL) in culture (150). TRAIL is also expressed in the synovial tissues of patients with RA (33). TRAIL is a TNF-related ligand that, on binding to its death domain containing receptors DR4 and DR5, induces apoptosis (150), and may have anti-inflammatory activity (151).

OPG has been added to cells in culture to demonstrate the activity of RANKL in assays for osteoclastogenic activity in cells and fluids from patients with peri-implant osteolysis. OPG inhibits the formation of osteo-clasts in cultures of cells isolated from peri-implant tissues of patients at revision (27). In addition, OPG inhibits the ability of joint fluid from patients with failed total hip arthroplasty to induce osteoclast formation in vitro (152). The rat adjuvant arthritis and serum induced arthritis models provide additional evidence for the role of RANKL in the pathogenesis of bone erosion in inflammatory arthritis (153,154). Arthritic rats treated with OPG early in the course of erosion demonstrate only minimal erosion of the cortical and trabecular bone compared with untreated (153). These studies indicate that low levels of OPG combined with elevated levels of bone resorbing cytokines may contribute to peri-implant osteolysis.

The ratios of the level of RANKL to OPG are likely to be important in regulating osteoclast formation in bone loss pathologies (28,33,133,135, 155,156). There is a significant correlation with RANKL:OPG mRNA ratios and the ability to form osteoclasts from the synovial tissue from patients with active RA (33). Furthermore, the ratio of the concentration of soluble RANKL to that of OPG was significantly higher in synovial fluid of RA patients than in synovial fluid of patients with OA or gout (135). Although similar findings are yet to be reported in patients with loose implants, our recent findings comparing the levels of mRNA expression of RANKL and OPG indicate that this is possible (28). We found that the ratio of RANKL to OPG mRNA was higher in the tissues retrieved from patients from which large numbers of osteoclasts rapidly formed ex vivo (28).

Figure 2F shows immunohistochemical staining for OPG in peri-implant tissues of patients undergoing joint revision. Studies of tissue from more than 20 patients consistently showed OPG protein is associated with endothelial cells in the small blood vessels. This is in agreement with several reports of endothelial cells expressing OPG by other investigators (157,158). We are yet to determine if OPG derived from endothelial cells affects implant loosening. If endothelial cells are a major source of OPG in peri-implant tissues, any reduction of OPG in the tissues may result in enhanced osteoclast formation. In addition, OPG is reported to be a survival factor for endothelial cells and may be involved in angiogenesis and tissue ingrowth (158), which is important for the granuloma formation in the peri-implant tissues (159). It appears that OPG has important roles in bone loss pathologies that are yet to be fully understood.

IL-4, IL-10, IL-12, and IL-18 are cytokines that may inhibit osteoclast formation (160–163). While it is possible they may have a role to play in peri-implant osteolysis, the relative levels of these cytokines have not been widely investigated in the peri-implant tissues.

TGF-β is abundant in bone and has also been found to be present in peri-implant tissues near loose hip implants that modulates bone metabolism (164). TGF-β may have ambivalent effects in bone loss pathologies as it has been reported to stimulate (165) and inhibit (166) osteoclast formation. Galvin et al. (167) demonstrated an increase in osteoclast differentiation induced by TGF-β in cultures of hematopoietic cells stimulated with RANKL and M-CSF. TGF-β1 can stimulate osteoclast fomation from isolated bone marrow cells of the monocyte/macrophage lineage and monocytic cell line RAW264.7 (168). It is clearly important in modulating the healing of bone and soft tissue. Its role in peri-implant loosening is uncertain and its activities may depend on the types of cells and cytokines present in the tissues.

Regulation of Essential Mediators of Osteoclastogenesis

While most studies have shown that RANK/RANKL interactions are the essential factors for osteoclast formation in health and disease, there are several reports that other cytokines may induce osteoclast formation in the absence of RANK stimulation. Notable exceptions are reports that TNF-α (140) and IL-1β (89) simulate osteoclastogenesis in the absence of RANKL. The relevance of these in vitro studies to in vivo situations needs to be assessed as concentrations of the cytokines may be significantly higher than that found in the tissues. As both IL-1β and TNF-α are seen in peri-implant tissues, osteoclast formation in the absence of RANKL remains a possibility. However, what may be more important in this pathology is the fact that these cytokines act in synergy with RANKL during osteoclast formation as well as stimulating RANKL expression.

The expression of RANKL in cultured osteoblastic cells is stimulated by both the local cytokines as well as systemic hormones. IL-1β, IL-6, PTH, PGE$_2$, IL-11, IL-17, and TNF-α increase the expression of membrane bound RANKL, as well as induce the release of soluble RANKL in osteoblastic cells (118,139). Many of these cytokines are known to be present in the peri-implant tissues.

TNF-α appears to act in synergy with RANKL to generate osteoclasts (141,169) and it is suggested that TNF-α may permit levels of RANKL normally too low to stimulate osteoclast production to promote osteoclast production (143). Other factors present in the peri-implant tissues are also involved in the cross talk between pre-osteoclasts and stromal cells expressing RANKL that is required for osteoclast formation (51,123,170). It is also possible that IL-1 and M-CSF enable osteoclasts to maintain their bone resorption activity by preventing apoptosis.

The natural inhibitor of RANKL, OPG, is also regulated by several cytokines present in the peri-implant tissues. IL-1β and PGE$_2$ were demonstrated by Hofbauer et al. (156) to stimulate OPG production. In contrast in studies with murine cells Nakashima (139) found IL-lβ suppressed OPG expression while at the same time stimulating RANKL expression. IL-1α has been reported to increase OPG mRNA expression when added to human osteosarcoma cells, human osteoblast-like cells (171), or human bone marrow cells (172–174) in culture, while Murakami et al. (175) reported a decrease in expression.

TGF-β has been shown to enhance RANKL-induced expression of TRAP in isolated bone marrow monocytes and the monocytic cell line RAW264.7 cells (168). TGF-β is also reported to stimulate OPG expression (176) and suppress expression of RANKL in bone marrow stromal cells and osteoblast cells (175,177). These effects are, at least in part, due to the effect of TGF-β on OPG as anti-OPG IgG reduces TGF-β induced decrease in the number of osteoclasts (175).

PTH may regulate RANKL expression (178). As the PTH-induced bone resorption in a fetal mouse long bone cultures could be abolished by the addition of anti-RANKL neutralizing antibody and OPG. PTH may have import effects on the RANKL:OPG ratio in osteoblastic cells (179). PTH may have important effects on osteoclast cell formation by not only dose dependently increasing RANKL mRNA expression but also decreasing OPG expression in cultured murine bone marrow, calvaria, and osteoblasts (180). This is further demonstrated by the observation that in parathyroidectomized rats, continuous infusion of PTH results in a dose-dependent increase in RANKL mRNA and a corresponding dose-dependent increase in OPG mRNA (101).

TNF-α, IL-6, IL-11, IL-17 (139), and PGE$_2$ have been shown to down regulate OPG mRNA expression in murine osteoblast cultures (175). These findings indicate that the regulation of OPG by cytokines is complex and may depend on the type of cells, the species, and tissues investigated. Although it is still not clear how OPG expression is controlled, its regulation in the peri-implant tissues is likely to be very important.

Far less research has been carried out on regulation of RANK expression. Stimulation and timing of RANK expression on the surface of cells of the monocyte/macrophage lineage is critical for osteoclast formation (18). It is significant to note that M-CSF stimulates RANK, expression on cells of the monocyte/macrophage lineage (18). Although this is yet to be shown in using human cells this finding is consistent with our discussions previously regarding the importance of M-CSF in osteoclast formation in the peri-implant tissues. This may explain why blocking of endogenous M-CSF production during the formation of osteoclasts from cells obtained from the peri-implant tissues of failed implants markedly reduces the numbers of osteoclasts that form (97).

PERI-IMPLANT FACTORS WHICH INFLUENCE OSTEOLYTIC MEDIATORS

Particles/Materials Effects on Osteoclastogenic Mediators

Pathological and experimental evidence now supports the hypothesis that particles of prosthetic material found in surrounding soft tissues, most often produced by wear of articulating joint components, are a major factor in osteolysis. In vivo studies have shown that these wear particles stimulate a chronic inflammatory-like response dominated by macrophages (84,181–185). Monocytes and macrophages are recruited to, and may proliferate within, the implant bed in response to prosthetic particles (84). Macrophages, including those that have phagocytosed particles, are stimulated to release pro-inflammatory products and mediators that stimulate osteoclastic differentiation and bone resorption (84,184,186).

Wear of some of the early design metal-on-metal implants was associated with peri-prosthetic osteolysis, and metal particles have been reported to stimulate pro-inflammatory responses in cells in culture (187). However, it is generally acknowledged that wear of PE components of metal-on-PE articulations and the associated osteolysis are also a major problem (57,188). Submicron PE particles have been identified as the dominant type of wear particle in peri-prosthetic tissues associated with uncemented implants (120). Analyses of retrieved metal-on-PE implants and surrounding peri-prosthetic tissues have shown a strong correlation between PE wear and peri-prosthetic osteolysis (189–191). Moreover, correlations found between peri-implant osteolysis and the number of PE particles in the surrounding tissues, but not other particles (189,190), are consistent with the more mild tissue responses that have been observed with metal particles in tissues retrieved from around metal-on-metal prostheses than with PE particles (192).

In vivo studies with canine (193) and rat pouch (194) models have investigated the differences between prosthetic wear particles of differing size and biochemistry in their effects on peri-implant tissue in terms of osteolytic cytokine release and cellular response. In vivo studies using a murine air pouch model have also shown that ultra high molecular weight PE particles stimulate high numbers of cells to infiltrate the pouch/synovial membrane, resulting in the highest increase in the density of cell in the membrane when compared with titanium 6-aluminium 4-vanadium alloy (TiAlV), cobalt chrome (CoCr), and polymethylmethacrylate (PMMA) particles (195).

Human peripheral blood monocytes phagocytose cellular debris causing the cells to enlarge as particles accumulate within their cytoplasm and appear like mature macrophages (196). These cells have been used in various studies to assess the biocompatibility of different alloys by studying differences in cellular response to particles of wear (93).

In vitro studies have shown that particles of different composition can elicit different biological responses when placed on macrophages. Many of these in vitro studies assessed particles in terms of toxicity and the ability to stimulate osteolytic cytokine release by incubating particles, such as TiAlV, ultra high molecular weight PE and CoCr particles with rat peritoneal macrophages or human monocytes (93,187,197–204). While CoCr particles were found to be toxic, TiAlV particles stimulated the release of PGE_2, IL-1, TNF, and IL-6. It is suggested that particles that are less toxic may be more detrimental in the long term as they could continually stimulate the release of mediators implicated in bone resorption (93).

Human monocytes have been used to study differences in toxicity and release of mediators in response to wear particles of different metal alloys of the same size and shape (187,197). Stainless steel (316 L S/S) and cobalt–chromium–molybdenum particles were toxic while TiAlV particles did not affect cell viability (197). Stainless steel particles were the strongest stimulator of IL-1β while TiAlV particles were the strongest stimulator of IL-6 and PGE_2. This is consistent with the study on effects on rat peritoneal cells (93). TiAlV particles have also been shown to stimulate higher levels of IL-1a, IL-1β, and PGE_2 when compared to PE (199).

Only slight differences in the chemical composition of prosthetic particles can cause differences in the biological response. For example, TiAlV particles are a stronger stimulator of osteolytic factors, PGE_2, IL-1, TNF, and IL-6, than titanium 6-aluminum 7-niobium (TiAlNb) particles at similar concentrations (187). The findings of studies like these may influence the choice of biomaterials used in articulating implants where wear particles may be produced.

In vitro studies show that the size of prosthetic particles may also influence the levels of osteoclastogenic mediators released from monocytes and macrophages (194,198,205). These effects may also depend on the shape and surface area of particles encountered (198). Studies of particles isolated from revision tissues show that most particles are less than 1 μm in diameter (58,182,206–208). This size of particle, approximately the same size as pathogenic bacteria, is easily phagocytosed by macrophages and can induce the release of many osteolytic cytokines.

Recently, we have investigated the direct effect of various metal particles on the expression of RANKL, RANK, OPG, M-CSF, and other mediators of osteoclast formation using reverse transcriptase polymerase chain reaction

(RT-PCR) (28). TiAlV and other particles stimulated mRNA expression of these mediators by monocytes that had phagocytosed particles. These mediators were also strongly expressed in peri-implant tissues obtained at revision (28).

Role of the Osteoblast

Osteoblasts near sites of peri-implant osteolysis may have an important role to play in regulating bone loss. Osteoblasts not only produce the surrounding bone marix but also provide support essential for osteoclast formation. A recent report has shown that there is high bone turnover around loose-cemented total hip joints (209). However, the bone that formed at these sites, frequently adjacent to macrophages/monocytes in granulomatous tissue, was described as immature and brittle due to poor mineralization. Weak bone near implants may be unable to support the implant and result in joint failure. The presence of poor quality bone at this site was thought to show that factors released from macrophages not only stimulated osteoclast activity but also adversely affected osteoblast bone formation.

Several studies report that osteoblast activity may be affected directly through contact with or even phagocytosis of wear particles (210–214). Heinemann et al. (215) suggested that human osteoblastic cells may change in culture to become cells that can phagocytose prosthetic particles and may express markers found on both osteoblasts and macrophages. Long-term cultures of human bone derived osteoblasts express bone-specific alkaline phosphatase as well as the macrophage marker CD68. Transmission EM on cultures of these human osteoblasts incubated with less than 3 µm in diameter cpTi, TiAlV, CoCr, or UHMWPE particles demonstrated particles intracellularly (212). A recent study found bone lining cells (osteoblasts) could remove bone particles from resorption sites left by osteoclasts in Howship's lacunae, which suggests a phagocytic role in vivo (216). It is important to establish whether phagocytosis of wear particles by osteoblasts is a major cause of prosthetic loosening.

Numerous in vivo studies of peri-implant tissues obtained at revision show that monocytes and macrophages phagocytose wear particles. It may be more likely that wear particles influence osteoblasts indirectly by first stimulating macrophages to release factors which then modulate the osteoclastogenic activity of osteoblasts (95,217–219). Studies using particles of orthopaedic cement (PMMA) (217,218) have demonstrated that osteoblasts may mediate osteoclastic bone resorption in the peri-implant tissues. Studies using human osteoblastic cells support this concept and show that IL-6, TNF-α, and PGE$_2$ can be released from human osteoblastic cells stimulated by particle-activated macrophages (95). IL-1β and TNF-α were identified as the major mediators released by the particle-activated macrophages that then stimulate the release of IL-6 and PGE$_2$ from human osteoblastic cells (95).

Wear particles may effect bone formation by osteoblasts by altering gene expression following phagocytosis of wear particles by osteoblasts (220). Studies using osteoblastic cell lines and human osteoblastic cells show that particulate wear debris induced NP-κB activation and IL-6 release (220,221) while decreasing collagen synthesis (220). Particles of titanium, titanium alloy, chromium orthophosphate, and polyethylene suppressed levels of pro-collagen α {I} and α {II} accompanied by reduced type I collagen synthesis. Osteoblast specific genes such as osteonectin and alkaline phosphatase were not altered. Phagocytosis of the particles by the cell line was shown to be crucial as inhibition of phagocytosis by cytochalasin D markedly reversed the particle-induced suppression of pro-collagen α1 {I} gene expression (220).

Particles of different size and chemical composition were shown to have different effects on macrophage responses and the same may be true for osteoblasts. The effect of particles too large to be phagocytosed on human bone cells from mature trabecular bone has also been investigated (222,223). Particles of UHMWPE of diameters up to 160 μm decreased cell growth while alumina particles of the same size did not. While both types of particle of less than 80 μm in diameter induced an inhibition in osteoblastic cell growth the inhibition induced by PE particles was greater.

The effect of particles on RANKL and OPG expression by osteoblasts is yet to be investigated. However, a recent study has attempted to determine if wear particles can affect the ability of osteoblasts to support osteoclast formation. Wear particles of CoCr, 316L SS, and TiAlV were cultured with PBMC and osteoblastic cells to determine their effect on osteoclast formation and bone resorption in vitro (26,97). Cells were characterized with macrophage associated markers [CD11b and CD14 positive and vitronectin (VNR)-negative] and osteoclast-associated markers (VNR) and lacunar bone resorption. Osteoclast formation and lacunar resorption were inhibited in a dose-dependent manner following phagocytosis of metal particles by monocytes in vitro. This effect occurred with all particles but the degree of response varied with different chemical and correlated with the degree of cell toxicity of the different alloys (97).

Infection

Joint failure due to infection may involve similar mechanisms to that seen in aseptic loosening. Histological diagnosis is usually based on the degree of acute inflammatory infiltrate, such as presence of neutrophil polymorphs per high power field (224). There is a strong correlation between the presence of acute inflammatory cells in peri-implant tissue and degree of bone loss in septic loosening. Infected cases usually involve inflamed granulomatous tissue and an inflammatory exudate covering arthroplasty tissues (224). Infection usually causes extensive and rapid osteolysis. Inflammatory cells are recruited into the area to engulf the bacteria and release chemokines and cytokines, such as IL-1β and TNF-α. These cytokines can then stimulate osteolysis as described in previous sections of this chapter. It is probable that endotoxin (lipopolysaccharide) released from bacteria activates cells, including tissue macrophages, which causes the release of TNF-α, IL-1β, and other osteolytic cytokines (225).

It has also been suggested that endotoxin may be involved in aseptic loosening due to wear particles (225). Endotoxin is known to adhere strongly to many materials and can readily adhere to the surface of wear particles. This would greatly affect the macrophage response to these particles and may contribute to the release of osteolytic cytokines from macrophages that have phagocytosed particles. It is not clear how wear particles that form in vivo would come into contact with endotoxin in the absence of infection. However, it does demonstrate that experiments with particles isolated from revision tissues or particles produced artificially need to be carefully analyzed for endotoxin contamination (226). This and other issues are discussed in greater detail in separate chapters later in this book.

Physical Effects

Mechanical factors have been suggested as potentially inducing peri-implant osteolysis prior to the production of wear particles (227). Pressure changes or fluid flow has been suggested as possible causes of peri-implant bone resorption and loosening (227–230). In one study the release of the osteolytic cytokines, IL-6 and TNF-α, IL-1β, from monocyte-derived macrophages was significantly increased when exposed to cyclic pressure regimes of different frequencies in culture (231). It has been suggested that the effects of cyclic pressure in conjunction with the presence of wear particles may synergistically stimulate the release of TNF-α, IL-6, and IL-1β (232).

Mechanical strain or fluid sheer stress is also reported to regulate PGE$_2$, TGF-β, OPG, and IL-11 expression (233–237). In addition, fluid sheer stress is reported to stimulate bone resorbing activity of osteoclasts in culture (234–236). This indicates that mechanical factors and peri-implant fluid pressure may regulate peri-implant osteolysis through cytokine-mediated activation of osteoclasts.

Immune Reactions

The involvement of specific immune responses directed against the prosthetic materials in peri-implant osteolysis remains controversial (237,238) and has been reviewed recently (239). In the tissues the foreign body reaction to prosthetic materials resembles that seen in the type IV hypersensitivity reaction in which T cells are thought to regulate macrophage functions. While few lymphocytes are usually seen in the peri-implant tissues, T lymphocyte modulation of macrophage function has been suggested to be important in peri-implant osteolysis (240). Activated T cells are known to directly induce osteoclastogenesis from human monocytes and have a role in bone destruction in other bone pathologies (135,241). The activated T cells seen in these pathologies may express RANKL and directly stimulate osteoclast formation (129,131). However, the degree of infiltration of lymphocytes seen in these other pathologies is rarely seen in aseptic loosening. Significantly, those lymphocytes that are present do not express markers normally found on activated lymphocytes (242). Our preliminary data shown in Figure 2E show that there are few, if any, cells with the appearance of lymphocytes that express RANKL in the peri-implant tissues of patients with failed prostheses.

SUMMARY AND OVERVIEW

Throughout this chapter we have identified numerous cytokines, chemicals, physical influences, and other factors that may cause peri-implant osteolysis. It is apparent that osteolysis is a complex process that involves cytokines and mediators at several stages. If we are to make use of this knowledge to improve the long-term stability of implants we must first assess which factors are the major regulators of this osteolytic process. While improvements may be made in implant design, therapies targeting the key cytokines and mediators that regulate peri-implant osteolysis are becoming a viable way of improving implant survival.

A very simplified view of osteoclast formation in the peri-implant tissues, based on our current knowledge, is summarized in Figure 3. The stimulation of the tissue macrophages, most likely after the phagocytosis of prosthetic wear particles, initiates the release of numerous cytokines and mediators in the peri-implant tissues. These include chemokines, which recruit precursor osteoclasts into the tissues. Importantly, M-CSF is also released which stimulates the recruited precursor osteoclast to express the receptor, RANK. In addition, TNF-α, IL-1$\beta\alpha$, and other cytokines activate surrounding cells and stimulate RANKL expression. The final step in peri-implant osteoclast formation is the production of RANKL by macrophages, osteoblast, and possibly other cells at the interface of bone and implant. This RANK–RANKL interaction results in the formation of mature osteoclasts, which cause the lysis of bone often seen in peri-implant loosening.

The formation of osteoclasts may be an ideal target of therapy because it relies on relatively few factors and it is a point at which numerous pathways for osteolysis converge. Therapies based on the inhibition of TNF-α (243,244) or RANKL (245), by its natural inhibitor OPG (27,152,246) have been used in vivo and in vitro in experimental models. The results of these studies have shown that these approaches to the treatment of peri-implant osteolysis are promising. Our understanding of the cytokines and mediators

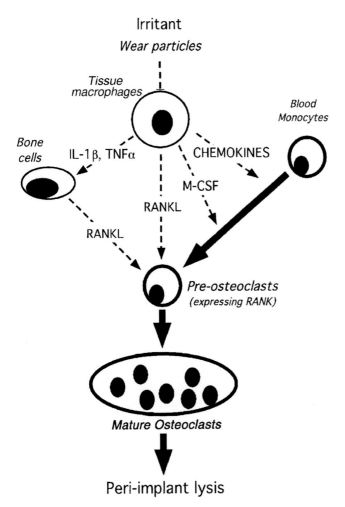

Figure 3 Diagram representing the major cytokines and mediators involved in the process of osteoclast formation in the peri-implant tissues near failed prostheses. This is described in more detail in the text.

that cause peri-implant osteolysis is still evolving. However, therapies based on regulating the mediators and cytokines of osteolysis may soon be used to enhance the long-term survival of implants.

The rapid advance of research in bone metabolism has meant that several new factors and intracellular signaling pathways have been identified during preparation of this manuscript. Although these factors are likely to influence peri-implant osteolysis their exact role(s) is yet to be determined.

ACKNOWLEDGMENTS

The authors would like to thank Dr. D. Findlay for his helpful advice and Mr. D. Caville for his photographic assistance.

REFERENCES

1. Suda T, Udagawa N, Nakamura I, Miyaura C, Takahashi N. Modulation of osteoclast differentiation by local factors. Bone 1995; 17:87S–91S.
2. Athanasou NA. Current concepts review: Cellular biology of bone-resorbing cells. J Bone Joint Surg 1996; 78-A:1096–1113.
3. Takahashi K, Udagawa N, Tanaka H, Murakami A, Owan TA, Tamura T, Suda T. Postmitotic osteoclast precursors are mononuclear cells which express macrophage-associated phenotypes. Dev Biol 1994; 163:212–221.
4. Conner JR, Dodds RA, James IE, Gowen M. Human osteoclast and giant cell differentiation: The apparent switch from non-specific esterase to tartrate resistant acid phosphatase activity coincides with the in situ expression of osteopontin mRNA. J Histochem Cytochem 1995; 43:1193–1201.
5. Fujikawa Y, Quinn JMW, Sabokbar A, McGee JOD, Athanasou NA. The human osteoclast precursor circulates in the monocyte fraction. Endocrinology 1996; 137:4058–4060.
6. Mundy GR. Bone resorption and turnover in health and disease. Bone 1987; 8:S9–S16.
7. Horton MA, Lewis D, McNulty K, Pringle JA, Chambers TJ. Monoclonal antibodies to osteoclastomas (giant cell bone tumours): definition of osteoclast-specific cellular antigens. Cancer Res 1985; 45:5663–5669.
8. Takeshita S, Kaji K, Kudo A. Identification and characterization of the new osteoclast progenitor with macrophage phenotypes being able to differentiate into mature osteoclasts. J Bone Miner Res 2000; 15:1477–1488.
9. Sherr CJ, Rettenmier CW, Sacca R, Roussel MF, Look AT, Stanley ER. The c-fms protooncogene is related to the receptor for the mononuclear phagocyte growth factor, CSF-1. Cell 1985; 41:665–676.
10. Rettenmier CW, Sacca R, Furman WL, Roussel MF, Holt JT, Nienhuis AW, Stanley ER, Sherr CJ. Expression of the human c-fms proto-oncogene product (colony stimulating factor-1 receptor) on peripheral blood mononuclear cells and choriocarcinoma cell lines. J Clin Invest 1986; 77:1740–1746.
11. Ashmun RA, Look AT, Roberts WM, Roussel MF, Seremetis S, Ohtsuka M, Sherr CJ. Monoclonal antibodies to the human CSF-1 receptor (c-fms protooncogene product) detect epitopes on normal mononuclear phagocytes and on human myeloid leukemic blast cells. Blood 1989; 73:827–837.
12. Hofstetter W, Wetterwald A, Cecchini MC, Felix H, Mueller C. Detection of the transcripts for the receptor for macrophage colony-stimulating factor, c-fms, in murine osteoclasts. Proc Natl Acad Sci USA 1992; 89:9637–9641.
13. Weir EC, Horowitz MC, Baron R, Centrella M, Kacinski B. Macrophage colony stimulating factor release and receptor expression in bone cells. J Bine Miner Res 1993; 8:1507–1517.

14. Yang S, Zhang Y, Rodriguiz RM, Ries WL, Key LLJ. Functions of the M-CSF receptor on osteoclasts. Bone 1996; 18:355–360.
15. Nakagawa N, Kinosaki M, Yamaguchi K, Shima N, Yasuda H, Yano K, Morinaga T, Higashio K. RANK is the essential signaling receptor for osteoclast differentiation factor in osteoclastogenesis. Biochem Biophys Res Commun 1998; 253:395–400.
16. Hsu H, Lacey DL, Dunstan CR, Solovyev I, Colombero A, Timms E, Tan H-L, Elliott G, Kelley MJ, Sarosi I, Wang L, et al. Tumor necrosis factor receptor family member RANK mediates osteoclast differentiation and activation induced by osteoprotegerin ligand. Proc Natl Acad Sci USA 1999; 96:3540–3545.
17. Burgess TL, Qoan Y-X, Kaufman S, Ring BD, Van G, Capparelli C, Kelley M, Hsu H, Boyle WJ, Dunstan CR, Hu S, Lacey DL. The ligand for osteoprotegerin (OPGL) directly activates mature osteoclasts. J Cell Biol 1999; 145: 527–538.
18. Aral F, Miyamoto T, Phneda O, Inada T, Sudo T, Brasel K, Miyata T, Anderson DM, Suda T. Commitment and differentiation of osteoclast precursor cells by the sequential expression of c-fms and receptor activator of nuclear factor κB (RANK) and receptors. J Exp Med 1999; 190:1741–1754.
19. Dougall WC, Glaccum M, Charrier K, Rohrbach K, Brasel K, De Smedt T, Daro E, Smith J, Tometsko ME, Maliszewski CR, et al. RANK is essential for osteoclast and lymph node development. Genes Dev 1999; 13:2412–2424.
20. Li J, Sarosi I, Yan X-Q, Morony S, Capparelli C, Tan H-L, McCabe S, Elliott R, Scully S, Van G, et al. RANK is the intrinsic hematopoietic cell surface receptor that controls osteoclastogenesis and regulation of bone mass and calcium metabolism. Proc Natl Acad Sci USA 2000; 97:1566–1571.
21. Neale SD, Athanasou NA. Cytokine receptor profile of arthroplasty macrophages, foreign body giant cells and mature osteoclasts. Acta Orthop Scand 1999; 70:452–458.
22. Kadoya Y, al-Saffar N, Kobayashi A, Revell PA. The expression of osteoclast markers on foreign body giant cells. Bone Miner Res 1994; 27:85–96.
23. Kadoya Y, Revell PA, al-Saffar N, Kobayashi A, Scott G, Freeman MAF. Bone formation and bone resorption in failed joint arthroplasties: histomorphometric analysis with histochemical and immunohistochemical technique. J Orthop Res 1996; 14:473–482.
24. Yanni G, Whelan A, Feighery C, Bresnihan B. Synovial tissue macrophages and joint erosion in rheumatoid arthritis. Ann Rheum Dis 1994; 53:39–44.
25. Sabokbar A, Fujukawa Y, Neale S, Murray DW, Athanasou NA. Human arthroplasty derived macrophages differentiate into osteoclastic bone resorbing cells. Ann Rheum Dis 1997; 56:414–420.
26. Neale SD, Sabokbar A, Fujikawa Y, Howie DW, Graves SE, Murray DW, Athanasou NA. Human bone stromal cells support osteoclast formation from arthroplasty-derived cells in vitro. In: Stein H, Suk S, Leung P-C, Thorngren KG, Akeson W, eds. Evidence for Prostaglandin Stimulation of bone Resorption SIROT. Sydney: Freund Publishing House Ltd, 1999:88–92.
27. Itonaga I, Sabokbar A, Murray DW, Athanasou NA. Effect of osteoprotegerin and osteoprotegerin ligand on osteoclast formation by arthroplasty membrane derived macrophages. Ann Rheum Dis 2000; 59:26–31.

28. Haynes DR, Crotti TN, Potter AE, Loric M, Atkins GJ, Howie DW, Findlay DM. The osteoclastogenic molecules RANKL and RANK are associated with periprosthetic osteolysis. J Bone Joint Surg Br 2001; 83-B:902–911.

29. Fujikawa Y, Shingu M, Torisu T, Itonaga I, Masumi S. Bone resorption by tartrate-resistant acid phosphatase-positive multinuclear cells isolated from rheumatoid synovium. Br J Rheumatol 1996; 192:97–104.

30. Fujikawa Y, Sabokbar A, Neale SD, Athanasou NA. Human osteoclast formation and bone resorption by monoytes and synovial macrophages in rheumatoid arthritis. Ann Rheum Dis 1996; 55:816–822.

31. Itonaga Y, Fujikawa Y, Sabokbar A, Murray DW, Athanasou NA. Rheumatoid arthritis synovial macrophage–osteoclast differentiation is osteoprotegerin ligand-dependent. J Pathol 2000; 192:97–104.

32. Suzuki Y, Tsutsumi Y, Nakagawa M, Suzuki H, Matsushita K, Beppu M, Aoki H, Ichikawa Y, Mizushima Y. Osteoclast-like cells in an in vitro model of bone destruction by rheumatoid synovium. Rheumatology 2001; 40:673–682.

33. Haynes DR, Crotti TN, Loric M, Bain GI, Atkins GJ, Findlay DM. Osteoprotegerin and receptor activator of nuclear factor kappa B ligand (RANKL) regulate osteoclast formation by cells in the human rheumatoid arthritic joint. J Rheumatol 2001; 40:623–630.

34. Udagawa N, Takahashi N, Akatsu T, Sasaki T, Yamaguchi A, Kodama H, Martin TJ, Suda T. The bone marrow-derived stromal cell lines MC3T3-G2/PA6 and ST2 support osteoclast-like cell differentiation in cocultures with mouse spleen cells. Endocrinology 1989; 125:1805–1813.

35. Quinn JMW, Fujikawa Y, McGee JOD, Athanasou NA. Rodent osteoblast-like cells support osteoclastic differentiation of human cord blood monocytes in the presence of M-CSF and 1,25 dihydroxyvitamin D_3. Int J Biochem Cell Biol 1997; 29:173–179.

36. Quinn JMW, McGee JOD, Athanasou NA. Human tumour-associated macrophages differentiate into osteoclastic bone-resorbing cells. J Pathol 1998; 184:31–36.

37. Quinn JMW, Elliott J, Gillespie MT, Martin TJ. A combination of osteoclast differentiation factor and macrophage-colony stimulating factor is sufficient for both human and mouse osteoclast formation in vitro. Endocrinology 1998; 139:4424–4427.

38. Hattersley G, Chambers TJ. Generation of osteoclastic function in mouse bone marrow cultures: multinuclearity and tartrate resistant acid phosphatase are unreliable markers for osteoclastic differentiation. Endocrinology 1989; 124:1689–1696.

39. Efstratiadis T, Moss DW. Tartrate-resistant acid phosphatase in human alveolar macrophages. Enzyme 1985; 34:140–143.

40. Bianco P, Costantini M, Dearden LC, Bonucci E. Expression of tartrate-resistant acid phosphatase in bone marrow macrophages. Basic Appl Histochem 1987; 31:433–440.

41. Chun L, Yoon J, Song Y, Huie P, Regula D, Goodman SB. The characterization of macrophages and osteoclasts in tissues harvested from revised total hip prostheses. J Biomed Mater Res 1999; 48:899–903.

42. Hattersley G, Chambers TJ. Calcitonin receptors as markers for osteoclast differentiation: correlation between generation of bone-resorptive cells and cells that express calcitonin receptors in mouse bone marrow cultures. Endocrinology 1989; 124:1689–1696.

43. Takahashi N, Akatsu T, Udagawa N, Sasaki T, Yamaguchi A, Moseley JM, Martin TJ, Suda T. Osteoblastic cells are involved in osteoclast formation. Endocrinology 1988; 123:2600–2602.

44. Akatsu T, Tamura T, Takahashi N, Udafawa N, Tanaka S, Sasaki T, Yamaguchi A, Nagata N, Suda T. Preparation and characterization of a mouse osteoclast-like multinucleated cell population. J Bone Miner Res 1992; 7:1297–1306.

45. Tsurakai T, Takahashi N, Jimi E, Nakamura I, Udagawa N, Nogimori K, Tamura M, Suda T. Isolation and characterization of osteoclast precursors that differentiate into osteoclasts on calvarial cells within a short period of time. J Cell Physiol 1998; 177:26–35.

46. Gravallese EM, Harada Y, Wang JT, Gom AH, Thornhill TS, Goldring SR. Identification of cell types responsible for bone resorption in rheumatoid arthritis and juvenile rheumatoid arthritis. Am J Pathol 1998; 152:943–951.

47. Wang W, Ferguson DJ, Quinn JMW, Simpson HRW, Athanasou NA. Biomaterial particle phagocytosis by bone-resorbing osteoclasts. J Bone Joint Surg Br 1997; 79-B:849–856.

48. Sabokbar A, Pandey R, Quinn JMW, Athanasou NA. Osteoclast differentiation by mononuclear phagocytes containing biomaterials. Arch Orthop Trauma Surg 1998; 117:136–140.

49. Quinn JMW, Neale SD, Fujikawa Y, McGee JOD, Athanasou NA. Human osteoclast formation from blood monocytes, peritoneal macrophages, and bone marrow cells. Calcif Tissue Int 1998; 62:527–531.

50. Quinn JMW, Sabokbar A, Athanasou NA. Cells of the mononuclear phagocyte series differentiate into osteoclastic lacunar bone resorbing cells. J Pathol 1996; 179:106–111.

51. Haynes DR, Atkins GJ, Loric M, Crotti TN, Geary SM, Findlay DM. Bidirectional signaling between stromal and hemopoietic cells regulates interleukin-1 expression during human osteoclast formation. Bone 1999; 25:269–278.

52. Udagawa N, Takahashi N, Akatsu T, Tanaka H, Sasaki T, Nishihara T. Origin of osteoclasts: mature monocytes and macrophages are capable of differentiating into osteoclasts under a suitable microenvironment prepared by bone marrow-derived stromal cells. Proc Natl Acad Sci USA 1990; 87:7260–7264.

53. Rodan GA, Martin TJ. Role of osteoblasts in hormonal control of bone resorption—a hypothesis. Calcif Tissue Int 1982; 34:311.

54. Martin TJ, Ng KW. Mechanisms by which cells of the osteoblast lineage control osteoclast formation and activity. J Cell Biochem 1994; 56:357–366.

55. Takayanagi H, Iizuka H, Juji T, Nakagawa T, Yamamoto A, Miyazaki T, Koshihara Y, Oda H, Nakamura K, Tanaka S. Involvement of receptor activator of nuclear factor kappa B ligand/osteoclast differentiation factor in osteoclastogenesis from synoviocytes in rheumatoid arthritis. Arthrisis Rheum 2000; 43:259–269.

56. Goldring SR, Schiller AL, Roelke MS, Rourke CM, O'Neil DA, Harris WH. The synovial-like membrane at the bone–cement interface in loose total hip

replacements and its proposed role in bone lysis. J Bone Joint Surg Am 1983; 65:575–584.

57. Vernon-Roberts B, Freeman MAR. The tissue response to total joint replacement prostheses. In: Swanson SAV, Freeman MAF, eds. The Scientific Basis of Joint Replacement. Tunbridge Wells, Kent: Pitman Medical Publishing, 1977:112–121.

58. Willert HG, Semlitsch M. Reactions of the articular capsule to wear products of artificial joint prostheses. J Biomed Mater Res 1977; 11:157–164.

59. Murphy PM, Baggiolini M, Charo IF, Herbert CA, Horuk R, Matsushima K, Miller LH, Oppenheim JJ, Power CA. International union of pharmacology. XXII. Nomenclature for chemokine receptors. Pharm Rev 2000; 52:145–176.

60. Lloyd C. Chemokines in allergic lung inflammation. Immunology 2002; 105: 144–154.

61. Ajuebor MN, Swain MG. Role of chemokines and chemokine receptors in the gastrointestinal tract. Immunology 2002; 105:137–143.

62. Lu B, Rutledge BJ, Gu L, Fiorillo J, Lukacs NW, Kunkel SL, North R, Gerard C, Rollins BJ. Abnormalities in monocyte recruitment and cytokine expression in monocyte chemoattractant protein 1-deficient mice. J Exp Med 1997; 185:1959–1968.

63. Gao JL, Wynn TA, Chang Y, Lee EJ, Broxmeyer HE, Cooper S, Tiffany HL, Kwon-Chung J, Murphy PM. Impaired host defense, hematopoiesis, granulo-matous inflammation and type 1–type 2 cytokine balance in mice lacking CC chemokine receptor 1. J Clin Invest 1997; 100:2552–2561.

64. Boring L, Gosling J, Chensue SW, Kunkel SL, Farese RVJ, Broxymeyer HE, Charo IR. Impaired monocyte migration and reduced type 1 (Th1) cytokine responses in C–C chemokine receptor 2 knockout mice. J Clin Invest 1997; 100:2552–2561.

65. Warmington KS, Boring L, Ruth JH, Sonstein J, Hogaboam CM, Curtis JL, Kunkel SL, Charo IR, Chensue SW. Effect of C–C chemokine receptor 2 (CCR2) knockout on type-2 (schistosomal antigen-elicited) pulmonary granu-loma formation: analysis of cellular recruitment and cytokine responses. Am J Pathol 1999; 154:1407–1416.

66. Hashimoto S, Nakayama T, Gon Y, Hata N, Koura T, Muruoka S, Matsumoto K, Hayashi S-I, Abe Y, Horie T. Correlation of plasma monocyte chemoa-ttractant protein-1 (MCP-1) and monocyte inflammatory protein-1 alpha (MIP-1alpha) levels with disease activity and clinical course of sarcoidosis. Clin Exp Immunol 1998; 111:604–610.

67. Chensue SW, Warmington KS, Allenspach EJ, Lu B, Gerard C, Kunkel SL, Lukacs NW. Differential expression and cross-regulatory function of RANTES during mycobacterial (type 1) and schistosomal (type 2) antigen-elicited granulomatous inflammation. J Immunol 1999; 163:165–173.

68. Petrek M, Pantelidis P, Southcott A, Lymphany P, Safranek P, Black CM, Kolek V, Weigl E, Du Booi RM. The source and role of RANTES in intersti-tial lung disease. Eur Respir J 1997; 10:1207–1216.

69. Hogaboam CM, Steinhauser ML, Chensue SW, Kunkel SL. Novel roles for chemokines and fibroblasts in interstitial fibrosis. Kidney Int 1998; 54: 2152–2159.

70. Friedland JS, Shattock RJ, Griffin GE. Phagocytosis of Mycobacterium tuberculosis or particulate stimuli by monocytic cells induces equivalent chemotactic protein-1 gene expression. Cytokine 1993; 5:150–160.

71. Desai A, Huang X, Warren JS. Intracellular glutathione redox status modulates MCP-1 expression in pulmonary granulomatous vasculitis. Lab Invest 1999; 79:837–847.

72. Conti P, Reale M, Feliciani C, Frydas S, Trakatellis M, Placido FC, Cataldo I, Di Gioacchino M, Barbacane RC. Augmentation of monocyte chemotactic protein-1 and mRNA transcript in chronic inflammatory states induced by potassium permangenate ($KMnO_4$) in vivo. Immunology 1997; 92:300–306.

73. Conti P, Feliciani C, Barbacane RC, Frydas S, Placido FC, Cataldo I, Reale M. Monocyte chemotactic protein-1 gene expression and translation in formed granulomatous calcified tissue in vivo. Calcif Tiss Int 1999; 64:57–62.

74. Kukita T, Nomiyama H, Ohmoto Y, Kukita A, Shuto T, Hotokebuchi T, Sugloka Y, Miura R, Iijima T. Macrophage inflammatory protein-1 alpha (LD78) expressed in human bone marrow: its role in regulation of hematopoiesis and osteoclast recruitment. Lab Invest 1997; 76:399–406.

75. Volejnikova S, Laskari M, Marks SC, Graves DT. Monocyte recruitment and expression of monocyte chemoattractant protein-1 are developmentally regulated in remodeling bone in the mouse. Am J Pathol 1997; 150:1711–1721.

76. Zheng MH, Fan Y, Smith A, Wysocki S, Papadimitriou JM, Wood DJ. Gene expression of monocyte chemoattractant protein-1 in giant cell tumors of bone osteoclastoma: possible involvement in CD68+ macrophage-like cell migration. J Cell Biochem 1998; 70:121–129.

77. Scheven BA, Milne JS, Hunter I, Robins SP. Macrophage-inflammatory protein-1 alpha regulates preosteoclast differentiation in vitro. Biochem Biohys Res Commun 1999; 254:773–778.

78. Ishiguro N, Kojima T, Ito T, Saga S, Anma H, Kurokouchi K, Iwahori Y, Iwase T, Iwata H. Macrophage activation and migration in interface tissue around loosening total hip arthroplasty components. J Biomed Mater Res 1997; 35:399–406.

79. Rhodes NP, Hunt JA, Williams DF. Macrophage subpopulation differentiation by stimulation with biomaterials. J Biomed Mater Res 1997; 37:481–488.

80. Nakashima Y, Sun DH, Trindade MCD, Chun LE, Song Y, Goodman SB, Schurman DJ, Maloney W, Smith RL. Induction of macrophage C–C chemokine expression by titanium alloy and bone cement particles. J Bone Joint Surg Br 1999; 81-B:155–162.

81. Shanbhag AS, Jacobs JJ, Black J, Galante JO, Glant TT. Cellular mediators secreted by interfacial membranes obtained at revision total hip arthroplasty. J Arthroplasty 1995; 10:498–506.

82. Lassus J, Waris V, Xu J-W, Li T-F, Hao J, Nietosvaara Y, Santavirta S, Konttinen TY. Increased interleukin-8 (IL-8) expression is related to aseptic loosening of total hip replacement. Arch Orthop Trauma Surg 2000; 120:328–332.

83. Rothe L, Collin-Osdoby P, Chen Y, Sunyer T, Chaudhary L, Tsay A, Goldring SR, Avioli L, Osdoby P. Human osteoclasts and osteoclast-like cells synthesize and release high basal and inflammatory stimulated levels of the potent chemokine interleukin-8. Endocrinology 1998; 139:4353–4363.

84. Jiranek WA, Machado M, Jasty M, Jevsevar D, Wolfe HJ, Goldring SR, Goldberg MJ, Harris WH. Production of cytokines around loosened cemented acetabular components. J Bone Joint Surg 1993; 75-A:863–879.

85. Appel AM, Sowder WG, Siverhus SW, Hopson CN, Herman JH. Prosthesis-associated pseudomembrane-induced bone resorption. Br J Rheumatol 1990; 29:32–36.

86. Chiba J, Schwendeman LJ, Booth JRE, Crossett LS, Rubash HE. A biochemical, histologic, and immunohistologic analysis of membranes obtained from failed cemented, and cementless total knee arthroplasty. Clin Orthop 1994; 299.

87. Perry MJ, Mortuza FY, Ponsford FM, Elson CJ, Atkins RM, Learmonth ID. Properties of tissue from around cemented joint implants with erosive and/or linear osteolysis. J Arthroplasty 1997; 12:670–676.

88. Gowen M, Wood DJ, Ihrie EJ, McGuire MK, Russell RG. An interleukin-1 like factor stimulate bone resorption in vitro. Nature 1983; 306:378–380.

89. Jimi EJ, Nakamura I, Duong LT, Ikebe T, Takahashi N, Rodan GA, Suda T. Interleukin 1 induces multinucleation and bone-resorbing activity of osteoclasts in the absence of osteoblast/stromal cells. Exp Cell Res 1999; 247:84–93.

90. Bertolini DR, Nedwin GE, Bringman TS, Smith DD, Mundy GR. Stimulation of bone resorption and inhibition of bone formation in vitro by human tumour necrosis factors. Nature 1986; 319:516–518.

91. Canalis E. Ihterleukin-1 has independent effects on deoxyribonucleic acid and collagen synthesis in cultures of rat calvarie. Endocrinology 1986; 118:74–81.

92. Smith DD, Gowen M, Mundy GR. Effects of interferon-gamma and other cytokines on collagen synthesis in fetal rat bone cultures. Endocrinology 1987; 120:2494–2499.

93. Haynes DR, Rogers SD, Hay S, Pearcy MJ, Howie DW. The differences in toxicity and release of bone-resorbing mediators induced by titanium and cobalt–chromium-alloy wear particles. J Bone Joint Surg Am 1993; 75-A:825–834.

94. Merkel KD, Erdmann JM, Mchugh KP, Abu-Amer Y, Ross FP, Teitelbaum SL. Tumor necrosis factor-α mediates orthopedic implant osteolysis. Am J Pathol 1999; 154:203–210.

95. Haynes DR, Hay SJ, Rogers SD, Ohta S, Howie DW, Graves SE. Regulation of bone cells by particle-activated mononuclear phagocytes. J Bone Joint Surg Br 1997; 79-B:988–994.

96. Devlin RD, Reddy SV, Savino R, Ciliberto G, Roodman GD. IL-6 mediates the effects of IL-1 or TNF, but not PTHrP or $1,25(OH)_2D_3$ on osteoclast-like cell formation in normal human bone marrow cultures. J Bone Miner Res 1998; 13:393–399.

97. Neale S, Sabokbar A, Howie DW, Murray DW, Athanasou NA. Macrophage colony-stimulating factor and interleukin-6 release by periprosthetic cells stimulates osteoclast formation and bone resorption. J Orthop Res 1999; 17: 686–694.

98. Quinn JMW, Sabokbar A, Denne M, de Vemejoul MC, McGee JO, Athanasou NA. Inhibitory and stimulatory effects of prostaglandins on osteoclast differentiation. Calcif Tiss Int 1997; 60:63–70.

99. Quinn JMW, McGee JOD, Athanasou NA. Cellular and hormonal factors influencing monocyte differentiation to osteoclastic bone-resorbing cells. Endocrinology 1994; 134:2416–2423.

100. Anderson DM, MacQuarrie R, Osinga C, Chen YF, Langman M, Gilbert R. Inhibition of leukotriene function can modulate particulate-induced changes in bone cell differentiation and activity. J Biomed Mater Res 2001; 58:406–414.

101. Ma YL, Cain RL, Halladay DL, Yang X, Zeng Q, Miles RR, Chandrasekhar S, Martin TJ, Onyia JE. Catabolic effects of continuous human PTH (1–38) in vivo is associated with sustained stimulation of RANKL and inhibition of osteoprotegerin and gene-associated bone formation. Endocrinology 2001; 142:4047–4054.

102. Fujita T. Parathyroid hormone in the treatment of osteoporosis. BioDrugs 2001; 15:721–728.

103. Athanasou NA. Clinical Radiological and Pathological Correlation of Diseases of Bone, Joint and Soft Tissue. London: Arnold Publishers, 2001:118–154.

104. Tanaka S, Takahashi N, Udagawa N, Tamura T, Akatsu T, Stanley ER, Kurokawa T, Suda T. Macrophage colony stimulatmg factor is indispensable for both proliferation and differentiation of osteoclast progenitors. J Clin Invest 1993; 91:257–263.

105. Suda T, Takahashi N, Martin TJ. Modulation of osteoclast differentiation. Endocr Rev 1992; 13:66–80.

106. Sarma U, Flanagan AM. Macrophage colony-stimulating factor induces substantial osteoclast generation and bone resorption in human bone marrow cultures. Blood 1996; 88:2531–2540.

107. Suda T, Takahashi N, Udagawa N, Jimi E, Gillespie MT, Martin TJ. Modulation of osteoclast differentiation and function by the new members of the tumor necrosis factor receptor and ligand families. Endocr Rev 1999; 20:345–357.

108. Fuller K, Owens JM, Jagger CJ, Wilson A, Moss R, Chambers TJ. Macrophage-colony-stimulating factor stimulates survival and chemotactic behaviour in isolated osteoclasts. J Exp Med 1993; 178:1733–1744.

109. Takei I, Takagi M, Ida H, Ogina T, Santavirta S, Konttinen YT. High macrophage-colony stimulating factor levels in synovial fluid of loose artificial hip joints. J Rheumatol 2000; 27:894–899.

110. Xu JW, Konttinen YT, Waris V, Patiala H, Sorsa T, Santavirta S. Macrophage-colony stimulating factor (M-CSF) is increased in the synovial-like membrane of the prosthetic tissues in the aseptic loosening of total hip replacement (THR). Clin Rheumatol 1997; 16:244–248.

111. al-Saffar N, Khwaja HA, Kadoya Y, Revell PA. Assessment of the role of GM-CSF in the cellular transformation and the development of erosive lesions around orthopaedic implants. Am J Clin Pathol 1996; 105:628–639.

112. Yang YC. Interleukin-11: an overview. Stem Cells 1993; 11:474–486.

113. Girasole G, Passeri G, Jilka RL, Manolagas SC. Interleukin-11: a new cytokine critical for osteoclast development. J Clin Invest 1994; 93:1516–1524.

114. Hill PA, Tumber A, Papaioannou S, Meikle MC. The cellular actions of interleukin-11 on bone resorption in vitro. Endocrinology 1998; 139:1564.

115. Lisignoli G, Piacentini A, Toneguzzi S, Grassi F, Cocchini B, Feruzzi A, Gualtieri G, Facchini A. Osteoblasts and stromal cells isolated from femora in rheumatoid arthritis (RA) and osteoarthritis (OA) patients express IL-11, leukaemia inhibitory factor and oncostatin M. Clin Exp Immunol 2000; 119:346–353.

116. Atkins GJ, Haynes DR, Geary SM, Loric M, Crotti TN, Findlay DM. Co-ordinated cytokine expression by stromal and hematopoietic cells during human osteoclast formation. Bone 2000; 26:653–661.

117. Xu JW, Li T-F, Partsch G, Ceponis A, Santavirta S, Konttinen YT. Interleukin-11 (IL-11) in aseptic loosening of total hip replacement (THR). Scand J Rheumatol 1998; 27:363–367.

118. Kotake S, Udagawa N, Takahashi N, Matsuzaki K, Itoh K, Ishiyama S, Saito S, Inoue K, Kamatani N, Gillespie MT, et al. IL-17 in synovial fluids from patients with rheumatoid arthritis is a potent stimulator of osteoclasto-genesis. J Clin Invest 1999; 103:1345–1352.

119. Chabaud M, Lubberts E, Joosten L, van den Berg W, Miossec P. IL-17 derived juxta-articular bone and synovium contributes to joint degradation in rheumatoid arthritis. Arthritis Res 2001; 3:168–177.

120. Jacobs JJ, Shanbhag AS, Glant TT, Black J, Galante JO. Wear debris in total joint replacements. J Am Acad Orthop Surg 1994; 2:212–220.

121. Takagi M, Santavirta S, Ida H, Ishii M, Mandelin J, Konttinen YT. Matrix metalloproteiases and tissue inhibitors of metalloproteinases in loose artificial hip joints. Clin Orthop 1998; 352:35–45.

122. Konttinen TY, Takagi M, Mandelin J, Lassus J, Salo J, Ainola M, Li T-F, Virtanen I, Liljestrom M, Sakai H, et al. Acid attack and cathepsin K in bone resorption around total hip replacement prosthesis. J Bone Miner Res 2001; 16:1780–1786.

123. Yasuda H, Shima N, Nakagawa N, Yamaguchi K, Kinosaki M, Mochizuki S-I, Tomoyasu A, Yano K, Goto M, Murakami A, et al. Osteoclast differentiation factor is a ligand for osteoprotegerin/osteoclast inhibitory factor and is identical to TRANCE/RANKL. Proc Natl Acad Sci USA 1998; 95:3597–3602.

124. Lacey DL, Timms E, Tan H-L, Kelley MJ, Dunstan CR, Burgess T, Elliot R, Colombero A, Elliot G, Scully S, et al. Osteoprotegerin ligand is a cytokine that regulates osteoclast differentiation and activation. Cell 1998; 93:165–176.

125. Wong BR, Josien R, Lee SY, Sauter B, Li H-L, Steinman RM, Choi Y. TRANCE [tumor necrosis factor (TNF)-related activation-induced cytokine], a new TNF family member predominantly expressed in T cells, is a dendritic cell-specific survival factor. J Exp Med 1997; 186:2075–2080.

126. Anderson DM, Marakovsky E, Billinglsey WL. A homologue of the TNF receptor and its ligand enhance T-cell growth and dendritic function. Nature 1997; 390:175–179.

127. Wong BR, Rho J, Arron J, Robinson E, Orlinick J, Chao M, Kalachikov S, Cayani E, Bartlett FS, Frankel WN, et al. TRANCE is a novel ligand of the tumor necrosis factor receptor family that activates c-Jun n-terminal kinase in T cells. J Biol Chem 1997; 272:25,190–25,194.

128. Matsuzaki K, Udagawa N, Takahashi N, Yamaguchi K, Yasuda H, Shima N, Morinaga T, Toyama Y, Yabe Y, Higashio K, et al. Osteoclast differentiation

factor (ODF) induces osteoclast-like cell formation in human peripheral blood mononuclear cell cultures. Biochem Biophys Res Commun 1998; 246:199–204.

129. Romas E, Bakharevski O, Hards DK, Kartsogiannis V, Quinn JMW, Ryan PFJ, Martin TJ, Gillespie MT. Expression of osteoclast differentiation factor at sites of bone resorption in collagen-induced arthritis. Arthritis Rheum 2000; 43:821–826.

130. Gravallese EM, Manning C, Tsay A, Naito A, Pan C, Amento E, Goldring S. Synovial tissue in rheumatoid arthritis is a source of osteoclast differentiation factor. Arthritis Rheum 2000; 43:250–258.

131. Teng Y-TA, Nguyen H, Gao X, Kong Y-Y, Gorcynski RM, Singh B, Ellen RP, Penninger JM. Functional human T-cell immunity and osteoprotegerin ligand control alveolar bone destruction in periodontal infection. J Clin Invest 2000; 106:R59–R67.

132. Horwood NJ, Kartsogiannis V, Quinn JMW, Romas Q, Martin TJ, Gillespie MT. Activated T lymphocytes support osteoclast formation in vitro. Biochem Biophys Res Commun 1999; 265:144–150.

133. Quinn JMW, Horwood NJ, Elliott J, Gillespie MT, Martin TJ. Fibroblastic stromal cells express receptor activator of NF-kappa B ligand and support osteoclast differentiation. J Bone Miner Res 2000; 15:1459–1466.

134. Sakai H, Jingushi S, Shuto T, Urbe K, Ikenoue T, Okazaki K, Kukita T, Kukita A, Iwamoto Y. Fibroblasts from the inner granulation tissue from hips at revision arthroplasty induce osteoclast differentiation, as do stromal cells. Ann Rheum Dis 2002; 61:103–109.

135. Kotake S, Udagawa N, Hakoda M, Mogi M, Yano K, Tsuda E, Takahashi K, Furuya T, Ishiyama S, Kim K-J, et al. Activated human T cells directly induce osteoclastogenesis from human monocytes. Arthritis Rheum 2001; 44:1003–1012.

136. Hakeda Y, Kobayashi Y, Yamaguchi K, Yasuda H, Tsuda E, Higashio K, Miyata T, Kumegawa M. Osteoclastogenesis mhibitory factor (OCIF) directly inhibits bone-resorbing activity of isolated mature osteoclasts. Biochem Biophys Res Commun 1998; 251:796–801.

137. Myers DE, Collier FML, Minkin C, Wang H, Holloway WR, Malakellis M. Expression of functional RANK on mature rat and human osteoclasts. FEBS Lett 1999; 463:295–300.

138. Fuller K, Wong B, Fox S, Choi Y, Chambers TJ. TRANCE is necessary and sufficient for osteoblast-mediated activation of bone resorption in osteoclasts. J Exp Med 1998; 188:997–1001.

139. Nakashima T, Kobayashi Y, Yamasaki S, Kawakami A, Eguchi K, Sasaki H, Sakai H. Protein expression and functional difference of membrane-bound and soluble receptor activator of NF-κB ligand: Modulation of the expression by osteotropic factors and cytokines. Biochem Biophys Res Commun 2000; 275:768–775.

140. Kobayashi K, Takahashi N, Jimi E, Udagawa N, Takami M, Kotake S, Nakagawa N, Kinosaki M, Yamaguchi K, Shima N, et al. Tumor necrosis factor α stimulates osteoclast differentiation by a mechanism independent of the ODF/RANKL–RANK interaction. J Exp Med 2000; 191:275–285.

141. Fuller K, Murphy PM, Kirstein B, Fox SW, Chambers TJ. TNF-alpha potently activates osteoclasts, through a direct action independent of and strongly synergistic with RANKL. Endocrinology 2002; 143:1108–1118.

142. Jimi EJ, Nakamura I, Duong LT, Ikebe T, Takahashi N, Rodan GA, Suda T. Interleukin-1 induces multinucleation and bone-resorbing activity of osteoclasts in the absence of osteoblasts/stromal cells. Exp Cell Res 1999; 247:84–93.

143. Lam J, Takeshita S, Barker JE, Kanagawa O, Ross FP, Teitelbaum SL. TNF-α induces osteoclastogenesis by direct stimulation of macrophages exposed to permissive levels of RANK ligand. J Clin Invest 2000; 106:1481–1488.

144. Akatsu T, Murakami T, Nishikawa M, Ono K, Shinomiya N, Tsuda E, Mochizuki S-I, Yamaguchi K, Kinosaki M, Higashio K, et al. Osteoclasto genesis inhibitory factor suppresses osteoclast survival by interfering in the interaction of stromal cells with osteoclast. Biochem Biophys Res Commun 1998; 250:229–234.

145. Galibert L, Tometsko ME, Anderson DM, Cosman D, Dougall WC. The involvement of multiple tumor necrosis factor receptor (TNFR)-associated factors in the signaling mechanisms of receptor activator of NF-κB, a member of the TNFR superfamily. J Biol Chem 1998; 273:34,120–34,127.

146. Wang W, Ferguson DJ, Quinn JMW, Simpson AH, Athanasou NA. Osteoclasts are capable of particle phagocytosis and bone resorption. J Pathol 1997; 182:92–98.

147. Simonet WS, Lacey DL, Dunstan CR, Kelley M, Chang M-S, Luthy R, Nguyen HQ, Wooden S, Bennett L, Boone T, et al. Osteoprotegerin: a novel secreted protein involved in the regulation of bone density. Cell 1997; 89: 309–319.

148. Tsuda E, Goto M, Mochizoki S-I, Yano K, Kobayashi F, Moringa T, Higashio K. Isolation of a novel cytokine from human fibroblasts that specifically inhibits osteoclastogenesis. Biochem Biophys Res Commun 1997; 234:137–142.

149. Hofbauer LC, Dunstan CR, Spelsberg TC, Riggs BL, Khosla S. Osteoprotegerin production by human osteoblast lineage cells is stimulated by vitamin D, bone morphogenetic protein-2, and cytokines. Biochem Biophys Res Commun 1998; 250:776–781.

150. Emery JG, McDonell P, Burke MB, Deen KC, Lyn S, Silverman C, Dul E, Appelbaum ER, Eichman C, Dirinzio R, et al. Osteoprotegerin is a receptor for the cytotoxic ligand TRAIL. J Biol Chem 1998; 273:14,363–14,367.

151. Song K, Chen Y, Goke R, Wilmen A, Seidel C, Goke A, Hilliard B, Chen Y. Tumor necrosis factor-related apoptosis-inducing ligand (TRAIL) is an inhibitor of autoimmune inflammation and cell cycle progression. J Exp Med 2000; 191:1095–1103.

152. Kim K-J, Kotake S, Udagawa N, Ida H, Ishii M, Takei I, Kudo T, Takagi M. Osteoprotegerin inhibits in vitro mouse osteoclast formation induced by joint fluid from failed total hip arthroplasty. J Biomed Mater Res 2001; 58:393–400.

153. Kong Y-Y, Feige U, Sarosi I, Bolon B, Tafuri A, Morony S, Capparelli C, Li J, Elliot R, McCabe S, et al. Activated T cells regulate bone loss and joint destruction in adjuvant arthritis through osteoprotegerin ligand. Nature 1999; 402: 304–309.

154. Pettit AR, Ji H, von Stechow D, Muller R, Goldring SR, Choi Y, Benoist C, Gravallese EM. TRANCE/RANKL knockout mice are protected from bone erosion in a serum transfer model of arthritis. Am J Pathol 2001; 159: 1689–1699.

155. Crotti TN, Potter AE, Atkins GJ, Findlay DM, Howie DW, Haynes DR. Bone lysis and inflammation. Inflamm Res 2004; 53:596–600.

156. Hofbauer LC, Lacey DL, Dunstan CR, Spelsberg TC, Riggs BL, Khosla S. Interleukin-1β and tumor necrosis factor-α, but not interleukin-6, stimulate osteoprotegerin ligand gene expression in human osteoblastic cells. Bone 1999; 25:255–259.

157. Collin-Osdoby P, Rothe L, Anderson F, Nelson M, Maloney W, Osdoby P. Receptor activator of NF-κB and osteoprotegerin expression by human microvascular endothelial cells, regulation by inflammatory cytokines, and role in human osteoclastogenesis. J Biol Chem 2001; 276:20,659–20,672.

158. Malyankar UM, Scatena M, Suchland KL, Yun TJ, Clark EA, Giachelli CM. Osteoprotegerin is an alpha vbeta 3-induced, NF-κB-dependent survival factor for endothelial cells. Biol Chem 2000; 275:20,959–20,962.

159. al-Saffar N, Mah JTL, Kadoya Y, Revell PA. Neovascularisation and the induction of cell adhesion molecules in response to degradation products from orthopaedic implants. Ann Rheum Dis 1995; 54:201–208.

160. Riancho JA, Zarrabeitia MT, Mundy GR, Yoneda T, Gonzales-Macias J. Effects of interleukin-4 on the formation of macrophages and osteoclast-like cells. J Bone Miner Res 1993; 8:1337–1344.

161. Owens JM, Gallagher AC, Chambers TJ. IL-10 modulates formation of osteoclasts in murine hematopoietic cultures. J Immunol 1996; 157:936–940.

162. Horwood NJ, Elliott J, Martin TJ, Gillespie MT. IL-12 alone and in synergy with IL-18 inhibits osteoclast formation in vitro. J Immunol 2001; 166:4915–4921.

163. Yamada N, Niwa S, Tsujimura T, Iwasaki T, Sugihara A, Futani H, Hayashi S-I, Okamura H, Akedo H, Terada N. Interleukin-18 and interleukin-12 synergistically inhibit osteoclastic bone-resorbing activity. Bone 2002; 30: 901–908.

164. Konttinen TY, Waris V, Xu JW, Jiranek WA, Sorsa T, Virtanen I, Santavirta S. Transforming growth factor-beta 1 and 2 in the synovial-like interface membrane between implant and bone in loosening of total hip arthroplasty. J Rheumatol 1997; 24:694–701.

165. Kaneda T, Nojima T, Nakagawa M, Ogasawara A, Kaneko H, Sato T, Mano H, Kumegawa M, Hakeda Y. Endogenous production of TGF-β is essential for osteoclastogenesis induced by a combination of receptor activator NF-κB ligand and macrophage-colony-stimulating factor. J Immunol 2000; 165:4254–4263.

166. Chenu C, Pfeilschifter J, Mundy GR, Roodman GD. Transforming growth factor β inhibits formation of osteoclast-like cells in long-term human marrow cultures. Proc Natl Acad Sci USA 1988; 85:5683.

167. Galvin RJS, Gatlin CL, Horn JW, Fuson TR. TGF-β enhances osteoclast differentiation in hematopoietic cell cultures stimulated with RANKL and M-CSF. Biochem Biophys Res Commun 1999; 265:233–239.

168. Koseki T, Gao Y, Okahashi N, Murase Y, Tsujisawa T, Sato T, Yamato K, Nishihara T. Role of TGF-β in osteoclastogenesis induced by RANKL. Cell Signal 2002; 14:31–36.

169. Komine M, Kukita A, Kukita T, Ogata Y, Hotokebuchi T, Kohashi O. Tumor necrosis factor-alpha cooperates with receptor activator of nuclear factor κB ligand in generation of osteoclasts in stromal cell-depleted rat bone marrow cell culture. Bone 2001; 28:474–483.

170. Wani MR, Fuller K, Kim NS, Choi Y, Chambers T. Prostaglandin E_2 cooperates with TRANCE in osteoclast induction from hemopoietic precursors: synergistic activation of differentiation, cell spreading, and fusion. Endocrinology 1999; 140:1927–1935.

171. Vidal NOA, Sjogren K, Eriksson BI, Ljunggren O, Ohlsson C. Osteoprotegerin mRNA is increased by interleukin-1α in the human osteosarcoma cell line MG-63 and in human osteoblast-like cells. Biochem Biophys Res Commun 1998; 248:696–700.

172. Brandstrom H, Jonsson KB, Ohlsson C, Vidal NOA, Ljunghall S, Ljunggren O. Regulation of osteoprotegerin mRNA levels by prostaglandin E_2 in human bone marrow stromal cells. Biochem Biophys Res Commun 1998; 247:338–341.

173. Brandstrom H, Bjorkman T, Ljunggren O. Regulation of osteoprotegerin secretion from primary cultures of human bone marrow stromal cells. Biochem Biophys Res Commun 2001; 280:831–835.

174. Brandstrom H, Jonsson K, Vidal O, Ljunghall S, Ohlsson C, Ljunggren O. Tumor necrosis factor-α and -β upregulate the levels of osteoprotegerin mRNA in human osteosarcoma MG-63 cells. Biochem Biophys Res Commun 1998; 248:454–457.

175. Murakami T, Yamamoto M, Yamamoto M, Ono K, Nishikawa M, Nagata N, Motoyoshi K, Akatsu T. Transfoiming growth factor-β1 increases mRNA levels of osteoclastogenesis inhibitory factor in osteoblastic/stromal cells and inhibits the survival of murine osteoclast-like cells. Biochem Biophys Res Commun 1998; 252:747–752.

176. Thirunavukkarasu K, Miles RR, Halladay DL, Yang X, Galvin RJS, Chandrasekhar S, Martin TJ, Onyia JE. Stimulation of osteoprotegerin (OPG) expression by transforming growth factor-β (TGF-β). J Biol Chem 2001; 276: 36,241–36,250.

177. Quinn JMW. Transforming growth factor β affects osteoclast differentiation via direct and indirect actions. J Bone Miner Res 2001; 16:1787–1794.

178. Tsukii K, Shima N, Mochizuki S-I, Yamaguchi K, Kinosaki M, Yano K, Shibata O, Udagawa N, Yasuda H, Suda T, Higashio K. Osteoclast differentiation factor mediates an essential signal for bone resorption induced by 1α,25 dihydroxyvitamin D_3, prostaglandin E_2 or parathyroid hormone in the microenvironment. Biochem Biophys Res Commun 1998; 246:337–341.

179. Horwood NJ, Elliot J, Martin TJ, Gillespie MT. Osteotropic agents regulate the expression of osteoclast differentiation factor and osteoprotegerin in osteoblastic stromal cells. Endocrinology 1998; 139:4743–4746.

180. Lee S-K, Lorenzo JA. Parathyroid hormone stimulates TRANCE and inhibits osteoprotegerin messenger ribonucleic acid expression in murine bone marrow

cultures: correlation with osteoclast-like cell formation. Endocrinology 1999; 140:3552–3561.

181. Howie DW, Vernon-Roberts B. Synovial macrophage response to aluminum oxide ceramic and cobalt–chrome alloy wear particles in rats. Biomaterials 1988; 9:442–448.

182. Howie DW. Tissue response in relation to type of wear particles around failed hip arthroplasties. J Arthrop 1990; 5:337–348.

183. Lerouge S, Huk O, Witvoet J, Sedel L. Ceramic–ceramic and metal–polyethylene total hip replacements; comparison of pseudomembranes after loosening. J Bone Joint Surg 1997; 79-B:135–139.

184. al-Saffar N, Revell PA, Khwaja HA, Bonfield W. Assessment of the role of cytokines in bone resorption in patients with total joint replacement. J Mater Science 1995; 6:762–767.

185. al-Saffar N, Revell A. Interleukin-l production by activated macrophages surrounding loosened orthopaedic implants: A potential role in osteolysis. Br J Rheumatol 1994; 33:309–316.

186. Glant TT, Jacobs JJ, Molnar G, Shanbhag AS, Valyon M, Galante JO. Bone resorption activitiy of particulate-stimulated macrophages. J Bone Miner Res 1983; 8:1071–1079.

187. Rogers SD, Howie DW, Graves SE, Pearcy MJ, Haynes DR. In vitro human monocyte response to wear particles of titanium alloy containing vanadium or niobium. J Bone Joint Surg Br 1997; 79-B:311–315.

188. Willert HG, Buchhom GH, Hess T. The significance of wear and material fatigue in loosening of hip prostheses. Orthopedics 1989; 18:350–369.

189. Kadoya Y, Kobayashi A, Ohashi H. Wear and osteolysis in total joint replacements. Acta Orthop Scand Suppl 1998; 278:1–16.

190. Wan Z, Dorr LD. Natural history of femoral focal osteolysis with proximal ingrowth smooth stem implant. J Arthroplasty 1996; 11:718–725.

191. Oparaugo PC, Clarke IC, Malchau H, Herberts P. Correlation of wear debris-induced osteolysis and revision with volumetric wear-rates of polyethylene: a survey of 8 reports in the literature. Acta Orthop Scand 2001; 72:22–28.

192. McGee MA, Howie DW, Costi K, Haynes DR, Wildernauer CI, Pearcy MJ, McLean JD. Implant retrieval studies of the wear and loosening of prosthetic joints: a review. Wear 2000; 241:158–165.

193. Dowd JE, Schwendeman LJ, Macaulay W, Doyle JS, Shanbhag AS, Wilson S, Hemndon JH, Rubash HE. Aseptic loosening in uncemented total hip arthroplasty in a canine model. Clin Orthop Rel Res 1995; 319:106–121.

194. Gelb H, Schumacher R, Cuclder J, Baker DG. In vivo inflammatory response to polymethylmethacrylate particulate debris: effect of size, morphology, and surface area. J Orthop Res 1994; 12:83–92.

195. Wooley PH, Morren R, Andary J, Sud S, Yang S-Y, Mayton L, Merkel D, Sieving A, Nasser S. Inflammatory response to orthopaedic biomaterials in the murine air pouch. Biomaerials 2002; 23:517–526.

196. Vernon-Roberts B. In: The Macrophage. Cambridge: Cambridge University Press, 1972.

197. Haynes DR, Boyle SJ, Rogers SD, Howie DW, Vernon-Roberts B. Variation in cytokines induced by particles from different prosthetic materials. Clin Orthop Rel Res 1998; 352:223–230.
198. Shanbhag AS, Jacobs JJ, Black J, Galante JO, Glant TT. Macrophage/ particle interactions: effect of size, composition and surface area. J Biomed Mater Res 1994; 28:81–90.
199. Shanbhag AS, Jacobs JJ, Black J, Galante JO, Glant TT. Human monocyte response to particulate biomaterials generated in vivo and in vitro. J Orthop Res 1995; 13:792–801.
200. Kubo T, Sawada K, Hirakawa K, Shimizu C, Takamatsu T, Hirasawa Y. Histiocyte reaction in rabbit femurs to UHMWPE, metal, and ceramic particles in different sizes. J Biomed Mater Res 1999; 45:363–369.
201. Horowitz MC, Purdon MA. Mediator interactions in macrophage/particle bone resorption. J Biomed Mater Res 1995; 29:477–484.
202. Giant TT, Jacobs JJ, Mikecz K, Yao J, Chubinskaja S, Williams JM, Urban RM, Shanbhag AS, Lee SH, Sumner DR. Participate induced, prostaglandin and cytokine-mediated bone resorption in an experimental system and in failed joint replacements. Am J Therap 1996; 3.
203. Catelas I, Petit A, Marchand R, Zukor DJ, Yahia LH, Huk OL. Cytotoxicity and macrophage cytokine release induced by ceramic and polyethylene particles in vitro. J Bone Joint Surg Br 1999; 81-B:516–521.
204. Chiba J, Maloney W, Inoue H, Rubash HE. Biochemical analysis of human macrophages activated by polyethylene particles retrieved from interface membranes after failed hip arthroplasty. J Arthroplasty 2001; 16:101–105.
205. Green TR, Fisher J, Stone M, Wroblewski BM, Ingham E. Polyethylene particles of a "critical size" are necessary for the induction of cytokines by macrophages in vitro. Biomaterials 1998; 19:2297–2303.
206. Shanbhag AS, Jacobs JJ, Glant TT, Gilbert JL, Black J, Galante JO. Composition and morphology of wear debris in failed uncemented total hip replacement. J Bone Joint Surg Br 1994; 76-B:60–67.
207. Milosev L, Antolic V, Minovic A, Cor A, Herman S, Pavlovcic V, Campbell P. Extensive metallosis and necrosis in failed prostheses with cemented titanium-alloy stems and ceramic heads. J Bone Joint Surg 2000; 82-B:352–357.
208. Lee J-M, Salvati EA, Betts F. Size of metallic and polyethylene debris particles in failed cemented total hip replacements. J Bone Joint Surg Br 1992; 74-B: 380–384.
209. Takagi M, Santavirta S, Ida H, Ishii M, Takei I, Nissalo S, Ogino T, Konttinen TY. High-turnover periprosthetic bone remodelling and immature bone formation around loose cemented total hip joints. J Bone Miner Res 2001; 16: 79–88.
210. Dean DD, Schwartz Z, Liu Y, Blanchard CR, Agrawai CM, Mabrey ID, Sylvia VL, Lohmann CH, Boyan BD. The effect of ultra-high molecular weight polyethylene wear debris on MG63 osteosarcoma cells in vitro. J Bone Joint Surg Am 1999; 81:452–461.
211. Rodrigo AM, Martinez ME, Martinez P, Escudero ML, Ruiz J, Saldana L, Gomez-Garcia L, Fernandez L, del Valle I, Munuera L. Effects of MA 956

superalloy and α-alumina particles on some markers of human osteoblastic cells in primary culture. J Biomed Mater Res 2000; 54:30–36.

212. Lohmann CH, Schwartz Z, Koster G, Jahn U, Buchhom GH, MacDougall MJ, Casasola D, Liu Y, Sylvia VL, Dean DD, Boyan BD. Phagocytosis of wear debris by osteoblasts affects differentiation and local factor production in a manner dependent on particle composition. Biomaterials 2000; 21:551–561.

213. Shida J, Trindade MCD, Goodman SB, Schurman DJ, Smith RL. Induction of interleukin-6 release in human osteoblast-like cells exposed to titanium particles in vitro. Calcif Tissue Int 2000; 67:151–155.

214. Vermes C, Chandrasekaren R, Jacobs JJ, Galante JO, Roebuck KA, Glant TT. The effects of particulate wear debris, cytokines, and growth factors on the MG-63 osteoblasts. J Bone Joint Surg A 2001; 83-A:201–211.

215. Heinemann DEH, Lohmann C, Siggelkow H, Alves F, Engel I, Koster G. Human osteoblast-like cells phagocytose metal particles that express the macrophage marker CD68 in vitro. J Bone Joint Surg Br 2000; 82-B:2883–2899.

216. Everts V, Delaisse JM, Korper W, Jansen DC, Tigchelaar-Gutter W, Saftig P, Beersten W. The bone lining cell: its role in cleaning Howship's lacunae and initiating bone formation. J Bone Miner Res 2002; 17:77–90.

217. Pollice PF, Silverton SF, Horowitz SM. Polymethacrylate-stimulated macrophages increase rat osteoclast precursor recruitment through their effect on osteoblasts in vitro. J Orthop Res 1995; 13:325–334.

218. Horowitz SM, Rapuano BP, Lane JM, Burstein AH. The interaction of the macrophages and the osteoblast in the pathophysiology of aseptic loosening of joint replacement. Calcif Tissue Int 1994; 54:320–324.

219. Horowitz SM, Gonzales JB. Inflammatory response to implant particulates in a macrophage/osteoblast coculture model. Calcif Tissue Int 1996; 59:392–396.

220. Vermes C, Roebuck KA, Chandrasekaren R, Dobai JG, Jacobs JJ, Giant TT. Particulate wear debris activates protein tyrosine kinases and nuclear factor kappaB, which down-regulates type I collagen synthesis in human osteoblasts. J Bone Miner Res 2000; 15:1756–1765.

221. Rodrigo AM, Martinez ME, Saldana L, Valles G, Martinez P, Gonzales-Carrasco JL, Cordero J, Munuera L. Effects of polyethylene and alpha-alumina particles on IL-6 expression and secretion in primary cultures of human osteoblastic cells. Biomaterials 2002; 23:901–908.

222. Martinez ME, Medina S, del Campo MT, Sanchez-Cabezudo MJ, Sanchez M, Munuera L. Effect of polyethylene on osteocalcin, alkaline phosphatase and procollagen secretion by human osteoblastic cells. Calcif Tissue Int 1998; 15: 1756–1765.

223. Martinez ME, Medina S, del Campo MT, Garcia JA, Rodrigo A, Munuera L. Effect of polyethylene particles on human osteoblastic cell growth. Biomaterials 1998; 19:183–187.

224. Pandey R, Berendt AR, Athanasou NA. Histological and microbiological findings in non-infected and infected revision arthroplasty tissues. Acta Orthop Trauma Surg 2000; 120:570–574.

225. Akisue T, Bauer TW, Farver CF, Mochida Y. The effect of wear particle debris on NF-κB activation and proinflammatory cytokine release in differentiated THP-1 cells. J Biomed Mater Res 2002; 59:507–515.

226. Hitchins VM, Merritt K. Decontaminating particles exposed to endotoxin (LPS). J Biomed Mater Res 1999; 46:434–437.

227. Van Der Vis HM, Aspenberg P, Kleine DK, Tigchelaar W, Van Noorden CJF. Short periods of oscillating fluid pressure directed at a titanium-bone interface in rabbits lead to bone lysis. Acta Orthop Scand 1998; 69:5–10.

228. Aspenberg P, Van Der Vis HM. Fluid pressure may cause periprosthetic osteolysis: Particles are not the only thing. Acta Orthop Scand 1998; 69:1–4.

229. Van Der Vis HM, Aspenberg P, Marti RM, Tigchelaar W, Van Noorden CJF. Fluid pressure causes bone resorption in a rabbit model of prosthetic loosening. Clin Orthop 1998; 350:201–208.

230. Skripitz R, Aspenberg P. Pressure-induced periprosthetic osteolysis: a rat model. J Orthop Res 2000; 18:481–484.

231. Ferrier GM, McEvoy A, Evans CE, Andrew JG. The effect of cyclic pressure on human monocyte-derived macrophages in vitro. J Bone Joint Surg Br 2000; 82-B:755–759.

232. McEvoy A, Jeyam M, Ferrier GM, Evana CE, Andrew JG. Synergistic effect of particles and cyclic pressure on cytokine production in human monocyte/macrophages: proposed role In periprosthetic osteolysis. Bone 2002; 1:171–177.

233. Ogasawara A, Arakawa T, Kaneda T, Takuma T, Sato T, Keaneko M, Hakeda Y. Fluid shear stress-induced cyclooxygenase-2 expression is mediated by C/EBP beta, cAMP-response element-binding protein, and AP-1 in osteoblastic MC3T3-E1 cells. J Biol Chem 2001; 276:7048–7054.

234. Kurata K, Uemura T, Nemoto A, Tateishi T, Murakami T, Higaki H, Iwamoto Y. Mechanical strain effect on bone-resorbing activity and messenger RNA expression of marker enzymes in isolated osteoclast culture. J Bone Miner Res 2001; 16:722–730.

235. Kobayashi Y, Hashimoto F, Miyamoto H, Kanaoka K, Miyazaki-Kawashita Y, Nakashima T, Shibata M, Kobayashi K, Kato Y, Sakai H. Force-induced osteoclast apoptosis in vivo is accompanied by elevation in transforming growth factor beta and osteoprotegerin expression. J Bone Miner Res 2000; 15:1924–1934.

236. Sakai K, Mohtai M, Shida J, Harimaya K, Benvenuti S, Brandi ML, Kukita T, Iwamoto Y. Fluid shear stress increases interleukin-11 expression in human osteoblast-like cells; its role in osteoclast induction. J Bone Miner Res 1999; 14:2089–2098.

237. Farber A, Chin R, Song Y, Huie P, Goodman SB. Chronic antigen-specific immune-system activation may potentially be involved in the loosening of cemented acetabular components. J Biomed Mater Res 2001; 55:433–141.

238. Hallab NJ, Mikecz K, Vermes C, Skipor A, Jacobs JJ. Orthopaedic implant related metal toxicity in terms of human lymphocyte reactivity to metal–protein complexes produced from cobalt-base and titanium-base implant alloy degradation. Mol Cell Biochem 2001; 222:127–136.

239. Hallab NJ, Merritt K, Jacobs JJ. Metal sensitivity in patients with orthopaedic implants. J Bone Joint Surg Am 2001; 83-A:428–436.

240. Goodman SB, Huie P, Song Y, Schurman D, Maloney W, Woolson S, Sibley R. Cellular profile and cytokine production at prosthetic interfaces. Study of tissues retrieved from revised hip and knee replacements. J Bone Joint Surg 1998; 80-B:531–539.

241. Taubman MA, Kawai T. Involvement of T-lymphocytes in periodontal disease and in direct and indirect induction ofboneresorption. Crit Rev Oral Biol Med 2001; 12:125–135.

242. Li TF, Santavirta S, Waris V, Lassus J, Lindroos L, Xu JW, Virtanen I, Konttinen TY. No lymphokines in T cells around loosened hip prostheses. Acta Orthop Scand 2001; 72:241–247.

243. Pollice PF, Rosier RN, Looney RJ, Puzus JE, Schwartz EM, O'Keefe RL. Oral pentoxifylline inhibits release of tumor necrosis factor-alpha from human peripheral blood monocytes: a potential treatment for aseptic loosening of total joint components. J Bone Joint Surg Am 2001; 83-A:1057–1061.

244. Trindade MC, Nakashima Y, Lind M, Sun DH, Goodman SB, Maloney W, Schurman DJ, Smith RL. Interleukin-4 inhibits granulocyte-macrophage colony-stimulating factor, interleukin-6, and tumor necrosis factor-alpha expression by human monocytes in response to polymethylmethacrylate particle challenged in vitro. J Orthop Res 1999; 17:797–802.

245. Childs LM, Eleftherios PP, Xing L, Dougall WC, Anderson D, Boskey AL, Puzus JE, Rosier RN, O'Keefe RL, Boyce BF, Schwarz EM. In vivo RANK signaling blockade using the receptor activator of NF-κB:Fc effectively prevents and ameliorates wear debris-induced osteolysis via osteoclast depletion without inhibiting osteogenesis. J Bone Miner Res 2002; 17:192–199.

246. Goater JJ, O'Keefe RJ, Rosier RN, Puzus JE, Schwartz EM. Efficacy of ex vivo OPG gene therapy in preventing wear debris induced osteolysis. J Orthop Res 2002; 20:169–173.

247. Wikaningnim R, Highton J, Parker A, Coleman M, Hessian PA, Roberts-Thomson PJ, Ahem MJ, Smith MD. Pathogenic mechanisms in the rheumatoid nodule: Comparison of pro-inflammatory cytokine production and cell adhesion molecule expression in rheumatoid nodules and synovial membranes from the same patient. Arthritis Rheum 1998; 41:1783–1797.

248. Kraan MC, Haringman JJ, Ahem MJ, Breedveld FC, Smith MD, Tak PP. Quantification of the cell infiltrate in synovial tissue by digital image analysis. Rheumatology 2000; 39:43–49.

13

Wear Debris Mediated Osteolysis: An Overview

Arun Shanbhag

Department of Orthopaedic Surgery, Massachusetts General Hospital, Harvard Medical School, Boston, Massachusetts, U.S.A.

INTRODUCTION

Improvements in surgical technique, prevention of infection, selection of materials, and refined methods of fixation have resulted in a total joint replacement procedure that is one of the most cost-effective means of restoring joint mobility and function (1). The vast majority of patients receiving joint replacements will have greater than 20 years of pain-free functional outcome and the success of this procedure has also increased societal expectations. Increasing numbers of joint replacements are being performed in a younger, more active patient population, which place higher demands on the components and need them to last for a longer life span. It is not surprising then that the survivorship of total hip replacements (THRs) in young, active patients is significantly reduced (2). There is thus a crucial need to understand the mechanisms by which joint replacements fail, and further to develop implant components, surgical procedures and therapies which improve the life span durable of these replacements.

Implant failure is associated with a localized granulomatous reaction resulting in resorption of the bone, which compromises bony anchors stabilizing the implant and leads to a painfully loose implant. In the absence of bacterial infection, this is termed aseptic loosening or osteolysis and is the most common mode of failure of total joint replacements. In the absence of therapeutic alternatives, revision surgery is required to debride the site and insert new components.

The underlying etiology of aseptic loosening has been explored for more than three decades and several mechanisms have been proposed as causative of aseptic loosening. These include wear debris-mediated osteolysis, mechanical factors such as increased fluid pressure and cement toxicity leading to bone necrosis, and a wear debris-driven adaptive immune response. These various mechanisms have been well documented in the following chapters (14–16) in this book, and are written by leading scientists who have investigated these mechanisms exhaustively. In this chapter, I will briefly summarize the evidence for wear debris as the primary cause of aseptic loosening and osteolysis.

HISTORICAL PERSPECTIVE

Charnley recognized loosening in joint replacements in the 1960s when the poly-tetrafluoroethylene (PTFE) acetabular components he used required revision within three years (3–6). Histopathological analysis of tissues retrieved during revision surgery demonstrated the presence of particulate debris surrounded by foreign body giant cells, forming a "caseating granulomata and sterile pus." To prove the hypothesis that particulate PTFE debris were causative of the granuloma, Charnley implanted finely divided PTFE subcutaneously in his thigh, and studied the increased size of the nodules, which he could palpate after three months (6). These findings provided Charnley the rationale to switch to a more wear resistant polyethylene for the articulating surface, which is used to this day with minor modifications (7).

Willert and Semlitsch extensively analyzed histopathological sections from around failed joint replacements and proposed that aseptic loosening of implants was caused by excessive wear debris generated from the polyethylene liner. The retrieved periprosthetic tissues contained sheets of macrophages laden with various types of particulate wear debris in a fibrous stroma, intermingled with multinucleated giant cells encapsulating larger debris (Figs. 1 and 2) (8–11). According to Willert's hypothesis, wear debris generated at the articulating surface would normally be cleared from the joint space by macrophage phagocytosis and transported via the lymphatic system (8,9). If the amount of wear debris generated were to exceed the clearance capacity of the local vasculature, the debris would be retained locally within the macrophages, stimulating them and leading to the formation of a periprosthetic granuloma (8,9). Granulomas initiate in the joint capsule and depending upon the amount of wear debris generated, the granulomatous reaction would extend distally into the bone–cement interface, sacrificing bone-implant anchors, resulting in component loosening (Fig. 3) (9).

While Willert and Semlitsch's original observations were made with cemented components, a similar process is believed to occur in uncemented implants (12–16). By carefully studying the tissues around failed components,

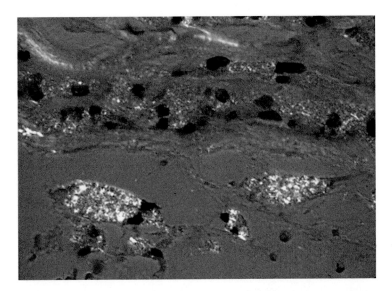

Figure 1 Histology of peri-implant interfacial tissue under polarization. Note the prominent macrophage in the left, laden with internalized birefringent polyethylene particles. The nuclei appear to be squished to the right edge of the cell. Birefringence is also observed in other cells in the membranous tissue. *Courtesy*: Photograph was kindly provided by Prof. Joshua J Jacobs, Rush University, Chicago, Illinois. (*See color insert.*)

Willert and Semlitsch further suggested that the "whole environment" of the joint participated in clearing prosthetic wear debris (9). Schmalzried et al. (15) elaborated further that wear debris generated at the articulating surface can be carried to all areas in the joint accessible to joint fluid. The joint fluid

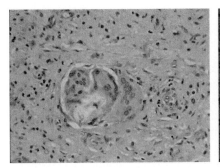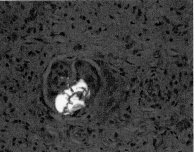

Figure 2 Histology of peri-implant interfacial tissue under normal (*left*) and polarization (*right*) conditions. A foreign body giant cell(s) has encapsulated a larger fragment of the birefringent polyethylene and isolated it from the surrounding tissue. Note the numerous nuclei in the giant cell. (*See color insert.*)

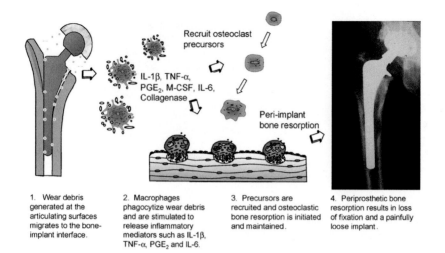

Recruit osteoclast precursors

IL-1β, TNF-α, PGE₂, M-CSF, IL-6, Collagenase

Peri-implant bone resorption

1. Wear debris generated at the articulating surfaces migrates to the bone-implant interface.

2. Macrophages phagocytize wear debris and are stimulated to release inflammatory mediators such as IL-1β, TNF-α, PGE₂ and IL-6.

3. Precursors are recruited and osteoclastic bone resorption is initiated and maintained.

4. Periprosthetic bone resorption results in loss of fixation and a painfully loose implant.

Figure 3 Schematic representation of the sequence of events leading to wear debris-mediated osteolysis. (*See color insert.*)

can carry wear debris generated at the articular surface, to the periprosthetic region, and the flow pattern would determine whether the wear debris was linearly dispersed along the component or accumulated in several focal areas (15). They further suggested that the pattern of debris deposition and subsequent localized biological response would determine whether bone loss was manifested as a focal lytic lesion, or as a linear lesion dissecting the bone–implant interface (15,17). Investigations of clinical materials during autopsies demonstrate the presence of wear debris at remote sites such as the lungs, kidneys, liver, spleen, and lymph nodes and confirms the clearance aspects of Willert's hypothesis (18–21).

ANALYSIS OF CLINICAL MATERIAL

Biochemical analyses of clinical materials harvested during revision surgery have been instrumental in providing the foundations of the pathogenesis of osteolysis. By placing retrieved tissues in organ culture, investigators can identify the cellular mediators released by cells in the peri-implant region, which in turn provide insight into the microenvironment of the cells. In their seminal work, Goldring et al. (22) used organ cultures techniques to demonstrate that peri-implant membranous tissues were capable of producing biological mediators such as collagenase and prostaglandin E_2 (PGE_2), which had the capacity to stimulate osteoclasts to resorb bone. Since then, numerous investigators have shown that this membranous tissue is capable of producing a variety of matrix degrading enzymes, prostaglandins, and potent pro-inflammatory cytokines such as interleukin (IL) -1α, IL-1β, IL-6, tumor necrosis factor-α (TNF-α), and platelet derived growth factor (PDGF) (23–26); matrix degrading enzymes such as gelatinase, stromelysins and various matrix metalloproteinases including MMP-1, MMP-9, MMP-10, MMP-12, and MMP-13 (27–30); and chemokines such as monocyte chemoattractant proteins MCP-1, MIP-1α, MIP-1β, and IL-8. This wider assortment of chemokines, growth factors, pro-inflammatory and anti-inflammatory cytokines, and mediators demonstrate a potent ability of the peri-prosthetic tissues to recruit and stimulate cells capable of stimulating osteoclastic bone resorption and fibrous tissue formation (22,23,25,26,31,32).

Immunohistochemistry and in situ hybridization have demonstrated that while a wide variety of cell types are present in the peri-prosthetic tissues (including fibroblasts, lymphocytes, eosinophils, and basophils), gene expression for inflammatory cytokines and mediators is specifically correlated with macrophages which have phagocytized wear debris (33,34). Haynes and Crotti in chapter 12 of this book have described the array of these cytokines and particularly the mediators of osteoclastogenesis receptor activator of NF-κB (RANK), receptor activator of NF-κB ligand (RANKL), and osteoprotegerin (OPG).

TYPES OF WEAR DEBRIS INVOLVED IN OSTEOLYSIS

Around total joint replacements, wear debris can arise from several sources. The predominant wear debris identified in osteolytic lesions and interfacial membranes, and representing 70–95% of the debris burden is particulate ultra high molecular weight polyethylene (UHMWPE) from the articulating surfaces (35–39). UHMWPE debris present around failed total hip, total knee, and total shoulder components has been retrieved and analyzed (35,37,38,40–44). These particles are predominantly spheroids 0.1–2.0 μm in size. Also present are fibrils interconnecting the spheroids forming larger aggregates (Fig. 4) (35,37,43). Wear also occurs at the convex, nonarticulating surface of the UHMWPE acetabular liner owing to motion of the liner against the metal backing and abrasion of the UHMWPE at the rim of the screw holes (45–47). Unfilled screw holes in the metal backing of the acetabular component are repositories of wear debris generated at the nonarticulating surfaces and may also house debris migrated from the articulating surfaces along the liner backing interface (Fig. 4) (40,45,48). Such UHMWPE debris are generally larger than those present around the femoral components (Fig. 5) (40,47). Unfilled screw holes also provide access for wear debris to migrate to the area behind the ingrowth cup potentially resulting in pelvic osteolysis, observed in clinical follow-up (49), and in autopsy retrievals (50). Metal screws which provide initial cup stability, can be the source of fretting and corrosion, causing metal debris and also abrasion with the liner resulting in additional UHMWPE shards and fibers.

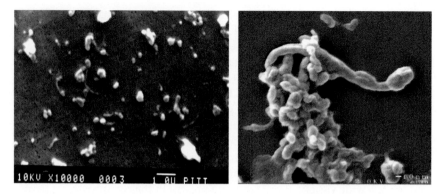

Figure 4 Particulate ultra high molecular weight polyethylene (UHMWPE) extracted from peri-implant interfacial tissues from around the femoral component (*left*) and from around acetabular screw holes (*right*). *Source*: From Refs. 35,40.

Metallic wear debris represents only a minor fraction of the debris burden in UHMWPE articulations and typically results from abrasion of the stem against bone or cement (35,37). Another important source of metallic debris in THRs is the junction at the modular femoral head and neck. The "morse taper" head connection permits fretting wear and introduces a crevice for subsequent generation of corrosion products (51–53). These corrosion products can be fragments of component oxides in various combinations including chromium orthophosphate, which has been identified in interfacial tissues (54,55). Metal debris can also be generated in other modular

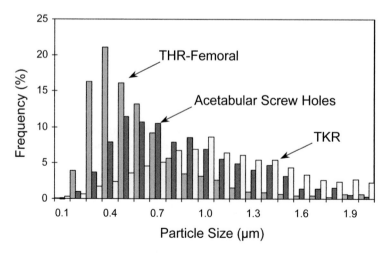

Figure 5 Frequency distribution of wear debris size from total joint replacements. *Source*: From Refs. 35,38,40.

components used to customize the prosthesis. Unusually, debris may also be introduced on the surface of the component as a result of polishing and lapping treatments (56). While metallic debris can lead to an especially aggressive cellular response (54,57–60), their smaller fraction yields them a minor role in causing implant failure. Of greater importance is the consequence of such harder debris driving between the head and UHMWPE articulating surfaces, where it can be the source of third-body wear, accelerating UHMWPE wear debris generation.

Considering that the periprosthetic tissues contain a large variety of types and sizes of particulate debris, it is not possible to ascertain which of the debris species is primarily involved in initiating the granulomatous reaction. In vitro and in vivo models are required to determine and confirm the incriminating particle species, as well as identify the sequence of events leading to implant loosening.

IN VITRO EVIDENCE OF WEAR MEDIATED OSTEOLYSIS

Based on histopathological analysis of clinical materials, macrophages with internalized debris appear to be the culprits in the initiation and propagation of the periprosthetic granuloma and associated bone resorption, leading eventually to implant loosening. Macrophages are the sentinels of the immune response, the primary cells at any site of inflammation and along with short-lived neutrophils, key participants in innate immunity. With their ability to degrade protein, process and present antigen, macrophages coordinate the recruitment and activity of T-cells and orchestrate the immune response (Fig. 3) (61,62). Macrophages cultured with wear debris in vitro have thus been used as crucial models for dissecting the sequence of events occurring at the bone–implant interface. In vitro macrophage-particle experiments permit us to study several variables individually, without interactions from confounding factors. In chapter 11 of this book, Professor Anderson has reviewed the central role of macrophages in inflammation and wound healing. In chapter 19, Puskas et al. have provided an overview of the different types of in vitro models and the unique issues of each. The primary goals of an in vitro model are to determine if particles can stimulate cells to release inflammatory mediators and if this inflammation is capable of causing bone resorption.

While there are advantages of using transformed or immortalized macrophage cell lines (see chapter 19), it is clinically more relevant to use primary cells for developing relevant models. Since macrophages in interfacial membranes are believed to be derived from the circulating monocytes, peripheral blood monocytes are the target cell of choice for studying and reproducing macrophage-particle interactions (57,63–67).

Early studies on macrophage-particle interactions have focused mainly on the toxicity of different particles. Co, Ni, and Co–Cr-alloy particles in phagocytizable sizes decreased phagocytic ability and damaged cell membranes extensively leading to cell death, while Ti-alloy particles were less deleterious (68–70). Polymethylmethacrylate (PMMA) and UHMWPE too caused varying levels of cell death, though far less than the metal particles (57,71,72). Shanbhag et al. (57,59) demonstrated that cell death increased with increasing dosage of challenging particles. Macrophages cultured with titanium particles for 24 hours were barely affected by particle concentrations representing one-tenth of the surface area of cells. Whereas, increasing the particle concentration 10-fold resulted in approximately a 50% decrease in cellular synthesis. A 100-fold increase in particle concentration, representing 10 times the surface area of particles as that of the cells, nearly abolished DNA synthesis. This cytotoxic effect is also dependent upon the composition of debris as polystyrene particles at comparable concentrations were not severely affected (59).

Particle toxicity directly impacts the ability of cells to initiate an inflammatory reaction. Haynes et al. (58) demonstrated that CoCr-alloy particles which caused extensive macrophage death very quickly, and thus could not synthesize and secrete inflammatory mediators (58). Ti-alloy particles were slightly less toxic and the resulting cell death occurred nearly 24 hour later, which provided sufficient time for the macrophages to synthesize and release large quantities of inflammatory mediators (58). To account for the varying densities of metallic and polymeric particles, Shanbhag et al. normalized for surface area of the wear debris and demonstrated that TiAlV and CpTi particles were the most stimulatory in eliciting a variety of inflammatory mediators such as PGE_2, IL-1α, IL-1β, and IL-6 (57,63). Two types of UHMWPE wear debris, either retrieved from patients with failed THR, or fabricated in the laboratory in a clinically relevant size, were both less stimulatory than metal particles, but significantly more stimulatory than nonstimulated cells (Fig. 6) (57,63). Numerous investigators using a variety of cell models have also demonstrated convincingly that particulate wear debris has a strong ability to stimulate macrophages to release significant levels of degradative enzymes and pro-inflammatory mediators (60,64,67,70,73–77).

Macrophages additionally release growth factors such a TGF-β_1 and stimulate fibroblast proliferation, both of which are essential for the fibrous scar formation in response to inflammation (63). This healing aspect of inflammation needs to go hand in hand in the peri-implant region, where not only is the bone resorbed, but the intervening space is refilled by a fibrous interfacing membrane (63,78–80).

In addition to cellular responses based on the composition and dose of particles, the size of the challenging particles can strongly influence the macrophage release of mediators (59,74,81). Investigators have demonstrated that particles small enough to be phagocytized (about 7 µm or less) will stimulate macrophages to a greater extent, whereas larger particles are

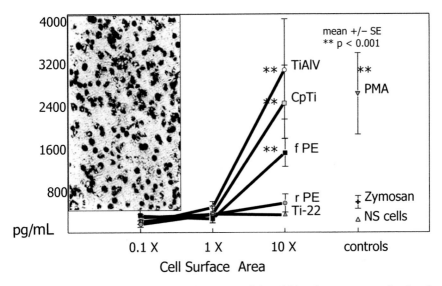

Figure 6 Interleukin-1β release by human peripheral blood monocytes stimulated with different types and doses of particles. Monocytes were cultured with the following particles—Ti-22: titanium particles, 22 μm in diameter; CpTi: submicron commercially pure titanium particles; TiAlV: submicron Ti–6Al–4V alloy particles (inset photo); rPE: retrieved UHMWPE particles; fPE: fabricated UHMWPE particles. *Source*: Adapted from Ref. 57.

less stimulatory, if at all (57,59,74,82,83). Within the phagocytozable range, finer particles are more inflammatory and culpable in the osteolytic process than are larger particles (8,81,84–88). Going one step further, investigators have demonstrated that mediators and enzymes released by macrophages are indeed capable of initiating and stimulating bone resorption. Wear debris-stimulated macrophage conditioned media increased bone resorption of ^{45}Ca-labeled murine calvaria (Fig. 7) (60,63). This confirmed that a particle culture with macrophages can set up a cascade of events resulting in bone resorption.

Cell types such as fibroblasts and osteoblasts present in the peri-implant region are also affected by wear debris. Particles directly stimulate fibroblasts to release high levels of collagenase and stromelysin, which can degrade the organic components of bone (42,89,90). Osteoblasts when exposed to particles are also compromised in their ability to synthesize collagen and make bone (91–93). This impacts their ability to compensate for the heightened macrophage-mediated bone resorption. Other cells in tissues likely are also involved in an autocrine–paracrine effect and may enhance activation of macrophages and osteoclasts to resorb adjacent mineralized tissue, but their role is secondary to the macrophage response.

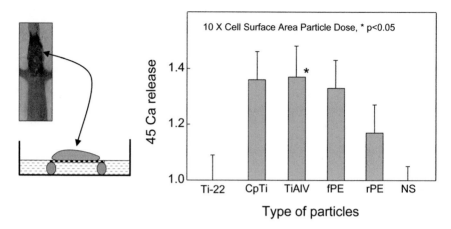

Figure 7 Spent medium from macrophages cultured with particles stimulate cells in calvaria to resorb bone. Human peripheral blood monocytes were cultured with the following particles— Ti-22: titanium particles, 22 μm in diameter; CpTi: submicron commercially pure titanium particles; TiAlV: submicron Ti–6Al–4V alloy particles; rPE: retrieved UHMWPE particles; fPE: fabricated UHMWPE particles. *Source*: From Ref. 63.

IN VIVO MODELS FOR OSTEOLYSIS

In vitro studies have demonstrated that particulate wear debris can stimulate cells to secrete multiple inflammatory cytokines and mediators dependent upon the size and concentration of wear debris. Both in vitro and in vivo cytokines and mediators interact in a complex cascade, wherein multiple mediators up- and down-regulate one another, and also modulate osteoclastic and perhaps, macrophage-related bone resorption (94,95). Due to the complex interactions of cytokines, mediators, receptors, and antagonist proteins, in vitro studies represent only a partial understanding of the consequences of cellular interactions with materials. In vivo studies are required to understand the overall effect of these cytokines and mediators released in response to wear debris.

In a simple yet effective proof of concept manner, Howie et al. (96) modeled the implantation of a bulk implant in an intramedullary cavity using a PMMA plug in the femoral condyle of rat knees. The osteolytic capacity of particulate wear debris was demonstrated by repeated injections of UHMWPE particles in the knee, resulting in the resorption of the bone surrounding the plugs. The loose cement plug was encased in a fibrous tissue composed of macrophages, foreign body giant cells, and UHMWPE particles which had replaced the interfacing bone (96). To reproduce a complete total joint, Dowd et al. (97) used a canine model. A clinically similar fiber metal-coated porous TiAlV femoral component articulated against an UHMWPE acetabular liner with a fiber-mesh-backed metal shell. Intraoperatively, particulate Ti-alloy, Co–Cr-alloy, or high density polyethylene were placed at the bone–implant interface. After 12 weeks post-operative, a granulomatous tissue was observed at the bone implant interface. This membrane consisted of macrophages and foreign-body giant cells with intra- and extra-cellular wear debris, and histologically resembled the tissues from around clinically loosened components (10,16,23). Furthermore, when these membranous tissues were placed in organ culture, they released IL-1, PGE_2, collagenase, and gelatinase (97). Enhancing this model by using submicron UHMWPE particles in clinically similar sizes and shapes, and extending the post-operative period to 24 weeks, resulted in the clinically analogous radiographic evidence of peri-implant bone loss. The pattern of bone loss and associated periosteal

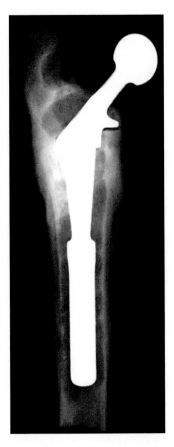

Figure 8　UHMWPE wear debris-mediated osteolysis in a canine uncemented total hip replacement model. UHMWPE particles were introduced intraoperatively and osteolysis was observed 23 weeks after surgery. *Source*: From Refs. 97,98.

reaction was also similar to that observed in clinical patients (Fig. 8) (98,99). The striking similarity of radiographic manifestation, membrane histology and biochemistry of clinically loosened components confirmed the role of wear debris in leading to aseptic loosening and osteolysis. Such models are invaluable in further dissecting the biological mechanism of osteolysis and exploring therapeutic options to stall and reverse the process (99).

SUMMARY

In this chapter, the case of wear debris leading to osteolysis and aseptic loosening of total joint replacements is clearly made. Clinical investigations as well as in vitro and in vivo models confirm that wear debris by itself is sufficient to initiate an inflammatory response leading to bone resorption. While there are other mechanisms, these are likely overlaid in specific cases on top of the primary wear debris driven inflammation. The evidence is sufficiently convincing that most new developments of implant systems and materials are made to reduce the rate of wear and the wear debris burden. This has indeed improved the useful life and extended the durability of an already very successful surgical procedure.

REFERENCES

1. Bozic KJ, Rosenberg AG, Huckman RS, Herndon JH. Economic evaluation in orthopaedics. J Bone Joint Surg Am 2003; 85-A(1):129–142.
2. Older J. Charnley low-friction arthroplasty: a worldwide retrospective review at 15 to 20 years. J Arthroplasty 2002; 17(6):675–680.
3. Charnley J. Anchorage of the femoral head prosthesis to the shaft of the femur. J Bone Joint Surg 1960; 42-B:28–30.
4. Charnley J, Follacci FM, Hammond BT. The long-term reaction of bone to self-curing acrylic cement. J Bone Joint Surg 1968; 50-B:822–829.
5. Charnley J. Tissue reaction to implanted plastics. In: Charnley J, ed. Acrylic Cement in Orthopedic Surgery. Edinburgh: E & S Livingstone, 1970:1–9.
6. Charnley J. Tissue reactions to polytetrafluorethylene: Letter to the editor. Lancet 1963; 1963:1379.
7. Shanbhag AS. What experimental approaches (tissue retrieval, in vivo, in vitro, etc) have been used to investigate the biologic effects of particles? In: Wright TM, Goodman SB, eds. Implant Wear in Total Joint Replacements. Rosemont: American Academy of Orthopaedic Surgeons, 2001:114–123.
8. Willert HG, Semlitsch M. Tissue reactions to plastic and metallic wear products of joint endoprostheses. In: Gschwend N, Debrunner HU, eds. Total Hip Prosthesis. Baltimore: Williams & Wilkins, 1976:205–239.
9. Willert HG. Reactions of the articular capsule to wear products of artificial joint prostheses. J Biomed Mater Res 1977; 11(2):157–164.
10. Mirra JM, Amstutz HC, Matos M, Gold R. The pathology of the joint tissues and its clinical relevance in prosthesis failure. Clin Orthop 1976; 117:221–240.

11. Mirra JM, Marder RA, Amstutz HC. The pathology of failed total joint arthroplasty. Clin Orthop 1982; 170:175–183.

12. Jacobs JJ, Urban RM, Schajowicz F, Gavrilovic J, Galante JO. Particulate-associated endosteal osteolysis in titanium-base alloy cementless total hip replacement. In: St John KR, ed. Particulate Debris from Medical Implants: Mechanisms of Formation and Biological Consequences, ASTM STP 1144. Philadelphia: American Society for Testing and Materials, 1992:52–60.

13. Willert HG, Bertram H, Buchhorn GH. Osteolysis in alloarthroplasty of the hip. The role of bone cement fragmentation. Clin Orthop Relat Res 1990; 258:108–121.

14. Willert HG, Bertram H, Buchhorn GH. Osteolysis in alloarthroplasty of the hip. The role of ultra-high molecular weight polyethylene wear particles. Clin Orthop Relat Res 1990; 258:95–107.

15. Schmalzried TP, Jasty M, Harris WH. Periprosthetic bone loss in total hip arthroplasty. Polyethylene wear debris and the concept of the effective joint space. J Bone Joint Surg Am 1992; 74(6):849–863.

16. Maloney WJ, Jasty M, Harris WH, Galante JO, Callaghan JJ. Endosteal erosion in association with stable uncemented femoral components. J Bone Joint Surg Am 1990; 72(7):1025–1034.

17. Shanbhag AS, Hasselman CT, Jacobs JJ, Rubash HE. Biologic response to wear debris. In: Callaghan JJ, Rosenberg AG, Rubash HE, eds. The Adult Hip. Philadelphia: Lippincott-Raven, 1998:279–288.

18. Jacobs JJ, Patterson LM, Skipor AK, Hall DJ, Urban RM, Black J, Galante JO. Postmortem retrieval of total joint replacement components. J Biomed Mater Res 1999; 48(3):385–391.

19. Urban RM, Jacobs JJ, Tomlinson MJ, Gavrilovic J, Black J, Peoc'h M. Dissemination of wear particles to the liver, spleen, and abdominal lymph nodes of patients with hip or knee replacement. J Bone Joint Surg Am 2000; 82(4):457–476.

20. Gray MH, Talbert ML, Talbert WM, Bansal M, Hsu A. Changes seen in lymph nodes draining the sites of large joint prostheses. Am J Surg Pathol 1989; 13:1050–1056.

21. Hicks DG, Judkins AR, Sickel JZ, Rosier RN, Puzas JE, O'Keefe RJ. Granular histiocytes of pelvic lymph nodes following total hip arthroplasty. The presence of wear debris, cytokine production, and immunologically activated macrophages. J Bone Joint Surg 1996; 78-A:482–496.

22. Goldring SR, Schiller AL, Roelke M, Rourke CM, O'Neill DA, Harris WH. The synovial-like membrane at the bone–cement interface in loose total hip replacements and its proposed role in bone lysis. J Bone Joint Surg Am 1983; 65-A:575–584.

23. Shanbhag AS, Jacobs JJ, Black J, Galante JO, Glant TT. Cellular mediators secreted by interfacial membranes obtained at revision total hip arthroplasty. J Arthroplasty 1995; 10(4):498–506.

24. Goodman SB, Chin RC, Chiou SS, Schurman DJ, Woolson ST, Masada MP. A clinical-pathologic-biochemical study of the membrane surrounding loosened and nonloosened total hip arthroplasties. Clin Orthop 1989; 244:182–187.

25. Kim KJ, Rubash HE, Wilson SC, D'Antonio JA, McClain EJ. A histologic and biochemical comparison of the interface tissues in cementless and cemented hip prostheses. Clin Orthop 1993; 287:142–152.

26. Dorr LD, Bloebaum R, Emmanual J, Meldrum R. Histologic, biochemical and ion analysis of tissue and fluids retrieved during total hip arthroplasty. Clin Orthop 1990; 261:82–95.

27. Takagi M, Santavirta S, Ida H, Ishii M, Mandelin J, Konttinen YT. Matrix metalloproteinases and tissue inhibitors of metalloproteinases in loose artificial hip joints. Clin Orthop 1998; 352:35–45.

28. Pap T, Pap G, Hummel KM, Franz JK, Jeisy E, Sainsbury I, Gay RE, Billingham M, Neumann W, Gay S. Membrane-type-1 matrix metalloproteinase is abundantly expressed in fibroblasts and osteoclasts at the bone–implant interface of aseptically loosened joint arthroplasties in situ. J Rheumatol 1999; 26(1):166–169.

29. Takei I, Takagi M, Santavirta S, Ida H, Ishii M, Ogino T, Ainola M, Konttinen YT. Messenger ribonucleic acid expression of 16 matrix metalloproteinases in bone–implant interface tissues of loose artificial hip joints. J Biomed Mater Res 2000; 52(4):613–620.

30. Konttinen YT, Ainola M, Valleala H, Ma J, Ida H, Mandelin J, Kinne RW, Santavirta S, Sorsa T, Lopez-Otin C, Takagi M. Analysis of 16 different matrix metalloproteinases (MMP-1 to MMP-20) in the synovial membrane: different profiles in trauma and rheumatoid arthritis. Ann Rheum Dis 1999; 58(11):691–697.

31. Chiba J, Rubash HE, Kim KJ, Iwaki Y. The characterization of cytokines in the interface tissue obtained from failed cementless total hip arthroplasty with and without femoral osteolysis. Clin Orthop 1994; 300:304–312.

32. Goodman SB, Chin RC. Prostaglandin E2 levels in the membrane surrounding bulk and particulate polymethylmethacrylate in the rabbit tibia. A preliminary study. Clin Orthop 1990; 257:305–309.

33. Jiranek WA, Machado M, Jasty M, Jevsevar D, Wolfe HJ, Goldring SR, Goldberg MJ, Harris WH. Production of cytokines around loosened cemented acetabular components. Analysis with immunohistochemical techniques and in situ hybridization. J Bone Joint Surg Am 1993; 75(6):863–879.

34. Goodman SB, Knoblich G, O'Connor M, Song Y, Huie P, Sibley R. Heterogeneity in cellular and cytokine profiles from multiple samples of tissue surrounding revised hip prostheses. J Biomed Mater Res 1996; 31(3):421–428.

35. Shanbhag AS, Jacobs JJ, Glant TT, Gilbert JL, Black J, Galante JO. Composition and morphology of wear debris in failed uncemented total hip replacement. J Bone Joint Surg Br 1994; 76(1):60–67.

36. Abb J, Zander H, Abb H, Albert E, Deinhardt F. Association of human leucocyte low responsiveness to inducers of interferon alpha with HLA-DR2. Immunology 1983; 49:239–244.

37. Maloney WJ, Smith RL, Schmalzried TP, Chiba J, Huene D, Rubash HE. Isolation and characterization of wear particles generated in patients who have had failure of a hip arthroplasty without cement. J Bone Joint Surg 1995; 77-A:1301–1310.

38. Shanbhag AS, Bailey HO, Hwang DS, Cha CW, Eror NG, Rubash HE. Quantitative analysis of ultrahigh molecular weight polyethylene (UHMWPE) wear debris associated with total knee replacements. J Biomed Mater Res 2000; 53(1):100–110.

39. Friedman RJ, Black J, Galante JO, Jacobs JJ, Skinner HB. Current concepts in orthopaedic biomaterials and implant fixation. J Bone Joint Surg Am 1993; 75-A: 1086–1109.

40. Shanbhag AS, Bailey HO, Hwang DS, Eror NG, Woo SL-Y, Rubash HE. Chemical and morphological characterization of wear debris associated with acetabular screw holes. Trans Soc Biomater 1995; 18:325.

41. Margevicius KJ, Bauer TW, McMahon JT, Brown SA, Merritt K. Isolation and characterization of debris in membranes around total joint prostheses. J Bone Joint Surg Am 1994; 76-A:1664–1675.

42. Horikoshi M, Dowd J, Maloney WJ, Crossett L, Rubash HE. Activation of human fibroblasts and macrophages by particulate wear debris from failed total hip and total knee arthroplasty. Trans Orthop Res Soc 1994; 19:199.

43. Campbell P, Ma S, Yeom B, McKellop HA, Schmalzried TP, Amstutz HC. Isolation of predominantly submicron-sized UHMWPE wear particles from periprosthetic tissues. J Biomed Mater Res 1995; 29:127–131.

44. Klimkiewicz JJ, Iannotti JP, Rubash HE, Shanbhag AS. Aseptic loosening of the humeral component in total shoulder arthroplasty. J Shoulder Elbow Surg 1998; 7(4):422–426.

45. Huk OL, Bansal M, Betts F, Rimnac CM, Lieberman JR, Huo MH, Salvati EA. Polyethylene and metal debris generated by non-articulating surfaces of modular acetabular components. J Bone Joint Surg 1994; 76-B:568–574.

46. Doehring TC, Saigal S, Shanbhag AS, Rubash HE. Micromotion of acetabular liners: Measurements comparing the effectiveness of locking mechanisms. Trans Orthop Res Soc 1996; 21:427.

47. Shanbhag AS, Bailey HO, Eror NG, Woo SL-Y, Rubash HE. Characterization and comparison of UHMWPE wear debris retrieved from total hip and total knee arthroplasties. Trans Orthop Res Soc 1996; 21:467.

48. Macaulay W, Hasselman CT, Shanbhag AS, Dowd JE, Woel S, Rubash HE. Bone ingrowth and particulate debris in a canine acetabular arthroplasty model. Trans Orthop Res Soc 1996; 21:93.

49. Maloney WJ, Smith RL. Periprosthetic osteolysis in total hip arthroplasty: the role of particulate wear debris. Instr Course Lect 1996; 45:171–182.

50. Urban RM, Jacobs JJ, Sapienza CI, Hall DJ, Infanger S, Sumner DR, Berzins A, Turner TM, Galante JO. Interface tissues and modes of particulate debris infiltration in 25 cementless acetabular components retrieved at autopsy. Trans Orthop Res Soc 1996; 21:45.

51. Gilbert JL, Buckley CA, Jacobs JJ. In vivo corrosion of modular hip prosthesis components in mixed and similar metal combinations. The effect of crevice, stress, motion, and alloy coupling. J Biomed Mater Res 1993; 27(12):1533–1544.

52. Collier JP, Surprenant VA, Jensen RE, Mayor MB, Surprenant HP. Corrosion between the components of modular femoral hip prostheses. J Bone Joint Surg Br 1992; 74(4):511–517.

53. Mevellec C, Burleigh TD, Shanbhag AS. Corrosion in modular femoral hip prostheses: A study of 22 retrieved implants. Proceedings of the 15th Southern Biomedical Engineering Conference, Dayton, OH, March 29–31, 1996:3–4.

54. Jacobs JJ, Urban RM, Gilbert JL, Skipor AK, Black J, Jasty M, Galante JO. Local and distant products from modularity. Clin Orthop 1995; 319:94–105.

55. Urban RM, Jacobs JJ, Gilbert JL, Galante JO. Migration of corrosion products from modular hip prostheses. Clin Orthop 1994; 76-A(September):1345–1359.

56. Merchant KK, Rohr WL, Lintner WP, Bhambri SK. Orthopaedic implant surface debris. Trans Orthop Res Soc 1995; 20:164.

57. Shanbhag AS, Jacobs JJ, Black J, Galante JO, Glant TT. Human monocyte response to particulate biomaterials generated in vivo and in vitro. J Orthop Res 1995; 13(5):792–801.

58. Haynes DR, Rogers SD, Hay S, App B, Pearcy MJ, Howie DW. The differences in toxicity and release of bone-resorbing mediators induced by titanium and cobalt–chromium-alloy wear particles. J Bone Joint Surg Am 1993; 75-A:825–834.

59. Shanbhag AS, Jacobs JJ, Black J, Galante JO, Glant TT. Macrophage/particle interactions: effect of size, composition and surface area. J Biomed Mater Res 1994; 28(1):81–90.

60. Glant TT, Jacobs JJ, Molnar G, Shanbhag AS, Valyon M, Galante JO. Bone resorption activity of particulate-stimulated macrophages. J Bone Miner Res 1993; 8(9):1071–1079.

61. Morrissette N, Gold E, Aderem A. The macrophage—a cell for all seasons. Trends Cell Biol 1999; 9(5):199–201.

62. Solbach W, Moll H, Rollinghoff M. Lymphocytes play the music but the macrophage calls the tune. Immunol Today 1991; 12(1):4–6.

63. Shanbhag AS, Jacobs JJ, Black J, Galante JO, Glant TT. Effects of particles on fibroblast proliferation and bone resorption in vitro. Clin Orthop 1997; 342: 205–217.

64. Ingham E, Green TR, Stone MH, Kowalski R, Watkins N, Fisher J. Production of TNF-alpha and bone resorbing activity by macrophages in response to different types of bone cement particles. Biomaterials 2000; 21(10):1005–1013.

65. Matthews JB, Besong AA, Green TR, Stone MH, Wroblewski BM, Fisher J, Ingham E. Evaluation of the response of primary human peripheral blood mononuclear phagocytes to challenge with in vitro generated clinically relevant UHMWPE particles of known size and dose. J Biomed Mater Res 2000; 52(2):296–307.

66. Lind M, Trindade MC, Nakashima Y, Schurman DJ, Goodman SB, Smith L. Chemotaxis and activation of particle-challenged human monocytes in response to monocyte migration inhibitory factor and C–C chemokines. J Biomed Mater Res 1999; 48(3):246–250.

67. Lind M, Trindade MC, Schurman DJ, Goodman SB, Smith RL. Monocyte migration inhibitory factor synthesis and gene expression in particle-activated macrophages. Cytokine 2000; 12(7):909–913.

68. Rae T. A study on the effects of particulate metals of orthopaedic interest on murine macrophages *in vitro*. J Bone Joint Surg 1975; 57-B:444–450.

69. Garrett R, Wilksch J, Vernon-Roberts B. Effects of cobalt–chrome alloy wear particles on the morphology, viability and phagocytic activity of murine macrophages in vitro. Aust J Exp Biol Med Sci 1983; 61(3):355–369.

70. Rae T. The biological response to titanium and titanium–aluminum–vanadium alloy particles I. Tissue culture studies. Biomaterials 1986; 7:30–36.

71. Horowitz SM, Gautsch TL, Frondoza CG, Riley L, Jr. Macrophage exposure to polymethyl methacrylate leads to mediator release and injury. J Orthop Res 1991; 9:406–413.

72. Horowitz SM, Frondoza CG, Lennox DW. Effects of polymethylmethacrylate exposure upon macrophages. J Orthop Res 1988; 6:827–832.

73. Glant TT, Jacobs JJ. Response of three murine macrophage populations to particulate debris: Bone resorption in organ cultures. J Orthop Res 1994; 12: 720–731.

74. Horowitz SM, Doty SB, Lane JM, Burstein AH. Studies of the mechanism by which the mechanical failure of polymethylmethacrylate leads to bone resorption. J Bone Joint Surg 1993; 75-A:802–813.

75. Nakashima Y, Sun DH, Trindade MC, Chun LE, Song Y, Goodman SB, Schurman DJ, Maloney WJ, Smith RL. Induction of macrophage C–C chemokine expression by titanium alloy and bone cement particles. J Bone Joint Surg Br 1999; 81(1):155–162.

76. Nakashima Y, Sun DH, Trindade MC, Maloney WJ, Goodman SB, Schurman DJ, Smith RL. Signaling pathways for tumor necrosis factor-alpha and interleukin-6 expression in human macrophages exposed to titanium-alloy particulate debris in vitro. J Bone Joint Surg Am 1999; 81(5):603–615.

77. Ingham E, Fisher J. Biological reactions to wear debris in total joint replacement. Proc Inst Mech Eng [H] 2000; 214(1):21–37.

78. Diegelmann RF, Cohen IK, Kaplan AM. The role of macrophages in wound repair: a review. Plast Reconstr Surg 1981; 68(1):107–113.

79. Diegelmann RF, Cohen IK, Kaplan AM. Effect of macrophages on fibroblast DNA synthesis and proliferation. Proc Soc Exp Biol Med 1982; 169(4):445–451.

80. Takemura R, Werb Z. Secretory products of macrophages and their physiological functions. Am J Physiol 1984; 246(1 Pt 1):C1–C9.

81. Gelb H, Schumacher HR, Cuckler J, Baker DG. In vivo inflammatory response to polymethylmethacrylate particulate debris: Effect of size, morphology, and surface area. J Orthop Res 1994; 12:83–92.

82. Rae T. The toxicity of metals used in orthopaedic prostheses. An experimental study using cultured human synovial fibroblasts. J Bone Joint Surg 1981; 63-B:435–440.

83. Rae T. The action of cobalt, nickel and chromium on phagocytosis and bacterial killing by human polymorphonuclear leucocytes; its relevance to infection after total joint arthroplasty. Biomaterials 1983; 4:175–180.

84. Vernon-Roberts B, Freeman MAR. Morphological and analytical studies of the tissues adjacent to joint prostheses: investigations into the causes of loosening prostheses. In: Schaldach M, Hohmann D, eds. Advances in Artificial Hip and Knee Joint Technology. Berlin: Springer, 1976:148–186.

85. Sullivan PM, MacKenzie JR, Callaghan JJ, Johnston RC. Total hip arthroplasty with cement in patients who are less than fifty years old. J Bone Joint Surg 1994; 76-A(6):863–869.

86. Forest M, Carlioz A, Vacher Lavenu MC, Postel M, Kerboull M, Tomeno B, Courpied JP. Histological patterns of bone and articular tissues after orthopaedic reconstructive surgery (artificial joint implants). Pathol Res Pract 1991; 187: 963–977.

87. Howie DW. Tissue response in relation to type of wear particles around failed hip arthroplasties. J Arthroplasty 1990; 5:337–348.

88. Wright TM, Astion DJ, Bansal M, Rimnac CM, Green T, Insall JN, Robinson RP. Failure of carbon-fiber-reinforced polyethylene total knee-replacement components. J Bone Joint Surg Am 1988; 70-A:926–932.

89. Yao J, Glant TT, Lark MW, Mikecz K, Jacobs JJ, Hutchinson NI, Hoerrner LA, Kuettner KE, Galante JO. The potential role of fibroblasts in periprosthetic osteolysis: Fibroblast response to titanium particles. J Bone Miner Res 1995; 10:1417–1427.

90. Maloney WJ, Smith RL, Castro F, Schurman DJ. Fibroblast response to metallic debris in vitro. Enzyme induction, cell proliferation, and toxicity. J Bone Joint Surg Am 1993; 75-A:835–844.

91. Vermes C, Chandrasekaran R, Jacobs JJ, Galante JO, Roebuck KA, Glant TT. The effects of particulate wear debris, cytokines, and growth factors on the functions of MG-63 osteoblasts. J Bone Joint Surg Am 2001; 83-A(2):201–211.

92. Vermes C, Roebuck KA, Chandrasekaran R, Dobai JG, Jacobs JJ, Glant TT. Particulate wear debris activates protein tyrosine kinases and nuclear factor kappaB, which down-regulates type I collagen synthesis in human osteoblasts. J Bone Miner Res 2000; 15(9):1756–1765.

93. Yao J, Cs-Szabo G, Jacobs JJ, Kuettner KE, Glant TT. Suppression of osteoblast function by titanium particles. J Bone Joint Surg Am 1997; 79-A(1): 107–112.

94. Athanasou NA, Quinn J, Bulstrode CJK. Resorption of bone by inflammatory cells derived from the joint capsule of hip arthroplasties. J Bone Joint Surg 1992; 74B:57–62.

95. Quinn J, Joyner C, Triffitt JT, Athanasou NA. Polymethylmethacrylate-induced inflammatory macrophages resorb bone. J Bone Joint Surg 1992; 74-B: 652–658.

96. Howie DW, Vernon-Roberts B, Oakeshott R, Manthey B. A rat model of resorption of bone at the cement–bone interface in the presence of polyethylene wear particles. J Bone Joint Surg Am 1988; 70-A:257–263.

97. Dowd JE, Schwendeman LJ, Macaulay W, Doyle JS, Shanbhag AS, Wilson S, Herndon JH, Rubash HE. Aseptic loosening in uncemented total hip arthroplasty in a canine model. Clin Orthop 1995; (319):106–121.

98. Hasselman CT, Shanbhag AS, Kovach C, Marinelli R, Rubash HE. Osteolysis and aseptic loosening in a canine uncemented total hip arthroplasty (THA) model. Trans Orthop Res Soc 1997; 22:22.

99. Shanbhag AS, Hasselman CT, Rubash HE. The John Charnley Award. Inhibition of wear debris mediated osteolysis in a canine total hip arthroplasty model. Clin Orthop 1997; 344:33–43.

14

Role of the Immune Response in Implant Loosening

Paul H. Wooley

Department of Orthopaedic Surgery, Immunology, and Biomedical Engineering, Wayne State University, Detroit, Michigan, U.S.A.

INTRODUCTION

The influence of immunology pervades all aspects of medicine, from the vast numbers of diagnostic tests that employ antibody-mediated reactions to the treatment of organ graft rejection with T cell specific pharmaceutical agents. The direct effects of immunology upon the practice of orthopaedic surgery may not be immediately obvious, but the consequences of immune responses to implanted materials are requiring greater consideration with the evolution of the specialty towards advanced tissue engineering. Problems due to immunological effects upon orthopaedic implants and grafts are less obvious than those encountered in the early years of organ transplantation, but recent studies suggest that the immune system may readily undermine the benefits of skilled surgery. One casualty of the advance of immunology is the concept of "inert." It is accepted that no foreign material can be implanted in the body without a biological response. The precise factors that determine whether the response becomes essentially benign or aggressively destructive remain to be elucidated, but these factors are becoming more understood with advances in immunological science. In this chapter, we will examine the mechanisms of normal immunity, and investigate how hypersensitivity to metal and polymer biomaterials, and responses to bone allografts which can contribute to the biological responses that result in implant loosening.

THE NORMAL IMMUNE RESPONSE

The primary function of the immune system is considered to be host defense against invasion by pathogens. The immune system must be able to discriminate between the normal components of the body, or "self," and foreign matter (nonself). Tolerance to self, but an aggressive reaction to eliminate nonself, is the hallmark of a successful immune system. To achieve this balance, the immune system constantly monitors the status of the body through a variety of cells, particularly leucocytes (white blood cells) and accessory cells, either distributed throughout the circulatory system or resident within tissues and lymphoid organs, notably the spleen, lymph nodes, bone marrow, and thymus. The nature of the immune reaction against the presence of nonself in the body depends upon the stimulus provided by the foreign matter and the "perceived threat" received by the immune system. Foreign material may be simply removed from the system by macrophages, a minor inflammatory reaction can occur, or a specific cellular or antibody response may be provoked. The differing specialized reactions have allowed the immune response to be broadly divided into two interrelated parts. Humoral immunity is concerned with the production of antibodies, while cellular immunity is concerned with the development of reactive cells, and the regulation of immune functions.

At the initiation of the immune response, foreign material or "antigen" must first be recognized (Fig. 1). This recognition is achieved through an interaction between phagocytic (antigen presenting) cells and T lymphocytes. Antigen-presenting cells provide the initial level of immune regulation, since the majority of responses start with these cells ingesting antigens via phagocytosis. Antigens are partially digested by enzymatic degradation within the phagosome, and then processed within the cytoplasm. Antigen processing results in the embedding of antigens in the groove between the alpha and beta chains of the class II major histocompatibility (MHC) molecule (the HLA-DR molecule in humans), and this hybrid structure is then expressed upon the surface of the antigen-presenting cell. T lymphocytes recognize the dual signal of foreign antigen in association with the "self" class II molecule, by virtue of the T cell receptor (TCR). In addition to antigen presentation, the phagocytic cells promote immune responsiveness through the secretion of the immunological hormone interleukin-1 (IL-1). IL-1 is a soluble factor with a number of immune and pro-inflammatory effects, which include the activation of lymphocytes, and increased expression of receptors for the lymphocyte autocrine IL-2. The recognition of antigen alone is insufficient for the initiation of T cell activation. Additional receptors, such as B7 and CD28, must be engaged to provide a second signal prior to cytokine responsiveness. The consequence of a single signal (antigen recognition alone) is apoptosis, or programmed cell death, of the stimulated T cell. It has recently been realized that the overall outcome of the single signal is

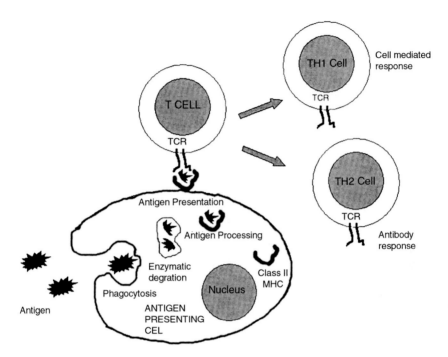

Figure 1 Antigen is phagocytozed and partially digested by macrophages, and epitopes assembled within the groove of the MHC class II molecule. This complex is expressed on the cell surface and recognized by the T cell receptor of CD4+ T lymphocytes. Activation occurs following secondary surface receptor binding and cytokine signaling. The T cell orchestrates the response towards cellular immunity via THl pathways, or humoral immunity via predominantly TH2 pathways.

immune tolerance, and the thymus can utilize this apoptotic response to eliminate "self" reactive immune cells and maintain the discrimination between self and nonself.

T cells that recognize antigen and commence the cellular response are usually CD4+ T "helper" cells, and produce the autocrine interleukin-2 (IL-2), which mediates the activation and replication of the T cells. These T cells orchestrate the immune response, provoking the generation of cytotoxic cells which attack foreign or virally infected cells, secreting interleukins, stimulating the differentiation of B cells into plasma cells, and providing feedback to phagocytic cells via cytokines. T helper cells can be differentiated into two functional types: TH1 and TH2 cells. TH1 cells promote cell-mediated responses, while TH2 cells mediate serological responses via B cell activation and differentiation. The subclasses of TH1 and TH2 may be identified by their cytokine profile, with THI cells generating IL-2 and gamma interferon, and TH2 cells secreting IL-4 and IL-5. Each T cell is specific for only one antigen (in context with HLA-DR) due its unique T cell receptor, which is constructed from two associated receptor chains (alpha and beta) and acquired by the T cell during the thymic education process. TCR are derived from the immunoglobulin "supergene" family, and bear a structural relationship to the antibody molecule (see below). They are comprised of constant regions (Cα and Cβ) and variable regions (Vα and Vβ), with the antigen-combining region (CDR3) residing within the variable portion of the molecule. Conserved sections within the V-region chains permit the division of T cells into Vα and Vβ "families," but this assignment of T cell subsets does not reflect antigen specificity.

In addition to antigen recognition and response, T cells can serve as effector cells to attack foreign antigens. Classic cytotoxic T lymphocytes are CD8+, and have evolved to recognize viral antigens expressed on the surface of infected target cells in context of the MHC class I molecule (HLA-A, B, and C in humans). Since class I (HLA-A, HLA-B, and HLA-C) antigens are expressed on the majority of tissues, a virally transfected cell can alert the immune system by embedding viral antigens in the class I molecular complex and provoking recognition and destruction by cytotoxic T effector cells. Nonself antigens present on noncompatible grafted tissue also provide recognition signals for cytotoxic T cells. In particular, nonself class I and class II MHC antigens (on allogeneic donor tissues) appear to be particularly provocative of T cell responses, probably due to their close structural relationship to the self-MHC antigens that restrict the immune response. The original concept that CD4+ T cells recognize allograft antigens in context of class II MHC, and elicit CD8+ cytotoxic cells that attack allograft antigens in context with class I MHC is a viable notion to consider in cellular immune responses; however, the complexity of the response now suggests that this may be an oversimplification.

Subsequent to antigen recognition by T cells, particularly CD4+ TH2 lymphocytes, the immune system can produce antibodies specific for the foreign antigen. Antibodies are secreted by plasma cells, the terminally differentiated form of the B lymphocyte. B cells, which bear immunoglobulin on the cell surface, also express the differentiation marker CD 19, and Class II MHC antigens. B cells differentiate into antibody secreting plasma cells on receipt of multiple intracellular signals, which are typically (i) binding of antigen to surface immunoglobulin, and (ii) a cascade of lymphocyte hormone (interleukin) signals, including IL-4, IL-5, IL-6, IL-10, and IL-12. B cells may also serve as antigen-presenting cells since they express both antigen specific surface receptors (antibody) and class II MHC antigens (Fig. 2). Similar to T cells, the B cell is specific for only one antigen due to selection of antibody genes that occurs during the educational process. Antibody secreted from a plasma cell is thus monoclonal in nature, although a complex foreign body such as a bacterium expresses a multitude of antigenic epitopes, all of which can elicit specific responses, resulting in a polyspecific immune

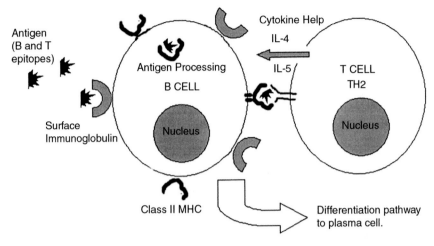

Figure 2 B cells can recognize antigen directly by virtue of surface immunoglobulins. Antigenic epitopes can be internalized and re-expressed in context of the MHC class II molecule. CD4+ T lymphocytes can form the tri-molecular complex and provide immune help by the secretion of cytokines, notably IL-4 and IL-5. Under these circumstances, the B cell can clonally expand and then differentiate to plasma cells, which secrete immunoglobulin.

response. The term antibody (or immunoglobulin, Ig) refers to five classes of serum proteins. They are comprised of two identical heavy (H) polypeptide chains and two identical light (L) chains, which are joined by disulphide bonds. The molecule is subdivided into various regions. The constant regions (CHl, CH2, CH3, and CL) provide the backbone of the molecule, the hinge region, and domains that mediate functions including complement fixation, Fc receptor binding, cell membrane attachment, and mast cell degranulation (IgE). The variable regions (V_H and V_L) contain the hypervariable domains. Hypervariability, which is under immunogenetic regulation, provides the tremendous diversity in the antigen-binding site on the immunoglobulin molecule. It is this variability that provides the enormous number of different specificities that are required for antibodies to react with the diverse range of antigens that are encountered in the environment. The hypervariability of the molecule also provides "idiotypic" markers for immunoglobulin. Each antibody is unique due to the variable portion of the molecule, and this property (idiotype) provides a point of recognition that is used to regulate the production of individual specific antibodies. Immunoglobulins are classified into five classes: IgM, IgG, IgA, IgD, and IgE. IgM is considered as the primordial antibody, since it is a pentamer of the Ig molecule and is the product of a primary immune response. IgM fixes and activates the complement cascade. IgG is the major serum immunoglobulin, and is the product of the secondary immune response to most antigens. IgG molecules are further divided into subclasses, from IgGl to IgG4, and the subclasses IgGl, IgG2, and IgG3 fix complement. IgA is the major Ig class in secretions, and may be joined to form a dimer by a transport protein. The function of IgD is unclear; it is found at very low levels in serum, but at a high frequency on the surface of B cells. IgE mediates the type 1 hypersensitivity (immediate allergic) response, by interacting with the Fc receptor on mast cells and basophils, and provoking degranulation and the release of mediators such as histamine.

Variability in the different soluble factors, receptors, variable regions of the immunoglobulin molecule, and cell surface antigens provides genetic mechanisms for the control of the immune response. Conversely, abnormal regulation offers clues to the origin of the autoimmune diseases. The human leukocyte antigen (HLA) system is a polymorphic gene system on Chromosome 6 that has evolved as a mechanism by which an individual inherits a variety of cell surface antigens from the gene pool in a codominant manner. This provides the lymphocytes of a heterozygous individual with the advantage of multiple "immune response" genes, and ensures a selective advantage should a response deficiency be associated with a specific HLA antigen. Nevertheless, a number of diseases such as ankylosing spondylitis and rheumatoid arthritis are associated with the possession of particular HLA types. HLA antigens are divided into three classes: Class I (HLA-A, HLA-B, and HLA-C) antigens are expressed on the majority of tissues, and provide recognition signals for cytotoxic T effector cells. Class II antigens are restricted to cells of the immune system, particularly B cells, activated T cells, and antigen-presenting cells. Class III antigens are involved in the control of complement components. Polymorphic systems are the key to the broad specificity generated throughout the immune system. They occur in genes encoding the T cell receptors and the variable regions of the immunoglobulin molecule. This variability is believed to arise from a common genetic source, and this system is referred to as the immunoglobulin supergene family (Fig. 3). Cell surface receptors are typically comprised of two polypeptide chains (alpha and beta), and the diversity of the variable (antigen specific) portion of the molecule is generated (in immunoglobulin) by the combination of the products of three (Variable, Diversity, and Joining) genes together at random to generate the receptor site. Self-reactive elements of the immune system are eliminated during the neonatal period, leaving individuals with an immune response repertoire that is genetically inherited, but modified by somatic cell events.

HYPERSENSITIVITY—THE ALLERGIC RESPONSE

The term hypersensitivity denotes an excessive immune response that results in some degree of tissue damage. Hypersensitivity reactions have been historically

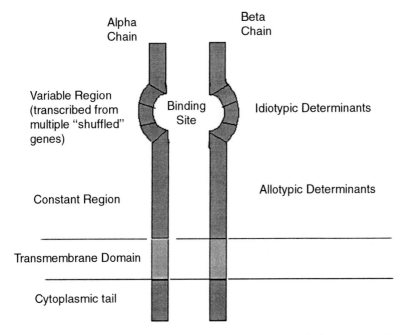

Figure 3 A stereotypical representation of the immunoglobulin supergene family of molecules. These structures are comprised of at least two sub-chains (alpha and beta), which are usually linked by disulphide bonds. Multiple genes are "shuffled" by deletion of intervening sequencing to generate a functional variable region gene, which encodes the binding site. The random selection of the variable region genes permits the vast repertoire of specificity in the immunoglobulin molecule and the T cell receptor, which in turn provides idiotypic determinants on the variable portion of the molecule. The framework of the molecule is provided by a constant region, which also expressed limited allotypic determinants. The constant region also included a transmembrane portion of the molecule, and a cytoplasmic tail responsible for cellular signaling.

classified as one of four types: Type I = immediate hypersensitivity mediated by IgE antibody responses, Type II = antibody-mediated cell cytotoxicity, Type III = immune complex-mediated tissue damage, and Type IV = delayed type hypersensitivity or T cell mediated reactions. Each of these groups can be subcategorized to some extent. However, the majority of allergic responses can usually be defined as either Type I or Type IV hypersensitivity, and we will examine the response to orthopaedic biomaterials in context of these two types. It is important to remember that patients only develop "allergic" responses following secondary or chronic exposure to an antigen. The patient must first experience a primary immune response, in which the antigen is processed by macrophages (or related cells) and presented in the context of the individual's tissue antigen (Class II MHC antigens) to CD4+ T helper cells. The T cells will subsequently recruit B cells to differentiate into antibody (IgM) secreting plasma cells or (dependant upon the nature of the antigen) other T cells (effector cells) that eliminate target cells expressing the antigen. The primary response is rapid (7–10 days) and there are no obvious adverse responses in the patient during this initial phase of immunity. At the conclusion of the primary response, T cells and B cells differentiate into "memory" cells that retain the specificity for this antigen, and enable a rapid response on repeated contact. On subsequent or chronic exposure to the antigen, an elevated immune response occurs that is designed to eliminate a pathogen due to heightened activity and increased specificity against the antigens. On occasions, the secondary immune response can lead to adverse patient reactions. Immediate (Type I) hypersensitivity arises due the differentiation of B cells into plasma cells that secrete IgE. The induction of IgE appears to require the binding of allergen by B cells (via surface immunoglobulin), internal antigen processing by the B cell, and the production of both IL-4 and IL-13. The switch from IgM to IgE occurs due to sequential deletional events at the B cell gene level, and may transpire following a switch from IgM to IgG rather than a direct switch. IgE antibody bound to antigen engages mast cells via the epsilon receptor, and causes degranulation with the release of histamine, giving rise to symptoms typical of hay fever. Type I hypersensitivity appears to have evolved as a weapon against parasite antigens, since local histamine release appears to perturb the attachment of skin parasites such as ticks, and reduce colonization by helminths (worms).

Chronic exposure to antigen can also result in delayed (Type IV) hypersensitivity, which is T cell mediated, and (as the name implies) produces tissue reactions after a minimum of 12 hour and usually peaks by 72 hour. The most common clinical problem that arises from Type IV hypersensitivity is contact dermatitis, which usually presents as an epidermal phenomenon. Antigens that provoke contact reactions are frequently chemical in nature such as nickel and latex compounds, and components of poison ivy and poison oak. These low-molecular weight chemical entities are not freestanding antigens, but are classified as haptens. Haptens are compounds that can bind to (native) proteins such as albumin, and modify the conformational structure so that the hapten–carrier conjugate is recognized as foreign by the immune system. Langerhans' cells predominate in the presentation of antigens that provoke contact sensitivity both within the skin and following migration of these sensitized dendritic cells to the lymph node. T cells that recognize haptens migrate to sites that contain the sensitizing antigen (usually skin), where they mediate inflammatory reactions that result in tissue damage. These cytotoxic T cells are frequently CD4+, although CD8+ T cells are also seen at the reaction sites. The local tissue reaction frequently results in expression of class II MHC antigens on keratinocytes, which may be indicative of abnormal antigen presentation during the response.

EFFECTS OF POLYMERS ON THE IMMUNE RESPONSE

The structure of orthopaedic polymers suggests that they do not possess the properties that permit the immune reactivity against typical protein antigens. Phagocytes are not believed to possess enzymes that can readily degrade most polymers, and it is uncertain that linear portions of the polymer molecule can be processed to associate with the class II MHC groove, and hence be recognized as antigens by CD4+ T cells. However the vast majority of immunology research to date has focused upon the study of protein-based antigens, and other means of immune response induction may exist beyond our current state of knowledge. Until recently, it was widely held that lipid molecules were nonantigenic, but the discovery of anti-cardiolipin antibodies and an associated clinical syndrome has broadened the concept of antigenic activity. Polymers may influence immunity through two mechanism—the induction of a direct response, and adjuvant activity. While there is overwhelming evidence that wear debris particles of polymethylmethacrylate (PMMA) and ultra high molecular weight polyethylene (UHMWPE) can provoke tissue inflammatory reactions, it is less clear whether chronic inflammation leads to direct immunity in orthopaedic patients. Nevertheless, positive skin reactions to PMMA have been reported in 25% of cemented total joint arthroplasty patients (1), and hypersensitivity can clearly result due to exposure to PMMA (2,3). We have investigated T cell responses to polymers using in vitro culture techniques to examine cellular activation and cytokine responses, using standard immune methodologies (4,5). When PMMA was cultured with peripheral blood mononuclear cells from either normal subjects or cemented total joint arthroplasty patients, we were surprised to detect dose-dependant cellular activation in both groups. Cellular activation was associated with the production of the cytokines IL-1 and IL-2, suggesting the participation of T cells in the response. Patients with stable arthroplasties were observed to have lower responses to PMMA than the responses in patients with loose or painful prostheses. A follow-up study in osteoarthritis (6) indicated that the cellular response to PMMA was significantly higher in revision arthroplasty patients with a diagnosis of aseptic loosening compared with a pre-operative primary surgery group. The response in patients undergoing revision surgery due to mechanical failure or infection did not show elevated responses. When patients from the primary surgery group were re-evaluated after a minimum of 10 months, a significant elevation in the cellular response to PMMA was observed, while the response in patients with successful revision surgery was significantly decreased from the pre-operative level. These findings suggest that arthroplasty patients do develop cellular responses to PMMA, and elevated levels of reactivity are associated with prosthesis failure. In comparison with response to PMMA, UHMWPE did not provoke a cellular reaction in this study. However, there are technical difficulties using UHMWPE in tissue culture, as its buoyant density prevents it maintaining contact with cultured cells. Nevertheless, we have seen a number of patients with a stimulation index indicative of positive response to UHMWPE. Cellular reactivity of orthopaedic polymers have been reported by Gil-Albarova et al. (7), who demonstrated both positive skin patch reactions and proliferative responses to PMMA in patients with aseptic loosening. Using similar culture techniques to our laboratory, Santavirta et al. (8) reported that two major markers of immune T cell activation (HLA-DR antigens and IL-2 surface receptors) were increased by PMMA particle stimulation, although proliferation of peripheral blood mononuclear cells was not observed, possibly due to the shorter exposure of the cells to antigen in culture. Boynton et al. (9) cultured T cells extracted from periprosthetic tissue, and determined that T cell amplification of the innate macrophage inflammatory reaction to particulate debris may play a role in the inflammatory response. Other studies (10) have demonstrated that both CD4+ and CD8+ T cells frequently accumulate in periprosthetic tissue associated with loosened joint replacements. However, none of these investigations can say with certainty that the responses observed are directed against a polymer antigen. Other implanted polymers are reported to cause immune reactions in certain recipients, notable PTFE, Dacron, and silicone (11–13). The recent controversy concerning silicone breast implants serves to highlight the gaps in knowledge when evaluating immune responses to polymers. Orthopaedic surgeons are quite familiar with the capacity of silicone to provoke adverse reactions, since the term "silicone synovitis" was coined to describe a reactive synovitis occurring in a number of patients with silicone elastomer prostheses (14–17) characterized by a hypertrophic villous synovitis with marked synovial membrane thickening, and infiltration by macrophages, giant cells, lymphocytes, and plasma cells. Particulate silicone debris was implicated in this synovitis, since particles ranging in size from 6 to 100 μm were visible in histological sections. Particles were also found distal to the affected joints, notably in the lymphatic system and in the bone marrow (18–20). Several studies stress the similarities between a flare-up of rheumatoid arthritis and the inflammatory reaction to a silicone joint implant, and there is some experimental evidence for de novo joint reactions to silicone in rodents, since the intra-articular injection of silicone in rabbit knees causes an inflammatory synovitis (17). Despite these investigations, the overall mechanism of the response to silicone and other polymers is still poorly understood. A hypothesis that has gained recent acceptance is the concept that polymers may provide an adjuvant-like activity to native macromolecules, which adhere to hydrophobic surfaces and subsequently become irnmunogenic (21). We investigated this idea in aseptic loosening, by examining proteins that adhere to failed hip and knee arthroplasty, and the occurrence of autoantibodies to these bound proteins in revision surgery patients (22). Polyacrylamide gel electrophoresis (PAGE) revealed a broad variety of proteins adherent to failed

UHMWPE components, with 21 different proteins present in extracts from 42 prostheses. Western blotting showed a high incidence of autoantibodies to UHMWPE-bound proteins in revision arthroplasty patients, with over 60% of sera testing positive to one or more adherent antigens. Type I collagen was a frequent target of the antibody reactivity, but antibodies to collagen (particularly denatured type I collagen) have been reported in osteoarthritis (23), and it cannot be held for certain that the collagen binding to UHMWPE leads to antibody formation in all cases. Antibodies binding denatured collagen are common in orthopaedic patients (24), although operative procedures do not appear to elevate the titers to any significant degree (25). However, since the incidence of antibodies to collagen in operative revision patients is very high, it appears likely that the implantation of UHMWPE, followed by the deposition of collagen, may contribute to elevated antibody levels. Antibodies that form immune complexes by binding with polyethylene-adherent protein may have the capacity to fix complement, and the complement cascade may, in turn, attract inflammatory cells to the polyethylene surface. Immunoglobulin (IgG) bound to polymer implants has been shown to activate human neutrophils in vitro and attract murine phagocytes when implanted in vivo (26). Since UHMWPE particles are generated due to the motion and wear of orthopaedic prosthetic components, the presence of polyethylene-bound proteins could be significant when phagocytes in the tissue adjoining the prosthesis site engulf the particulate debris. This stimulating effect may extend to the lymph nodes, since Hicks et al. (27) noted intense immunohisto-chemical staining of histiocytes for HLA-DR antigens, and elevated levels of pro-inflammatory cytokines in pelvic lymph nodes from patients with failed arthroplasties. At this point, the potential adjuvant capacity of UHMWPE debris may be realized. The phagocytosis of particles may result in activated macrophages that secrete both pro-inflammatory cytokines and proteolytic enzymes, and provide activation signals to lymphocytes. Proteins bound to UHMWPE may have altered conformational structures, and the combination of strong stimulation from the nondegradable particle and the altered form of the self-protein could be sufficient to break self-tolerance and initiate autoantibody generation. It must be recognized that the production of autoantibodies is not synonymous with autoimmune disease, and there is no evidence of an adverse systemic effect of antibodies to UHMWPE-bound proteins in arthroplasy patients. However, chronic immunologically mediated inflammation could result from this reaction to protein-coated prosthesis debris and the resulting immune complexes, and thus contribute to damage of tissues in the periprosthetic region. It has been reported that the inflammatory tissue response to implanted material may have an adverse effect upon the chemical integrity of the polymer (28), which could result in damage that broadens the range of antigenic targets. Notably, it has been suggested that responses to *N,N*-dimethylparatoluidine (DMT), an accelerator used in bone cement, could be responsible for hypersensitivity reactions to fixatives. In a study of patients that developed aseptic loosening less than two years after total hip replacement, nearly half were found to exhibit skin test positive reactions to DMT (29). Further research is clearly required to define both the chemical entities that are released from orthopaedic polymers over time, and the role of the immune response in the recognition and adverse reactions to polymers and adherent proteins.

IMMUNE RESPONSE TO METALS

Solid metal alloy components of orthopaedic prostheses are clearly beyond the size range of entities expected to generate classic immune responses. It requires four factors to occur in order to develop metal sensitivity: (i) the release of metallic ions from the metal due to the corrosive action of plasma or sweat, (ii) the coupling of the ions to an endogenous protein or cell to form a hapten, (iii) the accumulation of the hapten-carrier complex to a threshold level that can trigger a primary immune response, and (iv) continued chronic exposure to the hapten-carrier complex. Metals are subject to corrosion due to the chemical nature of body fluids. Metal ions may also act directly upon cells of the immune system, and mediate abnormal sensitivity due to toxic or stimulatory effects. The capacity of several metals to elicit contact hypersensitivity responses is well recognized, and nickel appears to be the most common sensitizing allergen. Studies suggest that nickel reactivity affects between 5% and 15% of women and 1–2% of men in the North American population (30,31). There appears to be a mild genetic regulation to nickel allergy, with a relative risk around 2.83 in first-degree relatives of sensitive patients (32). The marked sex variation between nickel sensitivity is believed to be associated with jewelry (33), particularly the practice of body piercing (34). As this phenomenon is becoming more common in men, it will be interesting to observe whether the incidence of male metal sensitivity rises in the future.

Metal sensitivity appears to be high in arthroplasty patients, and may be further elevated in candidates for revision surgery. Elves et al. (35) examined 50 patients and reported a 38% positive skin patch reaction to one or more of an allergen library consisting of chromium, cobalt, nickel, molybdenum, vanadium, and titanium. The incidence in revision surgery patients was elevated to 65%, while only 15% of patients with stable arthroplasties were contact sensitive, and the positive reactions were limited to nickel and cobalt. Evans et al. (36) also reported an incidence of metal sensitivity of 65% in patients with loose prostheses, with no sensitivity in 24 patients with intact joint implants. The specificity of the response to the individual metals is important, since broadened metal sensitivity does not usually arise due to cross-reactivity (37). It should be noted that it is uncertain whether aseptic loosening causes metal sensitization, or is the result of elevated ion exposure due to particles shed from a failing metal component. Thus, it is controversial as to whether metal hypersensitivity can contribute to the pathology of aseptic loosening (36,38–41).

There is a reasonable association between positive skin tests and lymphocyte proliferative responses to nickel salts (42), and phenotypical analysis of the nickel-specific T cell lines indicated that the response is predominantly mediated by CD8+ T lymphocytes bearing the alpha beta T cell receptor (43). This suggests that metal sensitivity is mediated via classical immune response mechanisms, and indicates that metal haptens are recognized by standard antigen processing systems using normal transporter associated antigen processing (TAP) gene mechanisms, although an increased prevalence of the TAP2B allele has been identified in nickel allergic patients (44). Reports confirm that the regulation of the nickel-specific T cell response is mediated by CD4+ T lymphocytes (45) and that class II MHC antigens restrict the response (46). Recent reports (47–49) indicate that T cell receptor subsets may be bias in CD4+ T cells from hypersensitive individuals responding to nickel, with over-representation of the Vβ17, Vβ13, Vβ20, Vβ2, or Vβ14 phenotypes. These observations suggest that classic immunogenetic regulation applies to nickel hypersensitivity, and therefore patients at risk may possibly be identified via HLA phenotyping and T cell subset analysis. Further, regulatory nickel-specific CD4+ T cells with the potential to downregulate nickel reactivity via IL-10 secretion have been identified, indicating potential immunotherapeutic approaches to the control of metal contact hypersensitivity.

Peripheral blood cells from patients with aseptic loosening do exhibit elevated in vitro responses to metals. Granchi et al. (50) reported that a chromium extract significantly increased the expression of the activated T cell (CD3/CD69) phenotype. A chromium-induced "activation index" was higher in patients with loosening of hip prostheses than in healthy donors and pre-operative patients, while lymphocyte activation due to chromium stimulation was higher in implant recipients (irrespective of the prosthesis status) when compared with healthy donors. In vitro studies have also suggested that metal ions released from implants may have direct effects on immune function and lymphocyte surface antigens. Fe^{+3}, Ni^{+2}, and Co^{+2} have been shown to cause inhibition of the T cell antigen CD2, which may interfere with T cell activation since both CD2 and CD3 are involved in the antigen recognition process (51). The development of responses to metal ions has been detected in 26% of patients postoperatively using cell migration assays (52), and we have used cell proliferation techniques to examine cellular responses to orthopaedic alloys (5,6). Our finding indicated that the response to Co–Cr (but not Ti-6-4) was significantly higher in revision surgery patients compared with a pre-operative primary surgery group ($p < 0.05$). Further analysis revealed that elevated responses to Co-Cr were observed in patients undergoing revision surgery due to painful prostheses or aseptic loosening ($p < 0.05$ and $p < 0.01$, respectively), while responses to Co-Cr in patients undergoing revision surgery due to mechanical failure or infection were similar to the responses in the pre-operative primary surgery group.

In addition to cellular reactivity to metals, there is evidence that hapten-carrier complexes containing metals may lead to antibody formation. Yang and Merritt (53) conjugated Cr, Co, and Ni ions to albumin bound on an ELISA plate, and found antibody reactive with these complexes in sera from arthroplasty patients. Remarkably, all patients examined developed IgE antibodies (the hallmark of Type I immediate hypersensitivity) against at least one metal, and a high incidence of IgM, IgG, and IgA antibodies was also recorded. The potential for hapten–carrier stimulation using these metal ions was confirmed by the injection of rabbit albumin–glutathione–metal complexes into mice, which resulted in strong serum antibody reactions (54). However, the presence of an antibody response to metal–protein complexes has not been associated with a poor surgical outcome. Reactivity to metals may be enhanced by the inflammatory reaction to periprosthetic wear debris. Elevated levels of IL-1 and GM-CSF have been seen in cells stimulated in vitro with prosthetic metal particulate material, to a level comparable to mitogen activation (55). Cobalt–chromium particles have been shown to induce histiocytic responses and the production of IL-1 and PGE2 in a canine model of aseptic loosening (56).

There is agreement among several laboratories that differences exist in cellular reactivity induced by titanium–aluminum–vanadium alloy and by cobalt–chromium alloy. Haynes et al. (57) noted that TiAlV increased the release of PGE_2, IL-1, TNF, and IL-6, while Co–Cr was associated with a decreased release of PGE_2 and IL-6. Wang et al. (58) found that Ti, Cr, and Co enhanced the release of IL-1 from monocytes, Ti and Cr enhanced the release of TNF, and Ti alone enhanced the release of IL-6. It also appears that the morphology of the cellular response in the periprosthetic region of the loosened implant varies between Co–Cr and TiAlV (59).

Given the specificity of the immune system, this suggests that the selection of a different alloy in a presensitized patient may be a useful strategy to circumvent any potential adverse effects that might arise due to immune reactivity to orthopaedic metals.

IMMUNE RESPONSE TO BONE

The use of bone allografts is not an uncommon practice in primary total joint replacement, occurring in approximately 4% of patients at our institution. The incidence of grafting rises to 46% in our revision surgery patients, and thus we must consider the significance of the immune response to bone in the development of prosthesis loosening. Bone tissue was among the earliest of human transplanted tissues, with early procedures including the report of Meekeren in 1668 describing the reconstruction of a cranium using xenografted bone from a canine skull (60). Between 1908 and 1925 Lexer performed hemi-joint allograft transplant with an approximately 50% long-term success rate (61). Despite this history, the literature concerning transplantation immunology of bone remains subdued and ambiguous compared with the vast body of information published on soft tissue transplantation. Bone does appear to enjoy a considerable measure of transplantation tolerance, and tissue matching of bone between donors and recipients is considered an unnecessary, difficult, and expensive procedure in clinical practice. Nevertheless, it is recognized that immunological reactions to bone allografts do occur in both patients and experimental animal models, and several preoperative procedures have been used to reduce the antigenicity of bone allografts. Currently, the most common preparative procedure is allograft freezing, which serves the function to render passenger cells within the graft nonviable. However, while dead cells are less provocative of a strong immunological response than live cells, bone allografts represent a substantial introduction of a foreign protein into the recipient. Over 700,000 bone grafts are performed yearly in North America, and there is considerable clinical use of allogenic bone in reconstructive orthopaedic surgery. The failure rate for frozen allografts has been in the order of 11–20% (62), and these failures have been attributed to a combination of factors. Many researchers have investigated immune responses to allografts, but despite intensive work, in both animal and humans, the significance of the immune response on the fate of bone allografts remains controversial. It is generally believed that matching for MHC antigens, a procedural requirement for all major organ transplants is unnecessary for the successful transplantation of bone, and the clinical results of bone allografting tend to support this claim. However, experimental models using genetically disparate strains from several species indicate that cellular and serological immune responses may influence the fate of bone allografts, although the immunological reaction does not appear to be manifested as a classical graft rejection episode. Musculo (63) evaluated the influence of HLA matching in 46 patients receiving frozen bone allografts, and observed that patients who matched for class I or II human leukocyte antigens with the donor scored higher than patients totally mismatched, although the differences in the radiological score were not significant. Interesting, matching for class II human leukocyte antigens alone seemed not to influence outcome of allografts. Patients who showed evidence of an anti-graft immune response scored significantly lower on outcome than those who did not. The authors concluded that frozen bone allografts could trigger an indirect pathway of alloantigen recognition in the recipient that did not correlate with human leukocyte antigen blood tests, which may explain the lack of correlation between HLA mismatches and bone allograft outcomes. However, the spectrum of immune reactivity was not assessed, and the possibility of reactivity with non-MHC antigens within the allograft was not evaluated. Popkirov (64) analyzed clinical and immunological data in 66 frozen bone graft patients, and identified an immune reaction due to the transplantation in 10% of patients, with the development of anti-lymphocyte antibodies. Cytotoxic antibodies reactive against allogeneic cells were detected in patients' sera after transplantation of frozen grafts, and grafting of human cancellous bone appeared to induce specific cellular and serological responses to lymphocyte antigens in recipients (65). This suggested that serological responses are important in the transplantation of large bone grafts, and implied that the immunological response to the graft could modify the pathological resorption of the graft, possibly due to bone antigenicity possessing an inductive action that can influence new bone formation. Strong et al. (66) investigated immunological responses to frozen bone allografts using sera obtained pre-operatively and at various time points after surgery. After grafting, 58% of allograft recipients showed evidence of sensitization to class I antigens and 55% recipients showed evidence to sensitization to class II antigens using the microcytotoxicity assay. They also observed that the anti-HLA response evoked in allograft recipients was a real phenomenon (67), but adverse effects on bone allografts were not obvious.

Due to the outbred genetic nature of the human population, precise histocompatibility responses can only be evaluated using animal models of bone grafting. Shigetomi (68) used immunohistochemistry and radioimmunoassay to study the rejection of bone allografts in rats mediated via MHC antigen expression on osteocytes and serum alloantibody (anti-allotype) levels in graft recipients. Osteocytes in normal rat bone tissue expressed MHC class I antigen to a varying degree, and this cell surface antigen increased post-transplantation. A marked decrease in the number of osteocytes was observed in DA recipients, and surviving osteocytes strongly expressed MHC class I antigens in the graft. F344 strain rat recipients with DA strain rat bone grafts showed high titers of anti-class I alloantibody. Thus, MHC class I antigens on osteocytes appear to be involved in bone allograft rejection. The investigation of specific cytotoxic antibody responses after vascularized and nonvascularized bone allografting implantation in rats and dogs revealed that donor specific antibody responses were elicited by MHC mismatched grafts, directed primarily at class I antigens (69). The antibody response was transient and less frequent in animals receiving frozen grafts, and the clinical implications of the response were unclear. In a second study (70), this group evaluated fresh and frozen cortical bone grafts either matched or mismatched for both major and non-major MHC antigens in rats. The immune response, the histological incorporation of the graft, biomechanical testing, and quantitative isotopic kinetics were used to assess outcome. Both MHC antigens and the pretreatment of the graft had profound effects on the incorporation of the graft. Anti-donor antibodies were only present in the serum of animals with a major mismatch, and freezing markedly attenuated the antibody response. Re-vascularization was profoundly affected by histocompatibility antigen matching, with syngeneic grafts revascularized more quickly and to a greater degree than the mismatched grafts. Freezing reduced the re-vascularization of syngeneic grafts but had no discernible effect on the grafts with a minor mismatch. Other animal studies in dogs, rats and rabbits (71–75) have showed either histological or immunological evidence of an immune response against bone allograft (by the demonstration of cytotoxic antibodies and cell-mediated immunity to allografts), and suggested that graft incorporation was most successful biologically and biomechanically when histocompatibility difference was minimized by matching. Using rabbits, Frielaender et al. (76) demonstrated both cellular and serological responses to fresh allografts and deep-frozen corticocancellous bone, while freeze-dried cortical bone allografts failed to sensitize recipients and were apparently less antigenic. However, Bos et al. (77) showed that frozen grafts in rats had the same fate regardless of histocompatibility relations between donors and recipients, and all grafts were inferior to fresh syngeneic grafts. Further, fresh allografts were inferior to the fresh syngeneic grafts and similar to the frozen grafts. Thus, the animal studies support the observation that the immunological response to histocompatibility antigens cannot completely account for the outcome of bone allografts, and observations vary quite markedly in terms of the association of the immunological responses to MHC antigens and the graft outcome.

It appears that other bone antigens besides the histocompatibility antigens expressed on cells may be relevant in the immunological reaction to allografts. Immunological reactions to bone extracted proteins in allograft recipients have been reported. Ahos et al. (78) identified moderate to weak cellular reactivity to antigens extracted from donor bone, although allograft incorporation was not different in reactive patients compared with bone antigen unresponsive patients, and long-term degenerative joint and sclerotic density bone changes were not correlated with the immune responses. The specificity of these responses was not evaluated, but the authors hypothesized that an immune reaction to graft components might hinder bone healing. No evaluation of concomitant anti-MHC immunity was evaluated in this study. Others have studied the effects of allograft pretreatment, particularly freezing, upon bone antigens. Langer et al. (79,80) studied the behavior of frozen allografts to assess the immunological effects of freezing on antigenicity, and concluded that no alteration of immunogenicity occurs. However Burwell (81) suggested that freezing markedly impairs antigenicity, and several others (82–84) support this claim. Frozen and freeze dried allograft has been shown to remodel and survive in functional form, despite the demonstration in vitro of immune response to these types of grafts. While there is little published evidence in patients beyond these observations, several animal studies concur with the concept of adverse reactions to bone antigens during allografting. Examination of the incorporation and immune response towards sterilized bone allografts in inbred rats, and comparison of irradiated, autoclaved, and cryo-preserved bone indicated that irradiated grafts incorporated at a slower rate than cryo-preserved transplants, while autoclaved bone was not incorporated (85). A cell-mediated response against cryo-preserved grafts was demonstrated, and while irradiated grafts induced a major immune response, cryo-preserved grafts were essentially nonantigenic. The results suggest a correlation between loss of antigenicity and failure of graft incorporation, suggesting bone antigens may provoke the induction of cellular mechanisms during graft incorporation. Frielaender et al. (86,87) investigated the effect of immunization with cartilage matrix components on rabbits, and concluded that the immunogenicity of proteoglycan and collagen components may play a role in the outcome of allogeneic and xenogeneic osteochondral grafts, and contribute to progression of degenerative joint disease. Rodrigo et al. (88) demonstrated that solvent irrigation of subchondral bone with Triton-X may inhibit or prevent the immune response to fresh bone allografts in rats and sheep. There was a significant improvement in allograft outcome over control (Betadine) irrigation, although the allograft groups were not equivalent to autografts. The healing patterns of frozen foreign allografts, frozen syngeneic allografts, and fresh cortical autografts in rats suggested that new bone formation started earlier in autografts than in allografts or syngeneic grafts compared with autografts, and antigen-mismatched allografts exhibited retarded formation of new bone throughout the union process (89). The mRNA levels of type I collagen were elevated in autografts compared with allografts, and type I collagen mRNA expression was more sustained in the healing tissue than in antigen-mismatched allografts. No apparent differences were seen between allografts and autografts in the expression of type III collagen. No cartilage-specific type II collagen mRNA was observed, indicating that antigen mismatching or preservation by freezing did not alter the basic mechanism of the interface healing process, although it did slow down the beginning of the process. The experiments suggest that an antigen mismatch between donor and recipient affects the temporal gene expression of extracellular bone matrix and delays new bone formation at the graft–host interface of cortical bone allografts. Irnmunologic responses against defatted frozen bone allografts appear to be reduced, and de-fatting increased the rate of bone formation rate (90). However, during an investigation of the immunological effects of de-fatting using autografts (91), where pairs of grafts were frozen, and one graft from each pair was defatted with chloroform/methanol, there was no difference in bone formation rate between defatted and nondefatted implants. These data suggest that the increased bone formation rate in defatted allografts is caused by the removal of allograft antigens, possibly specific cell surface antigens.

   One consideration that is rarely considered during the evaluation of the allograft outcome is the immunological status of the patient due to the underlying connective tissue disease, although the response to bone matrix components is considered as a factor in allograft rejection (92). While the immunological aspects of OA are rarely considered central to the pathology of the arthritis, the immune reactivity against connective tissue antigens, particularly those bound to prosthesis components (discussed above) or directed against antigens released from damaged joint tissues, may contribute to the chronicity of the disease process (23). Jasin (93) reported that osteoarthritic cartilage samples obtained during arthroplasty contained sequestered immune complexes containing antibodies to type I collagen, suggesting that a response to connective tissue antigens is not an uncommon finding in the patient population undergoing joint replacement operations. Minor antigenic variations in connective tissue components occur between individuals; therefore, it is conceivable that certain allograft recipients may respond to foreign or autologous bone antigens due to their arthritic condition. To date, the cumulative effects of an immunological response to histocompatibility antigens expressed upon the allograft and a reaction to connective tissue antigens present in the foreign bone have not been examined in the outcome of allograft procedures. The situation is complicated when allografts are used in arthroplasty procedures, since the inflammatory response initiated by the generation of wear debris could increase the exposure of allograft antigens to antigen-presenting cells, with adverse outcomes upon the integration of the graft and the security of the implant.

THE IMMUNE RESPONSE IN CLINICAL PRACTICE

An immune response to orthopaedic biomaterials that results in an adverse outcome of joint arthroplasty is a relatively infrequent occurrence. While this is fortunate for the practice of orthopaedic surgery, the low prevalence has led to poor diagnostic procedures and prophylactic activity. Surgeons should be familiar with the warning of known adverse reactions to materials that is included in the package insert, and obtain a pre-operative history that could alert them to potential problems in all patients. The early opinion by Rooker and Wilkinson (40) that "there is little evidence of a direct causal relationship between metal sensitivity and subsequent loosening" should not be interpreted to read that an allergic response to orthopaedic is a trivial consideration for the orthopaedic surgeon. It is now acknowledged that it is unclear whether metal sensitivity is a contributing factor to implant failure (41). A relationship between reactivity to chromium, cobalt, or nickel and complications due to dental devices has been well established (94), with a convincing subsidence of clinical reactions associated with the removal of the suspected biomaterial. These findings stand as a cautionary note for the use of all implanted devices. The minimum consideration in the orthopaedic patient is to enquire concerning allergic reactions to jewelry, dental amalgams, and methacrylate-based glues. Since jewelry reactions are not uncommon, the self-identified positive patient should be further assessed to evaluate whether there is a pre-existing response to orthopaedic alloys. First, many self-identified jewelry responders do not prove positive to classic skin tests with either metals or salts, and do not exhibit unusual in vitro cellular responses to biomaterials. This information may provide a degree of re-assurance to both the patient and the surgeon, and can be determined by any competent allergist or immunologist. However, it should be noted that skin sensitivity to metals can be a subtle response and the classic "wheal and flare" skin reaction is rarely seen. Some patients do show a strong contact reaction, with a marked pruritic, erythematous rash extending beyond the test area. This type of response is hard to ignore, and certainly raises several flags for the selection of materials. The typical patient reaction is shown in Figure 4, with a moderate inflammatory reaction in close contact with Co–Cr dust, and negative reaction to Ti-6-4 and the control patch. This response is usually mildly pruritic, but the sensation reported by the patient is commonly transient. We recommend metal alloy dust to perform this type of skin test, as the use of nickel-sized metal disks is prone to poor contact with the patients' skin. However, reactivity has also been detected with titanium-containing ointment (95) and nickel salts (35). Alloy dust should be liberally applied to a $3\,mm^2$ area on the patients' forearm, and secured in place by hypo-allergic tape. Separate alloys should be placed at least 3 cm apart, and preferably separated by a control (no metal dust) tape patch. The patient should be instructed to keep the test area as dry as possible, and ensure contact by the addition of band-aid tape or wrapping if necessary. The reaction sites should normally be scored after one week of contact. However, the patient should contact the immunologist immediately should the sensation beneath the tape, become irritating. In patients with strong contact sensitivity, a clearly positive reaction may be

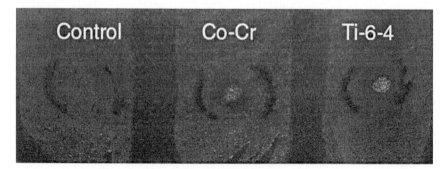

Figure 4 A typical skin reaction to orthopaedic alloys in a metal sensitive patient. The response is shown one week after the application of alloy dust. There is a moderate inflammatory reaction surrounding the Co–Cr, and a negative reaction to both the Ti-6–4 and the control patch. The patient reported a mildly pruritic sensation to the Co–Cr patch prior to the removal of the tape, and the reaction resolved within 48 hours of flushing the alloy dust from the skin.

present between 48 and 72 hours, and this response can progress to ulceration if the allergen is not removed promptly. If the skin becomes broken, the removal of the dust can be problematic, but topical application of cortisone ointment usually prevents any severe reactivity from the skin test. Before removal of the tape, patients should be asked to identify any apparent reactions to the specific test sites. The reaction site should be examined for signs of inflammation, and then alloy dust flushed from the site using cool water, and the contact area re-inspected closely for erythema and papular reactions. The control patch should also be assessed for responses. In the advent of a negative response to the alloy dust, the patient should be instructed to return should a subsequent reaction occur at the site. In rare instances, skin reactions can suddenly arise as late as 48 hours after inspection, even with normal flushing to remove all visible dust. The assessment of contact sensitivity reactions (both positive and negative) are particularly useful in conjunction with in vitro cellular responses assessed in peripheral blood cells, although this test is not commonly available in clinical practice. Our laboratory and others (42) have found a good correlation between positive skin tests and hyper-proliferation of cells cultured in the presence of a specific biomaterial. However, this association is by no means absolute, and discordance between the tests can occur. Most investigators agree that it is more common to see a negative skin test and a positive in vitro reaction than vice versa (96). As in all immunological tests, the current pharmacological profile of the patient should be evaluated to note any medications that can disrupt cellular responses to antigenic stimulation. During the evaluation of the in vitro response to biomaterials, the immunologist should be particularly concerned by a toxic reaction to the biomaterial at high dose that evolves to a marked proliferative reaction at low doses. This pattern of responsiveness is common in revision patients with complications that can be attributed to biomaterial responses.

The influence of the immunology findings upon the clinical decisions is highly dependent upon the individual situations. Trauma surgeons are rarely able to avail themselves of a history of metal responses, let alone the services of a specialized immunology lab. In routine joint arthroplasty surgery, the input from an immunology evaluation can prove valuable when a selection of materials (such as a choice of stainless steel, titanium, or cobalt–chrome alloys) is available. Although the value of the hypersensitivity test in predicting an adverse outcome is controversial (97), we feel that this information should be part of the global surgical decision making. The most common situation where immune reactivity becomes an issue is retrospective to the surgical procedure. The usual presentation to the orthopaedic immunologist is a patient with a poor postoperative course, a painful prosthesis, and chronic drainage from the implantation site. Invariably these patients have been extensively worked-up for an infectious etiology, with a string of negative findings. The fluid draining from the site is frequently rich in lymphocytes, and polymorphonuclear leucocytes (PMNs) are less well represented than would be expected in infection. A review of the immediate postoperative course can prove useful, particularly if the patient exhibited any inflammatory reaction to surgical staples (98). Skin clips may contain chromium, nickel, molybdenum, cobalt, and titanium in concentrations high enough to cause contact reactions, which may delay wound healing. Should a reaction to staples be noted, the surgeon should have concerns for the prosthesis, since this reaction is indicative of pre-existing metal sensitivity. The patient may experience febrile episodes, with or without local inflammation at the implant site, since fever is consistent with a hypersensitivity response. Another useful criterion is the appearance of skin rashes, which are not necessarily close to the wound site. Rashes on the arms, legs, and trunk can occur when the metal hapten-carrier complex becomes trapped in the capillaries of the skin, or metal ions become directly coupled to keratinocytes and dendritic cells (99,100) or concentrated within skin cells (101). T cells then migrate to these sites and cause inflammatory tissue damage, resulting in the appearance of a rash. However, the problematic patient may have a normal postoperative recovery and only present with a painful prosthesis with poor fixation after a considerable time period (six months to two years). In this instance, it is possible that an immune response has developed to the prosthesis itself. Several processes must occur for this to happen. First, for metal allergy to develop there must be sufficient ion release from the metal components to generate a hapten-carrier complex. Then the hapten-carrier complex must accumulate to a threshold level in order to trigger the primary immune response. The threshold level for a response in humans has not been accurately determined, and is predicted to vary widely among different individuals. Based mainly on animal studies, antigen threshold levels are usually considered to be around 1 µg, with the caveat that typical (protein) antigens have been used for this determination. Since the rate of metallic ion dissociation from 316L stainless steel has been determined to be $0.03\,\mu g/cm^2/wk$ (102,103), this suggests that at least eight weeks would be required to provide sufficient ion release from a femoral component to stimulate the primary immune response in a worst case scenario. This hypothesis is consistent with the observation by Cramers (104) that contact sensitivity took 3–3.5 months to develop in patients implanted with plates and screws made of 316L stainless steel. Ion leakage may be accelerated by a number of factors, such as crevice corrosion, so the implant design may influence the potential for a device to stimulate an immunological response. Implant wear may be particularly important for typical orthopaedic alloys, since the production of small particles increases the surface area for ion leakage and promotes the exposure to phagocytic cells and their corrosive products. Agins et al. (105) conducted retrieval analysis on eight periprosthetic (dry) tissues from titanium alloy implants using atomic absorption spectrophotometry, and reported a mean accumulation of 1047 µ/gm titanium, 115 µ/gm aluminum, and 67 µ/gm vanadium. The accumulation increased with time after implantation, but all values were significantly elevated over normal tissue levels as early as 11 months postsurgery. These metal levels are clearly high enough to have deleterious effects upon cells in the local area, although the development of immune responses was not documented in these patients. Membranes from the titanium–alloy implants tend to contain more metal debris than those from the cobalt–chromium-alloy implants, although levels of inflammatory cytokines and tissue metalloproteinases were not significantly different between the two orthopaedic alloys (106). Since metal-on-metal implants are enjoying renewed interest in orthopaedic surgery, it will be valuable to follow these patients for the development of immune sensitivity. Reports concerning early devices suggested that up to half of the surgical failures might be attributed to metal allergy (107). More recent findings indicate that Co–Cr wear particles from metal-on-metal bearings may be considerably smaller than the typical particle size range reported for UHMWPE particles, but apparently result in a less severe tissue reaction (108). It was suggested that metal particles may corrode and disseminate from local tissue sites to a higher degree than UHMWPE particles, and there is evidence to support this concept from atomic absorption spectrophotometry conducted upon lymphoreticular tissues (109), a case report of lymphadenopathy (110), and an extensive examination of debris in para-aortic lymph nodes and spleens (111). It should be considered that this resolution of metal from the periprosthetic area may be accompanied by a higher systemic exposure to metal ions, and hence a greater potential to elicit metal sensitivity.

The time frame for an immune response to polymers is far less predictable, and may be more closely tied to the generation of particulate wear debris. It is reasonable to predict that a high volume of particulate debris will stimulate macrophages and instigate a local inflammatory reaction. Since the main cytokine mediators of inflammation, IL-1 and TNF, have deleterious effects upon bone growth via signaling of osteoclastic activity, a chronic reaction to debris might be expected to adversely impact upon the fixation of an implant. While the inflammatory aspects of the response to particulate debris are now well accepted, few investigators have extended their studies to examine whether chronic inflammatory reactions progress towards increased immune reactivity to biomaterials in aseptic loosening. Since contact sensitivity testing to PMMA and UHMWPE are not well established, no strong information is available on the clinical application of hypersensitivity responses to polymers on the prediction of prosthesis loosening. While the in vitro cellular responses to PMMA (reviewed above) appear to be associated with poor clinical outcomes, insufficient follow-up data is currently available to define the sensitivity and specificity of this assay. However, where an equivalent surgery decision can be made between cemented and uncemented components, we suggest the avoidance of cement in the strongly PMMA reactive patient.

SUMMARY

The future of orthopaedic surgery appears to be intricately involved with the development of novel biomaterials and the application of tissue engineering, cytokine modulation, and gene therapy. These rapidly advancing fields hold great promise to revolutionize the approach to connective tissue diseases, with a long-term goal of the restoration of bone and joints to near original structure and function. Orthopaedic surgeons are not timid in embracing new technology, as the widespread acceptance of bone morphogenic proteins (BMPs) indicates, and most surgeons hold a positive approach to the application of advances in biology to the surgical field. It is rarely the role of the investigative immunologist to sound a note of caution, but there are some obvious gaps in our current state of knowledge on the immune response to biomaterials. While the immune response appears to result in infrequent adverse reactions to metals, polymers, and allografts, we currently have only a limited capacity to diagnose the contribution of these reactions to aseptic loosening, and an even weaker ability to identify patients at risk prior to the selection of appropriate prosthetic components. Part of the problem is the complexity of joint replacements; while it is relatively easy to investigate immunotoxicological reactions to individual components in virgin form, it is a completely different problem to interpret the inflammatory and immune interactions in tissue chronically exposed to particulate debris from a variety of biomaterials. It can be argued that research for the near term should be focused upon revision arthroplasty patients. This unfortunate group may provide the key to identifying both risk factors and the mechanisms of adverse responses associated with prosthesis loosening. Data generated in the patients may permit the selection of the least provocative components in terms of generation of wear debris and stimulation of cellular reactions, and ultimately improve the biocompatibility of all orthopaedic devices.

REFERENCES

1. Clementi D, Surace A, Celestini M, Pietrogrande V. Clinical investigations of tolerance to materials and acrylic cement in patients with hip prostheses. Ital J Orthop Traumatol 1980; 6:97–104.
2. Fisher AA. Reactions to acrylic bone cement in orthopaedic surgeons and patients. Cutis 1986; 37:425–426.
3. Fousssereau J, Cavelier C, Protois JP, Deviller J. Contact dermatitis from methyl methacrylate in an above-knee prosthesis. Contact Dermat 1989; 20: 69–70.
4. Pacifici R, Rifas L, McCracken R, Vered I, McMurtry C, Avioli LV, Peck WA. Ovarian steroid treatment blocks a postmenopausal increase in blood interleukin-1 release. Proc Natl Acad Sci USA 1989; 86:2398–2402.
5. Wooley PH, Nasser S, Fitzgerald RH, Jr. The immune response to implant materials in humans. Clin Orthop Relat Res 1996; 326:63–70.

6. Wooley PH, Petersen S, Song Z, Nasser S. Cellular immune responses to orthopaedic implant materials following cemented total joint replacement. J Orthop Res 1997; 15:874–880.
7. Gil-Albarova J, Lacleriga A, Barrios C, Canadell J. Lymphocyte response to polymethylmethacrylate in loose total hip prostheses. J Bone Joint Surg–Br Vol 1992; 74:825–830.
8. Santavirta S, Konttinen YY, Bergroth V, Gronblad M. Lack of immune response to methyl methacrylate in lymphocyte cultures. Acta Orthop Scand 1991; 62:29–32.
9. Boynton EL, Henry M, Morton J, Waddell JP. The inflammatory response to particulate wear debris in total hip arthroplasty. Can J Surg 1995; 38:507–515.
10. Greitemann B, Mues B, Polster J, Pauly T, Sorg C. Inflammatory reactions in primary osteoarthritis of the hip and total hip prosthesis loosening. Arch Orthop Trauma Surg 1992; 111:138–141.
11. Lodi M, Cavallini G, Susa A, Lanfredi M. Biomaterials and immune system: cellular reactivity towards PTFE and Dacron vascular substitutes pointed out by the leukocyte adherence inhibition (LAI) test. Int Angiol 1988; 7:344–348.
12. Zippel R, Wilhelm L, Marusch F, Koch A, Urban G, Schlosser M. Antigenicity of polyester (Dacron) vascular prostheses in an animal model. Eur J Vasc Endovasc Surg 2001; 21:202–207.
13. Jimenez DF, Keating R, Goodrich JT. Silicone allergy in ventriculoperitoneal shunts. Childs Nervous Syst 1994; 10:59–63.
14. Christie AJ, Pierret G, Levitan J. Silicone synovitis. Semin Arthritis Rheum 1989; 19:166–171.
15. Bansal M, Goldman AB, Bullough PG, Mascarenhas B. Case report 706: Silicone-induced reactive synovitis. Skeletal Radiol 1992; 21:49–51.
16. Bogoch ER. Silicone synovitis. J Rheumatol 1987; 14:1086–1088.
17. Worsing RA Jr, Engber WD, Lange TA. Reactive synovitis from particulate silastic. J Bone Joint Surg Am Vol 64; 581–585, 1982.
18. Lazaro MA, Garcia Morteo D, de Benyacar MA, Paira SO, Lema B, Garcia Morteo O, Maldonado Cocco JA. Lymphadenopathy secondary to silicone hand joint prostheses. Clin Exp Rheumatol 1990; 8:17–22.
19. Paplanus SH, Payne CM. Axillary lymphadenopathy 17 years after digital silicone implants: study with x-ray microanalysis. J Hand Surg 1988; 13:399.
20. Bernstein SA, Strickland RW, Lazarus E. Axillary lymphadenopathy due to Swanson implants. J Rheumatol 1993; 20:1066–1069.
21. Kossovsky N, Heggers JP, Robson MC. Bioreactivity of silicone. CRC Crit Rev Biocompatibility 1987; 3:53–85.
22. Wooley PH, Fitzgerald RH Jr, Song Z, Davis P, Whalen JD, Trumble S, Nasser S. Proteins bound to polyethylene components in patients who have aseptic loosening after total joint arthroplasty. A preliminary report [see comments]. J Bone Joint Surg Am 1999; 81:616–623.
23. Stuart JM, Huffstutter EH, Townes AS, Kang AH. Incidence and specificity of antibodies to types I, II, III, IV, and collagen V in rheumatoid arthritis and other rheumatic diseases as measured by 1251-radioimmunoassay. Arthritis Rheum 1983; 26:832–840.

24. Adelmann B, Schoning B. Binding of native and denatured collagen to immunoglobulins and cold insoluble globulin in serum of patients undergoing orthopaedic surgery. Klinische Wochenschrift 1980; 58:625–629.

25. Bujia J, Alsalameh S, Naumann A, Wilmes E, Sittinger M, Burmester GR. Humoral immune response against minor collagens type IX and XI in patients with cartilage graft resorption after reconstructive surgery. Ann Rheum Dis 1994; 53:229–234.

26. Tang L, Lucas AH, Eaton JW. Inflammatory responses to implanted polymeric biomaterials: role of surface-adsorbed immunoglobulin G. J Lab Clin Med 1993; 122:292–300.

27. Hicks DG, Judkins AR, Sickel JZ, Rosier RN, Puzas JE, RJ O'Keefe. Granular histiocytosis of pelvic lymph, nodes following total hip arthroplasty. The presence of wear debris, cytokine production, and immunologically activated macrophages.. J Bone Joint Surg Am 1996; Vol 78:482–496.

28. Ali SA, Doherty PJ, Williams DF. Molecular biointeractions of biomedical polymers with extracellular exudate and inflammatory cells and their effects on the biocompatibility, in vivo. Biomaterials 1994; 15:779–85.

29. Haddad FS, Cobb AG, Bentley G, Levell NJ, Dowd PM. Hypersensitivity in aseptic loosening of total hip replacements. The role of constituents of bone cement. J Bone Joint Surg Br 1996; 78:546–549.

30. Liden C. Occupational contact dermatitis due to nickel allergy. Sci Total Environ 1994; 148:283–285.

31. Black J. Biological Performance of Materials. New York, Marcel Dekker, 1999.

32. Fleming CJ, Burden AD, Forsyth A. The genetics of allergic contact hypersensitivity to nickel. Contact Dermat 1999; 41:251–253.

33. Arikan A, Kulak Y. A study of chromium, nickel and cobalt hypersensitivity. J Marmara Univ Dent Fac 1992; 1:223–229.

34. McDonagh AJ, Wright AL, Cork MJ, Gawkrodger DJ. Nickel sensitivity: the influence of ear piercing and atopy. Br J Dermatol 1992; 126:16–18.

35. Elves MW, Wilson JN, Scales JT, Kemp HB. Incidence of metal sensitivity in patients with total joint replacements. BMJ 1975; 4:376–378.

36. Evans EM. Metal sensitivity as a cause of bone necrosis and loosening of the prosthesis in total joint replacement. J Bone Joint Surg-British Volume 1974; 56(B):626.

37. Liden C, Wahlberg JE. Cross-reactivity to metal compounds studied in guinea pigs induced with chromate or cobalt. Acta Derm Venereol 1994; 74:341–343.

38. Benson MK, Goodwin PG, Brostoff J. Metal sensitivity in patients with joint replacement arthroplasties. BMJ 1975; 4:374–375.

39. Gawkrodger DJ. Nickel sensitivity and the implantation of orthopaedic prostheses. Contact Dermat 1993; 28:257–259.

40. Rooker GD, Wilkinson JD. Metal sensitivity in patients undergoing hip replacement. A prospective study. J Bone Joint Surg 1980; 62-B:502–505.

41. Hallab N, Merritt K, Jacobs JJ. Metal sensitivity in patients with orthopaedic implants. J Bone Joint Surg Am 2001; 83-A:428–436.

42. Basketter DA, Lea LJ, Cooper KJ, Ryan CA, Gerberick GF, Dearman RJ, Kimber I. Identification of metal allergens in the local lymph node assay. Am J Contact Dermat 1999; 10:207–212.

43. Bour H, Nicolas JF, Garrigue JL, Demidem A, Schmitt D. Establishment of nickel-specific T cell lines from patients with allergic contact dermatitis: comparison of different protocols. Clin Immunol Immunopathol 1994; 73:142–145.
44. Silvennoinen-Kassinen S, Ikaheimo I, Tiilikainen A. TAP1 and TAP2 genes in nickel allergy. Int Arch Allergy Immunol 1997; 114:94–96.
45. Cavani A, Mei D, Guerra E, Corinti S, Giani M, Pirrotta L, Puddu P, Girolomoni G. Patients with allergic contact dermatitis to nickel and nonallergic individuals display different nickel-specific T cell responses. Evidence for the presence of effector CD8+ and regulatory CD4+ T cells. J Invest Dermatol 1998; 111:621–628.
46. Sinigaglia F. The molecular basis of metal recognition by T cells. J Invest Dermatol 1994; 102:398–401.
47. Vollmer J, Weltzien HU, Moulon C. TCR reactivity in human nickel allergy indicates contacts with complementarity-determining region 3 but excludes superantigen-like recognition. J Immunol 1999; 163:2723–2731.
48. Vollmer J, Fritz M, Dormoy A, Weltzien HU, Moulon C. Dominance of the BV17 element in nickel-specific human T cell receptors relates to severity of contact sensitivity. Eur J Immunol 1997; 27:1865–1874.
49. Werfel T, Hentschel M, Kapp A, Renz H. Dichotomy of blood- and skin-derived IL-4-producing allergen-specific T cells and restricted V beta repertoire in nickel-mediated contact dermatitis. J Immunol 1997; 158:2500–2505.
50. Granchi D, Ciaperti G, Savarino L, Stea S, Filippini F, Sudanese A, Rotini R, Giunti A. Expression of the CD69 activation antigen on lymphocytes of patients with hip prosthesis. Biomaterials 2000; 21:2059–2065.
51. Bravo I, Carvalho GS, Barbosa MA, De Sousa M. Differential effects of eight metal ions on lymphocyte differentiation antigens in vitro. J Biomed Mater Res 1990; 24:1059–1068.
52. Merritt K, Rodrigo JJ. Immune response to synthetic materials. Sensitization of patients receiving orthopaedic implants. Clin Orthop 1996; 10:71–79.
53. Yang J, Merritt K. Detection of antibodies against corrosion products in patients after Co–Cr total joint replacements. J Biomed Mater Res 1994; 28:1249–1258.
54. Yang J, Merritt K. Production of monoclonal antibodies to study corrosion products of CO–CR biomaterials. J Biomed Mater Res 1996; 31:71–80.
55. Al-Saffar N, Khwaja HA, Kadoya Y, Revell PA. Assessment of the role of GM-CSF in the cellular transformation and the development of erosive lesions around orthopaedic implants. Am J Clin Pathol 1996; 105:628–639.
56. Thornhill TS, Ozuna RM, Shortkroff S, Keller K, Sledge CB, Spector M. Biochemical and histological evaluation of the synovial-like tissue around failed (loose) total joint replacement prostheses in human subjects and a canine model. Biomaterials 1990; 11:69–72.
57. Haynes DR, Rogers SD, Hay S, Pearcy MJ, Howie DW. The differences in toxicity and release of bone-resorbing mediators induced by titanium and cobalt–chromium–alloy wear particles. J Bone Joint Surg Am Vol 1993; 75:825–834.
58. Wang JY, Wicklund BH, Gustilo RB, Tsukayama DT. Titanium, chromium and cobalt ions modulate the release of bone-associated cytokines by human monocytes/macrophages in vitro. Biomaterials 1996; 17:2233–2240.

59. Witt JD, Swann M. Metal wear and tissue response in failed titanium alloy total hip replacements. J Bone Joint Surg Vol 1991; 73:559–563.

60. van Meekeren J. Heel- en geneeskonstige aanmerkingen. Commelijin. 1668. Amersterdam.

61. Kossovsky N, Freiman CJ. Physicochemical and immunological basis of silicone pathophysiology. J Biomater Sci Polym Ed 1995; 7:101–113.

62. Oakeshott RD, McAuley JP, Gross AE, Morgan DA, Zukor DJ, Rudan JF, Brooks PJ. Allograft reconstruction in revision total hip surgery. In: Regazzoini P, Aebi M, eds. Bone Transplantation. Berlin: Springer, 1989:265–273.

63. Muscolo DL, Ayerza MA, Calabrese ME, Redal MA, Santini AE. Human leukocyte antigen matching, radiographic score, and histologic findings in massive frozen bone allografts. Clin Orthop Relat Res 1996; 326:115–126.

64. Popkirov S, Minev M. Clinical importance of the immunoserological data on the bone allotransplantation. Arch Orthop Unfallchir 1976; 85:289–298.

65. Hofmann GO, Falk C, Wangemann T. Immunological transformations in the recipient of grafted allogeneic human bone. Arch Orthop Trauma Surg 1997; 116:143–50.

66. Strong DM, Friedlaender GE, Ahmed A, Sell KW. Immunogenicity of freeze-dried and deep-frozen bone allografts. In: Simatos D, Strong DM, Turc JM, eds. Cryoimmunologie/Cryoimmunology. INSERM, Paris, 1976; 209–215.

67. Friedlaender GE, Strong DM, Sell KW. Studies on the antigenicity of bone. II. Donor-specific anti-HLA antibodies in human recipients of freeze-dried allografts. J Bone Joint Surg Am 1984; 66:107–112.

68. Shigetomi M, Kawai S, Fukumoto T. Studies of allotransplantation of bone using immunohistochemistry and radioimmunoassay in rats. Clin Orthop Relat Res 1993:345–51.

69. Stevenson S, Shaffer JW, Goldberg VM. The humoral response to vascular and nonvascular allografts of bone. Clin Ortho Relat Res 1996:86–95.

70. Stevenson S, Li XQ, Davy DT, Klein L, Goldberg VM. Critical biological determinants of incorporation of non-vascularized cortical bone grafts. Quantification of a complex process and structure. J Bone Joint Surg Am 1997; 79:1–16.

71. Larsson S, Thelander U, Friberg S. C-reactive protein (CRP) levels after elective orthopaedic surgery. Clin Orthop Relat Research 1992:237–242.

72. Waterman AH, Schrik JJ. Allergy in hip arthroplasty. Contact Dermat 1985; 13:294–301.

73. Kossovsky N, Gornbein JA, Zeidler M, Stassi J, Chun G, Papasian N, Nguyen R, Ly K, Rajguru S. Self-reported signs and symptoms in breast implant patients with novel antibodies to silicone surface associated antigens [anti- SSAA(x)]. J Appl Biomater 1995; 6:153–160.

74. Rudzki Z, Otfinowski J, Stachura J. The histological appearance of the periprosthetic capsule in failed total hip arthroplasty differs depending on the presence of polyethylene acetabulum destruction, iliac bone damage and presence of infection. Pol J Pathol 1996; 47:19–25.

75. Brautbar N, Campbell A, Vojdani A. Silicone breast implants and autoimmunity: causation, association, or myth?. J Biomater Sci Polym Ed 1995; 7:133–145.

76. Friedlaender GE, Strong DM, Sell KW. Studies on the antigenicity of bone. I. Freeze-dried and deep-frozen bone allografts in rabbits. J Bone Joint Surg 1976; 58:854–858.
77. Bos GD, Goldberg VM, Gordon NH, Dollinger BM, Zika JM, Powell AE, Heiple KG. The long-term fate of fresh and frozen orthotopic bone allografts in genetically defined rats. Clin Orthop 1985:245–254.
78. Aho AJ, Eskola J, Ekfors T, Manner I, Kouri T, Hollmen T. Immune responses and clinical outcome of massive human osteoarticular allografts. Clin Orthop 1998:196–206.
79. Langer F, Czitrom A, Pritzker KP, Gross AE. The immunogenicity of fresh and frozen allogeneic bone. J Bone Joint Surg Am 1975; 57:216–220.
80. Langer F, Gross AE, West M, Urovitz EP. The immunogenicity of allograft knee joint transplants. Clin Orthop 1978:155–162.
81. Burwell RG. The fate of freeze-dried bone allograft. Transplant Proc 1976; 8:95–111.
82. Bos GD, Goldberg VM, Zika JM, Heiple KG, Powell AE. Immune responses of rats to frozen bone allografts. J Bone Joint Surg Am 1983; 65:239–246.
83. Burchardt H, Enneking WF. Transplantation of bone. Surg Clin North Am 1978; 58:403–427.
84. Horowitz MC, Friedlaender GE. Immunologic aspects of bone transplantation. A rationale for future studies. Orthop Clin North Am 1987; 18:227–233.
85. Schratt HE, Spyra JL. Experimental studies of healing and antigenicity of sterilized bone transplants. Chirurg 1997; 68:77–83.
86. Friedlaender GE, Ladenbauer-Bellis IM, Chrisman OD. Imnmnogenicity of xenogeneic cartilage matrix components in a rabbit model. Yale J Biol Med 1983; 56:211–217.
87. Friedlaender GE. Immune responses to osteochondral allografts. Current knowledge and future directions. Clin Orthop 1983:58–68.
88. Rodrigo JJ, Heiden E, Hegyes M, Sharkey NA. Immune response inhibition by irrigating subchondral bone with cytotoxic agents. Clin Orthop 1996: 96–106.
89. Virolainen P, Vuorio E, Aro HT. Different healing rates of bone autografts, syngeneic grafts, and allografts in an experimental rat model. Arch Orthop Trauma Surg 1997; 116:486–491.
90. Thoren K, Aspenberg P. Increased bone ingrowth distance into lipid-extracted bank bone at 6 weeks. A titanium chamber study in allogeneic and syngeneic rats. Arch Orthop Trauma Surg 1995; 114:167–171.
91. Thoren K, Aspenberg P, Thorngren KG. Lipid extraction decreases the specific immunologic response to bone allografts in rabbits. Acta Orthop Scandi 1993; 64:44–6.
92. Burchardt H. The biology of bone graft repair. Clin Orthop 1983:28–42.
93. Jasin HE. Autoantibody specificities of immune complexes sequestered in articular cartilage of patients with rheumatoid arthritis and osteoarthritis. Arthritis Rheum 1985; 28:241–248.
94. Hildebrand HF, Veron C, Martin P. Biocompatibility of Co–Cr–Ni alloys. New York: Plenum Press, 1998:201–223.

95. Lalor PA, Revell PA, Gray AB, Wright S, Railton GT, Freeman MA. Sensitivity to titanium. A cause of implant failure?. J Bone Joint Surg 1991; 73:25–28.

96. Lisby S, Hansen LH, Skov L, Menne T, Baadsgaard O. Nickel-induced activation of T cells in individuals with negative patch test to nickel sulphate. Arch Dermatol Res 1999; 291:247–252.

97. Milavec-Puretic V, Orlic D, Marusic A. Sensitivity to metals in 40 patients with failed hip endoprosthesis. Arch Orthop Trauma Surg 1998; 117:383–386.

98. Lhotka CG, Szekeres T, Fritzer-Szekeres M, Schwarz G, Steffan I, Maschke M, Dubsky G, Kremser M, Zweymuller K. Are allergic reactions to skin clips associated with delayed wound healing?. Am J Surg 1998; 176:320–323.

99. Sosroseno W. The immunology of nickel-induced allergic contact dermatitis. Asian Pac J Allergy Immunol 1995; 13:173–181.

100. Van Den Broeke LT, Heffler LC, Tengvall LM, Nilsson JL, Karlberg, AT, Scheynius A. Direct $Ni2^+$ antigen formation on cultured human dendritic cells. Immunology 1999; 96:578–585.

101. Lansdown AB. Physiological and toxicological changes in the skin resulting from the action and interaction of metal ions. Crit Rev Toxicol 1995; 25:397–462.

102. Haudrechy P, Foussereau J, Mantout B, Baroux B. Nickel release from nickel-plated metals and stainless steels. Contact Dermat 1994; 31:249–255.

103. Haudrechy P, Mantout B, Frappaz A, Rousseau D, Chabeau G, Faure M, Claudy A. Nickel release from stainless steels. Contact Dermat 1997; 37: 113–117.

104. Cramers M, Lucht U. Metal sensitivity in patients treated for tibial fractures with plates of stainless steel. Acta Orthop Scand 1977; 48:245–249.

105. Agins HJ, Alcock NW, Bansal M, Salvati EA, Wilson PD, Jr, Pellicci PM, Bullough PG. Metallic wear in failed titanium-alloy total hip replacements. A histological and quantitative analysis. J Bone Joint Surg 1988; 70-A:347–356.

106. Kim KJ, Chiba J, Rubash HE. In vivo and in vitro analysis of membranes from hip prostheses inserted without cemeat. J Bone Joint Surg 1994; 76-A:172–180.

107. Munro-Ashman D, Miller AJ. Rejection of metal to metal prosthesis and skin sensitivity to cobalt. Contact Dermat 1976; 2:65–67.

108. Doom PF, Campbell PA, Worrall J, Benya PD, McKellop HA, Amstutz HC. Metal wear particle characterization from metal on metal total hip replacements: transmission electron microscopy study of periprosthetic tissues and isolated particles. J Biomed Mater Res 1998; 42:103–111.

109. Langkamer VG, Case CP, Heap P, Taylor A, Collins C, Pearse M, Solomon L. Systemic distribution of wear debris after hip replacement. A cause for concern? J Bone Joint Surg 1992; 74-B:831–839

110. Shinto Y, Uchida A, Yoshikawa H, Araki N, Kato T, Ono K. Inguinal lymphadenopathy due to metal release from a prosthesis. A case report. J Bone Joint Surg Br 1993; 75:266–269.

111. Urban RM, Jacobs JJ, Tomlinson MJ, Gavrilovic J, Black J, Peoc'h M. Dissemination of wear particles to the liver, spleen, and abdominal lymph nodes of patients with hip or knee replacement. J Bone Joint Surg Am 2000; 82: 457–476.

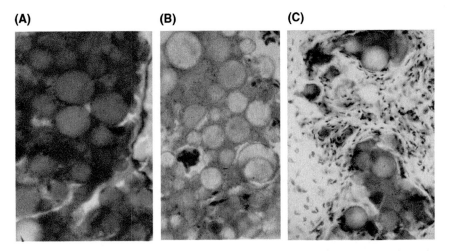

Figure 3.2 Microfissures in PMMA bone cement, implants and disintegration of the cement implant. (*See p. 57.*)

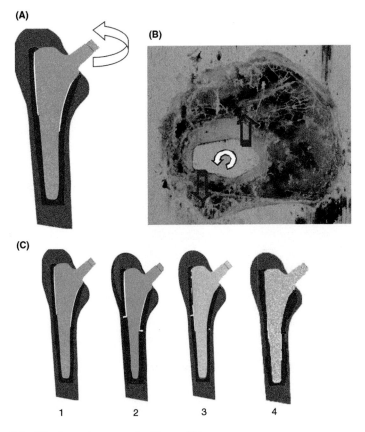

Figure 3.3 The loosening cascade. (*See p. 59.*)

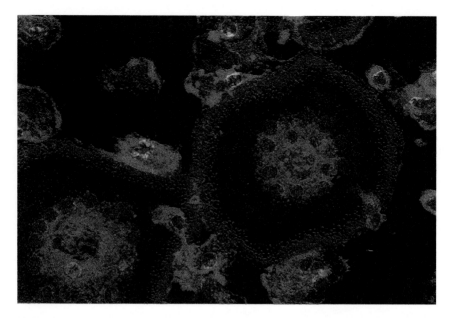

Figure 11.4 Macrophage fusion and foreign body giant cell formation in vitro. (*See p. 269.*)

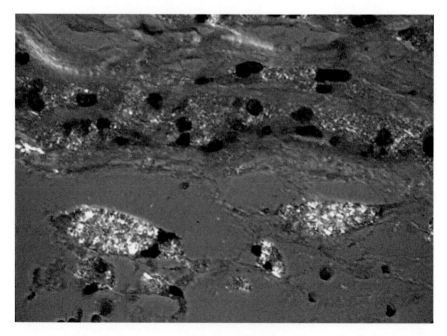

Figure 13.1 Histology of peri-implant interfacial tissue under polarization. (*See p. 329.*)

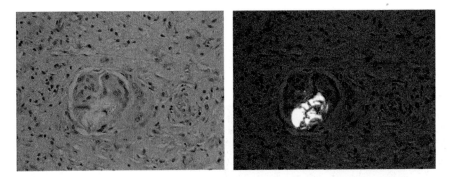

Figure 13.2 Histology of peri-implant interfacial tissue under normal (*left*) and polarization (*right*) conditions. (*See p. 329.*)

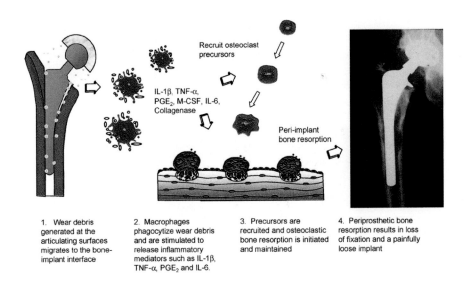

| 1. Wear debris generated at the articulating surfaces migrates to the bone-implant interface | 2. Macrophages phagocytize wear debris and are stimulated to release inflammatory mediators such as IL-1β, TNF-α, PGE₂ and IL-6. | 3. Precursors are recruited and osteoclastic bone resorption is initiated and maintained | 4. Periprosthetic bone resorption results in loss of fixation and a painfully loose implant |

Figure 13.3 Schematic representation of the sequence of events leading to wear debris-mediated osteolysis. (*See p. 330.*)

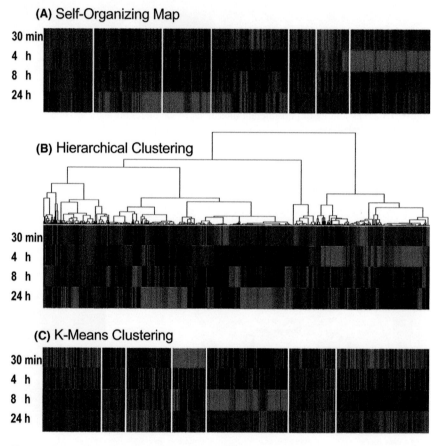

Figure 30.4 Clustering algorithms. (*See p. 770.*)

15

Stress-Related Bone Resorption

J. D. Bobyn and M. Tanzer

Division of Orthopaedics, Montreal General Hospital, McGill University, Montreal, Canada

A. H. Glassman

The Ohio State University College of Medicine, The Halley Orthopaedic Clinic, Columbus, Ohio, U.S.A.

INTRODUCTION

It has long been recognized that the placement of rigid metallic devices into bone alters peri-implant stress patterns, depriving bone of physiologic stress levels and causing bone resorption or disuse atrophy. A common example of this phenomenon is the loss of cortical bone density under fracture fixation plates fixed with screws, due to remodeling that can cause bone fracture after plate removal because of structural weakening. This problem has stimulated the development of more flexible plates that allow more physiologic bone loading, an engineering approach that has also been pursued in hip and knee joint implant design, as discussed later in this chapter.

In both fracture management and joint reconstruction, the primary source of the adverse remodeling is the stiffness mismatch between implant and bone. Contributing factors are also the rigidity of mechanical attachment between implant and bone as well as the direction of loading. The extent of this problem was graphically demonstrated in the mid-1970s with a canine femoral segmental replacement model (Fig. 1) (51). Since then, many other examples with different implants have been described in the literature. A fundamental of solid mechanics is that when two materials are joined, the stiffer material or structure bears the majority of the load.

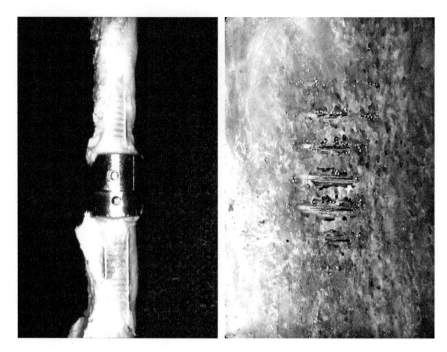

Figure 1 Explanted canine femur with porous coated, threaded segmental implant illustrating extensive bone resorption because of stress shielding due to stiffness mismatch. *Source*: From Ref. 51.

This is particularly so when the composite structure is loaded axially or in parallel; the stiffer material prevents the adjacent material from deforming, as it would on its own. With less deformation (strain) there is less material load (stress). In general, the extent of preferential stress transfer through the implant increases with increasing differences between bone and implant stiffness and increasing rigidity of connection between them. Load direction can also play an important role in stress shielding. When an implant is connected to bone and load is directed purely in compression, such as in some regions of the tibial plateau of a knee replacement, stress shielding can be reduced because load is more efficiently transferred to bone through the implant material, regardless of its stiffness.

Loss of bone mass adjacent to an implant from stress shielding has an entirely different etiology and radiographic appearance than the cystic bone loss known as osteolysis that occurs as an inflammatory reaction to accumulated wear particles (Fig. 2) (37). This latter type of bone loss is addressed in a separate chapter. The loss of bone due to stress shielding is mechanically induced and typically manifests as either cortical thinning or a more diffuse decrease in peri-implant bone density. In contrast, osteolysis typically

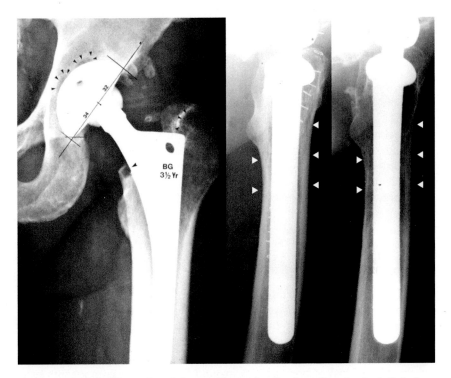

Figure 2 *Left*: Radiograph at 3.5 years illustrating focal, scalloped osteolytic lesions behind the acetabular cup and in the proximal femur that are characteristic of wear debris-mediated bone loss. *Right*: Postoperative and five-year lateral radiographs of a case with an extensively porous coated cobalt–chromium stem illustrating cortical thinning and the diffuse type of bone loss that is characteristic of stress shielding.

appears as one or more radiographically obvious, localized lesions with well-defined borders, sometimes sharply scalloped.

In the field of joint replacement the problem of implant stiffness and stress shielding has been studied for over two decades, particularly on the femoral side of hip replacement and knee replacement, and less so in the acetabulum and the proximal tibia.

BONE RESORPTION IN THE HIP–FEMUR

From an engineering standpoint, it is a simple matter to consider stiffness differences between an implant and bone by examining material and cross-sectional properties (20). The bending stiffness of any construct is calculated by the mathematical product of the material elastic modulus (E) and a geometric factor known as the second area moment of inertia (I) that is based on cross-sectional shape and size (stiffness $= EI$). The elastic modulus is an inherent material property that is independent of geometry. The moment of inertia varies with the fourth power of the cross-sectional dimensions, thus small changes in implant size cause profound changes in the overall stiffness calculation. In an analogous manner, torsional implant stiffness is governed by the shear modulus of the material and the polar moment of inertia, which varies with the fourth power of cross-sectional dimensions. Given these relationships, stem stiffness can be adjusted through simple manipulation of E and/or I (3). Thus, stems made of titanium alloy ($E = 110$ GPa) are about half as stiff as stems made of cobalt–chromium alloy ($E = 205$ GPa). Design features such as slots or flutes reduce the moment of inertia according to the previously mentioned fourth power relationship. For any given femur, a cementless stem is typically larger and therefore stiffer than a cemented stem and thus would be expected to cause more stress shielding.

Conventional Metal Stem Designs

The aforementioned mechanical relationships generally bear the most consequence in the hip, where high-stiffness femoral stems that are rigidly connected to the femur by bone ingrowth tend to stress shield bone and cause resorption. The initial studies of stress-related bone remodeling were only semi-quantitative in nature and involved inspection of serial radiographs for evidence of loss of bone density around femoral stem components such as the Anatomic Medullary Locking® stem (AML®, Depuy, Warsaw, IN) (18–20). Plain radiographs are quite insensitive for detecting bone density change, with differences of up to 30% required before being reliably detectable (24,26). As such, the studies of Engh and Bobyn were unable to quantitate the extent of bone mineral change. Nonetheless, their studies revealed important relationships among patient and implant factors, and the radiographic appearance of bone loss (19–21).

Bone resorption increases demonstrably with increasing stem size and stiffness. In the study of Engh and Bobyn (21), resorption distal to the level of the lesser trochanter was five-fold more prevalent in cases with cobalt–chromium AML stems that were 13.5 mm or larger in diameter than in cases with smaller stems. Cases demonstrating radiographic signs of bone ingrowth showed greater resorption than those with signs of fibrous tissue fixation. This represented clinical confirmation of theoretical predictions that the stronger the mechanical bond between implant and bone, the greater the extent of stress shielding (33,34). The more rigidly bone is connected to metal, the more its strain (deformation) is governed by the stiffness of the metal. A less rigid connection, as exists with a fibrous interface, enables bone to deform more independently of the adjacent implant and to therefore experience higher loads. The extent of porous coating on the stem also affects the amount and distribution of peri-implant bone resorption.

Extensively porous coated stems funnel load more distally and result in loss of bone density over a greater length of the bone–implant interface. Stems with porous coating confined to the metaphyseal region tend to preserve more bone distal to the level of bone ingrowth but the amount of bone loss within the region of ingrowth can be as much or more than occurs with extensively porous coated stems (50).

Dual energy X-ray absorptiometry (DXA) represents a more sensitive means of detecting and quantifying adaptive remodeling about total hip femoral stems. DXA studies of cadaver retrievals demonstrate losses of bone mineral density ranging from 7% to 52% compared with their contralateral controls, with the greatest losses occurring in association with larger diameter, extensively coated prostheses (22,23,40). These studies also emphasize the important relationship between initial bone mineral content and subsequent remodeling, namely, the lower the initial bone mass the greater is the degree of stress-related bone resorption. This is explained by the direct relationship between bone density and bone stiffness. A femur with less bone mineral density is less stiff relative to the implanted stem. Quantitative analysis of bone remodeling patterns around cemented stems confirms this relationship, demonstrating reductions in bone density approaching the same levels noted with noncemented stems (48). Studies of titanium stems using DXA have generally shown lesser amounts of resorption compared with cobalt–chromium stems, supporting the theory that lower stiffness components attenuate stress shielding (41,80).

Both implant and femoral stiffness are key determinants of bone remodeling (3,6). The same implant placed into two femora of widely varying stiffness will cause different bone remodeling responses. Conversely, the same femur fitted with two implants of different stiffness would also be expected to remodel differently. Stiffness data on human femora have enabled identification of more acceptable ranges of stem/femur stiffness ratios (17). For instance, the original stainless steel Charnley cemented stem and the 10.5 mm diameter Co–Cr AML stem are both roughly 3–5 times less stiff in bending than the diaphysis of the average femur in which they are used. After more than 20 years follow-up with both implants, neither has been associated with exaggerated stress-related bone resorption, certainly not enough as to limit the function or longevity of the procedure. In contrast, AML stems (Co–Cr) 15.0 mm and larger are increasingly stiffer than the human femur in the diaphysis, by factors ranging from about 3 to 5 or more, and cause a relatively high incidence of pronounced peri-implant bone resorption (Fig. 2) (19–21).

The largest stiffness difference between stem and femur is proximal. As the stem flares, the stiffness parameters increase exponentially (because of the fourth power size relationship) and supersede the femur stiffness by factors of 5 to 20 or more, depending on the stem size and material. This disparity may help explain why peri-implant resorption tends to occur faster and is more extensive in the metaphysis. This has implications with regard to modular femoral prostheses designed for increased "fit and fill" of the femur. Large proximal implant segments used to fill the metaphysis will result in large proximal stiffness mismatches that may increase the extent of proximal femoral stress shielding and subsequent bone loss (70). This is true even in the case of a titanium implant, despite its lower elastic modulus.

Polymer and Carbon Composite Hip Stem Designs

The problems of implant stiffness and stress shielding of bone have stimulated interest in the development of more flexible hip stems. A common approach has been to coat metallic stems with low modulus polymers. It must be recognized however, that with increased implant flexibility, the shear stresses at the bone–implant interface can increase during loading (30,33), enabling differential motion between implant and bone and subsequent problems with loosening, pain, or mechanical abrasion/failure of the implant material.

Polymer-coated prostheses originated with the Isoelastic® design of Mathys, a stem with a stainless steel core and a thick casing of polyacetyl resin (53). Despite problems with loosening, stem fracture and polymer wear, the stem was used for many years with reasonable clinical success, primarily in Europe. Clinical results with stems coated with Proplast®, a spongy, porous polymer composite made of carbon fibers and polytetrafluoroethane were often associated with mechanical failure of the material and implant loosening (47,72). Similar results derived when porous polysulfone, a high strength thermoplastic material was applied to a titanium alloy (68). Reports of mechanical failure of the polymer coating, severe osteolysis, and a high revision rate led to its abandonment.

Carbon fiber and carbon–polymer composite materials have been under extensive study as candidates for a new generation of implants. Their potential advantage lies in the combination of high fatigue strength and elastic moduli closer to bone than metals. They can be fabricated to be non-homogeneous so that structural stiffness can be varied within different implant regions and more closely matched to bone. However, clinical trials with carbon–fiber composite femoral components have generally been disappointing, either because of inadequate fixation or problems with stem fracture (1). A fundamental problem with carbon composite implants is that they cannot be fabricated with conventional bone ingrowth surfaces and thus lack the ability for osseointegration. Also, their abrasion resistance to bone has not been fully characterized, leading to concern about the generation of particulate debris in the absence of osseointegration.

Most of the above implants featured either a rigid metal core with a polymeric coating, or a solid polymeric construct, and virtually all have failed mechanically and/or biologically. Mechanical failures occurred largely because the polymer involved did not have the structural integrity to withstand cyclic loading, resulting in either fracture of the implant, or shearing, fragmentation, and delamination of the coating. In either case, there was eventual loss of implant fixation. This often was accompanied by a pronounced inflammatory reaction, osteolysis, and dramatic bone loss in response to the particulate debris.

Extensively Porous Coated Low Stiffness Composite Hip Stem (Epoch®)

A more promising low stiffness composite hip stem design (Epoch®, Zimmer, Warsaw, IN) was recently developed to simultaneously achieve stable skeletal fixation, structural durability, and reduced femoral stress shielding (29,38). The prosthesis combines a thin, forged, cobalt–chromium core surrounded by polyaryletherketone, a thermoplastic polymeric adhesive that is molded between the core and an outer coating of commercially pure titanium fiber metal (Fig. 3). The resultant construct allows for proximal and distal canal filling, yet is significantly less rigid than all-metallic femoral stems crafted of either cobalt–chromium or titanium alloy across the entire range of stem diameters (Fig. 4). Mechanical testing has confirmed adequate

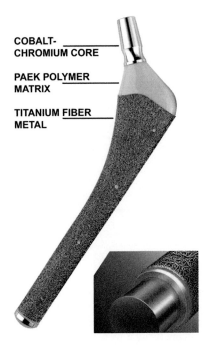

COBALT-CHROMIUM CORE

PAEK POLYMER MATRIX

TITANIUM FIBER METAL

Figure 3   Composite design of an extensively porous coated low stiffness hip stem.

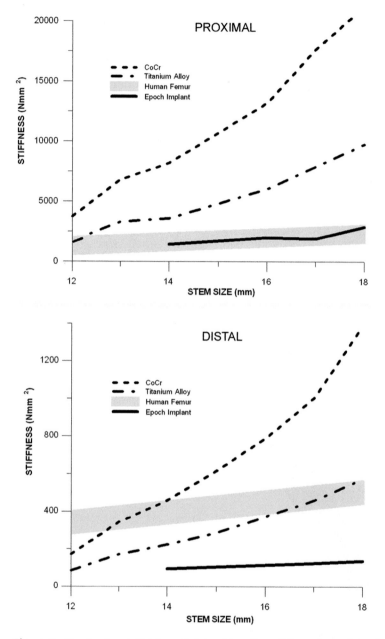

Figure 4 Proximal and distal mediolateral bending stiffness data of titanium stems, cobalt–chromium stems and low stiffness composite stems in different diameters (*measured distally*) compared with the stiffness range of human femora (*shaded band*). Note the high proximal stiffness of the stems relative to bone and the low, almost constant distal stiffness of the composite stems relative to bone.

fatigue strength and canine studies have revealed favorable biological fixation and stability (30,73).

Structured, multicenter clinical trials of the Epoch stem in the United States (171 hips) and 10 other countries (230 hips) were initiated in 1994 at 21 institutions (29). An independent radiographic review assessed implant fixation and osteolysis. Radiostereometric analysis (RSA) studies were performed on 18 cases in Sweden and serial DXA studies were conducted in several locations (31 hips). In addition, one of the participating surgeons conducted bilateral DXA studies on a cohort of patients in whom an Epoch stem was implanted subsequent to contralateral total hip replacement with a similarly sized, extensively porous coated cobalt–chromium AML stem (Depuy, Warsaw, IN).

Radiographically, the implants have consistently displayed signs of bone ingrowth and exhibited no progressive radiolucencies or osteolysis (29). The RSA studies have shown strong initial fixation and minimal stem micromotion in direct comparison with other metallic porous and cemented control implants (38). The DXA analysis revealed excellent periprosthetic bone mineral density (BMD) retention, with significant reduction in stress shielding compared to literature reports on other fully porous coated, all-metallic implants. The greatest average BMD loss of 15.1% was in Gruen zone 7. By comparison, McAuley et al. (50) demonstrated average losses of BMD in Gruen zone 7 of 62.2 and 35.4% about proximally and extensively porous coated AML stems, respectively. Of particular note is the DXA studies on the patients with bilateral hip replacement which indicate a three- to six-fold improvement in bone mineral retention about the proximal zones of the implant on the Epoch side compared with the AML side (Fig. 5).

Stems with Calcium Phosphate Coatings

Calcium phosphate coatings have been added to cementless total hip implants in an attempt to increase the extent and reliability of biologic fixation (42). The most commonly used coatings in clinical practice have been either hydroxyapatite (HA), which has a Ca/P ratio of 1.67, or tricalcium phosphate (TCP), which has a Ca/P ratio of 1.5. Various clinical studies and autopsy retrievals have demonstrated that HA-coated femoral components function equally, and in many cases, superiorly to non-HA-coated implants (2,16,27,39,42,61). However, like all well-fixed femoral components, osseointegration of an HA-coated femoral implant results in adaptive femoral remodeling over time (75).

Radiographic analysis of bone remodeling around proximally HA-coated femoral stems has generated contradictory results. While many studies have noted cancellous condensation at the distal extent of the HA coating as well as distal cortical hypertrophy (15,28,36,82), others have

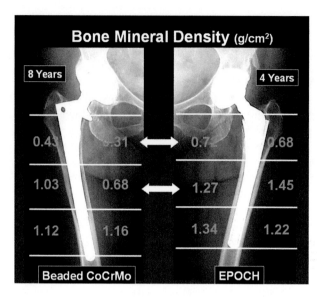

Figure 5 Anteroposterior radiograph of a bilateral case with an extensively porous coated low stiffness composite stem on the *left side* (four years) and an extensively porous coated cobalt–chromium stem on the *right side* (eight years). Superimposed on the radiograph are the BMD measurements in Gruen zones as measured by DXA. Note the marked retention of bone on the Epoch® stem side. *Abbreviations*: BMD, bone mineral density; DXA, dual energy X-ray absorptiometry.

found no effect of the coating on bone remodeling (64,65) These discrepant findings may result from the fact that radiographic examination only permits a subjective impression of femoral bone remodeling without accurate quantification as provided by DXA. As well, it is not clear from the majority of the studies evaluating calcium phosphate coatings how the postoperative femoral remodeling varies from that of uncoated implants. Few studies have actually compared the effect of using a femoral implant with and without HA coating on postoperative femoral remodeling or have used DXA to quantify the differences (16,61,63,66,69,82).

As measured with DXA, postoperative femoral bone loss has been found to be less with HA-coated cementless implants than with implants of the same shape without the HA coating (63,69). Scott and Jaffe (63) evaluated the effect of HA coating on femoral bone remodeling in three patients following bilateral cementless bipolar arthroplasties. In each patient, a proximally porous coated cobalt–chromium femoral component was implanted on one side while a proximally HA-coated titanium stem of identical geometry was implanted on the contralateral side. DXA analysis five to seven years postoperatively demonstrated that the cortical hypertrophy present in the HA-coated stems resulted in 22% and 36% more BMD in Gruen zones 2 and 6 than in the uncoated stems. Overall, the HA-coated implants averaged 4% to 21% greater BMD than the porous coated implants. Although the differences have been attributed to the HA coating, the differing degree and pattern of bone remodeling between the two stems may also have been affected by the different stem alloys (and hence different stiffness) and/or the presence or absence of porous coating.

There is one report of a prospective randomized trial that quantified with DXA the effect of calcium phosphate coating on femoral bone remodeling using identical proximally porous-coated femoral components (Multilock® stem, Zimmer, Warsaw, IN) (69). Twenty-two hips were randomized to a control group and 17 hips to a group with HA-TCP coating on the stem. Periprosthetic BMD measurements were compared at various intervals up to two years. Although alterations in BMD occurred with both stem designs, by two years hips in the HA–TCP group had greater BMD measurements than those hips with the identical uncoated stem. This difference reached statistical significance in Gruen zones 1–4, 6, and 7. The mean BMD loss was 20.0% for the control group and 9.3% for the group with HA–TCP coating. The improved retention most likely results from increased bone formation in the periprosthetic regions secondary to the osteogenic effects of the coating and/or increased load transfer between implant and bone because of enhanced osseointegration.

BONE RESORPTION IN THE HIP—ACETABULUM

There is very little information about periprosthetic bone remodeling in the pelvis, although mathematical modeling has predicted that because of altered load distribution after acetabular cup implantation, bone density will tend to hypertrophy at the periphery and diminish in the dome region (13,14,32,43). Wright et al. (81) recently published the only detailed report in the literature about the early natural history of changes in periprosthetic acetabular bone after hip replacement. Quantitative computed tomography was used to measure BMD in 26 patients with a cementless Trilogy component (Zimmer, Warsaw, IN). Baseline BMD was measured within the first five days of surgery and follow-up BMD was measured an average of 1.3 years after surgery. The region of interest was defined by a cylinder of cancellous bone centered within the ilium, directly cephalad to the acetabular dome. At follow-up, BMD was found to have diminished appreciably, more so closer to the implant than further away, with maximum average decreases of 26% to 33%.

The stiffness of the solid metal backing of an acetabular cup is much greater than that of the native subchondral bone and the mismatch in elasticity tends to direct loads toward the edges or periphery of the bone–implant interface (32,43). Because cancellous bone of the central part of

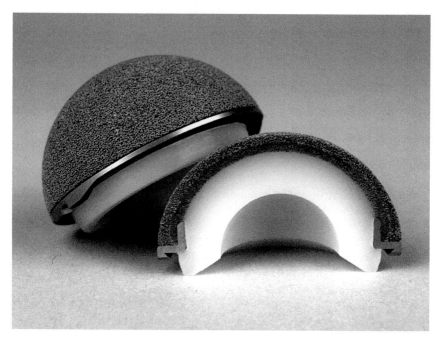

Figure 6 A low stiffness nonmodular acetabular cup construct in which polyethylene is compression molded directly into a porous tantalum metal backing.

the ilium is shielded from physiological stress it is prone to resorption, as documented by Wright et al. (81) Since there are no mid-term or long-term studies that have quantified the extent or progression of peri-acetabular implant bone resorption, it is not possible to predict whether stress shielding has an effect on implant fixation or implant migration (as could be measured by RSA). However, it is conceivable that, independent of frank aseptic loosening, progressive or extensive bone loss could, in the long term, diminish mechanical support of the implant and lead to progressive migration of an implant within the acetabular bed. This concern has led to the development of acetabular cup designs with increased flexibility through the use of lower stiffness porous metal backing constructs (Fig. 6), most notably those described by Morscher et al. (54,55,78) and Lewis et al. (7,45) Finite element studies predict that the acetabular stress pattern with a low stiffness porous tantalum cup design is more physiologic than with a traditional metal-backed design, closely approximating the situation with a cemented, all-polyethylene cup (58). Rationale for lower stiffness acetabular implant constructs is provided by the study of Böhler et al. (8) which found greater early vertical migration and a greater aseptic loosening rate with acetabular cups in which an alumina ceramic liner was used as opposed to a polyethylene liner. The much higher stiffness of the cups with the ceramic liners and the resulting altered peri-implant bone stress distribution was associated with the differences in migration and loosening. While stress-related bone resorption probably occurs to a lesser extent with cemented all-polyethylene cups than with metal-backed noncemented cups, the latter are currently preferred by most surgeons because of their potential for better long-term fixation.

BONE RESORPTION IN THE KNEE—FEMUR

Stress-related bone resorption in the knee has been studied much less than in the hip. The first recognition of the potential for resorption in the distal femur was by Bobyn et al. (4) who described a canine experiment with porous coated stemmed femoral implants in which substantial bone loss was documented within a few months of surgery. Changing the design by elimination of the stem noticeably reduced the extent of distal stress relief (5). The first clinical description of the problem was by Cameron and Cameron (12) who documented stress relief osteoporosis of the anterior femoral condyles in the vast majority of cases after total knee replacement. Because of the rigidity of the anterior flange of the femoral component of a knee replacement, patellar forces cannot load the anterior distal femur with consequent loss of bone density (Fig. 7). This phenomenon has been described several times in the literature (18,52,56,60,62,71,74,77).

Mintzer et al. (52) observed noticeable bone loss in about two-thirds of knee replacement patients independent of implant design or whether bone cement was used for fixation. Ebert et al. (18), in a minimum four-year follow-up of 121 cemented and noncemented total knee arthroplasties, observed osteopenia in the distal femur of each case within six months of surgery, without progression after one year. These earlier studies were retrospective and based on qualitative observations of roentgenographically detectable bone loss. A recent study by Petersen et al. (56) used dual-photon absorptiometry to quantitate distal femoral bone remodeling in patients with uncemented knee arthroplasties. Compared with measurements taken three months after surgery, BMD loss averaging 36% was documented behind the anterior flange two years postoperatively. Using finite element analyses, Tissakht et al. (71) and van Lenthe et al. (74), confirmed that reductions of bone stress and BMD of at least 30% are to be expected after knee replacement, particularly in the most antero-distal region of the femur. Moreover, the mathematical models predicted that the more complete the bonding of the bone–implant interface, the more extensive the stress shielding and the shorter the time required to reach a particular level of bone resorption. The suggestion from this latter finding is that debonding of the bone–implant interface, at least partially, may be an approach for reducing resorption. This of course is counterproductive to the surgical goal of establishing the best possible attachment of the implant to bone.

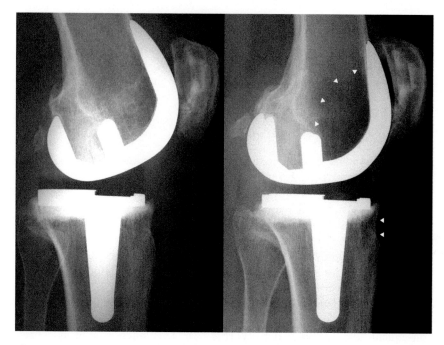

Figure 7 Postoperative (*left*) and five-year (*right*) radiographs of a knee replacement case illustrating marked anterodistal bone resorption in the femur because of stress shielding. There is also a small anterior zone of bone density loss in the proximal tibia but it is subtle and more evident on the actual plain films.

BONE RESORPTION IN THE KNEE—TIBIA

There are varying reports of stress-related bone resorption in the proximal tibia after knee replacement, depending on the type of implant studied and time period of examination (9). One of the earliest studies by Bohr and Lund utilized dual photon absorptiometry to measure BMD adjacent to uncemented PCA® implants (Howmedica, Rutherford, NJ) up to 3.5 years after surgery (10). They noted an average increase of BMD of about 15% for the first six months, followed by a gradual diminution after two years to levels slightly less than preoperatively. Hvid et al. (35) used computed tomography to study bone density changes around cemented tibial implants years postoperatively and noted an overall density loss, with the greatest change of about 30% occurring in rheumatoid arthritis patients. Petersen et al. (57), using dual photon absorptiometry in a more extensive study of 25 uncemented total knee replacements, noted the sensitivity of the medial and lateral tibial condyles to mechanical realignment of the knee soon after surgery, with unloaded areas losing BMD and newly loaded areas gaining BMD. Overall though, the density for all regions of interest underneath the tibial component showed a significant and progressive decrease in BMD that reached 22% at three years follow-up. In a recent study, Regner et al. (59) used triple-energy X-ray absorptiometry to examine changes in BMD in the medial tibial condyles of patients with Freeman–Samuelson hydroxyapatite-coated (DePuy, Warsaw, IN) and Miller–Galante II (Zimmer, Warsaw, IN) uncemented prostheses. The overall decrease in bone mineral at five years was 26%, with greater decreases noted in the cases with the Freeman–Samuelson implants. This design includes a larger, longer central stem that probably caused more proximal stress shielding because of more distal fixation. Li and Nilsson (46) studied 28 cases for two years using DXA and noted an initial average loss of BMD of 13% for the first three months followed by a return to initial levels out to the study endpoint. Although the average change in BMD between postoperative levels and those at two years was not statistically significant, the variation between individual patients was very large, ranging from a 44% increase to a 98% decrease. Levitz et al. (44) published the longest term analysis of bone density changes in the proximal tibia after knee replacement, with data on seven patients gathered postoperatively and eight years after surgery. The average density decrease was 36% as measured with dual photon absorptiometry and DXA.

The proximal tibia is clearly sensitive to changes in load distribution. Surgical realignment of the knee causes measurable changes in bone density in the lateral and medial compartments, with the once overstressed side tending to lose bone and the once understressed side tending to gain bone in the first few months of surgery. Bone remodeling resulting from surface replacement with an implant is variable and generally not as radiographically noticeable as in the distal femur (Fig. 7). It tends to be more pronounced in female patients and rheumatoid patients, those cohorts with lower initial bone stock. From a mechanical perspective, although the proximal tibia is loaded in compression there tends to be uneven distribution of stress transfer to bone. The stiffer the tibial implant the greater is the tendency for forces on the medial and lateral tibial condyles to be localized directly under the line of action of loading and the greater is the extent of peripheral stress shielding of bone. Also, central keels or stems are relatively stiff and tend to funnel load distally and stress shield the bone immediately beneath the implant, particularly if they are porous coated and become bone ingrown. This problem also pertains to peripheral porous coated pegs but less so with decreasing size and stiffness. Since stress-related bone resorption in the proximal tibia often reaches levels of 20–30% or more, it would seem prudent to adjust implant design to minimize the extent of stress shielding. One helpful approach, as just alluded to, is to avoid large and/ or long central stems where possible. As with acetabular implants, another approach is to reduce the mechanical rigidity of the implant using a material

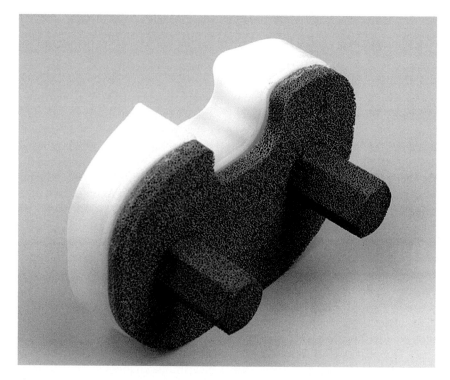

Figure 8 A low stiffness nonmodular tibial knee implant utilizing the same type of compression molded polyethylene construct depicted in Figure 6.

with lower stiffness properties than either titanium or cobalt–chromium alloy (Fig. 8) (7).

DISCUSSION AND CONCLUSIONS

It is clear from a review of the literature that stress-related bone resorption occurs to some extent around all hip and knee joint replacement implants. The rate of resorptive remodeling is quite rapid, with most of the change occurring within the first six months to two years. If there is progressive bone mineral loss beyond two years, it is relatively slight. The extent of resorption varies with different implant designs but it is often substantial, often reaching levels of 30% or more in certain peri-implant regions. From a radiographic standpoint, resorption is most easily recognized in the proximal femur adjacent to hip stems and much less so in other periprosthetic regions. As with wear debris-induced osteolysis, the actual extent of stress induced bone loss is always worse than can be perceived radiographically. Resorption is essentially a "silent" phenomenon in that it is not painful and patients are unaware of its progression.

In the case of the proximal femur, even in rather severe cases of stress shielding with large and stiff extensively porous coated hip stems, there do not appear to be identifiable clinical consequences to bone loss. Bugbee et al. (11) and more recently McAuley et al. (49) and Engh et al. (25) have closely reviewed cases with AML stems for long-term effects of stress shielding. Compared with cases showing little or no stress shielding, those with pronounced bone loss extending distal to the lesser trochanter actually tend to be associated with a lower revision rate and a higher likelihood of radiographic signs of bone ingrowth. Moreover, cases with pronounced bone loss do not show an increased propensity for the osteolytic type of bone resorption resulting from accumulated wear debris. This may in part be explained by patient-related differences. Patients with large femoral canals requiring larger, stiffer stems are often less active. Younger, more active patients with better bone and smaller canals develop less stress shielding, but are more prone to develop wear-related osteolysis. In any event, peri-implant bone that loses density because of stress shielding does not appear to be more susceptible to particle-induced osteolysis. Late term spontaneous bone fracture such as trochanteric avulsion does occur around porous coated implants but usually because of osteolysis from wear debris and not more so in cases with pronounced stress-related resorption than in cases with little or none. In this sense, stress shielding could be described as benign.

However, an argument always exists for preserving as much bone stock as possible. This is wise in both the shorter term, where implant support and stable fixation will benefit from mechanically sound host bone, and in the longer term, where it is helpful to have as much host bone as possible should a subsequent reconstruction be required. Germane to this issue is the study of Petersen et al. (57) who showed with RSA that tibial implant migration is less in patients with higher BMD, i.e., the stronger the bone foundation, the more stable the implant. A very important finding in the same study was that tibial component migration continued to progress between one and three years after surgery, but less so in patients with higher BMD. Böhler et al. (8) discussed similar findings in the acetabulum, with greater and progressive vertical cup migration occurring in patients with poorer quality bone stock. These results are probably somewhat dependent on the individual implant design and it is not known to what extent slow, continuous implant migration is related to aseptic loosening. However, the studies of Böhler et al. (8) and Petersen et al. (57) demonstrated that progressive implant migration is possible and is dependent on BMD. Thus, as supportive bone loses density through stress shielding, it may predispose to greater progressive implant migration in the absence of frank loosening (8). This is a strong argument for utilizing implants that are as mechanically compatible with bone as possible so as to minimize stress-related bone loss and maintain the best possible mechanical support. This is especially true with the advent of improved bearing technologies that promise very long-term wear-resistant articulations. Such considerations are the fundamental basis for the development and clinical testing of more compliant femoral stems, acetabular cups and tibial plateaus, as previously discussed. In this light, the mid-term radiographic and clinical data with the low stiffness stem design described by Glassman et al. are very encouraging (29,38). Given the well-documented history of femoral stress shielding around hip stems, it would seem reasonable to pursue any sound approach that can attenuate the problem. Recognition of stress-related bone resorption in the acetabulum and proximal tibia is more recent and lower stiffness implant designs require additional clinical follow-up to assess their effectiveness in alleviating periprosthetic BMD loss. For the moment there does not appear to be an implant design solution to the problem of bone loss in the anterior distal femur because of stress redistribution caused by knee implants.

A final note concerns recent information about managing periprosthetic bone loss through oral bisphosphonate therapy. Soininvaara et al. (67) showed in a one-year randomized, controlled trial that patients taking 10 mg of alendronate daily maintained distal femoral BMD values close to the baseline values while control patients showed significant bone loss. Similar findings in the hip have been noted by Venesmaa et al. (76) and Wilkinson et al. (79). Also of related interest is the report by Hilding et al. who showed with RSA that administration of clodronate reduces prosthetic migration in total knee patients. This is further support for the philosophy that preservation of bone stock about joint replacement implants is important to maximize implant stability in both the short and long term.

REFERENCES

1. Allcock S, Ali MA. Early failure of a carbon-fiber composite femoral component. J Arthroplasty 1997; 12:356–358.
2. Bloebaum RD, Bachus KN, Rubman MH, Dorr L. Postmortem comparative analysis of titanium and hydroxyapatite analysis of titanium and porous-coated femoral implants retrieved from the same patient. A case study. J Arthroplasty 1993; 8:203–211.
3. Bobyn JD, Glassman AH, Goto H, Krygier JJ, Brooks CE, Miller JE. The effect of stem stiffness on femoral bone resorption after canine porous-coated total hip arthroplasty. Clin Orthop 1990; 261:196–213.
4. Bobyn JD, Cameron HU, Abdulla D, Pilliar RM, Weatherly GC. Biologic fixation and bone modeling with an unconstrained canine total knee prosthesis. Clin Orthop Rel Res 1982; 166:301–312.
5. Bobyn JD, Abdulla D, Pilliar RM, Cameron HU. The effect of porous-surfaced knee prosthesis design on adaptive bone modeling. Proceedings of 2nd World Congress on Biomaterials, Washington, April, 1984.
6. Bobyn JD, Mortimer, ES, Glassman AH, Engh CA, Miller JE, Brooks CE. Producing and avoiding stress shielding: Laboratory and clinical observations of noncemented total hip arthroplasty. Clin Orthop 1992; 274:79–96.

7. Bobyn JD, Stackpool G, Toh K-K, Hacking SA, Tanzer M. Bone ingrowth characteristics and interface mechanics of a new porous tantalum biomaterial. J Bone Joint Surg Br 1999; 81-B:907–914.

8. Böhler M, Schachinger W, Wolfl G, Krismer M, Mayr G, Salzer M. Comparison of migration in modular sockets with ceramic and polyethylene inlays. Orthopaedics 2000; 23:1261–1266.

9. Bohr HH, Schaadt O. Mineral content of upper tibia assessed by dual photon densitometry. Acta Orthop Scand 1987; 58:557–559.

10. Bohr HH, Lund B. Bone mineral density of the proximal tibia following uncemented arthroplasty. J Arthroplasty 1987; 2:309–312.

11. Bugbee WD, Culpepper WJ, Engh CA Jr, Engh CA Sr. Long-term clinical consequences of stress-shielding after total hip arthroplasty without cement. J Bone Joint Surg Am 1997; 79–A:1007–1012.

12. Cameron HU, Cameron G. Stress relief osteoporosis of the anterior femoral condyles in total knee replacement. Orthop Rev 1987; 16:449–456.

13. Carter DR, Vasu R, Harris WH. Periacetabular stress distributions after joint replacement with subchondral bone retention. Acta Orthop Scand 1983; 54:29–35.

14. Carter DR, Fyhrie DP, Whalen RT. Trabecular bone density and loading history: regulation of connective tissue biology by mechanical energy. J Biomech 1987; 20:785–794.

15. D'Antonio JA, Capello WN, Manley MT. Remodeling of bone around hydroxyapatite-coated femoral stems. J Bone Joint Surg 1996; 78-A:1126–1234.

16. Dorr L, Zhinian W, Song M, Ranawat A. Bilateral total hip arthroplasty comparing hydroxyapatite coating to porous-coated fixation. J Arthroplasty 1998; 13:729–736.

17. Dujovne AR, Bobyn JD, Krygier JJ, Miller JE, Brooks CE. Mechanical compatibility of noncemented hip prostheses with the human femur. J Arthroplasty 1993; 8:7–22.

18. Ebert FR, Krackow KA, Lennox DW, Hungerford DS. Minimum 4-year follow-up of the PCA total knee arthroplasty in rheumatoid patients. J Arthroplasty 1992; 7:101–108.

19. Engh CA, Bobyn JD, Glassman AH. Porous coated hip replacement. The factors governing bone ingrowth, stress shielding, and clinical results. J Bone Joint Surg Br 1987; 69B:45–55.

20. Engh CA, Bobyn JD. Biological Fixation in Total Hip Arthroplasy. Thorofare: Slack Inc. 1985.

21. Engh CA, Bobyn JD. The influence of stem size and extent of porous coating on femoral bone resorption after primary cementless hip arthroplasty. Clin Orthop 1988; 231:7–28.

22. Engh CA, O'Connor D, Jasty M, McGovern TF, Bobyn JD, Harris WH. Quantification of implant micromotion, strain shielding, and bone resorption with porous-coated anatomic medullary locking femoral prostheses. Clin Orthop 1992; 285:13–29.

23. Engh CA, McGovern TF, Bobyn JD, Harris WH. A quantitative evaluation of periprosthetic bone-remodeling after cementless total hip arthroplasty. J Bone Joint Surg Am 1992; 74–A:1009–1020.

24. Engh CA Jr, McAuley JP, Sychterz CJ, Sacco ME, Engh CA Sr. The accuracy and reproducibility of radiographic assessment of stress-shielding. J Bone Joint Surg Am 2000; 82-A:1414–1420.
25. Engh CA Jr, Young AM, Engh CA Sr, Hopper RH Jr. Clinical consequences of stress-shielding after porous-coated hip arthroplasty: A mean 14 year follow-up. Clin Orthop, 2003, 417:157–163.
26. Finsen V, Anda S. Accuracy of visually estimated bone mineralization in routine radiographs of the lower extremity. Skeletal Radiol 1988; 17:270–275.
27. Furlong RJ, Osborn JF. Fixation of hip prostheses by hydroxyapatite ceramic coatings. J Bone Joint Surg 1991; 73-B:741–745.
28. Geesink RGT, Hoefnagels NHM. Six-year results of hydroxyapatite-coated total hip replacement. J Bone Joint Surg 1995; 77-B:534–547.
29. Glassman AH, Crowninshield RD, Schenck R, Herberts P. A low stiffness composite biologically fixed prosthesis. Clin Orthop 2001; 393:128–136.
30. Harvey EJ, Bobyn JD, Tanzer M, Krygier JJ. Effect of flexibility of the femoral stem on bone-remodeling and fixation of the stem in a canine total hip arthroplasty model without cement. J Bone Joint Surg Am 1999; 81-A:93–107.
31. Hilding M, Ryd L, Toksvig-Larsen S, Aspenberg P. Clodronate prevents prosthetic migration: a randomized radiostereometric study of 50 total knee patients. Acta Orthop Scand 2000; 71:553–557.
32. Huiskes R. Finite element analysis of acetabular reconstruction. Noncemented threaded cups. Acta Orthop Scand 1987; 58:620–625.
33. Huiskes R, Weinans H, van Rietbergen B. The relationship between stress shielding and bone resorption around total hip stems and the effects of flexible materials. Clin Orthop 1992; 274:124–134.
34. Huiskes R. Stress shielding and bone resorption in THA. clinical versus computer-simulation studies. Acta Orthop Belg 59 (Suppl) 1993; 1:118–129.
35. Hvid I, Bentzen SM, Jorgensen J. Remodeling of the tibial plateau after knee replacement: CT bone densitometry. Acta Orthop Scan 1988; 59:567–573.
36. Jaffe WL, Scott DF. Total hip arthroplasty with hydroxyapatite-coated prostheses. J Bone Joint Surg 1996; 78-A:1918–1934.
37. Jacobs JJ, Sumner DR, Galante JO. Mechanisms of bone loss associated with total hip replacement. Orthop Clin North Am 1993; 24:583–590.
38. Kärrholm J, Anderberg C, Snorrason F, Thanner J, Langeland N, Malchau H, Herberts. Evaluation of a femoral stem with reduced stiffness. A randomized study with use of radiostereometry and bone densitometry. J Bone Joint Surg 2002; 84A:1651–1658.
39. Kärrholm J, Malchau H, Snorrason F, Herberts P. Micromotion of femoral stems in total hip arthroplasty. A randomized study of cemented, hydroxyapatite-coated and porous-coated stems with roentgen stereophotogrammetric analysis. J Bone Joint Surg 1994; 76-A:1692–1705.
40. Kilgus DJ, Shimaoka EE, Tipton JS, Eberle RW. Dual energy x-ray absorptiometry measurement of bone mineral density around porous-coated cementless femoral implants: methods and preliminary results. J Bone Joint Surg 1993; 75:279–287.
41. Kiratli BJ, Heiner JP, McBeath AA, Wilson MA. Determination of bone mineral density by dual x-ray absorptiometry in patients with uncemented total hip arthroplasty. J Orthop Res 1992; 10:836–844.

42. Kroon PO, Freeman MAR. Hydroxyapatite coating of hip prostheses. Effect on migration into the the femur. J Bone Joint Surg 1992; 74-B:518–522.
43. Levenston ME, Beaupre GS, Carter DR, Schurman DJ. Skeletogenesis and bone remodeling theory applied to the peri-acetabular region. Trans Orthop Res Soc 1992:547.
44. Levitz CL, Lotke PA, Karp JS. Long-term changes in bone mineral density following total knee replacement. Clin Orthop December:1995; 68–72.
45. Lewis R, O'Keefe T, Unger A. Monobloc trabecular metal acetabulum—2 to 5 year results. Proc 70th Meet Am Acad Orthop Surg, 2003.
46. Li MG, Nilsson KG. Changes in bone mineral density at the proximal tibia after total knee arthroplasty: A 2-year follow-up of 28 knees using dual energy x-ray absorptiometry. J Orthop Res 2000; 18:40–47.
47. Maathuis PGM, Visser JD. High failure rate of soft-interface stem coating for fixation of femoral endoprostheses. J Arthroplasty 1996; 11:548–552.
48. Maloney WJ, Sychterz C, Bragdon C, McGovern T, Jasty M, Engh CA, Harris WH. Skeletal response to well fixed femoral components inserted with and without cement. Clin Orthop 1996; 333:15–26.
49. McAuley JP, Culpepper WJ, Engh CA. Total hip arthroplasty. Concerns with extensively porous coated femoral components. Clin Orthop 1998; 355:182–188.
50. McAuley JP, Sychterz CJ, Engh CA. Influence of porous coating level on proximal femoral remodeling. Clin Orthop 2000; 371:146–153.
51. Miller JE, Kelebay LC. Bone ingrowth-disuse osteoporosis. Orthop Trans 1981; 5:380.
52. Mintzer CM, Robertson DD, Rackemann S, Ewald FC, Scott RD, Spector M. Bone loss in the distal anterior femur after total knee arthroplasty. Clin Orthop 1990; 260:135–143.
53. Morscher E, Dick W. Cementless fixation of "Isoelastic" hip endoprostheses manufactured from plastic materials. Clin Orthop 1983; 176:77–87.
54. Morscher EW. Current status of acetabular fixation in primary total hip arthroplasy. Clin Orthop 1992; 274:172–193.
55. Morscher EW, Berli B, Jockers W, Schenk R. Rationale of a flexible press fit cup in total hip replacement. 5-year followup in 280 procedures. Clin Orthop 1997; 341:42–50.
56. Petersen MM, Olsen C, Lauritzen JB, Lund B. Changes in bone mineral density of the distal femur following uncemented total knee arthroplasty. J Arthroplasty 1995; 10:7–77.
57. Petersen MM, Nielsen PT, Lebech A, Toksvig-Larsen S, Lund B. Preoperative bone mineral density of the proximal tibia and migration of the tibial component after uncemented total knee arthroplasty. J Arthroplasty 1999; 14: 77–81.
58. Poggie RA, Brown TD, Pedersen DR. Finite element analysis of peri-acetabular stress of cemented, metal-backed, and porous tantalum backed acetabular components. Proc 45th Meet ORS, 1999:747.
59. Regnér LR, Carlsson LV, Kärrholm JN, Hansson TH, Herberts PG, Swanpalmer J. Bone mineral and migratory patterns in uncemented total knee arthroplasties: a randomized 5-year follow-up study of 38 knees. Acta Orthop Scand 1999; 70:603–608.

60. Robertson DD, Mintzer CM, Weissman BN, Ewald FC, LeBoff M, Spector M. Distal loss of femoral bone following total knee arthroplasty. Measurement with visual and computer-processing of roentgenograms and dual-energy x-ray absorptiometry. J Bone Joint Surg Am 1994; 76A:66–76.

61. Rothman RH, Hozack WJ, Ranawat A, Moriarty L. Hydroxyapatite-coated femoral stems. A matched-pair analysis of coated and uncoated implants. J Bone Joint Surg 1996; 78-A:319–324.

62. Seitz P, Ruegsegger P, Gschwend N, Dubs L. Changes in local bone density after knee arthroplasty: the use of quantitative computed tomography. J Bone Joint Surg Br 1987; 69:407–411.

63. Scott DF, Jaffe WL. Host-bone response to porous-coated cobalt-chrome and hydroxyapatite-coated titanium femoral components in hip arthroplasty. Dual-energy X-ray absorptiometry analysis of paired bilateral cases at 5 to 7 years. J Arthroplasty 1996; 11:429–437.

64. Smart RC, Barbagallo S, Slater GL. Measurement of periprosthetic bone density in hip arthroplasty using dual energy x-ray absorptiometry. J Arthroplasty 1996; 11:445–452.

65. Søballe K, Hansen ES, Rasmussen HB, Bünger C. Hydroxyapatite coating converts fibrous tissue to bone around loaded implants. J Bone Joint Surg 1993; 75-B:270–278.

66. Søballe K, Toksvig-Larsen S, Gelineck J, Fruensgaard S, Hansen ES, Ryd L, Lucht U, Bünger C. Migration of hydroxyapatite coated femoral prostheses. A roentgen stereophotogrammetric study. J Bone Joint Surg 1993; 75-B:681–687.

67. Soininvaara TA, Jurvelin JS, Miettinen HJA, Suomalainen OT, Alhava EM, Kroger PJ. Effect of alendronate on periprosthetic bone loss after total knee arthroplasty: A one-year, randomized, controlled trial of 19 patients. Calcif Tissue Int 2002; 71:472–477.

68. Spector M, Heyligers I, Roberson JR. Porous polymers for biological fixation. Clin Orthop 1988; 235:207–219.

69. Tanzer M, Kantor S, Rosenthall L, Bobyn JD. Femoral remodeling after a porous-coated total hip arthroplasty with and without hydroxyapatite–tricalcium phosphate coating. A prospective randomized trial. J Arthroplasty 2001; 16:552–558.

70. Tanzer M, Chan S, Brooks CE, Bobyn JD. Primary cementless total hip arthroplasty using a modular femoral component. A minimum 6-year follow up. J Arthroplasty 2001; 16(suppl):64–70.

71. Tissakht M, Ahmed AM, Chan KC. Stress shielding in the distal femur following TKR: Effect of bone/implant interface condition. Transactions of 39th Annual Meeting of ORS, San Francisco, 1993:426.

72. Tullos HS, McCaskill BL, Dickey R, Davidson J. Total hip arthroplasty with a low-modulus porous-coated femoral component. J Bone Joint Surg 1984; 66A:888–898.

73. Turner TM, Sumner DR, Urban RM, et al. Maintenance of proximal cortical bone with use of aless stiff femoral component in hemiarthroplasty of the hip without cement. J Bone Joint Surg Am 1997; 79A:1381–1390.

74. Van Lenthe GH, De Waal Malefijt MC, Huiskes R. Stress shielding after total knee replacement may cause bone resorption in the distal femur. J Bone Joint Surg Br 1997; 79-B1:117–122.

75. Van Rietbergen B, Huiskes R. Load transfer and stress shielding of the hydroxyapatite–ABG hip. J Arthroplasty 2001; 16:55–63.
76. Venesmaa PK, Kroger HP, Miettinen HJ, Jurvelin JS, Suomalainen OT, Alhava EM. Alendronate reduces periprosthetic bone loss after uncemented primary total hip arthroplasty: a prospective randomized study. J Bone Miner Res 2001; 16:2126–2131.
77. Whiteside LA, Pafford J. Load transfer characteristics of a noncemented total knee arthroplasty. Clin Orthop 1989; 239:168–177.
78. Widmer KH, Zurfluh B, Morscher EW. Load transfer and fixation mode of press–fit acetabular sockets. J Arthroplasty 2002; 17:926–935.
79. Wilkinson JM, Stockley I, Peel NF, Hamer AJ, Elson RA, Barrington NA, Eastell R. Effect of pamidronate in preventing local bone loss after total hip arthroplasty: a randomized, double-blind, controlled trial. J Bone Miner Res 2001; 16:556–564.
80. Wixson RL, Stulberg SD, Van Flandern GJ, Puri L. Maintenance of proximal bone mass with an uncemented femoral stem. Analysis with dual-energy x-ray absorptiometry. J Arthroplasty 1997; 12:365–373.
81. Wright JM, Pellicci PM, Salvati EA, Ghelman B, Roberts MM, Koh JL. Bone density adjacent to press-fit acetabular components. J Bone Joint Surg Am 2001; 83-A:529–536.
82. Yee AJM, Kreder HK, Bookman I, Davey JR. A randomized trial of hydroxyapatite coated prosthesis in total hip arthroplasty. Clin Orthop 1999; 366:120–132.

16

Pressure- and Motion-Induced Factors in Implant Loosening

Per Aspenberg

*Department of Neuroscience and Locomotion, Section for Orthopaedics,
Faculty of Health Science, Linköping University, Linköping, Sweden*

INTRODUCTION: A LESSON FROM THE DENTISTS

It is hard to imagine a greater challenge to a permanent osseous implant than to put it in an environment where one end of the implant is exposed to high concentrations of debris and bacteria while the opposite end maintains direct metal to bone contact without hydroxyapatite or a porous coating, and the entire implant is subjected to very high loads. Yet, this is done routinely by dentists using the so-called Brånemark concept (1). Such implants that have survived their first postoperative year have a 10-year survival comparable to the best total joint prostheses. How is this possible? When implanting a Brånemark implant, the use of an atraumatic operative technique is considered extremely important. Further, after the implant is in place, the mucosa is sutured and the implant allowed to osseointegrate under unloaded conditions before the outer end of the implant is exposed and attached to a load-bearing device. Immediate load bearing using this kind of implant in cancellous regions almost inevitably leads to failure. The superior result with unloaded osseointegration emphasizes the importance of the early postoperative period for the longevity of the implant. Some early biological processes have to proceed under unloaded conditions for these implants to be successful.

EARLY MIGRATION PREDICTS LATE LOOSENING

The lesson from the dentists suggests that the initial phase after implantation may be crucial. There is considerable evidence that this is also true for total joint implants. It has now been demonstrated for all components of total knee and hip prostheses that migration of the implant versus the bone bed during the first postoperative year predicts late loosening. This has been best shown using radiostereometric analysis (RSA), a method developed in Lund, Sweden, in the 1970s (2) and used in many academic orthopaedic centers in northern Europe. Unfortunately, this method has only recently been used in the United States and therefore, important findings using this method have not been sufficiently appreciated. For RSA, the patient receives 0.5 mm tantalum beads implanted in the bone bed at a distance from the total joint component. The total joint component also has similar markers fixed to it, and tantalum beads can also be implanted in the cement layer. Postoperatively and during follow-up visits, simultaneous X-ray exposures are produced in two different planes in a calibration set-up (Fig. 1). Using computerized trigonometric calculations it is then possible to measure changes in the position of the implant relative to the bone with an accuracy (95% confidence interval) down to 0.1–0.2 mm (3). For the tibial component of total knee implants, migration of the component versus the bone bed during the second postoperative year exceeding 0.2 mm has an 85% predictive power for implant failure, i.e., a patient with migration exceeding 0.2 mm has an 85% risk of needing a reoperation in the future (Fig. 2) (3). For hip prostheses the risk of loosening of femoral or acetabular components is also correlated to early migration, but the level of acceptable migration varies considerably between prosthesis designs (4,5). Also with conventional radiographic methods, postoperative migration of about 2 mm has been shown to predict failure (6–9).

Thus, it has been demonstrated beyond doubt that late loosening is strongly linked to events during the early postoperative period. Further, it is obvious from the literature that late loosening is related to various design variables of joint implants and also to surgical skill. In the Swedish Total Knee Register, surgeons performing less than 23 unicompartmental knee operations per year have a significantly higher risk of revision than surgeons doing 23 or more operations per year (10). This also indicates that late loosening to a large extent is a consequence of peri- or postoperatively events that are reflected by early component migration in relation to the bone bed. To a certain extent this migration is related to the biology of the bone bed. It is not only the consequence of micro fracture or mechanical settling, because when osteoclastic activity is diminished by bisphosphonate treatment, migration becomes significantly less (11).

The early loss of fixation theory for implant loosening has been advocated for over a decade by Mjöberg and others that have claimed that the

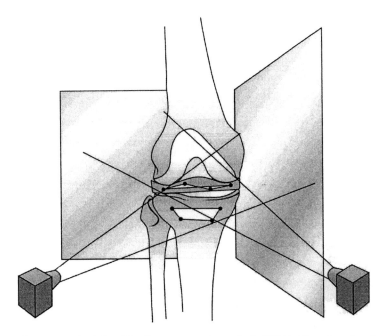

Figure 1 Principle of Radiostereometric analysis (RSA). Tantalum bead markers in the prosthesis form a "rigid body" whose position is defined in relation to a similar rigid body of markers in the bone and a calibration cage. This is done by using simultaneous X-ray exposures and computerized trigonometric calculations. The precision is dependent on the acquired bead configuration. Normally, a 0.1–0.2 mm change in position of a prosthesis versus the bone is significant (i.e., 0.1–0.2 mm migration from one examination to the next).

hypothesis of particle induced loosening includes a number of unnecessary ad hoc assumptions and further that it can neither explain the relation between early migration and late loosening, nor the relation between surgical experience or implant design and late results (12,13). Charnley showed in his pioneering work that the bone layer adjacent to a cemented implant becomes necrotic after the operation (14,15). Considering the trauma to the microvasculature it is hard to imagine that osteocytes close also to an uncemented implant would survive. Because osteocyte death is a strong signal for osteoclastic resorption, intense remodeling will start in the bone layer close to the fresh implant. However, as with remodeling of necrotic bone in other areas, this remodeling is unlikely to show the normal coupling between osteclastic and osteoblastic activity (16). Therefore, there is a risk that osteoclastic destruction of the necrotic bone bed will dominate over osteoblastic repair. This appears to be the case during implant migration, since it can be diminished with bisphosphonates (11). Thus, it appears that the ultimate fate of the prosthesis depends on the outcome of a race

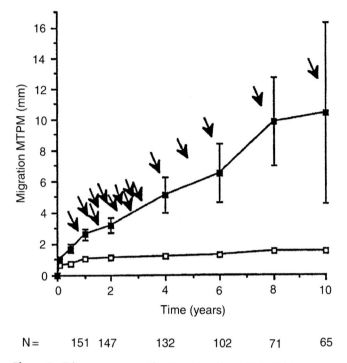

Figure 2 Diagram representing the migration of 143 tibial components (*open squares*) which were not revised and 15 tibial components (*filled squares*) which were revised for mechanical loosening. Arrows indicate the point in time when the arthroplasty became symptomatic. *Note*: None of the patients in this study who had a stable prosthesis during the second postoperative year has needed revision during the six or more years that have gone by since this was published; this is also the case for an extended material of nearly 1000 patients. (Ryd L. Personal communication; stable defined as not migrating more than 0.25 mm). *Source*: From Ref. 3.

between osteoclasts removing the necrotic bone in contact with the implant and osteoblasts making new bone to take over load bearing. If the osteoclasts win this race, early fixation will be lost and the patient will be at risk for late loosening (Fig. 3).

WHEN INITIAL FIXATION IS LOST, SECONDARY RESORPTIVE STIMULI APPEAR

Shear Forces

A total knee prosthesis that has migrated during the first postoperative year will show greater inducible displacement. This means that when RSA examinations are performed with and without rotatory stress upon the leg, they

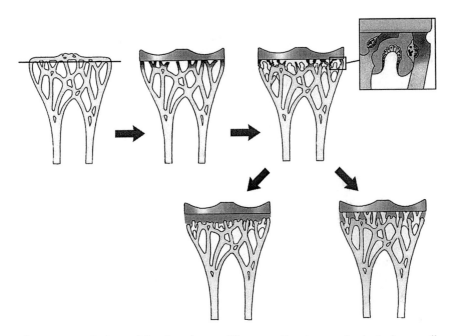

Figure 3 Early loss of fixation theory. The operation trauma leads to bone cell necrosis adjacent to the implant. This is a strong stimulus for osteoclastic resorption, coinciding with the regenerative response (*inset*). A race between bone resorption and formation will ensue, with two possible outcomes: either resorption of the layer of dead bone will undermine the mechanical support, rendering the implant unstable, or the regenerative response will produce sufficient bone to take over the load before the dead bone is lost. If the implant becomes unstable, a fibrous interface will form, which allows secondary resorptive mechanisms, such as reactions to particles or fluid pressure.

will show differences in position (17). This means that shearing displacement occurs, which requires a fibrous membrane at the interface. This membrane is subjected to both hydrostatic and shear loads. According to the mechanical tissue differentiation theory by Pauwels and Carter (18), shear forces will maintain fibrous composition of the membrane and inhibit bone formation whereas hydrostatic pressure will induce fibrocartilage. Claes and Heigele (19) have shown in an elegant study that intramembraneous bone formation requires strains to be smaller than approximately 5% and hydrostatic pressures below 0.15 MPa. Higher hydrostatic pressure still enables endochondral ossification as long as strains are less than approximately 15%. Larger strains in their sheep callus model lead to fibrous connective tissue only. A retrieval study of tibial components has shown fibrocartilage formation only in areas where hydrostatic pressure would be higher than 0.7 MPa according to FEM calculations (20). The maintenance of a fibrous membrane and inhibition of bone ingrowth into pores by shear displacements have been demonstrated in several models. Minor shear displacements might be overcome by bone formation stimulated by hydroxyapatite coating, but this of course depends on the magnitude of the shear forces (21). Shearing deformation only needs to be applied at rare occasions to be able to efficiently inhibit bone ingrowth into a 1 mm diameter pore in a titanium implant (22). On the other hand, very small deformation of a pore can stimulate bone ingrowth (23).

In summary, it appears clear that once a fibrous membrane is formed that allows significant shear displacement, the fixation is definitely lost. However, in different animal models (21,24,25) shear deformation has only induced fibrous membrane and no progressive osteolysis beyond that.

Fluid Pressure

Loading of the fibrous membrane will also result in fluid pressure changes. The normal (perpendicular) stress around a hip femoral component has been estimated by finite element calculations to be of the magnitude of 10 MPa (26). In osteolytic lesions in loosening, small passive joint movements can yield a pressure rise of about 200 mmHg (27). Patients with loose prostheses have a distension of their pseudocapsules compared to patients without loosening, and this distension correlates with intracapsular pressure rise in flexion and extension (28,29). Thus, pressures are increased in patients with loosening, and it is known for decades that hydrostatic fluid fluctuations are a strong osteolytic stimulus. One example is the bone erosions caused by arterial aneurisms and also the osteoarthritic cysts. A constant fluid pressure of 150 mmHg caused dramatic osteolytic lesions in rabbit cortical bone within a few days (30). Bone resorption appeared to be preceded by osteocyte death. A cyclic fluid pressure of 150 mmHg at 0.1 Hz applied 2 hr/day in a similar model also induced bone lysis although considerably less (31). Also in this case, osteolysis appeared to be preceded by osteocyte death. In this rabbit model, fluid pressure was applied using saline solution. The model has thereafter been developed to apply pressure via loading of a fibrous membrane adjacent to the bone surface with similar findings (32). A rat model has also been developed in which again a 1 mm fibrous membrane is allowed to form on top of the bone surface and thereafter this membrane is compressed to generate a fluid pressure (33). By applying 0.6 MPa during two daily 3 minute episodes of cyclical loadings (0.2 Hz) this leads to a dramatic osteolytic lesion within five days. Histologically, large numbers of osteoclasts appear within the bone and destruction starts internally rather than at the loaded surface, which is undermined and breaks down. The lytic lesion contains a granuloma. The mechanism for this dramatic osteoclast recruitment might involve osteocyte death and macrophage activation or both. It has recently been shown in vitro that fluid pressure fluctuations induce expression of IL-6 and TNF-α from cultured human monocyte derived macrophages (34). These cytokines are well known to induce osteoclast formation and activity.

Particles

Because the risk of loosening is determined pre- or postoperatively, wear particles cannot be the primary cause of prosthetic loosening. However, they may act as a secondary resorptive stimulus. If initial fixation is lost and a fibrous membrane forms at the interface, this can serve as a conduit allowing particles from the pseudojoint cavity to enter the interface. The well-described mechanisms whereby particles can activate osteoclasts can then work in concert with the effects of, e.g., fluid pressure. For understanding the loosening process it would be important to know the relative importance of particles versus physical factors such as fluid pressure. One way to get an impression of the relationship between these mechanisms is to compare the effects of particles alone with the effects of, e.g., fluid pressure. This requires that experiments be performed in models in which the effects of these various factors can be refined and isolated. Van der Vis et al. (35) implanted a polymethyl methacrylate (PMMA) rod into the rat femur together with submicron sized particles of various kinds and could not observe any bone resorption, although there was an inhibition of new bone formation adjacent to the implant. Aspenberg and Herbertsson (24) applied high density polythene (HDPE) particles to a stable interface between titanium and bone and could exclude even a minimal bone resorptive response.

Recently, the mouse calvarium model has been established for this kind of studies. Particles are applied subperiosteally on the dorsal surface of mouse calvaria. A bone resorptive response ensues, but lasts only for about a week. After that time point, there is instead increased bone formation, except in very old animals (36). The short duration of the effect of these particles is intriguing. The author recently tested the effect of HDPE particles that were deliberately contaminated with endotoxin (known to elicit inflammation, with TNF-α-production, etc.) at a stable titanium bone interface. A dramatic bone resorptive response ensued, but after about a week, the lesion became filled out with new-formed bone in spite of the continued presence of the particles (37). It appeared that the effects of the endotoxin were somehow overcome during that time period. This is a striking similarity with the mouse calvaria model. Considering the technical difficulties to achieve complete asepsis when operating on the head of a mouse, the short-time effects could perhaps be related to some kind of bacterial or endotoxin contamination also in that model.

Other studies of particles have used more complex models where the effects of an inflamed joint cavity or implant instability have been added. Kim et al. (38) used a cement rod in the rat femur, with contact with the knee joint cavity and applied particles continuously into the joint cavity via an osmotic mini-pump. They found an increased bone resorption. Although statistically significant, the extent of this resorption was minimal. Rushton and coworkers used an unstable tibial implant in rats and found increased and dose-dependent bone resorption at the implant–bone interface when particles were injected into the joint cavity (39). However, the unstable implants caused bone resorption by themselves and the added effect by the presence of particles was moderate (40). Finally, Shanbhag et al. (41) used an uncemented prosthesis in dogs where the particles were contained within the porous coating. These prostheses loosened with dramatic bone resorption. The interpretation of this experiment is difficult. Since the particles were applied within the porous coating it appears that they may have inhibited porous ingrowth and thereby prevented early fixation of the implant. The later resorptive phenomena might then be a consequence of micro-instability rather than the particles themselves. In a similar model with prolonged particle application into the joint cavity no loosening occurred, although the particles were shown to be present at the interface, (42).

PARTICLES APPEAR LESS IMPORTANT THAN PRESSURE AND INSTABILITY

In Vitro

Andrew et al. (43) recently reported that human macrophages produce the bone resorptive cytokines IL-1, IL-6, and TNF-α in response to fluid pressure fluctuations within a physiologic range (34). When phagocytosable particles were added, not only an additive, but a true synergistic effect was seen.

Animal Studies

In a rat model with sliding motion at a titanium–bone interface, the bone next to the titanium became resorbed and replaced by a fibrous membrane. There was no additive effect of 4 μm size HDPE particles that were added before or after the membrane had formed. If motion was discontinued, the particles however inhibited the reestablishment of a titanium–bone contact and tended to preserve the membrane (24). This negative effect upon new bone formation was found also in other models using the same and other kinds of particles (44). The author tested PMMA particles that induce bone resorption in vitro in the rat model for pressure osteolysis, described above. Although a slight osteolytic response was found by the particles alone, this was minimal compared to the effect of the five days, 4 min/day pressure regimen, and no additive effect was found (unpublished data).

Using a dog model with a porous coated cylinder in contact with the joint, polyethylene particles did not cause membrane formation if the implant was stable (45). In an unstable situation a membrane formed, and if particles were added it had a more "aggressive" appearance, but no increased bone resorption could be shown.

In a similar dog model, a bone cement rod in contact with the joint was inserted with or without 0.1 g of PMMA particles. The particles caused no osteolysis, whereas instability alone caused typical lytic lesions with cells expressing IL-1, IL-6, and TNF-α. No clear additive effect of adding particles to the unstable implant could be demonstrated although there may have been qualitative histological differences (46).

Clinical Observations

The importance of design (47), surgical skill (10,48), and postoperative stability (3) all indicate that early biologic events and mechanical factors such as fluid pressure are more important risk factors than particle production. For example, insufficient postoperative cement/bone contact cranially at the acetabulum increased the risk of loosening by a factor of 40 (4000%) (49).

One argument in favor of particle production being an important risk factor is the connection between wear and loosening. However, there is a problem of cause and effect. Once a prosthesis is loose, abrasion at the bone–implant interface will generate large amounts of bone, cement, or metal particles that will cause third body wear of the polyethene component. Thus, loosening is likely to cause wear, and the connection between wear and loosening cannot be used as support for the theory that particles are the main cause of loosening (12).

EARLY LOSS OF FIXATION THEORY IMPLIES NEW MEANS TO PREVENT LOOSENING

If in fact, the risk of late loosening were determined by the outcome of a race between osteoclasts and osteoblasts in the postoperative bone bed, this would have consequences for our attempts to prevent it. Postoperative stability becomes the number one priority in surgery and design, far more important than wear properties. This is in line with data from the Swedish hip and knee registers showing that surgical experience is clearly correlated to the risk of loosening. Furthermore, the theory of early loss of fixation implies that we can improve late results by influencing the early remodeling pharmacologically, e.g., by using bisphosphonates (Fig. 3).

In a prospective randomized double-blinded study, with complete follow-up of all patients, six months postoperative treatment with oral clodronate significantly improved the fixation of tibial total knee components as measured by RSA at one (11) and two years (unpublished data). The change in position versus the bone (migration) was diminished. This demonstrates the concept that migration is the result of biological processes involving osteoclastic resorption, and not only material failure of the bone bed.

Furthermore, it points at a possibility to decrease the risk of loosening. Increased postoperative migration has a strong predictive power for late loosening, and it appears likely that patients receiving postoperative bisphosphonate can have their migration lowered below the risk level. It would also be possible to achieve this early postoperative treatment by applying the bisphosphonate locally during the operation.

Finally, if fluid pressure turns out to be the most important factor, pressure drainage and bone grafting could perhaps sometimes replace revision surgery.

REFERENCES

1. Zarb GA, Albrektsson T. Consensus report: towards optimized treatment outcomes for dental implants. J Prosthet Dent 1998; 80(6):641.
2. Selvik G. Roentgen sterteophotogrammetry. Acta Orthop Scand 1974; 60(suppl 232).
3. Ryd L, Albrektsson BE, Carlsson L, Dansgard F, Herberts P, Lindstrand A, Regner L, Toksvig-Larsen S. Roentgen stereophotogrammetric analysis as a predictor of mechanical loosening of knee prostheses. J Bone Joint Surg Br 1995; 77(3):377–383.
4. Karrholm J, Borssen B, Lowenhielm G, Snorrason F. Does early micromotion of femoral stem prostheses matter? 4-7-year stereoradiographic follow-up of 84 cemented prostheses. J Bone Joint Surg Br 1994; 76(6):912–917.
5. Karrholm J, Herberts P, Hultmark P, Malchau H, Nivbrant B, Thanner J. Radiostereometry of hip prostheses. Review of methodology and clinical results. Clin Orthop 1997; 344:94–110.
6. Krismer M, Biedermann R, Stockl B, Fischer M, Bauer R, Haid C. The prediction of failure of the stem in THR by measurement of early migration using EBRA–FCA. Einzel–Bild–Roentgen-Analyse-femoral component analysis. J Bone Joint Surg Br 1999; 81(2):273–280.
7. Krismer M, Stockl B, Fischer M, Bauer R, Mayrhofer P, Ogon M. Early migration predicts late aseptic failure of hip sockets. J Bone Joint Surg Br 1996; 78(3):422–426.
8. Freeman MA. Acetabular cup migration: prediction of aseptic loosening. J Bone Joint Sure Br 1997; 79(2):342–343.
9. Stocks GW, Freeman MA, Evans SJ. Acetabular cup migration. Prediction of aseptic loosening. J Bone Joint Surg Br 1995; 77(6):853–861.
10. Robertsson O, Knutson K, Lewold S, Lidgren L. The routine of surgical management reduces failure after unicompartmental knee arthroplasty. J Bone Joint Surg Br 2001; 83(1):45–49.
11. Hilding M, Ryd L, Toksvig-Larsen S, Aspenberg P. Clodronate prevents prosthetic migration: a randomized radiostereometric study of 50 total knee patients. Acta Orthop Scand 2000; 71(6):553–557.
12. Mjoberg B. Theories of wear and loosening in hip prostheses. Wear-induced loosening vs loosening-induced wear—a review. Acta Orthop Scand 1994; 65(3):361–371.

13. Mjoberg B. The theory of early loosening of hip prostheses. Orthopedics 1997; 20(12):1169–1175.
14. Charnley J. The reaction of bone to self-curing acrylic cement. A long-term histological study in man. J Bone Joint Surg Br 1970; 52(2):340–353.
15. Charnley J. Proceedings: the histology of loosening between acrylic cement and bone. J Bone Joint Surg Br 1975; 57(2):245.
16. Glimcher MJ, Kenzora JE. Nicolas Andry award. The biology of osteonecrosis of the human femoral head and its clinical implications: 1. Tissue biology. Clin Orthoe 1979; 138:284–309.
17. Hilding MB, Yuan X, Ryd L. The stability of three different cementless tibial components. A randomized radiostereometric study in 45 knee arthroplasty patients. Acta Orthop Scand 1995; 66(1):21–27.
18. Carter DR, Beaupre GS, Giori NJ, Helms JA. Mechanobiology of skeletal regeneration. Clin Orthop 1998; 355(suppl):S41–S55.
19. Claes LE, Heigele CA. Magnitudes of local stress and strain along bony surfaces predict the course and type of fracture healing. J Biomech 1999; 32(3): 255–266.
20. Giori NJ, Ryd L, Carter DR. Mechanical influences on tissue differentiation at bone-cement interfaces. J Arthroplasty 1995; 10(4):514–522.
21. Soballe K. Hydroxyapatite ceramic coating for bone implant fixation. Mechanical and histological studies in dogs. Acta Orthop Scand 1993; 255 suppl:1–58.
22. Aspenberg P, Goodman S, Toksvig-Larsen S, Ryd L, Albrektsson T. Intermittent micromotion inhibits bone ingrowth. Titanium implants in rabbits. Acta Orthop Scand 1992; 63(2):141–145.
23. Goodman S, Aspenberg P. Effect of amplitude of micromotion on bone ingrowth into titanium chambers implanted in the rabbit tibia. Biomaterials 1992; 13(13):944–948.
24. Aspenberg P, Herbertsson P. Periprosthetic bone resorption. Particles versus movement. J Bone Joint Surg Br 1996; 78(4):641–646.
25. Aspenberg P, Van der Vis H. Migration, particles, and fluid pressure. A discussion of causes of prosthetic loosening. Clin Orthop 1998; 352:75–80.
26. Weinans H, Huiskes R, Grootenboer HJ. Quantitative analysis of bone reactions to relative motions at implant-bone interfaces. J Biomech 1993; 26(11): 1271–1281.
27. Anthony PP, Gie GA, Howie CR, Ling RS. Localised endosteal bone lysis in relation to the femoral components of cemented total hip arthroplasties. J Bone Joint Surg Br 1990; 72(6):971–979.
28. Robertsson O, Wingstrand H, Kesteris U, Jonsson K, Onnerfalt R. Intracapsular pressure and loosening of hip prostheses. Preoperative measurements in 18 hips. Acta Orthop Scand 1997; 68(3):231–234.
29. Kesteris U, Jonsson K, Robertsson O, Onnerfalt R, Wingstrand H. Polyethylene wear and synovitis in total hip arthroplasty: a sonographic study of 48 hips. J Arthroplasty 1999; 14(2):138–143.
30. Van der Vis HM, Aspenberg P, Marti RK, Tigchelaar W, Van Noorden CJ. Fluid pressure causes bone resorption in a rabbit model of prosthetic loosening. Clin Orthop 1998; 350:201–208.

31. van der Vis H, Aspenberg P, de Kleine R, Tigchelaar W, van Noorden CJ. Short periods of oscillating fluid pressure directed at a titanium-bone interface in rabbits lead to bone lysis. Acta Orthop Scand 1998; 69(1):5–10.

32. Van der Vis HM, Aspenberg P, Tigchelaar W, Van Noorden CJ. Mechanical compression of a fibrous membrane surrounding bone causes bone resorption. Acta Histochem 1999; 101(2):203–212.

33. Skripitz R, Aspenberg P. Pressure-induced periprosthetic osteolysis: a rat model. J Orthop Res 2000; 18(3):431–434.

34. Ferrier GM, McEvoy A, Evans CE, Andrew JG. The effect of cyclic pressure on human monocyte-derived macrophages in vitro. J Bone Joint Surg Br 2000; 82(5):755–759.

35. Van Der Vis HM, Marti RK, Tigchelaar W, Schuller HM, Van Noorden CJ. Benign cellular responses in rats to different wear particles in intra-articular and intramedullary environments. J Bone Joint Surg Br 1997; 79(5):837–843.

36. Kaar SG, Ragab AA, Kaye SJ, Kilic BA, Jinno T, Goldberg VM, Bi Y, Stewart MC, Carter JR, Greenfield EM. Rapid repair of titanium particle-induced osteolysis is dramatically reduced in aged mice. J Orthop Res 2001; 19(2):171–178.

37. Skoglund BL, Aspenberg LP. Bone resorptive effects of endotoxin contaminated HDPE particles spontaneously eliminatred in vivo. J Bone Joint Surg (Br) 2002. In press.

38. Kim KJ, Kobayashi Y, Itoh T. Osteolysis model with continuous infusion of polyethylene particles. Clin Orthop 1998; 352:46–52.

39. Brooks RA, Sharpe JR, Wimhurst JA, Myer BJ, Dawes EN, Rushton N. The effects of the concentration of high-density polyethylene particles on the bone-implant interface. J Bone Joint Surg Br 2000; 82(4):595–600.

40. Wimhurst JA, Brooks RA, Rushton N. The effects of particulate bone cements at the bone-implant interface. J Bone Joint Surg Br 2001; 83(4):588–592.

41. Shanbhag AS, Hasselman CT, Rubash HE. The John Charnley Award. Inhibition of wear debris mediated osteolysis in a canine total hip arthroplasty model. Clin Orthop 1997; 344:33–43.

42. Lalor PB, Snyder GJ, Toombs PW, Blevins JP, Aberman WE. Early osteolysis in a stable canine model of aseptic implant loosening. 44th Annual meeting, Orthopedic Research Society, New Orleans, LA, USA, 1998.

43. Andrew JGJ, Mcevoy M, Ferrier A, Evans G. Cyclic Pressure and Particles are Synergistic in Human Macrophage Activation. Orlando, FL: Orthopedic Research Society, 2000.

44. Goodman S, Aspenberg P, Song Y, Regula D, Lidgren L. Polyethylene and titanium alloy particles reduce bone formation. Dose-dependence in bone harvest chamber experiments in rabbits. Acta Orthop Scand 1996; 67(6):599–605.

45. Bechtold JES, Kubic K, Ovegaard V, Lewis S, Gustilo JL. Synergy between implant motion and particulate polyethylene in the formation of an aggressive periprosftietic membrane. 43rd Annual Meeting, Orthopedic Researh Society, San Fransisco, CA, USA, 1997.

46. Jones LC, Frondoza C, Hungerford DS. Effect of PMMA particles and movement on an implant interface in a canine model. J Bone Joint Surg Br 2001; 83(3):448–458.

47. Knutson K, Lewold S, Robertsson O, Lidgren L. The Swedish knee arthroplasty register. A nation-wide study of 30,003 knees 1976–1992. Acta Orthop Scand 1994; 65(4):375–386.
48. Herberts P, Malchau H. Long-term registration has improved the quality of hip replacement: a review of the Swedish THR Register comparing 160,000 cases. Acta Orthop Scand 2000; 71(2):111–121.
49. Ritter MA, Zhou H, Keating CM, Keating EM, Faris PM, Meding JB, Berend ME. Radiological factors influencing femoral and acetabular failure in cemented Charnley total hip arthroplasties. J Bone Joint Surg Br 1999; 81(6):982–986.

17

Role of Endotoxin in Implant Loosening

Fabian von Knoch, Harry E. Rubash, and Arun Shanbhag
*Department of Orthopaedic Surgery, Massachusetts General Hospital,
Harvard Medical School, Boston, Massachusetts, U.S.A.*

Steven R. Goldring and David R. Cho
*New England Baptist Bone and Joint Institute, Rheumatology and Metabolic Bone
Division, Beth Israel Deaconess Medical Center, Harvard Medical School, Boston,
Massachusetts, U.S.A.*

INTRODUCTION

Aseptic loosening is the major cause of long-term failure of orthopaedic
implants. Particulate wear debris released from the implants contributes to
the loosening process by activating macrophages, inducing peri-implant granulomatous inflammation, and subsequently leading to osteolysis. Numerous
in vitro models have demonstrated the capacity of wear particles to stimulate
the release of soluble proinflammatory cytokines with the ability to induce
local osteoclastic bone resorption. Recent observations have demonstrated
that the binding of bacterial endotoxins, or lipopolysaccharides (LPS) to particulate wear debris, can significantly modulate the pattern of cell responses in
in vitro models (1–4). These findings might suggest a potential role of LPS in
the pathogenesis of aseptic loosening after total joint replacements.

BASIC SCIENCE OF LPS

LPS, or bacterial endotoxin, is the principal component of the outer membrane
of gram-negative bacteria (5). LPS is a prototypical activator of the immune

system and is active at concentrations below 1 nM (6). A series of defense mechanisms are set into operation following infection by gram-negative bacteria, both in vertebrates and invertebrates. The complex immune response is based on both innate and acquired components. The innate immune response provides rapidly activated host defenses and is coordinated primarily by macrophages and polymorphonuclear leukocytes. These cells phagocytose and destroy the infectious agent, initiating additional inflammatory host defenses through the synthesis and release of proinflammatory cytokines.

In order to understand the sequence and mechanisms of the immune responses mediated by LPS, the chemical structure of these complex components has been studied extensively (6–8). LPS is a complex glycolipid consisting of three parts: a proximal hydrophobic lipid portion (lipid A) which anchors LPS to the bacterial outer membrane, the distal hydrophilic O-antigen polysaccharide which protrudes into the surrounding medium, and the core oligosaccharide that joins the lipid A and O-antigen structures. While O-antigen structures show considerable diversity in different gram-negative bacteria, the lipid A is highly conserved and consistently composed of a diglucosamine backbone containing ester-linked and amide-linked long-chain fatty acids. Lipid A is recognized to be the essential structural feature of LPS that governs its interactions with the innate immune system (7), and LPS is inactivated by treatments that remove the fatty-acid side chains from the lipid A moiety.

In the presence of gram-negative bacteria, the activation of host defenses requires the recognition of LPS by mechanisms involving an acute phase plasma protein called LPS-binding protein (LBP) and the glycosylphosphatidylinositol-anchored membrane protein *CD14* (6). LBP serves as an opsonin and CD14 an opsonic receptor for complexes of LPS and LBP. Several lines of evidence indicate that CD14 functions exclusively as a ligand-binding protein (6).

Most recently the mechanisms by which the LPS signal is transduced across the plasma membrane have been further elucidated. Toll-like receptors (TLRs) were identified as putative transmembrane proteins involved in the recognition of pathogen components such as LPS (6). Toll is a type 1 membrane protein. An extracellular domain with leucine-rich repeats characterizes this plasma membrane receptor, which is assumed to participate in ligand recognition. It also has an intracellular domain with sequence homology to the interleukin-1 receptor (IL-IR) called the Toll/IL-1R homology (TIR) domain (9). Mammals express an array of TLRs with structural similarity to Toll. Ten human types of TLRs have been identified to date (6). Certain TLRs are thought to interact with CD14 in order to generate a transmembrane signal linked to LPS-induced cell activation. Genetic studies strongly indicate that TLR4 might be the predominant receptor for the recognition of LPS. The findings in two murine strains which are hypo-responsive or nonresponsive to LPS have been linked to the genetic deficiency of TLR4 (10,11). In contrast, it was shown that Chinese hamsters carrying a null allele for TRL2 react normally to LPS (12). Furthermore, LPS responsiveness was unaffected in dominant-negative mutants of TLR2 (13). However, it remains uncertain whether the TLRs bind directly to LPS in mammalian cells. A recent study suggests that LPS and TLRs are indeed involved in a very close physical relationship during signal transduction (14).

ROLE OF LPS IN PARTICLE-INDUCED OSTEOLYSIS

It is believed that particle-induced activation of phagocytic cells at the bone–implant interface initiates an osteolytic cascade involving periprosthetic granulomatous inflammation and subsequent bone resorption (15–20). Three important observations support these conclusions. First, wear particles have been found within cells at sites of osteolysis in retrieval studies (21,22). Secondly, osteolysis can be induced by particles in vivo in different species including mouse, rat, rabbit, and dog (23–27). The third is the observed nature of in vitro particle internalization by phagocytic cells, which subsequently release a diversity of potent proinflammatory factors that are capable of inducing bone resorption (24,28–33).

In vitro cell culture models have significantly aided in the understanding of the mechanisms responsible for particle-induced modulation of cell activities. However, the observed patterns of cell response to particulate material have often shown discrepancies. Comparing the underlying study designs, it is clear that there is considerable heterogeneity in the experimental models, including the selection of cell type, the composition and structural features of the particulate material, and various culture-specific conditions. Selection of different cell types has been demonstrated to significantly modify the pattern of cell responses (34). Human peripheral blood monocytic cells respond differently depending on donor variables (35). In terms of the particulate material, numerous variables such as particulate shape, size, surface roughness, relative hydrophobicity or hydrophilicity, and composition are the critical determinants in defining the consequences of particle–cell interactions (29,35–38). Recent studies from our institutions, as well as from other groups, have specifically investigated the role of LPS in particle-induced cell responses and suggest that LPS contamination might be at least partially responsible for the discrepancy in results of various in vitro cell culture experiments (1–4).

LPS as a Likely Modulator of Particle–Cell Interactions

For several reasons, LPS constitutes a potential candidate which may modulate the particle–cell interactions both in vitro and in vivo. LPS is ubiquitously present and demonstrates a high affinity for implant materials, particularly titanium and titanium alloys (2,39,40). Without adequate precautions, LPS can be found in varying levels in tissue culture media and serum, as well as on plastic, glass, and metal particle surfaces (3). Moreover,

LPS initiates an intense stimulation of the proinflammatory cascade in macrophages, leading to the synthesis and release of soluble inflammatory mediators (41–44). The pattern of cell responses to LPS is similar to the effects of particles on phagocytic cell stimulation. These observations suggest that LPS contamination may contribute to the discrepant results in in vitro studies. Particle-associated LPS may also modify the biological properties of orthopaedic wear debris and therefore potentially could play a role in particle-induced peri-implant osteolysis.

EFFECTS OF LPS ON PARTICLE–CELL INTERACTIONS IN VITRO

In order to elucidate the potential role of LPS in in vitro particle–cell interactions, investigations have been performed using different cell culture models to evaluate relevant orthopaedic biomaterials. Ragab et al. originally suggested that LPS might be responsible for the stimulatory effects reported of certain particulate material on phagocytic cells. In support of their theory, they tested commonly used preparations of titanium particles as well as titanium alloy implants (as received from an industrial supplier) for the presence of LPS contamination (3). Using a highly sensitivity version of the limulus amoebocyte lysate (LAL) assay, both particles and implant surfaces as received from the industrial supplier tested positive for adherent LPS. From these findings, the authors concluded that "as received" titanium particles regularly exhibit contamination with adherent LPS, which might explain the discrepancy in reports regarding the potency of different particles in producing increases in cytokine levels.

The same research group developed a protocol for the cleaning of contaminated titanium particles. They used three different treatment protocols for removal of adherent LPS. The first method used 25% nitric acid at room temperature, the second a mixture of 0.1 N sodium hydroxide and 95% ethanol at 30°C for 18–20 hour. The third method used a combination of the first two methods (3). According to their results, the nitric acid method was insufficient for the removal of adherent LPS, while the alkali–ethanol method removed about 90% of the adherent LPS and the combination of both methods was more than 99.9% effective.

Subsequently, other investigators have suggested that LPS might play a role in particle-induced stimulation of macrophages. Others (2) and our laboratory utilized RAW 264.7 murine macrophages to investigate the effects of particle-associated LPS. This cell line was selected because it is capable of phagocytosis and is also extraordinarily sensitive to LPS (45). As part of our routine laboratory practice, all implant materials either obtained from outside vendors, or generated in-house are washed with 95% ethanol to remove potential manufacturing contaminants. When using "as received" particles under these standard laboratory conditions we observed that native particle species including CoCr, TiAlV, TiN, and silica, without any elaborate efforts to inactivate LPS, exhibited minimal capability to stimulate RAW 264.7 macrophages (1). Similarly, Daniels et al. (4) found minimal cell responses in murine macrophages after treatment with particles (high-density polyethylene and CoCr alloy) which were cleaned with ethanol and saline only. These observations are in sharp contrast to previous reports that metal particles can produce significant increases in cytokine levels (24,28,29,46–48). Although there is a potential risk of contaminating particles during routine handling in the laboratory environment, our experience suggests that significant contamination in "as received" particles per se does not occur.

Effects of LPS on Particle–Cell Interactions

In order to better understand the role of LPS in particle-mediated cell activation, it is useful to differentiate the effects of *soluble* LPS and material-associated *adherent* LPS (Fig. 1). To rigorously determine the effects of *soluble* LPS on phagocytic cells, we treated the murine macrophages with increasing concentrations of LPS (1 and 1000 ng/mL) (1) Treatment resulted in a dose-dependent increase in steady-state mRNA levels of the proinflammatory cytokmes, TNF-α IL-1α, IL-1β, and the chemokine MIP-2 as reported by others (2). In agreement with previous literature reports (2,6), murine macrophages were capable of responding to LPS at concentrations as low as 1 ng/ mL, while primary peripheral human macrophages respond to even lower levels of LPS, in the range of 0.1 ng/mL (35). To investigate the kinetics of LPS induction of cytokine mRNA levels we treated macrophages with LPS (100 ng/mL)

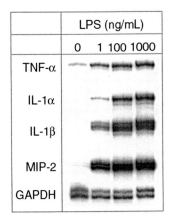

Figure 1 Upregulation of cytokine mRNA levels in RAW 264.7 macrophages treated with increasing concentrations of LPS at $t = 8$ hours GAPDH is used as a housekeeping gene. *Abbreviations*: LPS, lipropolysaccharides; GAPDH, glyceraldehyde-3-phosphate dehydrogenase. *Source*: From Ref. 1.

and extracted RNA at different time points (1). Interestingly, maximal expression of TNF-α (and MIP-2) mRNA levels was observed at 1 hour, with mRNA levels slowly decreasing over the remainder of the time course. In contrast, significant IL-1α and IL-1β expression did not occur until four hours after LPS treatment and levels remained elevated for 12 hours.

In further studies, we investigated the effects of *adherent* LPS (1). For this purpose, we pretreated particles with LPS at a known concentration (1 mg/mL). The particles were then washed extensively in 70% ethanol to remove any soluble or loosely adsorbed LPS. To exclude the presence of soluble LPS, we routinely analyzed conditioned media for LPS, using the LAL assay. All LPS values were less than or equal to the LAL assay negative control indicating that the enhanced activity of the LPS pretreated particles was mediated by particle-adherent LPS. Using different particle species (CoCr, TiAlV, TiN, and silica), the pretreatment with LPS resulted in substantial increase in TNF-α, IL-1α, and IL-1β release, measured using ELISA. RNase protection assays confirmed that in addition to the release of proteins, there was an upregulation of steady-state mRNA levels (Fig. 2).

Our results indicate that particles of different composition and surface chemistry exhibit the capacity to bind LPS and subsequently induce cell responses. Of importance, these cell responses were markedly enhanced compared to the results obtained with "as received" particles. Furthermore, the effects were not related to LPS released from the pretreated particles.

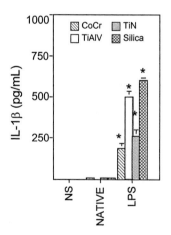

Figure 2 IL-1β release by RAW 264.7 macrophages treated with 4 different particle compositions (CoCr, TiAlV, TiN, and silica) and 2 different particle treatment conditions (NATIVE and LPS); NS = nonstimulated cells; NATIVE = as received particles washed with ethanol; LPS = particles pretreated with LPS and washed with ethanol. $p < 0.01$ compared to cells treated with corresponding native particles. *Source*: From Ref. 1.

The relative capacity of different materials to bind LPS has not been examined directly. To our knowledge, direct measurement of bound LPS on both cell and particle surfaces has not been accomplished. Thus, data concerning the effective local concentration of bound LPS is not immediately available. However, there is some evidence that different materials indeed show differential capacity to bind LPS, possibly related to differences in surface chemistry or structure. Daniels et al. (4) found that levels of cytokine release by IC-21 murine macrophages after LPS exposure were different for high-density polyethylene versus CoCr alloy.

Removal of Particle-Associated LPS

In order to more rigorously test different protocols for removal and inactivation of LPS, we as well as a group from the U.S. Food and Drug Administration (FDA) (2) intentionally contaminated different particles with a known LPS concentration, followed by treatment with differential washing procedures. The FDA group observed that washes with 70% ethanol for 48 hours at room temperature followed by repeated PBS washing were sufficient to abolish the effects of both soluble or polymethylmethacrylate (PMMA) particle-associated LPS (2). Our group deliberately contaminated different particles (CoCr, TiAlV, TiN, and silica) with a known concentration of LPS (1 mg/mL) for three days at room temperature with periodic vortexing and tested three cleaning protocols (1). These included washes in 70% ethanol for 24 hours repeated three times, or following three washes in 70% ethanol as described, either acetic acid treatment for three hours (49), or heat inactivation by autoclaving for one hour, and heating at 175°C for three hours (Fig. 3). To exclude the presence of soluble LPS, conditioned media were analyzed for LPS using the LAL assay. The latter two treatments significantly attenuated the stimulatory effects of adherent LPS. Autoclaving and baking was the most effective removal technique and almost completely abrogated the effects of LPS (Fig. 3). In contrast to the report from the FDA group (2) our findings indicate that even thorough washes in ethanol over the extended period of 72 hours do not completely inactivate particle-associated LPS. This discrepancy might be due in part to the different LPS treatment protocols used to contaminate the particles. The FDA group exposed the particles to a 100,000-fold lower concentration (10^{-5} mg/mL compared to 1 mg/mL in our studies) of LPS and for a considerably shorter period of time (one hour compared to three days).

A concern related to the LPS removal protocols is that the treatments might first alter the physico-chemical properties of the particles, and second remove molecules other than LPS, which could then change the particle–cell interactions. To address these questions Bi et al. (50) re-contaminated particles from which LPS had been previously removed. They found a restored ability of these particles to stimulate osteoclast differentiation (20,51).

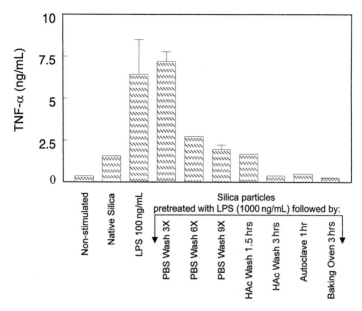

Figure 3   TNF-α release by RAW 264.7 macrophages is used as an indicator of the efficacy of different cleaning protocols following intentional treatment with LPS. The first 3 bars represent nonstimulated cells—cells stimulated with silica particles as received from vendor—as well as cells stimulated with LPS alone. The subsequent bars show the cell response to LPS pretreated silica particles after different cleaning procedures. *Abbreviation*: LPS, lipopolysaccharides.

This suggests that even after the application of removal treatments, with subsequent recontamination, the effects of LPS on particle–cell interactions are still effective.

Control of LPS Contamination in In Vitro Cell Culture Models

The above discussed findings demonstrate the importance of controlling for possible LPS contamination in studies examining the effects of wear debris in in vitro cell culture models. In most studies investigating in vitro cell–particle interactions, LAL assays are routinely utilized to rule out potential LPS contamination. However, cells are sensitive to soluble LPS concentration as low as 1 ng/mL and these levels are very near the limit of detection of even the most sensitive LAL assays. Thus, LAL assays might not be sufficiently sensitive to detect low but still biologically effective concentrations of soluble LPS. Because of the high affinity of LPS for particles, LPS contamination cannot be ruled out by a negative LAL assay of cell supernatants. In fact, Ragab et al. showed that supernatants of centrifuged particle suspensions showed only 1% of the LPS concentration bound to particles (3).

These findings stress the importance of employing measures to prevent LPS contamination.

Role of LPS in Signal Transduction in Particle–Cell Interactions

There is strong evidence that cells do not encounter particulate wear debris in a native state. Rather, serum-derived proteins rapidly adsorb onto the surface of wear particles as they are released from the implant surface (52). The substrate-specific cell responses might be mediated through interaction of the adsorbed proteins with specific cell surface receptors, followed by the activation of intracellular signaling pathways that transduce the cell responses. It is likely that similar effects are involved in in vitro cell culture systems. Additionally, factors other than those that are serum derived might also interact with the particle surface, and may modify the biological properties of the material.

Several lines of evidence indicate that wear particles and LPS activate similar, if not the same, signal transduction pathways. For both LPS and particles, these pathways have been reported to involve signaling molecules or systems, including nitric oxide (53), protein kinase C (54,55), tyrosine phosphorylation (54–56), NF-κB activation (54,57), and cAMP (58–60).

If LPS contamination is present, intracellular signal pathways involving interactions of the particle-bound LPS with LPS receptors on the cell surface could be activated (6,61). Without LPS contamination, serum proteins may adsorb and denature onto particulate surfaces and subsequently function as ligands with LPS-like activity. Similar to LPS, these proteins could then interact with cell surface receptors to induce cell response. If this is indeed the case, the stimulation with soluble LPS, particle-adherent LPS, or serum proteins denatured onto particles should result in the activation of similar signaling pathways and comparable proinflammatory cytokine profiles. This hypothesis is partly supported by a recent study from Hitchins and Merritt (2) which showed that deliberately contaminated PMMA particles resulted in stimulation of phagocytic cells (quantified by NO release) similar to that of LPS alone. It is also likely that different upstream signal pathways are involved, and these distinct pathways converge into common downstream signaling systems. Future investigations are necessary to further clarify these signaling pathways and the variables triggering their activation.

LPS IN CLINICAL OSTEOLYSIS

It has been previously established that LPS is a clinically relevant pathogen. LPS has been recognized to play a key role in the septic shock syndrome in humans related to its effects on the innate immune system (62). Additionally,

LPS has also been shown to be involved in the pathogenesis of chronic period-ontitis, reactive airway disease, and other inflammatory disorders involving cell–particle interactions (39,40,43,63). A potential role for LPS in the pathogenesis of peri-implant osteolysis (the major long-term complication of total joint replacements) is based primarily on the in vitro findings that LPS modifies particle–cell interactions, resulting in a marked enhancement in the release of proinflammatory cytokines such as IL-1α, IL-1β, or TNF-α. The important role that these mediators play in initiation and maintenance of inflammatory reactions and pathological bone resorption is well established (64–66). However, the definite role of LPS in particle-induced osteolysis around implants in humans needs to be further investigated.

LPS in Animal Models of Particle-Induced Osteolysis

There is some evidence that LPS when introduced intentionally can induce periprosthetic osteolysis in vivo. Different animal models were utilized for these purposes. One group developed a rat model by implanting titanium plates onto the proximal tibiae. They showed enhanced peri-implant osteolysis with LPS contaminated particles compared to clean particles (27). Another group studied a murine calvaria osteolysis model and found pronounced osteolysis in particles with adherent LPS compared to LPS free particles (50). However, it is noteworthy that these animal studies without exception rely on intentional LPS contamination.

Clinical Relevance of LPS to Periprosthetic Osteolysis in Humans

In order to explore the potential relevance of LPS in periprosthetic osteolysis in humans, it is essential to establish if LPS is present around orthopaedic implants in vivo. In one retrieval study, human total hip arthroplasty revision tissue was tested for the presence of LPS (67). After tissue collection and homogenization, the supernatants were evaluated by means of LAL assay. Tissue samples from primary total hip arthroplasty served as a control group. Interestingly, more LPS was found in the revision tissues as compared to the control tissues, which might indicate that in these cases LPS was involved in the pathogenesis of implant failure. However, there are many limitations in this study. In order to validate the LPS measurements, specific clinical data such as history of infection is needed. Finally, there is the concern of potential iatrogenic contamination during the retrieval procedure which might have confounded the results.

There are several different potential sources for LPS contamination of implanted orthopaedic devices. In cases of intra- or postoperative (gram-negative) wound infections, LPS contamination is possible. However, the risk of orthopaedic device-related infection (i.e., gram-negative and the more common gram-positive wound infections) is lower than 1–2% (68). Moreover, in the vast majority of cases of aseptic loosening, osteolysis around orthopaedic implants occurs without any clinically detectable infection. In the absence of overt infection, it is questionable if there are sufficient concentrations of LPS on bulky or particulate biomaterials. Despite this, LPS may be potentially derived from either subclinical infections around the implant or systemically, e.g., following oral manipulations such as eating and tooth brushing (69).

Therefore, in humans a role for LPS in periprosthetic bone resorption and subsequent aseptic loosening of the implant cannot be completely excluded. Further systematic investigations are required to elucidate the potential role of LPS in osteolysis around orthopaedic implants. If the adsorption of LPS proves to be relevant in the pathogenesis of periprosthetic osteolysis, then it is reasonable to consider the development of new implant materials that are more resistant to LPS adsorption or that interfere with the particle–cell interactions in order to prevent the initiation of the proinflammatory cascade. However, in light of two observations, it seems unlikely that LPS exists at biologically significant levels around orthopaedic implants in humans. First, the human body demonstrates a remarkable efficiency in its ability to rapidly remove LPS. Secondly, human LPS triggers massive immune reactions accompanied by severe systemic manifestations including septic shock, even when present in low levels. The observed effects of LPS in in vitro models may not be indicative of clinically relevant contribution to the pathogenesis of aseptic loosening of total joint replacements.

SUMMARY

There is very convincing evidence from recent in vitro cell culture studies that LPS is capable of markedly modulating particle–cell interactions leading to a marked enhancement in the release of proinflammatory cytokines. Therefore, stringent precautions need to be taken to avoid or eliminate any in vitro LPS contamination, in order to specifically investigate the reactive nature of wear debris. Although contamination in the laboratory environment may easily occur, in our experience particles "as received" are not contaminated per se. If extensive LPS contamination in vitro is still present it is very difficult to remove. Only rigorous treatment protocols such as autoclaving and baking might be sufficiently effective to abolish the effects of LPS. Consequently, prevention of LPS contamination by means of careful laboratory practice is of critical importance.

The presence of particle-associated LPS at the bone–implant interface in vivo could markedly enhance the adverse biological activity of particulate wear debris and may contribute to the pathogenesis of peri-implant osteolysis and loss of fixation. However, convincing evidence for a significant role of LPS in periprosthetic bone resorption in humans is still missing. Systematic studies are required to shed light on this important clinical question in order to determine the definite role of LPS in the pathology of particle-induced osteolysis.

REFERENCES

1. Cho DR, Shanbhag AS, Hong CY, Baran GR, Goldring SR. The role of adsorbed endotoxin in particle-induced stimulation of cytokine release. J Orthop Res 2002; 20:704–713.
2. Hitchins VM, Merritt K. Decontaminating particles exposed to bacterial endotoxin (LPS). J Biomed Mater Res 1999; 46:434–437.
3. Ragab AA, Van De MR, Lavish SA, Goldberg VM, Ninomiya JT, Carlin CR, Greenfield EM. Measurement and removal of adherent endotoxin from titanium particles and implant surfaces. J Orthop Res 1999; 17:803–809.
4. Daniels AU, Bames FH, Charlebois SJ, Smith RA. Macrophage cytokine response to particles and lipopolysaccharide in vitro. J Biomed Mater Res 2000; 49:469–478.
5. Rietschel ET, Brade H. Bacterial endotoxins. Sci Am 1992; 267:54–61.
6. Aderem A, Ulevitch RJ. Toll-like receptors in the induction of the innate immune response. Nature 2000; 406:782–787.
7. Darveau RP. Lipid A diversity and the innate host response to bacterial infection. Curr Opin Microbiol 1998; 1:36–42.
8. Raetz CR. Biochemistry of endotoxins. Annu Rev Biochem 1990; 59:129–170.
9. Heguy A, Baldari CT, Macchia G, Telford JL, Melli M. Amino acids conserved in interleukin-1 receptors (IL-lRs) and the Drosophila toll protein are essential for IL-1R signal transduction. J Biol Chem 1992; 267:2605–2609.
10. Poltorak A, He X, Smimova I, Liu MY, Huffel CV, Du X, Birdwell D, Alejos E, Silva M, Galanos C, Freudenberg M, Ricciardi-Castagnoli P, Layton B, Beutler B. Defective LPS signaling in C3H/HeJ and C57BL/10ScCr mice: mutations in Tlr4 gene. Science 1998; 282:2085–2088.
11. Qureshi ST, Lariviere L, Leveque G, Clermont S, Moore KJ, Gros P, Malo D. Endotoxin-tolerant mice have mutations in Toll-like receptor 4 (Tlr4). J Exp Med 1999; 189:615–625.
12. Heine H, Kirschning, CJ, Lien E, Monks BG, Rothe M, Golenbock DT. Cutting edge: cells that carry a null allele for toll-like receptor 2 are capable of responding to endotoxin. J Immunol 1999; 162:6971–6975.
13. Underhill DM, Ozinsky A, Hajjar AM, Stevens A, Wilson CB, Bassetti M, Aderem A. The Toll-like receptor 2 is recruited to macrophage phagosomes and discriminates between pathogens. Nature 1999; 401:811–815.
14. Poltorak A, Ricciardi-Castagnoli P, Citterio S, Beutler B. Physical contact between lipopolysaccharide and toll-like receptor 4 revealed by genetic complementation. Proc Natl Acad Sci USA 2000; 97:2163–2167.
15. Maloney WJ, Jasty M, Harris WH, Galante JO, Callaghan JJ. Endosteal erosion in association with stable uncemented femoral components. J Bone Joint Surg 1990; 72-A:1025–1034.
16. Goldrin SR, Schiller AL, Roelke M, Rourke CM, O'Neill DA, Harris WH. The synovial-like membrane at the bone–cement interface in loose total hip replacements and its proposed role in bone lysis. J Bone Joint Surg 1983; 65-A: 575–584.
17. Willert HG, Semlitsch M. Reactions of the articular capsule to wear products of artificial joint prostheses. J Biomed Mater Res 1977; 11:157–164.
18. Jones LC, Hungerford DS. Cement disease. Clin Orthop 1987; 225:192–206.

19. Vemon-Roberts B, Freeman MAR. In: Swanson SAV, Freeman MAR, eds. The tissue response to total joint replacement prostheses. New York, NY: John Wiley and Sons, 1977:86–129.

20. Bi Y, Van De Motter RR, Ragab AA, Goldberg VM, Anderso JM, Greenfield EM. Titanium particles stimulate bone resorption by inducing differentiation of murine osteoclasts. J Bone Joint Surg 2001; 83-A:501–508.

21. Goodman SB, Chin R, Chiou SS, Schurman DJ, Woolson ST, Masada MP. A clinical-pathologic-biochemical study of the membrane surrounding loosened and nonloosened total hip arthroplasties. Clin Orthop 1989; 244:182–187.

22. Shanbhag AS, Bailey HO, Hwang DS, Cha CW, Eror NG, Rubash HE. Quantitative analysis of ultrahigh molecular weight polyethylene (UHMWPE) wear debris associated with total knee replacements. J Biomed Mater Res 2000; 53:100–110.

23. Shanbhag AS, Hasselman CT, Rubash HE. The John Chamley Award. Inhibition of wear debris mediated osteolysis in a canine total hip arthroplasty model. Clin Orthop 1997; 344:33–43.

24. Howie DW, Vemon-Robert B, Oakeshott R, Manthey B. A rat model of resorption of bone at the cement–bone interface in the presence of polyethylene wear particles. J Bone Joint Surg 1988; 70-A:257–263.

25. Merkel KD, Erdmann JM, McHugh KP, Abu-Amer Y, Ross FP, Teitelbaun SL. Tumor necrosis factor-α mediates orthopaedic implant osteolysis. Am J Pathol 1999; 154:203–210.

26. Trindade MC, Song Y, Aspenberg P, Smith RL, Goodman SB. Proinflammatory mediator release in response to particle challenge: studies using the bone harvest chamber. J Biomed Mater Res 1999; 48:434–439.

27. Aspenberg P. Adherent endotoxins are necessary for particle-induced bone resorption in a rat model. Trans Orthop Res Soc 2000; 25:704.

28. Shanbhag AS, Jacobs JJ, Black J, Galante JO, Glant TT. Macrophage/particle interactions: effect of size, composition and surface area. J Biomed Mater Res 1994; 28:81–90.

29. Shanbhag AS, Jacobs JJ, Black J, Galante JO, Glant TT. Human monocyte response to particulate biomaterials generated in vivo and in vitro. J Orthop Res 1995; 13:792–801.

30. Shanbhag AS, Jacobs JJ, Black J, Galante JO, Glant TT. Effects of particles on fibroblast proliferation and bone resorption in vitro. Clin Orthop 1997; 342:205–217.

31. Glant TT, Jacobs JJ, Molnar G, Shanbhag AS, Valyon M, Galante JO. Bone resorption activity of particulate-stimulated macrophages. J Bone Miner Res 1993; 8:1071–1079.

32. Bennett NE, Wang JT, Manning CA, Goldring SR. Activation of human monocyte/macrophages and fibroblasts by metal particles: release of products with bone resorbing activities. Trans Orthop Res Soc 1991; 16:188.

33. Goodman SB, Fornasier VL, Lee J, Kei J. The histological effects of the implantation of different sizes of polyethylene particles in the rabbit tibia. J Biomed Mater Res 1990; 24:517–524.

34. Glant TT, Jacobs JJ. Response of three marine macrophage populations to particulate debris: bone resorption in organ cultures. J Orthop Res 1994; 12: 720–731.

35. Matthews JB, Besong AA, Green TR, Stone MH, Wroblewski BM, Fisher J, Ingham E. Evaluation of the response of primary human peripheral blood mononuclear phagocytes to challenge with in vitro generated clinically relevant UHMWPE particles of known size and dose. J Biomed Mater Res 2000; 52:296–307.

36. Shanbhag AS, Macaulay W, Stefanovic-Racic M, Rubash HE. Nitric oxide release by macrophages in response to particulate wear debris. J Biomed Mater Res 1998; 41:497–503.

37. Voronov I, Santerre JP, Hinek A, Callahan LW, Sandhu J, Boynton EL. Macrophage phagocytosis of polyethylene particulate in vitro. J Biomed Mater Res 1998; 39:40–51.

38. Ingham E, Green TR, Stone MH, Kowalski R, Watkins N, Fisher J. Production of TNF-alpha and bone resorbing activity by macrophages in response to different types of bone cement particles. Biomaterials 2000; 21:1005–1013.

39. Gagnon F, Knoernschild KL, Payant L, Tompkins GR, Litaker MS, Schnster GS. Endotoxin affinity for provisional restorative resins. J Prosthodont 1994; 3:228–236.

40. Nelson SK, Knoernschild KL, Robinson FG, Schuster GS. Lipopolysaccharide affinity for titanium implant biomaterials. J Prosthet Dent 1997; 77:76–82.

41. Fenton MJ, Golenbock DT. LPS-binding proteins and receptors. J Leukoc Biol 1998; 64:25–32.

42. Tobias PS, Gegner J, Tapping R, Orr S, Mathison J, Lee JD, Kravchenko V, Han J, Ulevitch RJ. Lipopolysaccharide dependent cellular activation. J Periodontal Res 1997; 32:99–103.

43. Dong W, Lewtas J, Luster MI. Role of endotoxin in tumor necrosis factor alpha expression from alveolar macrophages treated with urban air particles. Exp Lung Res 1996; 22:577–592.

44. Fujihara M, Muroi M, Muroi Y, Ito N, Suzuki T. Mechanism of lipopolysaccharide- triggered junB activation in a mouse macrophage-like cell line (J774). J Biol Chem 1993; 268:14,898–14,905.

45. Raschke WC, Baird S, Ralph P, Nakoinz I. Functional macrophage cell lines transformed by Abelson leukemia virus. Cell 1978; 15:261–267.

46. Goodman SB, Chin RC. Prostaglandin E2 levels in the membrane surrounding bulk and particulate polymethylmethacrylate in the rabbit tibia. A preliminary study. Clin Orthop 1990; 257:305–309.

47. Gelb H, Schumacher HR, Cuckler J, Baker DG. In vivo inflammatory response to polymethylmethacrylate particulate debris: effect of size, morphology, and surface area. J Orthop Res 1994; 12:83–92.

48. Haynes DR, Rogers SD, Hay S, App B, Pearcy MJ, Howie DW. The differences in toxicity and release of bone–resorbing mediators induced by titanium and cobalt–chromium-alloy wear particles. J Bone Joint Surg 1993; 75-A: 825–834.

49. Ha DK, Leung SW, Fung KP, Choy YM, Lee CY. Role of lipid A of endotoxin in the production of tumour necrosis factor. Mol Immunol 1985; 22:291–294.

50. Bi Y, Kaar SG, Stewart MC, Goldberg VM, Anderson JM, Greenfield EM. In vitro and in vivo studies of adherent endotoxin in orthopedic wear particle-induced osteolysis. Trans Orthop Res Soc 2000; 25:49.

51. Hirashima Y, Ishiguro N, Kondo S, Iwata H. Osteoclast induction from bone marrow cells is due to pro-inflammatory mediators from macrophages exposed to polyethylene particles: a possible mechanism of osteolysis in failed THA. J Biomed Mater Res 2001; 56:177–183.

52. Jenney CR, Anderson JM. Adsorbed serum proteins responsible for surface dependent human macrophage behavior. J Biomed Mater Res 2000; 49: 435–447.

53. Vallance P, Moncada S. Role of endogenous nitric oxide in septic shock. New Horiz 1993; 1:77–86.

54. Sweet MJ, Hume DA. Endotoxin signal transduction in macrophages. J Leukoc Biol 1996; 60:8–26.

55. Chow CW, Grinstein S, Rotstein OD. Signaling events in monocytes and macrophages. New Horiz 1995; 3:342–351.

56. Nakashima Y, Sun DH, Trindade MC, Maloney WJ, Goodman SB, Schurman DJ, Smith RL. Signaling pathways for tumor necrosis factor-alpha and interleukin-6 expression in human macrophages exposed to titanium-alloy particulate debris in vitro. J Bone Joint Surg Am 1999; 81:603–615.

57. Schwarz EM, Lu AP, Goater JJ, Benz EB, Kollias G, Rosier RN, Puzas JE, O'Keefe RJ. Tumor necrosis factor-alpha/nuclear transcription factor-kappaB signaling in periprosthetic osteolysis. J Orthop Res 2000; 18:472–480.

58. Blaine TA, Pollice PF, Rosier RN, Reynolds PR, Puzas JE, O'Keefe RJ. Modulation of the production of cytokines in titanium-stimulated human peripheral blood monocytes by pharmacological agents: the role of cAMP-mediated signaling mechanisms. J Bone Joint Surg 1997; 79-A:1519–1528.

59. Geng Y, Zhang B, Lotz M. Protein tyrosine kinase activation is required for lipopolysaccharide induction of cytokines in human blood monocytes. J Immunol 1993; 151:6692–6700.

60. Katakami Y, Nakao Y, Koizumi T, Katakami N, Ogawa R, Fujita T. Regulation of tumour necrosis factor production by mouse peritoneal macrophages: the role of cellular cyclic AMP. Immunology 1988; 64:719–724.

61. Ozinsky A, Underhill DM, Fontenot JD, Hajjar AM, Smith KD, Wilson CB, Schroeder JL, Aderem A. The repertoire for pattern recognition of pathogens by the innate immune system is defined by cooperation between toll-like receptors. Proc Natl Acad Sci USA 2000; 97:13,766–13,771.

62. Parrillo JE. Pathogenetic mechanisms of septic shock. N Engl J Med 1993; 328:1471–1477.

63. Jagielo PJ, Thorne PS, Kern JA, Quinn TJ, Schwartz DA. Role of endotoxin in grain dust-induced lung inflammation in mice. Am J Physiol 1996; 270: L1052–L1059.

64. Abu-Amer Y, Tondravi MM. NF-kappaB and bone: the breaking point [news; comment]. Nat Med 1997; 3:1189–1190.

65. Abu-Amer Y, Ross FP, Edwards J, Teitelbaum SL. Lipopolysaccharide-stimulated osteoclastogenesis is mediated by tumor necrosis factor via its P55 receptor. J Clin Invest 1997; 100:1557–1565.

66. Chiang CY, Kyritsis G, Graves DT, Amar S. Interleukin-1 and tumor necrosis factor activities partially account for calvarial bone resorption induced by local injection of lipopolysaccharide. Infect Immun 1999; 67:4231–4236.

67. Barnes F, Keiser D, Hardison A, Smith R. Testing revision tissue for presence of endotoxin. Trans Orthop Res Soc 2001; 26:956.
68. Widmer AF. New developments in diagnosis and treatment of infection in orthopedic implants. Clin Infect Dis 2001; 33(suppl 2):S94–106.
69. Robinson FG, Knoernschild KL, Sterrett JD, Tompkins GR. Porphyromonas gingivalis endotoxin affinity for dental ceramics. J Prosthet Dent 1996; 75: 217–227.

18

Signal Transduction and Gene Regulation in Cell–Material Interactions

Elizabeth A. Fritz and Kenneth A. Roebuck

Department of Immunology/Microbiology, Rush University Medical Center, Chicago, Illinois, U.S.A.

Tibor T. Giant

Departments of Biochemistry and Orthopaedic Surgery, Rush University Medical Center, Chicago, Illinois, U.S.A.

INTRODUCTION

Particulate wear debris is generated continuously at bone-cement and bone-implant interfaces by the normal wear and corrosion of the prosthesis. These nonbiodegradable particles pose a serious problem for the longevity of orthopaedic implants. High levels of ultra high molecular weight polyethylene (UHMWPE), polymethylmethacrylate (PMMA; bone cement), titanium (Ti), titanium alloy (TiAlV), and cobalt–chromium alloy (Co–Cr) are present within the interfacial tissues retrieved from implant failures associated with osteolysis and aseptic loosening (1–3). The accumulation of ultra fine particulate wear debris results in a chronic inflammatory condition involving the persistent activation of proinflammatory cytokines and chemotactic cytokines as well as increased production of prostaglandin E2 (PE2) and matrix metalloproteinases (4–21). However, the intracellular events and signaling pathways by which particulate wear debris activates these proinflammatory mediators are largely unknown and only now beginning to be studied.

The recent identification of possible intracellular signal transduction pathways elicited by particulate wear debris has opened an exciting new area within clinically oriented orthopaedic research (22). The ultimate aim of this new line of investigation is to delineate the fundamental cellular mechanisms of periprosthetic osteolysis induced by particulate wear debris and to establish strategies for the development of therapeutic agents to prevent, retard, or even reverse the adverse outcome of joint replacement procedures. Elucidation of how particulate species transmit cellular activation signals will prove to be essential for our understanding of the underlying mechanisms leading to implant failure by periprosthetic osteolysis and aseptic loosening. In this chapter, we review the major signal transduction pathways induced in the various cell types associated with periprosthetic osteolysis, with a focus on the regulatory role the different signaling pathways and their transcription factor targets play in the initiation and progression of the chronic inflammation associated with osteolysis.

INTRACELLULAR SIGNAL TRANSDUCTION

One of the most important recent advances in biomedical science is the identification of intracellular signaling events as part of cellular adaptive responses. These regulatory events are important for mammalian cells to deal with changes in their microenvironment, which are necessary to maintain homeostatsis. Cells receive external signals by way of surface membrane receptors and, as a consequence, certain amino acid residues (usually tyrosine, serine, or threonine) of the cytoplasmic tail of the receptor become phosphorylated. This initial biochemical event is amplified through a series of protein kinase-mediated phosphorylations that in the end trigger a defined set of long-term gene responses. Extracellular compounds in the form of lipids, hormones, growth factors, cytokines, chemokines, counter receptors of other cells, or other cellular mediators can bind to specific cell surface receptors. These cell surface interactions activate intracellular signal transduction cascades that result in the modification of nuclear transcription factor activities, which by changing the pattern of nuclear gene expression alter the genetic program of the cell.

Transcription factors are sequence-specific DNA binding proteins that activate gene expression by physically interacting with the promoter regions of transcriptionally responsive genes. Multiple signaling pathways activated by different receptors may functionally interact, either converging or diverging, to produce a highly specific cell response. For example, the proinflammatory cytokines TNF-α, IL-1, and IL-6 activate a complex network of intersecting signal transduction pathways that ultimately result in a well-defined inflammatory response that is characteristic for a given cell type. The inflammatory response is regulated primarily at the level of cytokine gene transcription through the promoter binding of the inducible transcription factors NF-κB, AP-1, NF-IL-6, and STAT (23–33). In many cases, these transcription factors act cooperatively through specific protein–protein and protein–DNA interactions to produce efficient gene transcription in response to different activation stimuli. For example, in the IL-8 gene promoter, NF-κB binds cooperatively with NF-IL-6 to a composite element in the IL-8 promoter to mediate the TNF-α response, but in response to respiratory syncytial virus infection, NF-κB cooperates with an upstream AP-1 site to activate IL-8 gene transcription (34). Thus, the differential cooperativity among transcription factors induced in a stimulus- and cell type-specific manner is what governs the transcriptional activity of gene promoters.

NF-κB/REL TRANSCRIPTION FACTOR FAMILY

Particulate wear debris has recently been shown to activate the inducible transcription factor NF-κB in cell types involved in osteolysis such as macrophages, osteoblasts, and fibroblasts (6,22,35,36). NF-κB is a member of the Rel family of transcription factors and is composed of two groups of structurally related interacting proteins that bind DNA recognition sites as dimers and whose activity is regulated by subcellular location (37). NF-κB/Rel family members of the first group include NF-κBl (p50) and NF-κB2 (p52), which are synthesized as precursor proteins of 105 (p105) and 100 (p100) kDa, respectively. The second group includes Rel A (p65), Rel B, and c-Rel, which are synthesized as mature proteins containing one or more potent activation domains. NF-κB typically exists as p65/p50 heterodimers, and dimerization of the different NF-κB subunits occurs via a 300 amino acid highly conserved Rel homology domain (RHD) that is also essential for nuclear localization and DNA binding. Functionally, each subunit possesses distinct DNA binding and transactivation properties, and when combined pair wise as heterodimers or heterodimers, they form NF-κB transcription factors with unique binding and transactivation characteristics (38,39).

In resting cells, latent NF-κB is complexed to a family of cytoplasmic retention proteins called inhibitors of NF-κB (I-κB) (Fig. 1). I-κBα, an ankyrin-rich protein, forms a complex with NF-κB subunits through interaction of the ankyrin repeats with the RHD of NF-κB, which blocks the nuclear localization signals of NF-κB preventing nuclear translocation (37). The release of I-κBα from NF-κB is signaled by I-κB kinase (IKK) phosphorylation of two conserved serine residues (Ser-32 and Ser-36) in the ammo-terminal domain of I-κBα (40). The serine phosphorylation of I-κB marks the protein inhibitor for polyubiquitination and subsequent proteolytic degradation by the ATP-dependent 26S proteosome complex, thereby exposing the nuclear localization signal (NLS) and permitting NF-κB to translocate to the nucleus and bind its recognition elements within

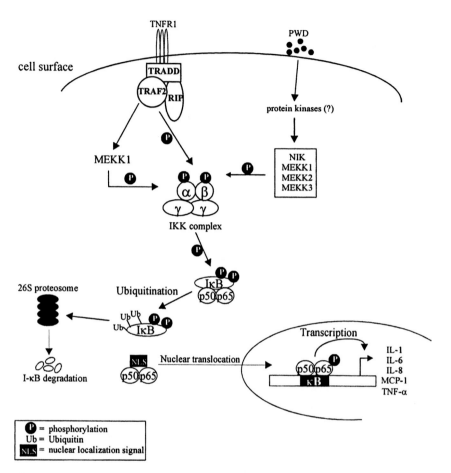

Figure 1 Comparison of TNF receptor (TNFRI) and PWD NF-κB signaling. TNFRI can activate the IKK complex either by direct phosphorylation or through activated MEKK1 Icinase activity. Although the precise pathway and kinase events are not known, it is thought that PWD can activate intracellular protein serine/ threonine or tyrosine kinases leading to activation of several MAPKKK signaling molecules and subsequent IKK activation. IKK phosphorylation of I-κB signals polyubiquitination and targeting of I-κB for proteosomal degradation, thereby permitting NF-κB (p65/p50 heterodimers) via the exposure of the NLS to translocate to the nucleus and activate cytokine and chemokine gene promoters. *Abbreviations*: PWD, potential particulate wear debris; MAPKKK, mitogen activated protein kinase kinases; NLS, nuclear localization signal; IKK, I-κB kinase.

the promoter regions of NF-κB-responsive genes such as IL-8 and MCP-1 (Fig. 1). Although NF-κB can bind target gene promoters, transactivation of the gene requires phosphorylation of the p65 transactivation domain on Ser-529 by casein kinase II (41).

The I-κB kinases coexist in a large complex consisting of a heterodimer of IKKα/IKKβ associated with a homodimer of IKKγ (Fig. 1). IKKα and IKKβ are the catalytic subunits involved in phosphorylation of I-κBα serine residues, and IKKγ serves as the regulatory subunit essential for the activation of IKK via upstream signaling components (40). Although phosphorylation of both IKKα and IKKβ subunits has been demonstrated in the activation of IKK, recent studies have shown that only IKKβ phosphorylation is critical for IKK kinase activity in response to proinflammatory stimuli (42). The activation of IKK has been linked to the recruitment of upstream signaling proteins, NIK (NF-κB inducible kinase) and adaptor proteins such as TRAF-2 and TRAF-6 (adaptor proteins that mediate TNF-α and IL-1 signaling, respectively) to the complex by the IKKγ regulatory subunit (40,43–45).

Particulate wear debris activates NF-κB signaling pathways in osteoblasts, fibroblasts, and macrophages (6,35,36). In osteoblasts, we showed that NF-κB was induced through a pathway involving the degradation of I-κBα, which occurred with delayed kinetics compared to the rapid degradation elicited by TNF-α, suggesting particulates may activate NF-κB via a distinct pathway that differs from the classical pathway activated by TNF-α (35). Nevertheless, both TNF-α and particulates induced similar DNA binding complexes composed of the same subunit components of NF-κB, namely Rel A (p65) and NF-κB1 (p50) (35). In macrophages, NF-κB activity correlated with the particle-mediated induction of TNF-α and IL-6 (6). Moreover, Ti particle challenge of macrophages resulted in the activation of both NF-κB and NF-IL6 transcription factors, which required protein serine/threonine and tyrosine kinase activity for enhanced DNA-binding activity (6).

AP-1 TRANSCRIPTION FACTOR FAMILY

Particulates can also activate the stress responsive transcription factor AP-1 (activator protein-1) (46). AP-1 is an inducible transcription factor of the basic leucine zipper (bZIP) family and consists of two subfamilies, Jun (whose members include cJun, JunB, and JunD) and Fos (whose members include cFos, FosB, Fral, and Fra2). AP-1 is critical for the expression of many genes involved in the inflammatory response, including cytokines and adhesion molecules (47,48). AP-1 binds to promoter elements as Jun homodimers or the more stable Jun/Fos heterodimers, which is the predominant form involved in activation of AP-1 responsive genes. However, AP-1 can also form cross heterodimer complexes with other bZIP family members, including the cAMP response element binding protein (CREB) and NF-IL6.

Numerous studies have shown that induction of AP-1 activity can be mediated by a variety of extracellular stimuli including growth factors, regulatory cytokines, and oxidant stress, through the activation of the three different mitogen activated protein kinase (MAPK) signaling pathways, ERK (extracellular-signal related kinases), JNK (Jun N-terminal kinase), and p38 kinase (49). MAPK activation of the AP-1 transcription factor occurs at two levels (Fig. 2). First, the transcription of the Jun and Fos genes is dependent on MAPK signaling. Second, once synthesized MAPK pathways are responsible for the phosphorylation of the newly formed AP-1 complexes, an event that is essential for their transactivation function.

Transcription of the c-Fos gene is mediated by the formation of a ternary complex on the serum response element (SRE) of the c-Fos promoter, which involves the cooperative interaction of Elk-1 with the serum response factor (SRF). This ternary complex on the SRE mediates c-Fos gene expression in response to cellular stress, growth factors, and cytokines (Fig. 2). Phosphorylation of Elk-1 by the JNK, ERK, and p38 MAPKs promotes interactions with SRF resulting in the activation of c-Fos gene transcription. Transcription of the c-Jun gene is mediated by AP-1 binding sites within the

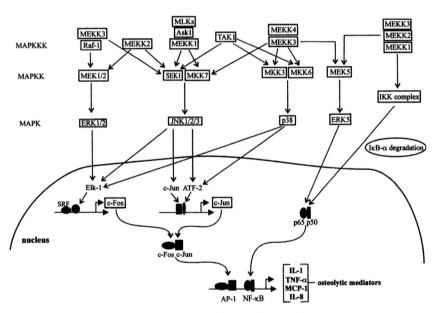

Figure 2 Regulation of AP-1 and NF-κB transcription factors by MAP kinase signaling pathways. Several MAPKKKs can activate MAPKK kinase activity, but only specific MAPKK components lead to MAPK activation. NF-κB activation occurs predominantly through MAPKKK activation of the IKK complex, but can be directly activated by the ERK5 pathway. MAPK activation of AP-1 is two tiered. The initial activation of the transcription factors Elk-1, ATF-2, and c-Jun is required for the transcriptional activation of the c-Jun and c-Fos genes, which combine to form newly synthesized AP-1 capable of cooperating with NF-κB to activate cytokine and chemokine gene promoters.

c-Jun promoter that are constitutively occupied by c-Jun and ATF-2 heterodimers. Phosphorylation of specific serine residues in the transactivation domains of the c-Jun/ATF-2 heterodimers by JNK and p38 MAP kinases mediates the activation of c-Jun gene transcription (Fig. 2). Once the c-Fos and c-Jun components have been synthesized, their functional activity depends on the phosphorylation of specific serine and threonine residues within their transactivation domains. JNK phosphorylates two serine residues (Ser-63 and Ser-73) of c-Jun, and FRK (fos-regitlating kinase) phosphorylates Thr-232 of c-Fos (50).

NF-IL6 TRANSCRIPTION FACTOR FAMILY

Nuclear factor-IL6 (NF-IL6; also known as C/EBPβ), is a bZIP transcription factor of the C/EBP family. NF-IL6 is involved in the transcriptional activation of many cytokines, chemokines, and acute phase protein genes, and was first identified as a DNA binding factor of the IL-1 responsive element in the human IL-6 promoter (51,52). NF-IL6 gene activation can occur via NF-IL6 alone or in cooperation with other transcription factors, such as NF-κB, AP-1, CREB, and STAT-3 (signal transducer and activation of transcription-3). A functional interaction of NF-IL6 withNF-κB, AP-1, or CREB has been observed; however, a synergistic induction of gene transcription is noticed with STAT-3 in the absence of protein–protein interaction (53). NF-IL6 is greatly enhanced in response to proinfiammatory stimuli such as LPS, IL-1, TNF-α, and IL-6 stimulation. The transcriptional activity of NF-IL6 is dependent on phosphorylation events involving three specific residues, Ser-231, Thr-235, and Ser-325. Phosphorylation of Thr-235 in the transactivation domain of NF-IL6 has been shown to be critical for the transactivation potential of NF-IL6, and studies suggest that Thr-235 phosphorylation occurs by a Ras-dependent MAPK signaling pathway. However, additional signaling molecules have also been shown to activate phosphorylation of NF-IL6. For instance, cAMP-mediated phosphorylation of NF-IL6 was associated with nuclear translocation and transactivation, and protein kinase C (PKC) phosphorylation was also demonstrated to activate NF-IL6 activity [reviewed in Ref. (53)].

STAT TRANSCRIPTION FACTOR FAMILY

STATs were first identified as a family of transcription factors activated by receptor ligation in interferon (IFN)-stimulated cells and are activated by tryrosine phosphorylation signals transmitted from activated cell-surface cytokine receptors (54). Cytokine receptor ligation and oligomeriztion signals the recruitment of Janus kinases (JAKs; JAK-1, JAK-2, JAK-3, and Tyk2) to the cytoplasmic domains of the receptors (Fig. 3). JAKs are the

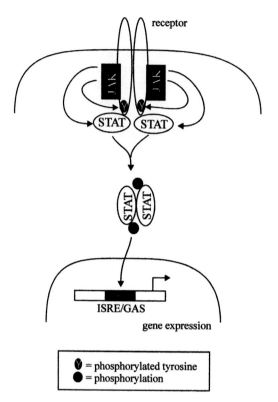

Figure 3 The JAK–STAT signaling pathway. Cytokines and interferons interact with their specific receptors on the cell surface. Receptor ligation causes the activation of JAK kinase activity resulting in the phosphorylation of receptor tyrosine residues, which serve as docking sites for the STAT transcription factors. Receptor-associated STATs are phosphorylated by JAKs, with subsequent formation of homo- or heterodimers, which allows the transcription factors to translocate to the nucleus where they bind to specific promoter elements, ISRE or GAS, to activate gene transcription. *Abbreviations*: STAT, signal transducer and activation of transcription; ISRE, IFN-stimulated response element; GAS, IFN-γ response sequence.

upstream signaling regulators of STAT activation and become activated by auto- or *trans*-phosphorylation in response to cell surface receptor–ligand interactions. Activated JAKs phosphorylate specific tyrosine residues of the cytoplasmic receptor tails which serve as docking sites for STAT transcription factors via interaction with their SH2 (Src homology-2) domains. The receptor-associated STATs then become phosphorylated by the kinase activity of JAKs (specific JAKs target specific STAT proteins) on specific tyrosine residues in their transactivation domains. The JAK–STAT

phosphorylation event allows dimerization of STAT proteins as either homo-
or heterodimers via their SH2 domains, and subsequent translocation to the
nucleus (Fig. 3). Nuclear localization of STAT permits binding of the protein
dimers to either the IFN-γ response sequence (GAS) or IFN-stimulated
response element (ISRE) in a sequence-specific manner with subsequent
transcriptional activation of cytokine-responsive genes (55).

MAP KINASE SIGNALING PATHWAYS

Transactivation of NF-κB, AP-1, and NF-IL6, a requirement for transcription factor activity, involves essential phosphorylation events mediated
by MAPK signaling (Fig. 2). MAPK signaling pathways are stimulated
by a variety of extracellular stimuli including growth factors, inflammatory
cytokines and chemokines, cellular stress, reactive oxygen species (ROS),
and UV irradiation, and transmit the cell-surface initiated signal to the
nucleus for transcriptional activation of responsive genes.

The MAPK family consists of four subclasses, each with their own
cascade of signaling events: the extracellular signal-related kinases 1 and 2
(ERK 1/2), Jun N-terminal kinases (JNK 1/2/3), p38 kinase, and Big
MAPKs (BMK/ERK5). MAPKs (i.e., ERK-1/2, JNK, or p38) are each activated through dual phosphorylation of conserved threonine and tyrosine residues in the kinase domain by specific MAPK kinases (MAPKK): ERK-1/2
activation occurs via MEK.-1/2, JNK activation by MKK-4/7, p38 activation by MKK-3/6, and ERK5 by MEK-5 (Fig. 2). In contrast, MAPKK
signaling proteins can be activated by multiple upstream MAPKK kinases
(MAPKKK). The ERK-1/2 pathway is primarily activated by growth
factor stimulation, whereas JNK and p38 signaling pathways are stimulated
by oxidative stress, cellular stress, and proinflammatory stimuli such as
LPS, IL-1, and TNF-α, as well as UV and gamma irradiation (56).

Although the MAPK pathways primarily lead to the activation of Jun
and Fos, recent studies have shown the involvement of the ERK 1/2 and JNK
signaling pathways in the activation of NF-κB (57). Moreover, upstream
members of the MAPK cascades, MEKK-1, MEKK-2, and MEKK-3, have
been associated with the phosphorylation of IKKα and IKKβ and activation of the IKK complex (58). MEKK-1 is an upstream regulator of the
JNK signaling pathway, MEKK-2 can activate the ERK1/2 and JNK cascades, and MEKK-3 signals lead to the activation of all MAPK pathways
(Fig. 2).

Particulate wear debris has been shown to activate multiple MAPK sig-
naling pathways. Nakashima et al. (6) demonstrated a potential role for the
ERK1/2 pathway in TiAlV induction of TNF-α and IL-6 by macrophages.
Recently, p38 MAPK was shown to participate in chromium (IV)-induced
NF-κB and AP-1 activation (46). Therefore, MAPK signaling pathways
appear to play a direct role in particulate activation of AP-1 and NF-κB.

PARTICLE-INDUCED SIGNAL TRANSDUCTION

Nakashima et al. (6) and Blaine et al. (15) have led the pioneering studies of signaling pathways possibly involved in the particulate-induced TNF-α and IL-6 secretion by monocytes/macrophages. The increased release of TNF-α and IL-6 following either TiAlV (6) or Ti (15) challenge was completely abrogated by both transcriptional and translational inhibitors, actinomycin D and cycloheximide, respectively, suggesting that the activation of these proinflammatory cytokine genes requires transcriptional activation and de novo protein synthesis. Induction of TNF-α and IL-6 gene expression is mediated by multiple signaling pathways involving the transcription factors NF-κB, AP-1, and NF-IL6, which act in combination to generate stimulus and cell-type specific gene expression (59,60). Indeed, NF-κB and NF-IL6 were activated in Ti-A stimulated macrophages, and consistent with the involvement of MAPK signaling in TNF-α and IL-6 gene activation, protein tyrosine and serine/threonine kinase activities were critical for the enhanced binding of NF-κB and NF-IL6 transcription factors (6). Moreover, activation of ERK was suggested by Western-blot detection of a 45 kDa band following TiAlV exposure (6). It was proposed that Ti-A particles activated cytokine gene expression in macrophages by a receptor-mediated signaling pathway following receptor ligation by particulate exposure. In support of this novel idea, cytochalasin B, an inhibitor of phagocytosis, had no effect on the particulate induction of IL-6 or TNF-α production, or activation of NF-κB and NF-IL6 (6).

The activation of TNF-α and IL-6 cytokine genes, as well as others, can also be mediated by the intracellular levels of cyclic AMP (cAMP) via a cAMP response element (CRE) within their gene promoters. cAMP is produced by adenylyl cyclase, a membrane-bound enzyme coupled to G-protein linked receptors, in response to extracellular stimuli, and serves as a second messenger in transmission of the cell surface initiated signal to gene activation in the nucleus. The primary target of cAMP is the activation of the serine/threonine protein kinase A (PKA), but this intracellular messenger affects multiple signal transduction pathways. Blaine et al. (15) examined the role of cAMP signaling in the Ti particle stimulation of IL-6 and TNF-α in human peripheral blood monocytes and found that agonists of cAMP (dibutyryl cAMP and Sp cAMP) downregulated TNF-α release, but upregulated the secretion of IL-6 in response to particle exposure. These results suggest that cAMP is an important modulator in the differential regulation of Ti-stimulated cytokine gene expression. A consistent suppressive role for cAMP was demonstrated by Blaine et al. (15) in the particulate induction of TNF-α. However, conflicting data was found for the stimulatory effect of cAMP on IL-6 secretion from particle challenged monocytes. Surprisingly, IL-6 release was not decreased by Rp cAMP, an inhibitor of cAMP-mediated signaling, and the phosphodiesterase inhibitor, ciprofloxacin, increased IL-6 production by Ti-stimulated monocytes. Since phosphodiesterases convert active cAMP into its inactive state, blocking their activity results in increased cAMP concentrations.

We have investigated the intracellular signaling mechanisms used by Ti particles to alter osteoblast gene expression (22). Specifically, we have focused on the identification of signaling pathways induced by Ti particles for the upregulation of the chemotactic cytokines IL-8 and MCP-1 and the downregulation of collagen type I in osteoblastic cells (4,35,36). Ti particles rapidly induced IL-8 and MCP-1 mRNA expression in MG-63 osteoblastic cells and bone marrow derived primary osteoblasts (Fig. 4). Inhibitor studies indicate that the Ti particle induction of IL-8 and MCP-1 gene expression is regulated at the level of gene transcription in the absence of de novo protein synthesis, consistent with a role for the latent transcription factor NF-κB (61). Indeed, DNA binding studies showed enhanced binding of the p65 and p50 subunits of NF-κB to the IL-8 promoter element following particle exposure (61). Ti particle activation of NF-κB was further demonstrated by the rapid degradation of I-kBα following particle exposure (35). Consistent with NF-κB activation, particle exposure of MG-63 osteoblast-like cells also resulted in the activation of protein tyrosine kinases (PTK)

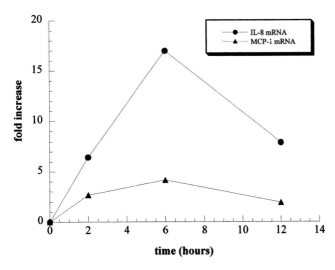

Figure 4 Titanium particles increase IL-8 and MCP-1 mRNA expression in human osteoblasts. Human bone marrow-derived osteoblasts were exposed to 0.5% (v/v) titanium particles and total mRNA isolated at the indicated times for analysis of chemokine mRNA ession using a chemokine specific RNase protection assay. Titanium particle challenge resulted in a time-dependent induction of IL-8 and MCP-1 mRNA expression, with peak expression observed at 6 hours post-treatment (17-fold induction for IL-8 and four fold induction for MCP-1).

and inhibition studies using genistein, a PTK inhibitor, and pyrrolidine dithiocarbamate (PDTC), an antioxidant known to inhibit NF-κB, demonstrated that PTK activity and NF-κB activation, respectively, were critical for the suppressive effects of Ti particles on the pro-collagen αl [I] mRNA synthesis (35,36). Taken together, these results indicate that Ti particles alter osteoblast gene expression through the activation of the PTK-mediated NF-κB signaling pathway.

Receptor-mediated signaling by particulate wear debris in the activation of cytokine genes is also supported by the requirement of G-protein activity in the particulate induction of IL-6 and MCP-1 release by fibroblasts (62). PMMA and Ti particles stimulated a dose-dependent increase in IL-6 and MCP-1 secretion that was decreased by pertussis toxin, a potent inhibitor of G-protein activity. G-proteins are coupled to cell-surface receptors, and are involved in the downstream activation of MAPK signaling pathways by activation of small-GTPase signaling molecules such as Ras, Rac, and Cdc42. Therefore, this study suggests that particulate wear debris may also activate receptor-mediated signaling in the induction of IL-6 and MCP-1 by fibroblasts.

SIGNALING MECHANISMS: PARTICLE PHAGOCYTOSIS VS. REDOX-REGULATION

Particulate wear debris is continually released into the periprosthetic space from the normal wear and corrosion of orthopaedic implants, and phagocytosis of the particulate matter is a natural host defense mechanism to signal an immune response against the foreign matter. However, nonbiodegradable particulates cannot be cleared from the bone-prosthesis microenvironment, resulting in continual particle phagocytosis by macrophages and the subsequent formation of granulamatous tissue (interfacial membrane) at the bone–cement or bone-implant interface. Several studies have shown the predominant presence of macrophages with intracellular particulates (Ti, TiAlV, UHMWPE, and PMMA) in the interfacial tissues harvested from implant failures associated with osteolysis and aseptic loosening (1,17,63–65). Furthermore, the presence of phagocytosable particles (1–12 μm) appeared to be the determining factor for bone resorption at bone-implant junction (66). Indeed, macrophage secretion of TNF-α, IL-1, and PGE2, all mediators of bone resorption, was dependent on phagocytosis of the particulate species. Large-sized PMMA particles beyond the phagocytosable diameter limit did not stimulate TNF-α expression, and internalization of Ti, PMMA, or polystyrene particulates was critical for IL-1 and PGE2 release. However, the studies by Nakashima et al. (6), as mentioned earlier, examined the role of phagocytosis in the induction of TNF-α and IL-6 gene expression and determined that secretion of these cytokines did not require Ti-A particle phagocytosis. These conflicting studies on the prerequisite of particulate phagocytosis for cytokine expression suggest that both phagocytosis and nonphagocytosis mechanisms may be operating in the generation of intracellular signaling. It is possible that each mechanism may elicit similar signaling pathways in the activation of macrophage proinflammatory cytokine genes.

Osteoblasts also have the ability to phagocytose particulates, which appears to contribute to alter gene expression (4,67). Human primary osteoblasts and MG-63 osteosarcoma cells have been reported to phagocytose a variety of particulate wear debris species such as Ti, TiAlV, Co–Cr alloy, and UHMWPE (18,67–69). Our studies demonstrate that MG-63 osteoblast-like cells phagocytose Ti particles, and this process is necessary for the Ti particle suppression of collagen type-I expression (4). Cytochalasin D, a potent inhibitor of phagocytosis, partially reversed the Ti particle inhibition of procollagen $\alpha 1[l]$ synthesis (36). In support of this finding large-sized Ti particles also could suppress procollagen $\alpha 1[I]$ expression, presumably due to the direct contact with membrane receptors as a part of frustrated phagocytosis (36). In addition, Shida et al. (18) reported the dependency of particle phagocytosis for the Ti induction of IL-6 release. They showed that pretreatment of MG-63 osteosarcoma cells with cytochalasin B, another inhibitor of phagocytosis, abolished the secretion of IL-6 in response to Ti exposure. Interestingly, however, we have shown that the activation of the transcription factor NF-κB does not appear to require phagocytosis of particulate matter, as large Ti particle exposure of MG-63 cells results in NF-κB nuclear translocation (36). Furthermore, kinetic studies of MG-63 particle phagocytosis suggest that the initial stimulation of chemokine gene expression by Ti particles also can occur in the absence of phagocytosis (61). Intracellular particulates were not observed until two hour postexposure (4), whereas increased IL-8 and MCP-1 mRNA expression was detected as early as one hour following Ti particle challenge (61). Taken together, these findings seem to point to the ability of particulates to elicit cellular signals prior to phagocytosis. Nevertheless, it appears that additional signals are also elicited during phagocytosis of the particles.

How do particles rapidly elicit cellular signals independent of phagocytosis? One possible mechanism may involve an oxidative stress interaction between the particles and cell membrane (Fig. 5). Particulate species are naturally associated with reactive oxidant species in vivo, and redox-regulated mechanisms are involved in the activation of many transcription factors including NF-κB. Initiation of redox signaling can occur by the generation of intracellular oxidants in response to extracellular stimuli, or via a redox reaction at the cell surface. Indeed, large particles, which cannot be phagocytosed, induce DNA-binding activity of NF-κB, suggesting that a cell surface–particle interaction may be sufficient for gene activation. Furthermore, a recent study reported activation of NF-κB

Particle phagocytosis   Cell surface/Receptor-mediated

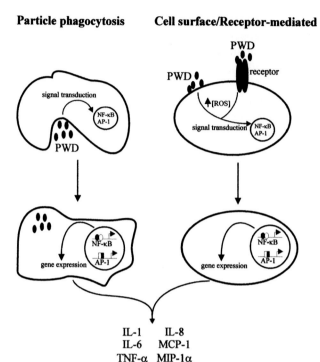

Figure 5 Potential signaling mechanisms activated by particulate wear debris. Particulate wear debris (PWD) may initiate intracellular signal transduction by particle phagocytosis and/or cell surface/receptor interactions that may involve the free radicals associated with the particulates. Activation of signal transduction leads to gene transcription in the nucleus by the transcription factors AP-1 and NF-κB with subsequent gene expression and secretion of osteolytic mediators.

by a nonpermeable redox active anion, suggesting that a plasma membrane redox reaction triggers the intracellular signaling cascade that targets NF-κB nuclear translocation (70). Similar to the large-sized particles, phagocytosable Ti particles may also initiate redox signaling at the cell surface prior to internalization due to their intrinsic free radical activity. Consistent with cell surface-mediated signaling Trindade et al. (62) demonstrated the requirement of G-proteins in the IL-6 and MCP-1 gene expression by Ti/PMMA particle challenged fibroblasts. This study suggests the potential involvement of cell surface receptors in the recognition of particulate matter, thereby leading to the activation of intracellular signaling cascades via receptor ligation. Moreover, H_2O_2, a reactive oxygen species known to be associated with Ti particles in vivo, has been shown to initiate redox activation of MAPK signaling through cell surface receptors (71,72).

REDOX MECHANISMS IN PARTICLE-MEDIATED SIGNALING

The inflammatory response is associated with the presence of reactive oxygen (ROS) and nitrogen (RNS) species. ROS, such as superoxide anion (O_2^-), hydrogen peroxide (H_2O_2 and hydroxyl radical ($^\bullet OH$), as well as RNS such as nitric oxide (NO) and peroxynitrite ($OONO^-$) have been recognized as important second messengers in the activation of signaling cascades and transcription factors such as AP-1, NF-κB, and STAT (73–77). Our laboratory demonstrated that exogenous H_2O_2 resulted in an upregulation of IL-8 gene expression via activation of the transcription factor AP-1 (33,47,59,60). In addition, separate studies have reported H_2O_2 and $^\bullet OH$ as messengers in the activation of NF-κB (78,79). Furthermore, both O_2^- and H_2O_2 have been shown to directly activate the MAPK signaling component ERIC 1/2 (80). As previously mentioned, particulates have been reported to be associated with free radical activity, which may provide a unifying mechanism by which particulate wear debris activates cellular signal transduction cascades (81).

Transcriptional activity of AP-1 is dependent on the nature of redox-sensitive cysteine residues within the DNA-binding domains of Fos and Jun which must be in the reduced state in order for AP-1 to bind to the DNA promoter element (77). The redox regulation of Fos and Jun is mediated by the nuclear redox factor-1, Ref-1/APE, a multifunctional enzyme that has distinct redox and DNA repair (apurinic/apryimidinic endonuclease) activities. The redox activity of Ref-1 is in turn modulated by the antioxidant thioredoxin, a redox-sensitive factor naturally residing in the cellular cytoplasm (82). Upon oxidative stress, thioredoxin becomes activated in the cytoplasm, and then translocates to the nucleus where it directly associates with and activates Ref-1. Casein kinase II phosphorylation of Ref-1 has also been demonstrated to be important in the redox regulation of AP-1 DNA-binding activity.

The proinflammatory cytokines TNF-α and IL-1 stimulate NF-κB activation by increasing the intracellular levels of ROS, with the ROS then serving as second messengers in the signaling cascades resulting in activation of NF-κB-regulated genes (73,78,83). In vitro studies have also demonstrated the activation of NF-κB by exogenous ROS, such as hydrogen peroxide (73,84). Similar to AP-1, NF-κB transcriptional activity is dependent on the redox status of specific cysteine residues for promoter binding, and both Ref-1 and thioredoxin have been shown, to stimulate the DNA-binding activity of NF-κB (85). Interestingly, although the anitoxidant properties of thioredoixn and Ref-1 lead to the transcriptional activation of NF-κB in the nucleus by allowing promoter binding, cytoplasmic antioxidants inhibit this transcription factor by blocking nuclear translocation of NF-κB. The intracellular thiol redox status of the potent antioxidant, glutathione (GSH), and ratio between GSH and its oxidized form, GSSG (gluthathione disulfide), are critical for the transcriptional activation of NF-κB (86). GSH inhibits the serine phosphorylation of I-kB, thereby preventing the dissociation of the inhibitor protein from NF-κB and resulting in the cytoplasmic retention of tins transcription factor. In addition, *N*-acetyl-L-cysteine (NAC), a synthetic precursor of GSH, has been shown to inhibit NF-κB activation in numerous studies (87). Moreover, high intracellular levels of GSSG also prevent NF-κB activity, suggesting that a sensitive balance between GSH and GSSG is required in order to effectively activate NF-κB.

Recently, studies have shown that the activity of the STAT transcription factors can be mediated by oxidative stress (88,89). Enhanced binding of STAT 1 and STAT 3 transcription factors was observed in response to exogenous H_2O_2 stimulation with the STAT 1/3 activation sensitive to the antioxidants NAC, GSH, PDTC, and catalase, the converting enzyme of H_2O_2 (89). H_2O_2 was also demonstrated to activate the tyrosine phosphorylation and nuclear translocation of STAT 3 (88,89). The authors suggest that H_2O_2, by inhibiting intracellular tyrosine phosphatases, increases the tyrosine phosphorylation of STAT 3 and thereby nuclear translocation. Moreover, increased phosphorylation of the tyrosine kinases JAK2 and Tyk2 was observed following H_2O_2 exposure. As mentioned earlier, JAK2 and Tyk2 are the receptor-associated upstream regulators of STAT transcription factor activation; therefore, these data suggest that H_2O_2 may initiate the intracellular JAK–STAT pathway at the cell surface via a receptor-mediated mechanism.

Recent studies have suggested a role for ROS and RNS in the development of osteolysis and implant failure. Hukkanen et al. (90) and Watkins et al. (91) demonstrated that macrophages, located in periprosthetic tissues and containing intracellular wear debris, expressed inducible nitric oxide synthase (iNOS) and cyclooxygenase-2 (cox-2). Immunohistochemical studies also suggested the presence of peroxynitrite, a product of the reaction of nitric oxide (NO) with superoxide anion, by increased levels of protein nitrosylation (90). Indeed, Shanbhag et al. (92) provided evidence of the release of NO from particulate wear debris stimulated macrophages, and showed that the NO release was dependent on the composition, concentration, and time of particle exposure, with TiAlV being the most stimulatory at 0.1% v/v, followed by Ti (0.05 or 0.1% v/v), then PMMA (0.1% v/v). Characterization of interfacial tissues harvested at revision surgery also revealed increased levels of hydrogen peroxide and decreased levels of catalase (93). H_2O_2, NO, and peroxynitrite can lead to the enhanced cytokine production of IL-1, TNF-α, and IL-6, as well as IL-8 and MCP-1 chemokine expression by activation of the redox-sensitive transcription factors NF-κB, NF-IL6, AP-1, and STAT (33,47,84,94).

CONCLUSIONS AND FUTURE DIRECTIONS

Despite the rapid progress made in our understanding of the underlying biological causes of osteolysis and implant loosening there remains much that we do not fully understand as we enter a new century of orthopaedic research. It is clear that particulate wear debris can have profound effects on cellular function by altering the pattern of nuclear gene expression. Ultra fine particles can either activate or suppress gene expression in cell types associated with osteolysis. In osteoblasts Ti particles increase IL-8 and MCP-1 chemokine gene expression while at the same time downregulating procollagen α1[I] gene expression. In macrophages TiAlV particles activate the cytokines IL-6 and TNF-α which can have adverse paracrine effects on both osteoclast and osteoblast function. Although in these cell types changes in gene expression correlate with NF-κB binding activity, the specific signaling events and pathways particulates target are largely unknown and appear to differ from proinflammatory cytokine signaling exemplified by TNF-α or IL-1. Future studies to advance the field will need to focus on defining the precise intracellular mechanisms by which particulates trigger signal transduction in all the relevant cell types. In that regard, it will be important to distinguish between the activation signals generated by ultra fine particulates mediated by phagocytosis and those initiated by the free radicals associated with particles. In addition, the specific protein kinases activated by particulate species that are critical for transmitting activation signals through the cytoplasm to the nucleus will need to be identified and characterized. Indeed, these kinase pathways or their functional end points may represent important therapeutic targets that could be clinically exploited to reduce or possibly reverse the osteolytic process.

ACKNOWLEDGMENTS

This work was supported by grants from the National Institutes of Health/National Institute of Arthritis and Musculoskeletal and Skin Diseases (AR 45835 to KAR) and Zimmer Inc.

REFERENCES

1. Jiranek WA, Machado M, Jasty M, Jevsevar D, Wolfe HJ, Goldring SR, Goldberg MJ, Harris WH. Production of cytokines around loosened cemented acetabular components. Analysis with immunohistochemical techniques and in situ hybridization. J Bone Joint Surg Am 1993; 75(6):863–879.
2. Margevicius KJ, Bauer TW, McMahon JT, Brown SA, Merritt K. Isolation and characterization of debris in membranes around total joint prostheses. J Bone Joint Surg Am 1994; 76(11):1664–1675.
3. Milosev L, Antolic V, Minovic A, Cor A, Herman S, Pavlovcic V, Campbell P. Extensive metallosis and necrosis in failed prostheses with cemented titanium-alloy stems and ceramic heads. J Bone Joint Surg Br 2000; 82-B:352–357.
4. Vermes C, Chandrasekaran R, Jacobs JJ, Galante JO, Roebuck KA, Glant TT. The effects of particulate wear debris, cytokines, and growth factors on the functions of MG-63 osteoblasts. J Bone Joint Surg Am 2001; 83(2):201–211.

5. Nakashima Y, Sun DH, Maloney WJ, Goodman SB, Schurman DJ, Smith RL. Induction of matrix metalloproteinase expression in human macrophages by orthopaedic particulate debris in vitro. J Bone Joint Surg Br 1998; 80(4): 694–700.

6. Nakashima Y, Sun DH, Trindade MC, Maloney WJ, Goodman SB, Schurman DJ, Smith RL. Signaling pathways for tumor necrosis factor-alpha and interleukin-6 expression in human macrophages exposed to titanium-alloy particulate debris in vitro. J Bone Joint Surg Am 1999; 81(5):603–615.

7. Manlapaz M, Maloney WJ, Smith RL. In vitro activation of human fibroblasts by retrieved titanium alloy wear debris. J Orthop Res 1996; 14(3):465–472.

8. Horowitz SM, Gonzales JB. Effects of polyethylene on macrophages. J Orthop Res 1997; 15(1):50–56.

9. Horowitz SM, Gonzales JB. Inflammatory response to implant particulates in a macrophage/osteoblast coculture model. Calcif Tissue Int 1996; 59(5):392–396.

10. Horowitz SM, Luchetti WT, Gonzales JB, Ritchie CK. The effects of cobalt chromium upon macrophages. J Biomed Mater Res 1998; 41(3):468–473.

11. Glant TT, Jacobs JJ, Molnar G, Shanbhag AS, Valyon M, Galante JO. Bone resorption activity of particulate-stimulated macrophages. J Bone Miner Res 1993; 8(9):1071–1079.

12. Glant TT, Jacobs JJ. Response of three murine macrophage populations to particulate debris: bone resorption in organ cultures. J Orthop Res 1994; 12(5):720–731.

13. Frokjaer J, Deleuran B, Lind M, Overgaard S, Soballe K, Bunger C. Polyethylene particles stimulate monocyte chemotactic and activating factor production in synovial mononuclear cells in vivo. An immunohistochemical study in rabbits. Acta Orthop Scand 1995; 66(4):303–307.

14. Dean DD, Schwartz Z, Blanchard CR, Liu Y, Agrawal CM, Lohmann CH, Sylvia VL, Boyan BD. Ultrahigh molecular weight polyethylene particles have direct effects on proliferation, differentiation, and local factor production of MG63 osteoblast-like cells. J Orthop Res 1999; 17(1):9–17.

15. Blaine TA, Pollice PF, Rosier RN, Reynolds PR, Puzas JE, O'Keefe RJ. Modulation of the production of cytokines in titanium-stimulated human peripheral blood monocytes by pharmacological agents. The role of cAMP-mediated signaling mechanisms. J Bone Joint Surg Am 1997; 79(10):1519–1528.

16. Pollice PF, Silverton SF, Horowitz SM. Polymethylmethacrylate-stimulated macrophages increase rat osteoclast precursor recruitment through their effect on osteoblasts in vitro. J Orthop Res 1995; 13(3):325–334.

17. Shanbhag AS, Jacobs JJ, Black J, Galante JO, Glant TT. Cellular mediators secreted by interfacial membranes obtained at revision total hip arthroplasty. J Arthroplasty 1995; 10(4):498–506.

18. Shida J, Trindade MC, Goodman SB, Schurman DJ, Smith RL. Induction of interleukin-6 release in human osteoblast-like cells exposed to titanium particles in vitro. Calcif Tissue Int 2000; 67(2):151–155.

19. Takei H, Pioletti DP, Kwon SY, Sung KL. Combined effect of titanium particles and TNF-alpha on the production of IL-6 by osteoblast-like cells. J Biomed Mater Res 2000; 52(2):382–387.

20. Trindade MC, Song Y, Aspenberg P, Smith RL, Goodman SB. Proinflammatory mediator release in response to particle challenge: studies using the bone harvest chamber. J Biomed Mater Res 1999; 48(4):434–439.

21. Yao J, Glant TT, Lark MW, Mikecz K, Jacobs JJ, Hutchinson NI, Hoerrner LA, Kuettner KE, Galante JO. The potential role of fibroblasts in periprosthetic osteolysis: fibroblast response to titanium particles. J Bone Miner Res 1995; 10(9):1417–1427.

22. Roebuck KA, Jacobs JJ, Glant TT. New horizons in orthopaedic research: elucidation of cellular signal transduction pathways. J Bone Joint Surg Am 1999; 81(5):599–602.

23. Grassl C, Luckow B, Schlondorff D, Dendorfer U. Transcriptional regulation of the interleukin-6 gene in mesangial cells. J Am Soc Nephrol 1999; 10(7): 1466–1477.

24. Georganas C, Liu H, Perlman H, Hoffmann A, Thimmapaya B, Pope RM. Regulation of IL-6 and IL-8 expression in rheumatoid arthritis synovial fibroblasts: the dominant role for NF-kappaB but not C/EBP beta or c-Jun. J Immunol 2000; 165(12):7199–7206.

25. Eickelberg O, Pansky A, Mussmann R, Bihl M, Tamm M, Hildebrand P, Perruchoud AP, Roth M. Transforming growth factor-beta1 induces interleukin-6 expression via activating protein-1 consisting of JunD homodimers in primary human lung fibroblasts. J Biol Chem 1999; 274(18):12933–12938.

26. Dendorfer U, Oettgen P, Libermann TA. Multiple regulatory elements in the interleukin-6 gene mediate induction by prostaglandins, cyclic AMP, and lipopolysaccharide. Mol Cell Biol 1994; 14(7):4443–4454.

27. Matsusaka T, Fujikawa K, Nishio Y, Mukaida N, Matsushima K, Kishimoto T, Akira S. Transcription factors NF-IL6 and NF-kappa B synergistically activate transcription of the inflammatory cytokines, interleukin 6 and interleukin 8. Proc Natl Acad Sci USA 1993; 90(21):10,193–10,197.

28. Ueda A, Ishigatsubo Y, Okubo T, Yoshimura T. Transcriptional regulation of the human monocyte chemoattractant protein-1 gene. Cooperation of two NF-kappaB sites and NF-kappaB/Rel subunit specificity. J Biol Chem 1997; 272(49):31,092–31,099.

29. Liu H, Sidiropoulos P, Song G, Pagliari LJ, Birrer MJ, Stein B, Anrather J, Pope RM. TNF-alpha gene expression in macrophages: regulation by NF-kappaB is independent of c-Jun or C/EBP beta. J Immunol 2000; 164(8):4277–4285.

30. Pope R, Mungre S, Liu H, Thimmapaya B. Regulation of TNF-alpha expression in normal macrophages: the role of C/EBPbeta. Cytokine 2000; 12(8): 1171–1181.

31. Ping D, Boekhoudt GH, Rogers EM, Boss JM. Nuclear factor-kappa B p65 mediates the assembly and activation of the TNF-responsive element of the murine monocyte chemoattractant-1 gene. J Immunol 1999; 162(2):727–734.

32. Hanazawa S, Takeshita A, Amano S, Semba T, Nirazuka T, Katoh H, Kitano S. Tumor necrosis factor-alpha induces expression of monocyte chemoattractant JE via fos and jun genes in clonal osteoblastic MC3T3-E1 cells. J Biol Chem 1993; 268(13):9526–9532.

33. Lakshminarayanan V, Drab-Weiss EA, Roebuck KA. H_2O_2 and tumor necrosis factor-alpha induce differential binding of the redox-responsive transcription

factors AP-1 and NF-kappaB to the interleukin-8 promoter in endothelial and epithelial cells. J Biol Chem 1998; 273(49):32,670–32,678.

34. Roebuck KA. Regulation of interleukin-8 gene expression. J Interferon Cytokine Res 1999; 19(5):429–438.

35. Roebuck KA, Vermes C, Carpenter LR, Fritz EA, Narayanan R, Glant TT. Down-regulation of procollagen alphal [I] messenger RNA by titanium particles correlates with nuclear factor kappaB (NF-kappaB) activation and increased rel A and NF-kappaBl binding to the collagen promoter. J Bone Miner Res 2001; 16(3):501–510.

36. Vermes C, Roebuck KA, Chandrasekaran R, Dobai JG, Jacobs JJ, Glant TT. Particulate wear debris activates protein tyrosine kinases and nuclear factor kappaB, which down-regulates type I collagen synthesis in human osteoblasts. J Bone Miner Res 2000; 15(9):1756–1765.

37. Siebenlist U, Franzoso G, Brown K. Structure, regulation and function of NF-kappaB. Annu Rev Cell Biol 1994; 10:405–455.

38. Phelps CB, Sengchanthalangsy LL, Malek S, Ghosh G. Mechanism of kappaB DNA binding by Rel/NF-kappaB dimers. J Biol Chem 2000; 275(32):24,392–24,399.

39. Kunsch C, Rosen CA. NF-kappaB subunit-specific regulation of the interleukin-8 promoter. Mol Cell Biol 1993; 13(10):6137–6146.

40. Karin M. The beginning of the end: IkappaB kinase (IKK) and NF-kappaB activation. J Biol Chem 1999; 274(39):27339–27342.

41. Bird TA, Schooley K, Dower SK, Hagen H, Virca GD. Activation of nuclear transcription factor NF-kappaB by interleukin-1 is accompanied by casein kinase II-mediated phosphorylation of the p65 subunit. J Biol Chem 1997; 272(51):32606–32612.

42. Janssen-Heininger YM, Poynter ME, Baeuerle PA. Recent advances towards understanding redox mechanisms in the activation of nuclear factor kappaB. Free Radic Biol Med 2000; 28(9):1317–1327.

43. Yin MJ, Christerson LB, Yamamoto Y, Kwak YT, Xu S, Mercurio F, Barbosa M, Cobb MH, Gaynor RB. HTLV-I Tax protein binds to MEKKl to stimulate IkappaB kinase activity and NF-kappaB activation. Cell 1998; 93(5):875–884.

44. Mercurio F, Zhu H, Murray BW, Shevchenko A, Bennett BL, Li J, Young DB, Barbosa M, Mann M, Manning A, Rao A. IKK-1 and IKK-2: cytokine-activated IkappaB kinases essential for NF-kappaB activation. Science 1997; 278(5339):860–866.

45. Nakano H, Shindo M, Sakon S, Nishinaka S, Mihara M, Yagita H, Okumura K. Differential regulation of IkappaB kinase alpha and beta by two upstream kinases, NF-kappaB-inducing kinase and mitogen-activated protein kinase/ERK kinase kinase-1. Proc Natl Acad Sci USA 1998; 95(7):3537–3542.

46. Chen F, Ding M, Lu Y, Leonard SS, Vallyathan V, Castranova V, Shi X. Participation of MAP kinase p38 and IkappaB ldnase in chromium (VI)-induced NF-kappaB and AP-1 activation. J Environ Pathol Toxicol Oncol 2000; 19(3):231–238.

47. Lakshminarayanan V, Beno DW, Costa RH, Roebuck KA. Differential regulation of interleukin-8 and intercellular adhesion molecule-1 by H_2O_2 and tumor

necrosis factor-alpha in endothelial and epithelial cells. J Biol Chem 1997; 272(52):32,910–32,918.

48. Roebuck KA, Rahman A, Lakshminarayanan V, Janakidevi K, Malik AB. H_2O_2 and tumor necrosis factor-alpha activate intercellular adhesion molecule 1 (ICAM-1) gene transcription through distinct cis-regulatory elements within the ICAM-1 promoter. J Biol Chem 1995; 270(32):18,966–18,974.

49. Whitmarsh AJ, Davis PJ. Transcription factor AP-1 regulation by mitogen-activated protein kinase signal transduction pathways. J Mol Med 1996; 74(10):589–607.

50. Karin M. The regulation of AP-1 activity by mitogen-activated protein kinases. J Biol Chem 1995; 270(28):16,483–16,486.

51. Akira S, Isshiki H, Sugita T, Tanabe O, Kinoshita S, Nishio Y, Nakajima T, Hirano T, Kishimoto T. A nuclear factor for IL-6 expression (NF-IL6) is a member of a C/EBP family. EMBO J 1990; 9(6):1897–1906.

52. Isshiki H, Akira S, Tanabe O, Nakajima T, Shimamoto T, Hirano T, Kishimoto T. Constitutive and interleukin-1 (IL-l)-inducible factors interact with the IL-1-responsive element in the IL-6 gene. Mol Cell Biol 1990; 10(6):2757–2764.

53. Akira S. IL-6-regulated transcription factors. Int J Biochem Cell Biol 1997; 29(12):1401–1418.

54. Schindler C. Cytokines and JAK-STAT signaling. Exp Cell Res 1999; 253(1): 7–14.

55. Rane SG, Reddy EP. Janus kinases: components of multiple signaling pathways. Oncogene 2000; 19(49):5662–5679.

56. Lewis TS, Shapiro PS, Ahn NG. Signal transduction through MAP kinase cascades. Adv Cancer Res 1998; 74:49–139.

57. Tuyt LM, Dokter WH, Birkenkamp K, Koopmans SB, Lummen C, Kruijer W, Vellenga E. Extracellular-regulated kinase 1/2, Jun N-terminal kinase, and c-Jun are involved in NF-kappa B-dependent IL-6 expression in human monocytes. J Immunol 1999; 162(8):4893–4902.

58. Zhao Q, Lee FS. Mitogen-activated protein kinase/ERK kinase kinases 2 and 3 activate nuclear factor-kappaB through IkappaB kinase-alpha and IkappaB kinase- beta. J Biol Chem 1999; 274(13):8355–8358.

59. Roebuck KA. Oxidant stress regulation of IL-8 and ICAM-1 gene expression: differential activation and binding of the transcription factors AP-1 and NF-kappaB (Review). Int J Mol Med 1999; 4(3):223–230.

60. Roebuck KA, Carpenter LR, Lakshminarayanan V, Page SM, Moy JN, Thomas LL. Stimulus-specific regulation of chemokine expression involves differential activation of the redox-responsive transcription factors AP-1 and NF-kappaB. J Leukoc Biol 1999; 65(3):291–298.

61. Fritz EA, Glant TT, Vermes C, Jacobs JJ, Roebuck KA. Titanium particles induce the immediate early stress responsive chemokines IL-8 and MCP-1 In osteoblasts. J Orthop Res 2002; 20(3):228–236.

62. Trindade MC, Schurman DJ, Maloney WJ, Goodman SB, Smith RL. G-protein activity requirement for polymethylmethacrylate and titanium particle-induced fibroblast interleukin-6 and monocyte chemoattractant protein-1 release in vitro. J Biomed Mater Res 2000; 51(3):360–368.

63. Kim KJ, Chiba J, Rubash HE. In vivo and in vitro analysis of membranes from hip prostheses inserted without cement. J Bone Joint Surg Am 1994; 76(2):172–180.

64. Chiba J, Schwendeman LJ, Booth RE Jr, Crossett LS, Rubash HE. A biochemical, histologic, and immunohistologic analysis of membranes obtained from failed cemented and cementless total knee arthroplasty. Clin Orthop 1994; (299):114–124.

65. Shanbhag AS, Jacobs JJ, Black J, Galante JO, Glant TT. Human monocyte response to particulate biomaterials generated in vivo and in vitro. J Orthop Res 1995; 13(5):792–801.

66. Horowitz SM, Doty SB, Lane JM, Burstein AH. Studies of the mechanism by which the mechanical failure of polymethylmethacrylate leads to bone resorption. J Bone Joint Surg Am 1993; 75(6):802–813.

67. Yao J, Cs-Szabo G, Jacobs JJ, Kuettner KE, Glant TT. Suppression of osteoblast function by titanium particles. J Bone Joint Surg Am 1997; 79(1):107–112.

68. Lohmann CH, Schwartz Z, Koster G, Jahn U, Buchhorn GH, MacDougall MJ, Casasola D, Liu Y, Sylvia VL, Dean DD, Boyan BD. Phagocytosis of wear debris by osteoblasts affects differentiation and local factor production in a manner dependent on particle composition. Biomaterials 2000; 21(6):551–561.

69. Heinemann DE, Lohmann C, Siggelkow H, Alves F, Engel I, Koster G. Human osteoblast-like cells phagocytose metal particles and express the macrophage marker CD68 in vitro. J Bone Joint Surg Br 2000; 82(2):283–289.

70. Kaul N, Choi J, Forman HJ. Transmembrane redox signaling activates NF-kappaB in macrophages. Free Radic Biol Med 1998; 24(1):202–207.

71. Kamata H, Shibukawa Y, Oka SI, Hirata H. Epidermal growth factor receptor is modulated by redox through multiple mechanisms. Effects of reductants and H_2O_2. Eur J Biochem 2000; 267(7):1933–1944.

72. Takeyama K, Dabbagh K, Jeong Shim J, Dao-Pick T, Ueki IF, Nadel JA. Oxidative stress causes mucin synthesis via transactivation of epidermal growth factor receptor: role of neutrophils. J Immunol 2000; 164(3):1546–1552.

73. Lum H, Roebuck KA. Oxidant stress and endothelial cell dysfunction. Am J Physiol Cell Physio 2001; 280(4):C719–C741.

74. Schoonbroodt S, Piette J. Oxidative stress interference with the nuclear factor-kappaB activation pathways. Biochem Pharmacol 2000; 60(8):1075–1083.

75. Gius D, Botero A, Shah S, Curry HA. Intracellular oxidation/reduction status in the regulation of transcription factors NF-kappaB and AP-1. Toxicol Lett 1999; 106(2–3):93–106.

76. Dalton TP, Shertzer HG, Puga A. Regulation of gene expression by reactive oxygen. Annu Rev Pharmacol Toxicol 1999; 39:67–101.

77. Abate C, Patel L, Rauscher FJD, Curran T. Redox regulation of fos and jun DNA-binding activity in vitro. Science 1990; 249(4973):1157–1161.

78. Schreck R, Rieber P, Baeuerle PA. Reactive oxygen intermediates as apparently widely used messengers in the activation of the NF-kappaB transcription factor and HIV-1. EMBO J 1991; 10(8):2247–2258.

79. Shi X, Dong Z, Huang C, Ma W, Liu K, Ye J, Chen F, Leonard SS, Ding M, Castranova V, Vallyathan V. The role of hydroxyl radical as a messenger in the

activation of nuclear transcription factor NF-kappaB. Mol Cell Biochem 1999; 194(1–2):63–70.

80. Milligan SA, Owens MW, Grisham MB. Differential regulation of extracellular signal-regulated kinase and nuclear factor-kappaB signal transduction pathways by hydrogen peroxide and tumor necrosis factor. Arch Biochem Biophys 1998; 352(2):255–262.

81. Donaldson K, Beswick PH, Gilmour PS. Free radical activity associated with the surface of particles: a unifying factor in determining biological activity?. Toxicol Lett 1996; 88(1–3):293–298.

82. Shau H, Huang AC, Faris M, Nazarian R, de Vellis J, Chen W. Thioredoxin peroxidase (natural killer enhancing factor) regulation of activator protein-1 function in endothelial cells. Biochem Biophys Res Commun 1998; 249(3): 683–686.

83. Takeuchi J, Hirota K, Itoh T, Shinkura R, Kitada K, Yodoi J, Namba T, Fukuda K. Thioredoxin inhibits tumor necrosis factor- or interleukin-1-induced NF-kappaB activation at a level upstream of NF-kappaB-inducing kinase. Antioxid Redox Signal 2000; 2(1):83–92.

84. Zouki C, Jozsef L, Ouellet S, Paquette Y, Filep JG. Peroxynitrite mediates cytokine- induced IL-8 gene expression and production by human leukocytes. J Leukoc Biol 2001; 69(5):815–824.

85. Matthews JR, Wakasugi N, Virelizier JL, Yodoi J, Hay RT. Thioredoxin regulates the DNA binding activity of NF-kappaB by reduction of a disulphide bond involving cysteine 62. Nucleic Acids Res 1992; 20(15):3821–3830.

86. Droge W, Schulze-Osthoff K, Mihm S, Galter D, Schenk H, Eck HP, Roth S, Gmunder H. Functions of glutathione and glutathione disulfide in immunology and immunopathology. FASEB J 1994; 8(14):1131–1138.

87. Schreck R, Albermann K, Baeuerle PA. Nuclear factor kappaB: an oxidative stress-responsive transcription factor of eukaryotic cells (a review). Free Radic Res Commun 1992; 17(4):221–237.

88. Carballo M, Conde M, El Bekay R, Martin-Nieto J, Camacho MJ, Monteseirin J, Conde J, Bedoya FJ, Sobrino F. Oxidative stress triggers STAT3 tyrosine phosphorylation and nuclear translocation in human lymphocytes. J Biol Chem 1999; 274(25):17580–17586.

89. Simon AR, Rai U, Fanburg BL, Cochran BH. Activation of the JAK–STAT pathway by reactive oxygen species. Am J Physiol 1998; 275(6 Pt 1):C1640–1652.

90. Hukkanen M, Corbett SA, Batten J, Konttinen YT, McCarthy ID, Maclouf J, Santavirta S, Hughes SP, Polak JM. Aseptic loosening of total hip replacement. Macrophage expression of inducible nitric oxide synthase and cyclo-oxygenase-2, together with peroxynitrite formation, as a possible mechanism for early prosthesis failure. J Bone Joint Surg Br 1997; 79(3):467–474.

91. Watkins SC, Macaulay W, Turner D, Kang R, Rubash HE, Evans CH. Identification of inducible nitric oxide synthase in human macrophages surrounding loosened hip prostheses. Am J Pathol 1997; 150(4):1199–1206.

92. Shanbhag AS, Macaulay W, Stefanovic-Racic M, Rubash HE. Nitric oxide release by macrophages in response to particulate wear debris. J Biomed Mater Res 1998; 41(3):497–503.

93. Tucci M, Baker R, Benghuzzi H, Hughes J. Levels of hydrogen peroxide in
    tissues adjacent to failing implantable devices may play an active role in cyto-
    kine production. Biomed Sci Instrum 2000; 36:215–220.
94. Hancock JT. Superoxide, hydrogen peroxide and nitric oxide as signalling mole-
    cules: their production and role in disease. Br J Biomed Sci 1997; 54(1):38–46.

In Vitro and In Vivo Models for Understanding Osteolysis

Brian L. Puskas, Mark J. Neavyn, and Arun Shanbhag

*Department of Orthopaedic Surgery, Massachusetts General Hospital,
Harvard Medical School, Boston, Massachusetts, U.S.A.*

INTRODUCTION

The success of total joint replacements (TJR) is due to extensive and systematic investigations into various clinical and biological aspects of the hip joint and materials replacing it. Despite the plethora of enhancements, peri-implant bone loss continues to be the primary cause for failure and revision of TJRs in both hips and knees (1–3). Detailed investigations by Charnley, Willert, and others (4–7), laid the foundation for the development of experimental models to understand this process of pathological bone loss. These models facilitated in-depth investigations into the biological environment contributing to implant failure and permitted the analysis of specific mechanisms leading to bone resorption. Experimental models allowed researchers to avoid the inherent challenges in clinical investigations and provided an opportunity to study the biological system within a relatively controlled environment. The integration of information gathered from in vitro and in vivo methods, as well as analyses of retrieved clinical materials, helps bridge the gap between laboratory investigations and clinical events occurring in the patient.

In this chapter, we will first examine the primary biological factors involved with osteolysis. Many studies that describe the cellular environment of failed prostheses use tissue specimens harvested from patients during revision surgery or autopsy. Next, we will discuss studies that have utilized in vitro models to elucidate the sequence of events leading to osteolysis and implant failure. The benefits and shortcomings of in vivo experimental models will be addressed in the context of the inflammatory response to particulate debris and bone biology concerning implant failure. Finally, we will discuss how in vitro and in vivo techniques have been used to evaluate hypotheses, provide insight into the inflammatory process, and have led to potential therapies for aseptic loosening and osteolysis.

TECHNIQUES IN ANALYZING CLINICAL MATERIAL

Histopathologic analysis of clinical material is the primary technique used to investigate the pathogenesis of osteolysis and aseptic loosening. During these analyses, cells, particulate debris, and biological mediators present are identified. The clinical materials analyzed may be harvested during biopsies, revision surgery (8–11), or autopsies (12,13). Investigators (14–16) have studied the synovial fluid, periprosthetic tissues, polyethylene and metal components and surfaces, as well as extra-articular tissues such as lymph nodes. During autopsies, the implant and surrounding soft tissues and bone are harvested; regional and distant lymph nodes and organ tissue from the lungs, liver, and spleen have also yielded critical information about the onset of osteolysis and aseptic loosening (12,13,17–20).

Depending on the focus of research, a variety of techniques are used to examine tissue specimens (Table 1). Light microscopy of hematoxylin and eosin (H&E) stained tissue sections is routine and provides valuable information on the general organization and morphology of the tissues and cells associated with periprosthetic bone loss. Confocal microscopy and electron microscopy have also been used to establish the intracellular spatial organization of wear debris particles in the context of the organelles and lysosomes of active inflammatory cells (21,22). Cellular mediators released by the peri-implant tissues can be identified by placing tissues in organ culture. Mediator profile can provide crucial insight into the microenvironment of the cells and potential autocrine and paracrine interactions (11,23,24). Investigators have confirmed the transcription and secretion of a variety of proinflammatory cytokines and chemokines, prostaglandins, and matrix-degrading enzymes within the periprosthetic membrane (8,24,25). This inflammatory environment has the capacity to stimulate osteoclastic bone resorption and peri-implant fibrous tissue formation leading to implant instability (23,25–27).

Peri-implant granulomatous tissues harvested during revision surgeries provide a unique opportunity to study the particulate wear debris causing osteolytic lesions. Various techniques have been used to digest the tissues and extract the particulate debris present (21,28–33). The morphological and physicochemical characteristics of retrieved particles are then determined using scanning electron microscopy, transmission electron microscopy, and atomic force microscopy (Table 1). These analyses have contributed to our

Table 1 Commonly Used Techniques to Analyze Clinically Obtained Materials

Tissues
Harvested during biopsy, revision surgery, and autopsy
Tissue collection sites
Peri-implant granuloma; interfacial membrane
Joint capsule
Bone and cartilage
Synovial or joint fluid aspiration
Extra-articular materials/samples
  lymph nodes
  spleen
  lungs
Peripheral blood cells
  monocytes
  neutrophils
  lymphocytes
Analysis
Histopathology
  light microscopy
  immunohistochemistry
  in situ hybridization
Confocal microscopy
Scanning electron microscopy
Transmission electron microscopy
Implant materials
Harvested during biopsy, revision surgery and, autopsy
Wear debris
  Digest and extract from tissues or fluids using KOH, NaOH, HCl, or enzymes
  Scanning electron microscopy
  Transmission electron microscopy
  Atomic force microscopy
  Particle size analysis
UHMWPE liners
  Optical microscopy
  Electron microscopy
  Fourier transform infrared spectroscopy
  Differential scanning calorimetry
  Wide angle X-ray diffraction
Metal components
  Stereo microscopy
  Scanning electron microscopy
  Energy dispersive X-ray
  Transmission electron microscopy
  Atomic force microscopy
  Coordinate measuring machine
  Metallurgical analysis
  Electrochemical analysis

understanding of the determinants of biologic reactivity (21,30,34) and have facilitated the development of clinically relevant experimental models discussed later in this chapter.

Material and metallurgic analyses of the retrieved implants identify important factors that increase the opportunities for lysis such as scratches on the femoral head, abrasion of the metal stem, delamination of the fiber-metal porous pad and metal beads, and fracture of wires and cables used during surgery (35,36). Techniques used to evaluate retrieved components include stereo microscopy, electron microscopy, and metallurgic analyses used to study metal grain structure, distribution, and corrosion (Table 1). Analyses of retrieved acetabular liners have yielded information on consolidation of the polyethylene base resin and sterilization and shelf storage of the liners (37–39). The techniques used in these cases include Fourier Transform Infrared Spectroscopy, differential-scanning calorimetry to identify the chemical species, and X-ray diffraction (wide and small angles) to study crystallinity (40,41).

IN VITRO MODELS

From the analysis of clinical specimens, various cell types and biological mediators involved in the chronic inflammatory process have been identified and the temporo-spatial relationship between tissues and cells established (Table 2). The role of macrophages and giant cells in phagocytosis and encapsulation of wear debris as well as the association of granulomas with bony erosions have been well documented (10,17,42–47). Furthermore, it is widely accepted that the macrophage–particle interaction within the fibrous tissue surrounding the prostheses is a key component of the inflammatory sequelae leading to osteolysis (1,27,48). Macrophages are the primary phagocytic cell at the bone-implant interface. These cells initiate an aggressive immunological response to foreign material which disrupts the homeostatic balance maintained by osteoblasts and osteoclasts (49–51).

Table 2   In Vitro Experimental Models

Cell types used (transformed and primary)	Analysis performed
Peripheral blood monocytes	Protein analysis
Macrophages (transformed and peritoneal)	Enzyme-linked immunosorbent assay (ELISA)
Osteoblasts	Western blots
Bone marrow stromal cells	
Osteoclasts	mRNA analysis
Fibroblasts	Northern blots
	RNase protection assay (RPA)
	cDNA microarrays

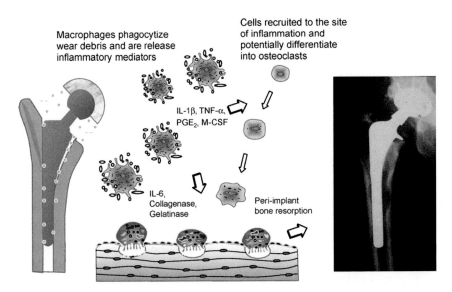

Macrophages phagocytize wear debris and are release inflammatory mediators

Cells recruited to the site of inflammation and potentially differentiate into osteoclasts

IL-1β, TNF-α, PGE$_2$, M-CSF

IL-6, Collagenase, Gelatinase

Peri-implant bone resorption

Figure 1 Schematic of wear debris-mediated osteolysis. Particulate debris generated at the articulating surfaces migrates to the bone–implant interface. Macrophages phagocytize the debris and are stimulated to release a variety of inflammatory mediators. These mediators stimulate osteoclast recruitment, maturation and stimulation to increase peri-implant bone resorption. Such localized resorptive process at the bone–implant interface results in the bone loss observed around implants and causes implant loosening.

In addition to being osteoclast precursors (52,53), macrophages secrete mediators involved in osteoclast recruitment, proliferation, differentiation, and maturation (54–56). During osteolysis, osteoclasts, which are large multinucleated catabolic cells responsible for bone resorption, overwhelm osteoblast-mediated bone formation leading to the degradation of the bone–implant anchor and loosening of the implant (Fig. 1).

Macrophages

Extensive research has been devoted to studying macrophage function and subsequent influences on the surrounding tissues. Macrophages provide a well-developed biological system to study the inflammatory response to foreign material. Here we will discuss the various approaches to studying this key orchestrator of inflammation.

Primary Monocytes and Macrophages

Human peripheral blood monocytes used in primary culture are clinically appropriate surrogates for in vivo macrophages (48). These mononuclear cells, found throughout the circulatory system, are precursors to macrophages involved in periprosthetic inflammation, and when used in in vitro models are representative of the genetically diverse human population. Mononuclear cells differentiate into macrophages at the site of inflammation and are responsible for the over-abundance of macrophages associated with particulate wear debris within the peri-implant tissue. They are easily isolated from whole blood donated by human patients and volunteers by centrifugation over discontinuous gradients, to exploit differences in specific gravity of different cell types (27,57). Investigators have traditionally used an overnight culture to select for adherent cells and to remove nonadherent contaminating cells and platelets (48,58,59).

In studying human cells, investigators are sensitive to the variability in the human monocyte response to biomaterials. Mathews et al. (60) demonstrated that cells isolated from different blood donors responded to identical stimuli with varying intensities. After incubating monocytes with ultra high molecular weight polyethylene (UHMWPE) particles at various doses, levels of IL-1β, IL-6, and granulocyte macrophage colony-stimulating factor (GM-CSF) remained low in 2/3 donors, but cytokine release was magnified in the remaining donor. A study by Herman et al. (61) demonstrated similar findings in the human monocyte response to identical stimuli as well as baseline production of inflammatory mediators among different donors. In a very recent study, Sethi et al. (62) demonstrated that human monocytes from different donors were sensitive to culture on biomaterial disks and released varying levels of inflammatory mediators. The genetic basis of individual variability may be the reason why only a subset of patients develop particle-mediated bone loss even though particulate wear debris is generated in all patients (62–64). In addition to genetic diversity among blood donors, individuals have a dynamic immune system and cultures from one time point may not represent a general biological response. In studying the biocompatibility of different materials with human peripheral blood monocytes, it is thus important to recognize the inherent challenges with human primary culture.

Rat or mouse peritoneal macrophages are also common forms of primary cell cultures used in studying macrophages (26,65). Cells can be isolated from the peritoneal cavity of the animal, then cultured and studied similarly to human peripheral blood monocytes. Although this model provides researchers an opportunity to study a large population of cells, the maintenance and ultimate sacrifice of animals can be resource intensive.

Transformed Macrophage Cell Lines

Many studies focusing on macrophage–wear debris interaction have utilized immortalized transformed cell lines as model systems (26,27,66–69). Immortalized cells are easily harvested in large numbers so that a wide variety of experimental conditions can be tested, and avoids contaminating cells such as lymphocytes, basophils and eosinophils. All cells are virtually identical, so experiments are consistent under similar conditions. In addition, this characteristic reproducibility of transformed cell lines permits researchers to compare the macrophage response to stimuli under multiple experimental conditions without concern for confounding variables such as genetic heterogeneity or immunological variation. Since most cell lines are readily available to the research community, it permits a better correlation of findings between different investigators. Despite its usefulness however, the genetic homogeneity of macrophage cell lines is a limiting factor in correlating experimental findings to the clinical environment. Some of the most commonly used murine macrophage cell lines used in studying osteolysis are RAW 264.7, P388D1, J774, and IC-21. Human cell lines include U937 and THP-1, although neither cell line adequately maintains the properties found in mature macrophages over long periods of time.

Transformed murine cells have been observed to maintain critical functions such as nonspecific phagocytosis, continual production of an array of cytokines and mediators, and adherence to tissue culture surfaces. As a cautionary note, Glant and Jacobs used (70) P388D1 and IC-21 murine macrophages in conjunction with a primary culture of mouse peritoneal macrophages to study the effects of titanium and polymethyl methacrylate (PMMA) particles on the secretion of interleukin (IL)-1 and prostaglandin E_2 (PGE$_2$) and convincingly demonstrated that different cell lines elicit significant differences from different macrophage populations. Peritoneal macrophages extracted from live mice tended to have increased bone-resorbing activity in response to titanium particles, whereas PMMA particles elicited greater activity in the two cell lines.

Fibroblasts

The main role of fibroblasts in the periprosthetic mileu is the formation of scar tissue, which encapsulates the site of inflammation (71). Increase in fibrous tissue at the bone–implant interface can lead to decreased bone ingrowth, ultimately leading to implant loosening. Fibroblasts are also involved in the degradation of organic components of bone and are facultative phagocytes, capable of responding to particulate wear debris (72,73). Thus, fibroblasts associated with interfacial tissue play an important role in the process of osteolysis and the development of aseptic loosening of TJR.

Maloney et al. (72) studied fibroblast–particle interaction and found a correlation between fibroblast proliferation and particle toxicity. When bovine synovial fibroblasts were cultured with titanium particles, phagocytosis was accompanied by membrane ruffling and filopodial extension. Conversely, when exposed to cobalt particles, fibroblasts underwent cytoplasmic shrinking and crenation, associated with cell death (72). They hypothesized that metallic wear debris may be instrumental in fibrous tissue formation around an implant. A succeeding study by Yao et al. (73) found that fibroblasts stimulated by metallic debris produced elevated levels of bone resorbing enzymes such as collagenase, stromelysin, and metalloproteinases. In conjunction with these findings, Shanbhag et al. (27) revealed that particle-free conditioned medium, collected from peripheral blood monocytes challenged with wear debris, stimulated fibroblast proliferation in vitro. Cellular mediators present in conditioned medium of the monocyte-particle cultures such as IL-1 induce fibrosis even if levels are insufficient to cause bone resorption (27). Therefore, the deleterious consequences of acute fibrosis at the bone-implant interface may have a synergistic role in osteolysis and aseptic loosening; fibrous tissue may impede initial bone ingrowth, and bone resorption may be further stimulated by mediators secreted from fibroblasts.

Osteoblasts

In normal physiology, bone resorption mediated by osteoclast catabolism is balanced by osteoblast-mediated bone formation (52). Osteoblasts are crucial in maintaining the structural integrity of bone. In the microenvironment of the bone–implant interface, bone formation may be diminished such that the system cannot compensate for pathologic bone loss surrounding the prosthesis. Consequently, the problem of osteolysis extends to osteoblast function, and it is important to study their interaction within the implant system.

As with many in vitro experimental models, transformed cell lines are constructive tools for studying the cellular response to specific stimuli. Cell lines used in studying the osteoblast response include mouse cells MC3T3-E1 (74,75) and the commonly used human osteoblastic cells SAOS-2 (76), and MG-63 (75–77). The MG-63 osteosarcoma cells retain unique functions of the osteoblast such as 1,25 di-hydroxy vitamin D3-induced collagen synthesis, parathyroid hormone-stimulated production of cyclic-adenosine monophosphate (c-AMP), and the production of both alkaline phosphatase and osteocalcin (78). Tests used to analyze the performance of these cells include alkaline phosphatase activity, osteocalcin production, collagen production, and proteoglycan sulfation. Using these techniques, Kieswetter et al. (79) observed that the activity of MG-63 cells was modulated by surface roughness of the culture dishes. This team also reported that MG-63 osteosarcoma cell activity was adversely affected by UHMWPE wear debris in a dose-dependent manner (78). Osteoblast culture with particle debris stimulated proliferation and prostaglandin E_2 production, while cell differentiation and matrix production were inhibited. In a similar study, Vermes et al. (80) demonstrated that the process of phagocytosis by osteoblasts stimulates the production of cytokines and inhibits type-I collagen synthesis. Thus, the presence of debris has a two-fold effect on osteolysis with respect to the osteoblasts: osteoblast function is inhibited, while osteoclast differentiation and activation is stimulated, through tumor necrosis factor (TNF)-α and IL-6 secretion by osteoblasts. Because of the diminished osteo-blast function, resorbed bone cannot be replaced in a timely manner. The process of osteolysis incorporates many facets of the dynamic bone system. In order to combat osteolysis in TJRs, these aspects of bone loss surround-ing the implant need to be fully understood.

Conducting Cell–Particle Interactions

As we have seen previously in this chapter, many in vitro studies have focused on the potential of clinically relevant particle species to initiate an inflammatory response leading to bone resorption. While particulate wear debris clearly have adverse affects on multiple cell types of the periprosthetic membrane, conducting cell–particle studies to isolate these findings requires a thorough understanding of the issues at play.

In an early in vivo study (1959), Cohen (81) investigated the subcuta-neous tissue response in rats to different forms and sizes of commonly used Co–Cr alloy and stainless steel particles. In a seminal report, Cohen recorded that larger particles (5–40 μm) provoked a limited inflammatory response that took the form of a fibrous tissue encapsulation. Finer particles (<1 μm) provoked an inflammatory reaction associated with tissue necrosis, acute inflammation, and extensive fibrosis (81). These findings have formed the basis of our understanding of particle inflammation associated with osteolysis and aseptic loosening.

There are different methodologies for developing an experimental design appropriate to investigating the cell–particle interaction. Limiting criteria for each method include density and size of particles. In Cohen's study, metallic particle dose was determined by the mass of the particles. Horowitz et al. (82) used a similar dosing method for challenging mononuc-lear cells with PMMA particles. Particles were grouped by diameter (1–300 and 1000–3000 μm) and the dose of challenging particles was determined by mass. This method of particle dosing was appropriate for the experimen-tal design because only one type of particle material (PMMA) was studied. Had the study expanded its focus and analyzed different materials, this method would not have been valid. This is because both the size of the particles and the density of the materials used would have to be taken into account. For example, if comparably sized titanium particles were also stu-died and a similar mass was used, the density differences between titanium ($\rho = 4.5\,\text{g/cm}^3$) and PMMA ($\rho = 1.0\,\text{g/cm}^3$) particles would translate in under dosing the Ti particles. Because each Ti particle has a mass 4.5 times greater than PMMA particles, for a given mass there would only be 22 particles of Ti for every 100 particles of PMMA (1.0/4.5), making the results meaningless.

This problem can be partially circumvented by using volume fraction as a measure of comparison. Volume fractions are independent of particle density and for a similar size of particles, the cells would still be challenged with the approximate same particle number of Ti and PMMA particles in the above example. Several investigators have used volume fraction and number of particles as a basis for conducting cell–particle interactions (72,83).

In periprosthetic tissues, a wide variety of particles are found of varying sizes ranging from 0.2 to 50μm, with widely varying density from UHMWPE ($\rho = 0.94\,\mathrm{g/cm^3}$) to Ti alloy ($\rho = 4.54\,\mathrm{g/cm^3}$), and Co–Cr ($\rho = 8.3\,\mathrm{g/cm^3}$), which makes the comparison very complicated. For such circumstances, Shanbhag et al. (48,69) demonstrated the appropriateness of dosing cells based on the surface area of the particles. In their studies, the dose of particles used to challenge macrophages was based on particle surface area. Because they used different types of materials, the surface area per unit weight varied, depending on the density of the particle species being used. For example, 0.147 mg of commercially pure titanium particles were used to achieve the same surface area as 0.016 mg of fabricated UHMWPE particles. Using this methodology, they demonstrated that when standardized for surface area, TiAlV particles were more stimulatory to human monocytes than UHMWPE particles (27,48). These results parallel the macrophage response to nonphagocytosable surfaces as well (62). Thus, surface area is a useful parameter to investigate the biologic interplay of foreign materials with varying size and composition. The challenges of this method are that a detailed particle analysis is required and assumptions regarding particle and cellular geometries must be made. These issues can be addressed using gas adsorption on particles and the Brunauer, Emmett, Teller (BET) (84) algorithm to calculate precise surface areas as is routinely done in engineering programs.

Limitations of In Vitro Models

The disadvantage of an in vitro model is the reduced ability to study the metabolic pathways acting in concert within the host. For instance, subculturing of cells can result in loss of specific properties active within a live animal. Further, since cultured cells are devoid of interactions with other cell types, they can only partially model what may be occurring in the body. Other issues include absorption and adsorption of drugs or media proteins on the surface of flasks containing cell cultures, which could possibly skew results. Similarly, the dedifferentiation of cultured cells may not accurately predict a tissue or organ's response. A confounding factor for dividing cell cultures is the stationary phase that is reached after confluence of the culture. In the stationary phase, cells are normally viable for only a few days in which cellular metabolism slows and many enzymatic processes are turned off. This could have a negative effect on the translation of experimental results. Despite these limitations, cell culture is an effective in vitro model for studying a specific aspect of a larger pathophysiological problem.

IN VIVO MODELS

An in vivo model can either be an animal model or a clinical study, and focuses on the integrated biological system. When in vivo models are designed creatively they can be effective tools to assess chronic human diseases. In vivo models involve multiple cell types interacting within the local environment and simultaneously responding to paracrine effects, and leads to a more relevant set of conditions. Factors that can affect immunological activity such as a particular environment, overall health of the individual, physical activity, and even genetic variability can be monitored and possibly controlled with in vivo models. Thus, an effective in vivo model permits us to understand the pathophysiology of osteolysis, most closely resembling actual events in the patient (Table 3).

Animal Care

Since in vivo studies rely primarily on the use of animal models, it is incumbent on researchers to follow ethical standards in animal studies, and minimize unnecessary harm or injury to animals. Experimental designs must be carefully developed to yield a clear and practical protocol relevant to the hypothesis being tested. Further, it should estimate the magnitude of any observed effects, as well as the amount of random variability present. Statistical power analysis is a useful tool required by most institutional review committees, which rationalizes the number of animals necessary to conduct an experiment. Appropriate training of staff is very important. Attention should also be paid to the physical and psychological health of the animals with proper animal facilities and veterinary support.

When correctly designed in conjunction with appropriate controls, in vivo experiments permit a generalized extrapolation to the human condition. For instance, where in vivo models are used to study failed THR, animal surgery is performed with the exacting standards and aseptic surgical

Table 3 In Vivo Experimental Models

Models to evaluate biocompatibility	*Models to study bone ingrowth/ongrowth*
Subcutaneous implantation	Surface coatings or modifications on rods
Intramuscular implantation	(intramedullary rod with coatings)
Air pouch model (rat)	
Bone site	
Models to study bone resorption	*Total joint replacement models*
Calvarial organ model	Canine model
Tibial defect model	Sheep model
Plug or rod in bone (rat, mice, rabbit)	Rat model
Bone harvest chamber	

principles as those used in patients. Key items to consider when operating on an animal for an experiment include: the type and dose of anesthesia, anatomic location of the surgical site, preparation of the incision site, specific instruments necessary, dressings, and perhaps most important, pain management and postsurgical recovery.

Biocompatibility of Materials

Since the 1950s, in vivo studies using rabbits, rats, and guinea pigs have been performed to investigate the biocompatibility of bulk and particulate biomaterials (4,81,85). Materials of various sizes, shapes, and compositions were implanted in different subcutaneous, intramuscular, or intra-articular locations. More recently, researchers have focused on the generation and the ensuing inflammatory reaction to fine wear debris associated with biomaterials used in TJR.

Edwards et al. (86) developed in vivo models in rats, in which repeated subcutaneous injections of air disrupted the connective tissue of the animal and created an air pouch. Based on histopathological studies, evaluation of various enzymatic activity, and electron microscopy, the air pouch resembled a synovial membrane (86). The rat air-pouch model helped characterize how specific biomaterials elicit a foreign body response to wear debris. Subsequently, the rodent air-pouch model has aided in the study of inflammatory mediators such as PGE_2 and TNF-α as well as responses to ceramics, PMMA, and particles of UHMWPE (87).

More recently, Gelb et al. (88) and Hooper et al. (89) have utilized the rodent subcutaneous air-pouch model to quantitatively assess the acute inflammatory response to biomaterials associated with THR. Hooper et al. (89) noted that within two days after implantation, macrophages were the predominant cell type recruited to the implant site and essentially confirmed earlier studies by Anderson (49,90) that the presence of a foreign material triggers an influx of inflammatory granulocytes and macrophages to the area and the intensity of the inflammatory response can depend on the characteristics of the material. Using the air-pouch model, Gelb et al. (88) reported that smaller, irregularly shaped particles of PMMA elicited significantly greater levels of inflammatory mediators than did smoother, spherical PMMA particles. The rodent air-pouch model thus allows the investigator to simulate the physiological conditions present clinically in a TJR patient. The primary shortcoming of this model is its nonosseous location, the absence of articulating implant, and the dissimilarity of the pseudomembrane seen around joint replacements.

Peri-Implant Bone Loss

Many investigators (91–93) have utilized neonatal rodent calvariae as easily accessible models to study bone biology. These models are also used in studying the nature of osteoclast-mediated bone resorption. Investigators have explored the process of osteoclast formation in hopes that this may lead to novel therapeutic strategies for their regulation. Merkel et al. (94) demonstrated that bone marrow macrophages cultured with implant particles express c-src, indicating their commitment to the osteoclast lineage. Because TNF-α induces the expression of the c-src protein, investigators developed knock-out mice lacking the p55 and p75 TNF receptors to examine if this cytokine was a reasonable target for the inhibition of osteoclastogenesis. Merkel et al. (94) observed that knock-out mice, while still developing a site of inflammation, were unable to develop osteoclasts, thus thwarting the onset of osteolysis. This in vivo model focused on a specific biochemical pathway that would not have been possible in a human study. At the same time, it has provided vital information to the understanding of osteoclast differentiation and a clear direction towards the development of nonsurgical methods to treat particle-induced ostelysis. While the inhibition of PGE_2 by indomethacin curtails bone resorption in mouse calvaria (95), it is essentially ineffective in long bones. This finding may highlight subtle variations in the catabolic pathways of bone resorption between flat bones (such as the calvaria) and long bones that are associated with joint replacements.

Other models have demonstrated the inflammatory response of particulate wear debris in a long bone location. For instance, Howie et al. (16,96) studied the inflammatory reaction to particulate high density polyethylene around a nonweight bearing bone cement plug in an in vivo rat model. Animals receiving a bone cement plug and no wear debris had a complete shell of new bone surrounding the cement plug two weeks after implantation. Repeated injections of polyethylene particles in the knee resulted in resorption of the bone surrounding the plugs. Bone loss around the plugs was associated with fibrous tissue containing macrophages, giant cells, and particles. This experimental model successfully demonstrated that the introduction of wear debris to a bone location leads to bone loss, similar to that seen in clinical TJR cases.

Goodman et al. (97) utilized a rabbit tibial-defect model to demonstrate that introduction of particulate debris can lead to the development of a florid fibrohistiocytic and giant cell reaction, as seen around loose implants. Goodman (98) exposed rabbits to different physical forms of PMMA; a bolus of doughy PMMA, a preformed PMMA plug, and commercially available particulate PMMA powder. Rabbits exposed to particulate PMMA mounted a heightened foreign body reaction compared to the thin, fibrous tissue membrane of the other groups. They noted that PGE_2 levels were approximately twice as high in animals receiving particulate PMMA (8). The rabbit tibial defect model effectively permitted an assessment of the histology and environment at the bone–cement interface and the development of aseptic loosening of cemented implants.

Modifying the rabbit tibial defect model with the bilateral implantation of a bone harvest chamber has allowed researchers to study spontaneous and gradual bone ingrowth (99). A bone harvest chamber permits investigations of the bone incorporation process under reproducible experimental conditions, and decreases intersample variability by utilizing specimens from the same location at different time points. Using this model, Trindade et al. (99) investigated the effects of UHMWPE and polystyrene (PS) particles on the levels of IL-1β, IL-6, and TNF-α at various intervals up to six weeks. They reported that UHMWPE particles stimulated the highest levels of cytokine release at four weeks.

Models of Total Hip Replacement

The anatomy of the dog, and the similarity of the implanted components has made the canine model of THR a popular model for studying TJR in humans. The in vivo canine model has promoted a better understanding of the pathophysiology of osteolysis and aseptic loosening, facilitated improvements in surgical methods for revision surgery, and helped investigate potential pharmaceutical agents for inhibiting and treating peri-implant bone loss. In order to parallel the clinical manifestations of aseptically loose implants, osteolytic activity is monitored through radiographic, histological, and biochemical techniques.

In order to investigate factors contributing to peri-implant bone loss, Spector et al. (100) developed a canine model of loose cemented femoral stems. Bone cement particles were introduced into the reamed medullary canal of eight dogs, and the cemented stem component was implanted in the femur. Four dogs were sacrificed four and seven months postoperatively, and radionuclide imaging was performed to observe bone turnover. They found a significant correlation between the radiographic characteristics associated with loosening, and the degree of canal fill of the stem. In the same study, Spector et al. isolated membranous tissue from the periprosthetic space for biochemical and histological observation. The interface tissues shared characteristics similar to those retrieved from clinical patients. Macrophages and foreign-body giant cells were intimately involved with fibrous tissues around the implanted material. Similarly, biochemical analysis demonstrated elevated levels of PGE_2 and IL-1 activity.

Turner et al. (101) designed a canine model replicating aseptic loosening of the stem component. Radiographic and histologic features of aseptic failure in this model paralleled those observed clinically. At revision surgery, stem components were implanted either without graft material, with hydroxyapatite/β-tricalcium phosphate within the medullary canal, with an autologous cancellous bone graft, or as a two-stage revision with implantation of the stem four months after an autologous cancellous bone graft (101). After revision surgery, investigators observed that bone ingrowth was best achieved using autologous bone graft (either one stage or two stage), where the osteogenic potential at the site of fixation was greatest. By using this in vivo model, Turner et al. were able to test the efficacy of different surgical methods in hopes of improving the longevity of revised implants.

Other investigators have found canine arthroplasty to be equally useful in determining relevant causative factors in the onset of osteolysis and aseptic loosening. Dowd et al. (102) studied 38 canines with cementless THR and investigated the contribution of micromotion of the stem as well as the contribution of wear debris [Co–Cr alloy, TiAlV, high density polyethylene (HDPE)] on the formation of periprosthetic tissues (102). One group of animals was implanted with a femoral stem allowing for motion between the distal and proximal portions of the component, and the remaining groups were given rigid implants dosed with particles (TiAlV, Co–Cr alloy, or HDPE) placed in a circumferential recessed gap around the femoral stem. Histological and biochemical analysis of induced membranes was found to be similar to those retrieved at revision surgery from human patients (102). Implants experiencing micromotion and those additionally challenged with wear debris had a larger macrophage infiltration within the periprosthetic membrane. In addition, canine implants challenged with wear debris triggered heightened inflammation, particularly with metal particle challenge.

Pharmaceutical Therapy

With a better understanding of the causative agents involved in osteolysis and aseptic loosening, Shanbhag et al. (45) examined a potential pharmacological treatment to attenuate bone resorption associated with aseptic loosening. Bisphosphonates, which are effective inhibitors of bone loss in patients with osteoporosis (103), were used in a canine THR model. Twenty-four adult male canines underwent THR surgery and were randomized into three groups. Group I served as a control, and the bone–implant system was not challenged with wear debris. One billion particles (a mixture of UHMWPE—90% by number; TiAlV—5%, and Co–Cr alloy—5%) were fabricated in vitro and added intraoperatively to the proximal femoral gap for Group II and III animals. This mixture replicated the morphology and composition of wear debris in clinically failed hip arthroplasties (2,21 104–106). One week postoperatively, daily oral alendronate treatment (Fosamax, Merck, Rahway, NJ, 5 mg on an empty stomach at start of each day) was initiated in Group III animals. After 24 weeks, the animals were sacrificed and radiographic analysis performed. In canines with wear debris alone, Shanbhag et al. found radiolucencies around the implant, bearing striking similarity to the peri-implant bone loss seen clinically in humans with THR. Histological analysis revealed a granulomatous response and when placed in organ culture, the peri-implant tissue samples released elevated levels of PGE_2 (45). This indicated that the particle-induced inflammation continued unabated in all groups with wear debris. Without bisphosphonate treatment, this inflammation propagated the osteoclastic bone-resorbing activity, leading to implant loosening. In the treatment group, despite the ongoing inflammation, bisphosphonates inhibited osteoclasts and implant loosening was prevented (Fig. 2). The use of this model which simulated the clinical condition found in humans has greatly enhanced our understanding of the pathophysiology of osteolysis and demonstrated the feasibility of pharmacological treatments in joint replacements. These findings have also led to a clinical trial investigating the efficacy of bisphosphonates in treating rapidly expanding osteolysis. Other pharmaceutical agents are also being investigated to reverse peri-implant bone loss and are discussed extensively in a separate chapter.

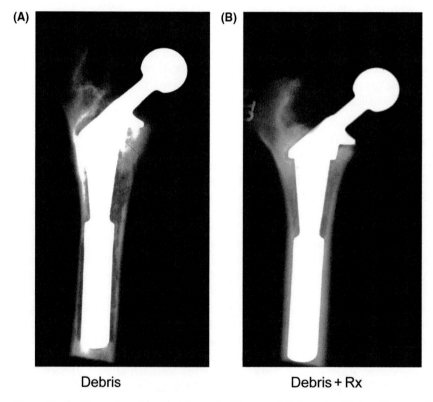

(A) Debris   **(B)** Debris + Rx

Figure 2   Radiographs of canines treated with wear debris and additionally treated with oral alendronate. After a 26-week postoperative period (**A**) peri-implant bone loss is observed around the joint replacements in untreated animals, (**B**) while no bone loss was observed in animals treated with oral alendronate.

SUMMARY

The current understanding of the complex pathophysiology of the bone–implant interface has been evolving since the inception of TJR four decades ago. In vitro and in vivo experimental models have played a significant role in the identification of biological and biomechanical factors leading to osteolysis and aseptic loosening. Since the work of John Charnley and Hans Willert, in vitro and in vivo models have helped to delineate that the generation of particulate wear debris is a primary causative factor leading to osteolysis. In vitro analyses of retrieved clinical materials has helped to focus investigations on the macrophage as a key mediator of the inflammatory response and the activity of osteoclasts. In vivo experiments have allowed researchers to study the bone–implant system in an environment more representative of human TJRs. The rat air-pouch model has confirmed in vitro inflammatory findings, while different rabbit and canine models have elucidated the pathophysiology of particle-induced osteolysis and aseptic loosening.

Over the years, clinicians and basic scientists alike have made progressive advancements in the understanding of osteolysis and aseptic loosening. Many improvements in surgical technique, implant design, material longevity, and biocompatibility, as well as the advent of novel pharmaceutical agents, are a direct result of research utilizing the models and techniques described in this chapter.

Today, in vitro and in vivo techniques are mainstays in research regarding the failure of TJR. In vitro and in vivo experimental models, each

Table 4 Comparison of In Vivo and In Vitro Experimental Models

In vitro models	In vivo models
Easy to setup and get started	Significant experience, planning and resources required
Study individual cell types	Study effects of all associated cell types
Dissect signaling pathways	Study complex interactions; holistic systems approach
Explore feasibility of pharmaceutical agents	Evaluate efficacy and complications of pharmaceutical agents thoroughly
Minimize confounding variables	Explore all unintended consequences
Not affected by paracrine effects	Effect on remote organs
Exclude third body wear	Autocrine and paracrine effects
	Effect of third body wear
Acute effects of materials and drugs	Long-term effects of materials and drugs
May not translate to clinical findings	Preclinical testing
Approval required for using human cells and materials	Approval required for Institutional Animal Care and Utilization Committee
Relatively inexpensive ($)	Very expensive ($$$$$)

with their own strengths and limitations, are used to complement each other in order to prove or disprove an experimental hypothesis (Table 4). In the hands of skilled investigators, these models also provide creative insights for new approaches to prevention and treatment. While clinical investigation has provided us with a layout of the basic clinical and radiographic features involved in osteolysis and aseptic loosening, in vitro studies have delved deeper into the cellular microenvironment and biochemical sequelae associated with the problem. Animal models have provided a bridge between the clinical pathology and the cellular response, enhancing the clinical relevance of scientific findings. The synergy between in vitro and in vivo models allows investigators to continue to move forward in revealing the events responsible for TJR failure. Only by incorporating variations of these different scientific methods in our investigations can we hope to significantly reduce the prevalence of osteolysis and aseptic loosening and extend the durability of joint replacements.

REFERENCES

1. Implant Wear in Total Joint Replacement. Rosemont, IL: American Academy of Orthopaedic Surgeons, 2001.
2. Friedman RJ, Black J, Galante JO, Jacobs JJ, Skinner HB. Current concepts in orthopaedic biomaterials and implant fixation. J Bone Joint Surg 1993; 75-A: 1086–1109.
3. Goldring SR, Clark CR, Wright TM. Editorial: The problem in total joint arthroplasty: aseptic loosening. J Bone Joint Surg 1993; 75-A:799–801.
4. Charnley J. Tissue reactions to polytetrafluorethylene: Letter to the editor. Lancet 1963; 1963:1379.
5. Charnley J. Arthroplasty of the hip. Lancet 1961:1129–1132.
6. Willert HG, Semlitsch M. Tissue reactions to plastic and metallic wear products of joint endoprostheses. In: Gschwend N, Debrunner HU, eds. Total Hip Prosthesis. Baltimore: Williams and Wilkins, 1976:205–239.
7. Willert HG, Semlitsch M. Reactions of the articular capsule to wear products of artificial joint prostheses. J Biomed Mater Res 1977; 11:157–164.
8. Goodman SB, Chin RC, Chiou SS, Schurman DJ, Woolson ST, Masada MP. A clinical-pathologic-biochemical study of the membrane surrounding loosened and nonloosened total hip arthroplasties. Clin Orthop 1989; 244: 182–187.
9. Berger RA, Quigley LR, Jacobs JJ, Sheinkop MB, Rosenberg AG, Galante JO. The fate of stable cemented acetabular components retained during revision of a femoral component of a total hip arthroplasty. J Bone Joint Surg Am 1999; 81(12):1682–1691.
10. Kadoya Y, Revell PA, Al Saffar N, Kobayashi A, Scott G, Freeman MA. Bone formation and bone resorption in failed total joint arthroplasties: histomorphometric analysis with histochemical and immunohistochemical technique. J Orthop Res 1996; 14(3):473–482.

11. Kim KJ, Rubash HE, Wilson SC, D'Antonio JA, McClain EJ. A histologic and biochemical comparison of the interface tissues in cementless and cemented hip prostheses. Clin Orthop 1993; 287:142–152.

12. Jacobs JJ, Patterson LM, Skipor AK, Hall DJ, Urban RM, Black J, et al. Postmortem retrieval of total joint replacement components. J Biomed Mater Res 1999; 48(3):385–391.

13. Jasty M, Jiranek W, Harris WH. Acrylic fragmentation in total hip replacements and its biological consequences. Clin Orthop 1992; 285:116–128.

14. Gray MH, Talbert ML, Talbert WM, Bansal M, Hsu A. Changes seen in lymph nodes draining the sites of large joint prostheses. Am J Surg Pathol 1989; 13:1050–1056.

15. Hicks DG, Judkins AR, Sickel JZ, Rosier RN, Puzas JE, O'Keefe RJ. Granular histiocytes of pelvic lymph nodes following total hip arthroplasty. The presence of wear debris, cytokine production, and immunologically activated macrophages. J Bone Joint Surg 1996; 78-A:482–496.

16. Howie DW, Vernon-Roberts B. The synovial response to intraarticular cobalt–chrome wear particles. Clin Orthop 1988; 232:244–254.

17. Urban RM, Jacobs JJ, Tomlinson MJ, Gavrilovic J, Black J, Peoc'h M. Dissemination of wear particles to the liver, spleen, and abdominal lymph nodes of patients with hip or knee replacement. J Bone Joint Surg Am 2000; 82(4):457–476.

18. Engh CA, Hooten JP Jr, Zettl-Schaffer KF, Ghaffarpour M, McGovern TF, Bobyn JD. Evaluation of bone ingrowth in proximally and extensively porous-coated anatomic medullary locking prostheses retrieved at autopsy. J Bone Joint Surg Am 1995; 77(6):903–910.

19. Bloebaum RD, Mihalopoulus NL, Jensen JW, Dorr LD. Postmortem analysis of bone growth into porous-coated acetabular components. J Bone Joint Surg 1997; 79-A:1013–1022.

20. Wasielewski RC, Parks N, Williams I, Surprenant H, Collier JP, Engh G. Tibial insert undersurface as a contributing source of polyethylene wear debris. Clin Orthop 1997; 345:53–59.

21. Shanbhag AS, Jacobs JJ, Glant TT, Gilbert JL, Black J, Galante JO. Composition and morphology of wear debris in failed uncemented total hip replacement. J Bone Joint Surg Br 1994; 76(1):60–67.

22. Kobayashi A, Bonfield W, Kadoya Y, Yamac T, Freeman MA, Scott G, et al. The size and shape of particulate polyethylene wear debris in total joint replacements. Proc Inst Mech Eng [H] 1997; 211(1):11–15.

23. Jiranek WA, Machado M, Jasty M, Jevsevar D, Wolfe HJ, Goldring SR, et al. Production of cytokines around loosened cemented acetabular components. Analysis with immunohistochemical techniques and in situ hybridization. J Bone Joint Surg Am 1993; 75(6):863–879.

24. Dorr LD, Bloebaum R, Emmanual J, Meldrum R. Histologic, biochemical and ion analysis of tissue and fluids retrieved during total hip arthroplasty. Clin Orthop 1990; 261:82–95.

25. Shanbhag AS, Jacobs JJ, Black J, Galante JO, Glant TT. Cellular mediators secreted by interfacial membranes obtained at revision total hip arthroplasty. J Arthroplasty 1995; 10(4):498–506.

26. Glant TT, Jacobs JJ, Molnar G, Shanbhag AS, Valyon M, Galante JO. Bone resorption activity of particulate-stimulated macrophages. J Bone Miner Res 1993; 8(9):1071–1079.

27. Shanbhag AS, Jacobs JJ, Black J, Galante JO, Glant TT. Effects of particles on fibroblast proliferation and bone resorption in vitro. Clin Orthop 1997; 342:205–217.

28. Campbell P, Ma S, Yeom B, McKellop HA, Schmalzried TP, Amstutz HC. Isolation of predominantly submicron-sized UHMWPE wear particles from periprosthetic tissues. J Biomed Mater Res 1995; 29:127–131.

29. Schmalzried TP, Jasty M, Rosenberg A, Harris WH. Histologic identification of polyethylene wear debris using Oil Red O stain. J Appl Biomater 1993; 4(2):119–125.

30. Maloney WJ, Smith RL, Schmalzried TP, Chiba J, Huene D, Rubash HE. Isolation and characterization of wear particles generated in patients who have had failure of a hip arthroplasty without cement. J Bone Joint Surg 1995; 77-A: 1301–1310.

31. Doorn PF, Campbell PA, Worrall J, Benya PD, McKellop HA, Amstutz HC. Metal wear particle characterization from metal on metal total hip replacements: transmission electron microscopy study of periprosthetic tissues and isolated particles. J Biomed Mater Res 1998; 42(1):103–111.

32. Schmalzried TP, Campbell P, Schmitt AK, Brown IC, Amstutz HC. Shapes and dimensional characteristics of polyethylene wear particles generated in vivo by total knee replacements compared to total hip replacements. J Biomed Mater Res (Appl Biomater) 1997; 38:203–210.

33. Shanbhag AS, Bailey HO, Hwang DS, Cha CW, Eror NG, Rubash HE. Quantitative analysis of ultra high molecular weight polyethylene (UHMWPE) wear debris associated with total knee replacements. J Biomed Mater Res 2000; 53(1):100–110.

34. Klimkiewicz JJ, Iannotti JP, Rubash HE, Shanbhag AS. Aseptic loosening of the humeral component in total shoulder arthroplasty. J Shoulder Elbow Surg 1998; 7(4):422–426.

35. Gilbert JL, Buckley CA, Jacobs JJ. In vivo corrosion of modular hip prosthesis components in mixed and similar metal combinations. The effect of crevice, stress, motion, and alloy coupling. J Biomed Mater Res 1993; 27(12): 1533–1544.

36. Jacobs JJ, Urban RM, Gilbert JL, Skipor AK, Black J, Jasty M, et al. Local and distant products from modularity. Clin Orthop 1995; 319:94–105.

37. Sutula LC, Collier JP, Saum KA, Currier BH, Currier JH, Sanford WM, et al. The Otto Aufranc Award. Impact of gamma sterilization on clinical performance of polyethylene in the hip. Clin Orthop 1995; 319:28–40.

38. Kurtz SM, Muratoglu OK, Evans M, Edidin AA. Advances in the processing, sterilization, and crosslinking of ultra-high molecular weight polyethylene for total joint arthroplasty. Biomaterials 1999; 20(18):1659–1688.

39. Wright TM, Rimnac CM, Faris PM, Bansal M. Analysis of surface damage in retrieved carbon fiber-reinforced and plain polyethylene tibial components from posterior stabilized total knee replacements. J Bone Joint Surg 1988; 70-A:1312–1319.

40. Bellare A, Cohen RE. Morphology of rod stock and compression-moulded sheets of ultra-high- molecular-weight polyethylene used in orthopaedic implants. Biomaterials 1996; 17(24):2325–2333.

41. Ries MD, Bellare A, Livingston BJ, Cohen RE, Spector M. Early delamination of a Hylamer-M tibial insert. J Arthroplasty 1996; 11(8):974–976.

42. Coleman DL, King RN, Andrade JD. The foreign body reaction: a chronic inflammatory response. J Biomed Mater Res 1974; 8(5):199–211.

43. Steinman RM, Mellman IS, Muller WA, Cohn ZA. Endocytosis and the recycling of plasma membrane. J Cell Biol 1983; 96:1–27.

44. Maloney WJ, Jasty M, Harris WH, Galante JO, Callaghan JJ. Endosteal erosion in association with stable uncemented femoral components. J Bone Joint Surg Am 1990; 72(7):1025–1034.

45. Shanbhag AS, Hasselman CT, Rubash HE. The John Charnley Award. Inhibition of wear debris mediated osteolysis in a canine total hip arthroplasty model. Clin Orthop 1997; 344:33–43.

46. Al Saffar N, Khwaja HA, Kadoya Y, Revell PA. Assessment of the role of GM-CSF in the cellular transformation and the development of erosive lesions around orthopaedic implants. Am J Clin Pathol 1996; 105(5):628–639.

47. Jacobs JJ, Urban RM, Schajowicz F, Gavrilovic J, Galante JO. Particulate-associated endosteal osteolysis in titanium-base alloy cementless total hip replacement. In: St John KR, ed. Particulate Debris from Medical Implants: Mechanisms of Formation and Biological Consequences, ASTM STP 1144. Philadelphia: American Society for Testing and Materials, 1992:52–60.

48. Shanbhag AS, Jacobs JJ, Black J, Galante JO, Glant TT. Human monocyte response to particulate biomaterials generated in vivo and in vitro. J Orthop Res 1995; 13(5):792–801.

49. Anderson JM, Miller KM. Biomaterial biocompatibility and the macrophage. Biomaterials 1984; 5(1):5–10.

50. Morrissette N, Gold E, Aderem A. The macrophage—a cell for all seasons. Trends Cell Biol 1999; 9(5):199–201.

51. Solbach W, Moll H, Rollinghoff M. Lymphocytes play the music but the macrophage calls the tune. Immunol Today 1991; 12(1):4–6.

52. Vaes G. Cellular biology and biochemical mechanism of bone resorption. A review of recent developments on the formation, activation, and mode of action of osteoclasts. Clin Orthop 1988; 231:239–271.

53. Udagawa N, Takahashi N, Akatsu T, Tanaka H, Sasaki T, Nishihara T, et al. Origin of osteoclasts: mature monocytes and macrophages are capable of differentiating into osteoblasts under a suitable microenvironment prepared by bone marrow-derived stromal cells. Proc Natl Acad Sci USA 1990; 87: 7260–7264.

54. Lacey DL, Timms E, Tan HL, Kelley MJ, Dunstan CR, Burgess T, et al. Osteoprotegerin ligand is a cytokine that regulates osteoclast differentiation and activation. Cell 1998; 93(2):165–176.

55. Lum L, Wong BR, Josien R, Becherer JD, Erdjument-Bromage H, Schlondorff J, et al. Evidence for a role of a tumor necrosis factor-α (TNF-α)-converting enzyme-like protease in shedding of TRANCE, a TNF family member involved

in osteoclastogenesis and dendritic cell survival. J Biol Chem 1999; 274(19): 13,613–13,618.

56. Kobayashi K, Takahashi N, Jimi E, Udagawa N, Takami M, Kotake S, et al. Tumor necrosis factor alpha stimulates osteoclast differentiation by a mechanism independent of the ODF/RANKL–RANK interaction. J Exp Med 2000; 191(2):275–286.

57. Roos D, de Boer M. Purification and cryopreservation of phagocytes from human blood. Meth Enzymol 1986; 132:225–243.

58. Miller KM, Anderson JM. In vitro stimulation of fibroblast activity by factors generated from human monocytes activated by biomedical polymers. J Biomed Mater Res 1989; 23(8):911–930.

59. Trindade MC, Nakashima Y, Lind M, Sun DH, Goodman SB, Maloney WJ, et al. Interleukin-4 inhibits granulocyte-macrophage colony-stimulating factor, interleukin-6, and tumor necrosis factor-alpha expression by human monocytes in response to polymethylmethacrylate particle challenge in vitro. J Orthop Res 1999; 17(6):797–802.

60. Matthews JB, Green TR, Stone MH, Wroblewski BM, Fisher J, Ingham E. Comparison of the response of primary human peripheral blood mononuclear phagocytes from different donors to challenge with model polyethylene particles of known size and dose [in process citation]. Biomaterials 2000; 21(20):2033–2044.

61. Herman JH, Sowder WG, Anderson D, Appel AM, Hopson CN. Polymethylmethacrylate-induced release of bone-resorbing factors. J Bone Joint Surg 1989; 71-A:1530–1541.

62. Sethi RK, Neavyn MJ, Rubash HE, Shanbhag AS. Macrophage response to cross-linked and conventional UHMWPE. Biomaterials 2003; 24(15): 2561–2573.

63. Danis VA. Cytokine production by normal human monocytes: inter-subject variation and relationship to an IL-1 receptor antagonist (IL-1Ra) gene polymorphism. Clin Exp Immunol 1995; 99:303–310.

64. Matthews JB, Besong AA, Green TR, Stone MH, Wroblewski BM, Fisher J, et al. Evaluation of the response of primary human peripheral blood mononuclear phagocytes to challenge with in vitro generated clinically relevant UHMWPE particles of known size and dose. J Biomed Mater Res 2000; 52(2): 296–307.

65. Daniels AU, Barnes FH, Charlebois SJ, Smith RA. Macrophage cytokine response to particles and lipopolysaccharide in vitro. J Biomed Mater Res 2000; 49(4):469–478.

66. Rae T. A study on the effects of particulate metals of orthopaedic interest on murine macrophages in vitro. J Bone Joint Surg 1975; 57-B:444–450.

67. Heekin RD, Callaghan JJ, Hopkinson WJ, Savory CG, Xenos JS. The porous-coated anatomic total hip prosthesis, inserted without cement. J Bone Joint Surg 1993; 75-A:77–91.

68. Ingham E, Green TR, Stone MH, Kowalski R, Watkins N, Fisher J. Production of TNF-alpha and bone resorbing activity by macrophages in response to different types of bone cement particles. Biomaterials 2000; 21(10): 1005–1013.

69. Shanbhag AS, Jacobs JJ, Black J, Galante JO, Glant TT. Macrophage/particle interactions: effect of size, composition and surface area. J Biomed Mater Res 1994; 28(1):81–90.
70. Glant TT, Jacobs JJ. Response of three murine macrophage populations to particulate debris: bone resorption in organ cultures. J Orthop Res 1994; 12:720–731.
71. Diegelmann RF, Cohen IK, Kaplan AM. The role of macrophages in wound repair: a review. Plast Reconstr Surg 1981; 68(1):107–113.
72. Maloney WJ, Smith RL, Castro F, Schurman DJ. Fibroblast response to metallic debris in vitro. Enzyme induction, cell proliferation, and toxicity. J Bone Joint Surg 1993; 75-A:835–844.
73. Yao J, Glant TT, Lark MW, Mikecz K, Jacobs JJ, Hutchinson NI, et al. The potential role of fibroblasts in periprosthetic osteolysis: fibroblast response to titanium particles. J Bone Miner Res 1995; 10:1417–1427.
74. Quarles LD, Yohay DA, Lever LW, Caton R, Wenstrup RJ. Distinct proliferative and differentiatied stages of murine MC3T3-E1 cells in culture: an in vitro model of osteoblast development. J Bone Miner Res 1992; 7(6):683–692.
75. Shanbhag AS, Kenney JK, Manning CA, Flannery M, Rubash HE, Goldring SR. Mitogenic effect of bisphosphonates on osteoblastic cells. Trans Orthop Res Soc 2000; 25:688.
76. Zhu J, Valente AJ, Lorenzo JA, Carnes D, Graves DT. Expression of monocyte chemoattractant protein 1 in human osteoblastic cells stimulated by proinflammatory mediators. J Bone Miner Res 1994; 9(7):1123–1130.
77. Lajeunesse D, Frondoza C, Schoffield B, Sacktor B. Osteocalcin secretion by the human osteosarcoma cell line MG-63. J Bone Miner Res 1990; 5(9): 915–921.
78. Dean DD, Schwartz Z, Liu Y, Blanchard CR, Agrawal CM, Mabrey JD, et al. The effect of ultra-high molecular weight polyethylene wear debris on MG63 osteosarcoma cells in vitro. J Bone Joint Surg Am 1999; 81(4):452–461.
79. Kieswetter K, Schwartz Z, Hummert TW, Cochran DL, Simpson J, Dean DD, et al. Surface roughness modulates the local production of growth factors and cytokines by osteoblast-like MG-63 cells. J Biomed Mater Res 1996; 32(1):55–63.
80. Vermes C, Chandrasekaran R, Jacobs JJ, Galante JO, Roebuck KA, Glant TT. The effects of particulate wear debris, cytokines, and growth factors on the functions of MG-63 osteoblasts. J Bone Joint Surg Am 2001; 83-A(2): 201–211.
81. Cohen J. Assay of foreign-body reaction. J Bone Joint Surg 1959; 41-A: 152–166.
82. Horowitz SM, Doty SB, Lane JM, Burstein AH. Studies of the mechanism by which the mechanical failure of polymethylmethacrylate leads to bone resorption. J Bone Joint Surg 1993; 75-A:802–813.
83. Lee SH, Brennan FR, Jacobs JJ, Urban RM, Ragasa DR, Glant TT. Human monocyte/macrophage response to cobalt–chromium corrosion products and titanium particles in patients with total joint replacements. J Orthop Res 1997; 15(1):40–49.
84. Brunauer S, Emmett PH, Teller E. Adsorption of gases in multimolecular layers. J Am Chem Soc 1938; 60:309–319.

85. Vernon-Roberts B, Freeman MAR. Morphological and analytical studies of the tissues adjacent to joint prostheses: investigations into the causes of loosening prostheses. In: Schaldach M, Hohmann D, eds. Advances in Artificial Hip and Knee Joint Technology. Berlin: Springer, 1976:148–186.

86. Edwards JC, Sedgwick AD, Willoughby DA. The formation of a structure with the features of synovial lining by subcutaneous injection of air: an in vivo tissue culture system. J Pathol 1981; 134(2):147–156.

87. Nagase M, Baker DG, Schumacher HR Jr. Prolonged inflammatory reactions induced by artificial ceramics in the rat air pouch model. J Rheumatol 1988; 15(9):1334–1338.

88. Gelb H, Schumacher HR, Cuckler J, Baker DG. In vivo inflammatory response to polymethylmethacrylate particulate debris: effect of size, morphology, and surface area. J Orthop Res 1994; 12:83–92.

89. Hooper KA, Nickolas TL, Yurkow EJ, Kohn J, Laskin DL. Characterization of the inflammatory response to biomaterials using a rodent air pouch model. J Biomed Mater Res 2000; 50(3):365–374.

90. Anderson JM. Multinucleated giant cells. Curr Opin Hematol 2000; 7(1): 40–47.

91. Reynolds JJ, Dingle JT. A sensitive in vitro method for studying the induction and inhibition of bone resorption. Calcif Tissue Res 1970; 4:339–349.

92. Lubin RA, Wong GL, Cohn DV. Biochemical characterization with parathormone and calcitonin of isolated bone cells: provisional identification of osteoclasts and osteoblasts. Endocrinology 1976; 99:526–534.

93. Beresford JN, Gallagher JA, Gowen M, Couch M, Poser J, Wood DD, et al. The effects of monocyte-conditioned medium and interleukin-1 on the synthesis of collagenous and non-collagenous proteins by mouse bone and human bone cells in vitro. Biochim Biophys Acta 1984; 801:58–65.

94. Merkel KD, Erdmann JM, McHugh KP, Abu-Amer Y, Ross FP. Tumor necrosis factor-α mediates orthopedic implant osteolysis. Am J Pathol 1999; 154(1):203–210.

95. Lerner UH, Ransjö M, Ljunggren O. Prostaglandin E_2 causes a transient inhibition of mineral mobilization, matrix degradation, and lysosomal enzyme release for mouse calvarial bones in vitro. Calcif Tissue Int 1987; 40:323–331.

96. Howie DW, Vernon-Roberts B, Oakeshott R, Manthey B. A rat model of resorption of bone at the cement–bone interface in the presence of polyethylene wear particles. J Bone Joint Surg 1988; 70-A:257–263.

97. Goodman SB, Fornasier VL, Kei J. The effects of bulk versus particulate ultra-high-molecular-weight polyethylene on bone. J Arthroplasty 1988; 3(suppl): S41–S46.

98. Goodman SB, Fornasier VL, Kei J. The effects of bulk versus particulate polymethylmethacrylate on bone. Clin Orthop 1988; 232:255–262.

99. Trindade MC, Song Y, Aspenberg P, Smith RL, Goodman SB. Proinflammatory mediator release in response to particle challenge: studies using the bone harvest chamber. J Biomed Mater Res 1999; 48(4):434–439.

100. Spector M, Shortkroff S, Hsu HP, Lane N, Sledge CB, Thornhill TS. Tissue changes around loose prostheses. A canine model to investigate the effects of an antiinflammatory agent. Clin Orthop 1990; (261):140–152.

101. Turner TM, Urban RM, Sumner DR, Galante JO. Revision, without cement, of aseptically loose, cemented total hip prostheses. J Bone Joint Surg 1993; 75-A: 845–862.

102. Dowd JE, Schwendeman LJ, Macaulay W, Doyle JS, Shanbhag AS, Wilson S, et al. Aseptic loosening in uncemented total hip arthroplasty in a canine model. Clin Orthop 1995; (319):106–121.

103. Rodan GA, Fleisch HA. Bisphosphonates: mechanisms of action. J Clin Invest 1996; 97(12):2692–2696.

104. Shanbhag AS, Rubash HE. Wear: the basis of particle disease in total hip arthroplasty. Tech Orthop 1994; 8(4):269–274.

105. Hasselman CT, Kovach C, Keys B, Rubash HE, Shanbhag AS. Macrophage response to synergistic challenge with prosthetic wear debris. Trans Orthop Res Soc 1997; 22:739.

106. Shanbhag AS, Hasselman CT, Rubash HE. Technique for generating submicrometer ultra high molecular weight polyethylene particles. J Orthop Res 1996; 14(6):1000–1004.

20

Surgical Techniques: Modern Cementing Techniques

Craig J. Della Valle and Richard A. Berger

*Department of Orthopaedic Surgery, Rush University
Medical Center, Chicago, Illinois, U.S.A.*

When Charnley first introduced his concept of low friction arthroplasty of the hip, he advocated fixation of both the femoral and acetabular components with polymethylmethacrylate bone cement (1). While the initial results were good, a higher rate of failure has been seen on the acetabular side when fixation with cement is utilized, and thus the majority of surgeons in North America presently use a cementless acetabular component (2). However, there continues to be considerable controversy surrounding fixation of the femoral component in total hip arthroplasty. Despite advancements in cementless femoral components, cementing the femoral component with polymethylmethacrylate arguably remains the long-term standard for fixation. The performance of a cemented femoral component is dependent upon multiple variables: patient selection, stem size, canal preparation, cement preparation and strength, as well as cementing techniques including achieving a continuous cement mantle. It is clear that the results of total hip arthroplasty performed with a cemented femoral component are related to the quality of the cement mantle. Other factors such as geometry of the stem, its surface finish probably also play a role; however, the best design is still heavy debated. The aim of this chapter is to review the evolution of modern cementing techniques and how the surgical techniques employed effect the durability of total hip arthroplasty performed with a cemented femoral component.

RADIOGRAPHIC ANALYSIS

The first step in analyzing cement technique is a thorough understanding of the radiographic hallmarks of a good cement mantle and the markers of cemented femoral component loosening.

Cement Mantle Grading

The most commonly utilized classification of femoral component cement mantles describes mantles as either A, B, C-1, C-2, or D (3–5). The rating of an "A" cementing technique refers to complete filling of the proximal portion of the diaphyseal canal such that no distinction between the cortex and cement can be made; a so-called "white out" (Fig. 1). A "B" cementing mantle refers to a near complete distribution of cement in the proximal diaphysis with a distinguishable interface between cortex and cement. The rating of a "C-1" cement mantle refers to incomplete filling of the proximal portion of the diaphyseal canal such that more than 50% of the cement bone interface shows radiolucencies or the presence of voids in the cement. A "C-2" cementing technique is assigned if either the mantle has an area of cement that measures less than 1 mm in thickness or if the femoral component is in direct contact with bone (Fig. 2). Finally, "D" cementing technique refers to gross deficiencies in the mantle such as no cement below the stem, major defects in the mantle, or multiple large voids in the mantle (Fig. 3).

Although cement mantle grading is dependent upon the adequacy of the radiographs reviewed and the number of views obtained (6), as well as issues of interobserver and intraobserver variability (7), the most important differentiation seems to be between a cement mantle grading of A, B, or C-1, which are generally considered optimal, compared to a grading of C-2 or D which are generally considered suboptimal and more prone to failure. Clinical studies support this notion (4,6,8) and many of the surgical techniques utilized today are aimed at assisting the surgeon in reproducibly achieving an optimal cement mantle.

Radiographic Criteria for Femoral Component Loosening

The most commonly utilized criteria for loosening of a cemented femoral component were described by Harris et al. (9). These authors described femoral components as loose if there is evidence of femoral component subsidence of more than 2 mm, a change in implant position of more than 2° on serial radiographs, evidence of a cement mantle fracture, or a fracture of the femoral component itself (Fig. 4). Implants are considered to be probably loose if there is a continuous radiolucent line at the cement–bone interface and possibly loose if there is a radiolucent line present at the cement–bone interface of more than 50%. Although the significance of radiolucent lines at the prosthesis–bone interface has been called into question, and may be

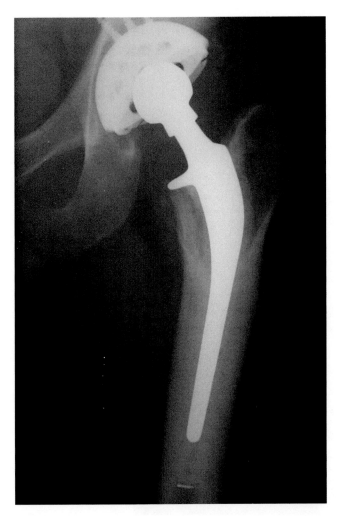

Figure 1 Radiograph of a grade "A" cement mantle; there is complete filling of the proximal portion of the diaphyseal canal such that no distinction between the cortex and cement can be made.

attributable to bony remodeling at this interface, this classification remains the most commonly used to evaluate the radiographic results of cemented femoral components.

A zonal analysis as described by Gruen (10) is also routinely utilized in reporting the results of cemented femoral components in total hip arthroplasty. In this analysis, the femoral component is divided into seven zones on the AP radiograph and seven zones on the lateral radiograph (Fig. 5). Radiolucent lines at the bone–cement and prosthesis–cement interface are

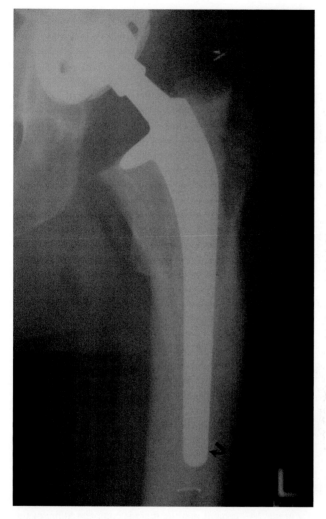

Figure 2   Radiograph of a grade "C-2"cement mantle; the femoral component is in direct contact with the femoral diaphysis (*arrow*).

recorded and progression in the number of zones involved is typically considered evidence of loosening.

EVOLUTION OF CEMENT TECHNIQUE

First Generation Cement Technique

First generation cement technique refers to hand or finger packing of polymethylmethacrylate bone cement into the femoral canal when it is in

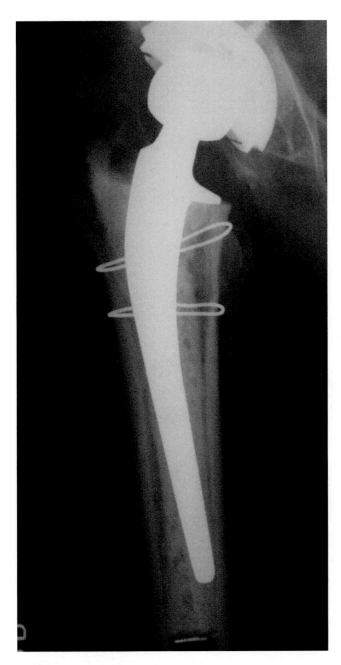

Figure 3 Radiograph of a grade "D" cement mantle; there are major defects in the cement mantle along with multiple areas where the prosthesis is in contact with cortical bone.

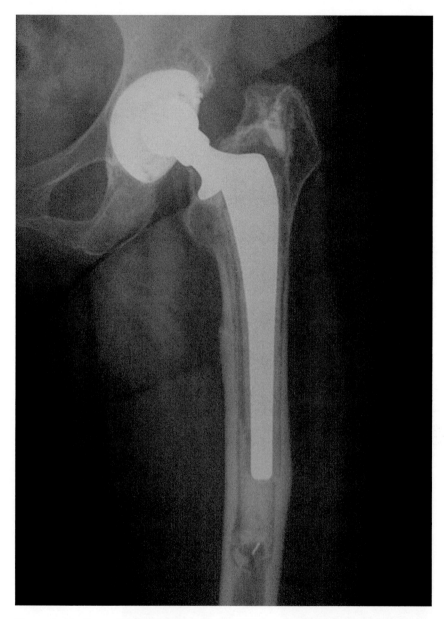

Figure 4   Radiograph of a cemented femoral component with definite radiographic signs of loosening including a fracture of the cement mantle and clear evidence of femoral component subsidence; there is a complete radiolucent line at the cement–bone interface.

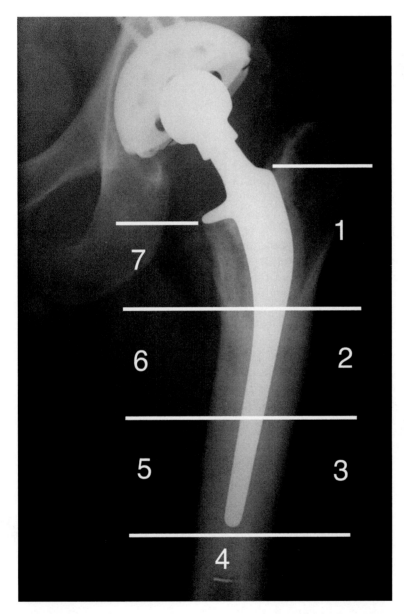

Figure 5 Zonal analysis as described by Gruen with the femur divided into seven zones on the AP radiograph as shown; seven zones are also analyzed on the lateral radiograph.

a doughy state. Femoral components used at this time were often made of stainless steel or cast cobalt–chromium alloys with substantial rates of implant fractures being reported. In addition, the geometry of many first generation implants had narrow medial margins as well as sharp corners that lead to localized areas of high stress within the cement mantle. The results of total hip arthroplasty when this technique was utilized have been variable and may be in part dependent on the prosthetic design employed and on the skill of the surgeon. Sutherland et al. (11) reported that 40 of 100 consecutive Muller curved stems had failed by 10 years when first generation cementing techniques were employed. Although this high failure rate may be attributable in part to the design of this component (with multiple sharp edges) the results were almost certainly also affected by the cement mantle achieved with first generation cement techniques. Stauffer (12) reported the results of 300 Charnley total hip replacements performed between 1960 and 1970 and found that by 10 years, the rate of failure of the femoral component was nearly 30%. Callaghan et al. (13) however, reported a much lower rate of cemented femoral component failure among 330 total hips performed between 1970 and 1972 using first generation cementing techniques. At a minimum of 25 years, 59 hips were available for evaluation; only four hips were revised secondary to loosening of the femoral component (7%). When the entire cohort was considered, the prevalence of revision for aseptic loosening of the femoral component was 3%. Based on these disparate results using the same prosthesis, it became apparent that surgical techniques needed to improve in order to enhance the surgeon's ability to effectively deliver cement into the proximal femur, to ensure that an adequate cement mantle could be achieved.

Second Generation Cement Technique

Secondary generation cementing technique refers to the placement of a bone, cement, or plastic plug into the proximal diaphysis of the femoral canal to allow for some degree of cement pressurization and the use of a cement gun to introduce the cement into the femoral canal in a retrograde fashion. Pulsatile lavage is also used to cleanse the femoral canal of loose cancellous bone, blood, fat, and marrow contents, and dried prior to cementing. This process has been shown to increase the depth of cement preparation and increase the shear strength at the bone–cement interface (14). The goal of these changes was to improve the interdigitation of the cement in the surrounding cancellous bone and to obtain a circumferential cement mantle more reliably (15). Femoral component designs changed as well, with implants made of stronger forged superalloys with rounded edges and broader medial borders to decrease stresses in the cement mantles.

    Klapach et al. (16) compared the results of cemented total hip arthroplasty performed by the same surgeon, with the same femoral component among two cohorts of patients using first and second generation cementing techniques. At a minimum of 20 years, the rate of femoral component failure (defined as radiographic loosening or revision for loosening) among the 330 femoral components inserted with first generation cementing techniques was 6.3% compared to 4.8% for the 357 total hip arthroplasties where second generation cementing techniques were utilized. Although this difference was not statistically significant, adequate filling of the femoral canal and the cement mantle grade were statistically associated with improved femoral component survival. The authors did find that the ability to achieve an adequate cement mantle was more predictable with the use of second generation cementing techniques.

Smith et al. (6) reported on the results of 161 hips in 140 patients who underwent total hip arthroplasty with second generation cementing techniques at a mean of 18 years. Eight femoral components (5%) required revision for loosening and 10 hips (6%) had definite radiographic evidence of loosening. Failure was associated with a thin (<1 mm) or deficient cement mantle; all hips that required revision for femoral component loosening had a C-2 cement mantle and none of the hips with a grade A or B cement mantle required revision or were radiographically loose. The predicted survivorship for the component was 88% at 20 years. Although not the focus of the chapter, it should be noted that the failure rate of the cemented acetabular components used in this study was still high, with a 59% rate of revision or radiographic evidence of loosening, and the improved cementing techniques employed thus did not improve the durability of the acetabular reconstruction. Barrack et al. (5) in a similar study, evaluated the results of second generation cementing techniques in a cohort of 50 hips in 44 patients who were less than 50 years old at the time of surgery. No patient required revision for loosening and one stem met criteria for definite loosening at a mean of 12 years.

Third Generation Cementing Technique

Third generation cementing technique refers to pressurization of the cement during insertion, porosity reduction of the cement, and surface modifications of the implant itself. Pressurization is utilized to increase the amount of cement interdigitation into the cancellous bone in an attempt to increase the strength of the bone–cement interface (17). Porosity reduction includes vacuum mixing of cement and/or centrifugation. Bone cement fails in fatigue and it was felt that by reducing or eliminating pores in the cement, increased strength would be achieved and would lead to a decreased rate of failure as cement voids have been implicated as the initiating and/or propagating points for fractures in the cement mantle. Burke et al (18) studied the effects of centrifugation in a canine model and found that the ultimate tensile strength increased by 24%, the ultimate tensile strain increased by 54% and most importantly that the fatigue life was improved by 136%.

Wixson et al. (19) found similar beneficial effects when a vacuum mixing device was utilized to prepare bone cement.

Surface modifications of the implant itself have been very controversial with regard to their effects on the in vitro strength of the cement–prosthesis interface (which have shown beneficial effects) and the in vivo clinical results (which have been much more variable). Surface modifications of the implant can include both micro texturing and macro texturing of the implant or the precoating of polymethylmethacrylate to the prosthesis itself. While the clinical results of surface modifications have been variable, it is clear that the effect of surface finish is highly dependent upon the geometry of the implant utilized. Both smooth and rough finishes can perform well in different designs. The process of precoating with polymethylmethacrylate must be done on a rougher finish or the coating will not adhere. In general, implants with a higher surface roughness are much more strongly bonded to the cement and increased stresses are transmitted to the cement–bone interface; therefore, loosening typically occurs at the bone–cement interface. In general, implants with a smooth surface are not bonded to the cement which decreases stresses transmitted to the cement–bone interface; therefore, loosening typically occurs at the prosthesis–cement interface.

An excellent example of the effects of implant surface finish on clinical results was seen with the Exeter primary femoral stem. This double tapered implant was originally designed with a polished surface. Clinical results were excellent, however, small amounts of implant subsidence were generally identified. In an effort to improve the outcomes with this implant, the surface finish was changed from a polished to a matte surface. This surface design change was associated with higher rates of clinical and radiographic loosening and it was felt that with this particular stem design, the rougher surface greatly accelerated the process of loosening when subsidence occurred (20,21).

In a similar study with a femoral component of a different geometry, Collis and Mohler (22) examined the results of 244 consecutive hybrid total hip arthroplasties; the first 122 employed a roughened femoral component inserted with cement and in the subsequent 122, a polished stem of the same geometry was utilized. This stem has a cobra shaped proximal segment and an oval shaped distal geometry. Third generation cementing techniques were utilized in both cohorts of patients including the use of vacuum mixed cement. Four of the hips in the grit blasted stem group required revision compared to none of the stems in the polished group. The failures were associated with substantial osteolysis. The survivorship for the grit blasted stems was 91.9% at seven years compared to 100% at the same time interval for the polished stems. Other studies have corroborated these results and in general it is believed that while smoother implant surfaces are associated with a higher degree of micromotion within the cement mantle, they generate less particulate debris; in contrast, rougher stems have higher cement–metal interface fixation strengths and loosen less often. However, if they do migrate, a higher amount of debris is generated (23). However, excellent results have been reported, however, with rough finish stems (24,25). These variable results may be the result of different cementing techniques.

The results of a rough stem with polymethylmethacrylate precoating have also varied according to the cementing technique achieved. Berger et al. (8) reported on 150 consecutive hybrid total hip arthroplasties. The femoral component was precoated with polymethylmethacrylate and the cementing techniques utilized included pressurization of the cement but vacuum mixing or centrifugation of the cement was not utilized. Aseptic loosening occurred in only two hips (1.3%) at a mean of 103 months; both hips were associated with poor cement mantles (C-2 or D). Dowd et al. (26) reported much poorer results using the same acetabular and femoral components as described in the study by Berger et al. with third generation cementing techniques. At a mean of 6.3 years, 23 of 154 hips reviewed had failed (15%); failures were associated with Grade C or D cement mantles. These authors felt that a poor cement mantle may predispose to failure at the cement–bone interface with this rough and precoated stem Oishi et al. (27) reported excellent results with this same stem inserted with third generation cementing techniques. Ong et al. (28) also reported higher failure rates when the precoated version of a stem was compared to a non-precoated version of the same stem. These studies demonstrate that the effects of surface finish are very design and technique sensitive.

Fourth Generation Cement Technique

Fourth generation cementing techniques include the use of proximal and distal centralizers in an attempt to make the achievement of a uniform cement mantle more reproducible (Figs. 6–8). Stem centralizers can either be applied by the manufacturer or be added to the stem by the surgeon prior to insertion. Berger et al. (29) studied the effects of a distal stem centralizer in a randomized study of 450 hips. These authors found that the group in whom a centralizer has been used have significantly fewer hips with cement mantle deficiencies and a higher proportion of hips with neutral as opposed to varus alignment. Hanson et al. (30) found similar results among a group of 100 hips, 50 with and 50 without distal centralization. The stems inserted with a distal centralizer were more neutrally aligned and had improved cement mantles. Another study suggested, however, that even with the use of centralizers, straight stems are at high risk for areas of thin cement mantles, and advocated the use of anatomic stem designs to decrease this risk (5). However, care should be taken when using certain centralizer designs, as voids in the cement mantle can be caused as the stem is inserted and the centralizer is dragged through the cement mantle (32,33).

Goldberg et al. (33) reported the results of 100 primary total hip arthroplasties in which both proximal and distal centralizers were utilized. At a mean of 5.7 years, no stems had failed. The authors' radiographic analysis

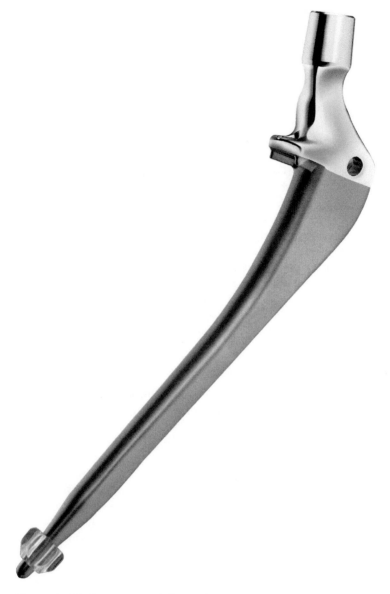

Figure 6 Modern cemented femoral component with both distal and proximal centralizers. The proximal centralizer is manufactured as part of the stem in this particular design.

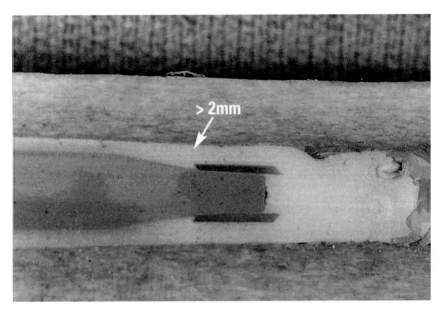

Figure 7 Longitudinal cross section of a cemented femoral component with a distal centralizer. The distal centralizer helps the surgeon to achieve a cement mantle of greater than 2 mm.

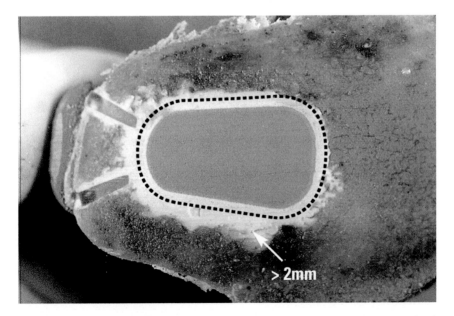

Figure 8 Transverse section of a cemented femoral component with a proximal centralizer. The proximal centralizer helps the surgeon to achieve a cement mantle of greater than 2 mm.

showed that 91 of the 100 hips were implanted in a neutral alignment with a cement mantle that was considered optimal. These authors noted that six of the distal and one of the proximal centralizers fractured at the time of stem insertion and that voids in the cement mantle were seen around the distal centralizer.

Effect of a Collar

The inclusion of a collar in the design of cemented femoral components has also been controversial. Proponents of a collar state that it assists with load transfer to the proximal femur that may prevent stress shielding and potentially protect the proximal cement mantle (34,35). Others feel that the collar is unnecessary and may be detrimental if the implant is expected to subside within the cement mantle (36). From a functional perspective, the most useful function of the collar may be to ensure that the stem is cemented at the same level as the broaches that were used to trial.

Meding et al. (37) in a prospective randomized study of 437 hips randomized patients to the identical femoral component with or without a collar. At an average of 76 months, no clinical or radiographic differences were noted. Another similar prospective randomized series of 84 hips that compared the same femoral component with and without a collar found no clinical difference at a mean of 9.6 years (38). Thus, with the majority of femoral component designs (excluding designs such as a double tapered stem which is known and expected to subside) the use of a collar is based on surgeon preference.

Stem Preheating

Another technique that has been utilized in an attempt to strengthen the bond between the femoral component and the surrounding cement mantle is the preheating of the femoral component. Although preheating of the stem was first utilized in an attempt to speed cement polymerization and thus operative time (39), it was later found that preheating the femoral stem to 44°C led to porosity reduction at the cement–stem interface. In a more detailed analysis, Iesaka et al. (40) studied the effects of preheating the femoral stem to 37, 44, or 50°C prior to insertion in the cement mantle. These authors confirmed not only porosity reduction at the stem–cement interface but also reported increased interface shear strengths and fatigue lifetimes when the preheated stems were compared to stems inserted at room temperature and biomechanically tested. Unfortunately, no clinical studies assessing the effect of stem preheating on component survivorship is yet available in the literature.

PRESENT TECHNIQUE FOR THE INSERTION OF CEMENTED FEMORAL COMPONENTS

In our current practice, we utilize fourth generation cement technique, however the stem that we currently utilize is not precoated, but has a satin finish. Following acetabular preparation and component insertion, the proximal femur is exposed. A box osteotome is utilized to remove the remaining femoral neck laterally and then a canal finder is manually inserted into the femoral canal. Care is taken to remove adequate bone from the superior femoral neck remnant and medial aspect of the greater trochanter to ensure that neutral alignment of the femoral component is achieved. The femoral canal is then sequentially broached (not reamed) from the smallest sized broach to the largest one that can be easily seated in the proximal femur. Trialing of the hip is then performed to ensure that adequate stability and restoration of femoral offset and leg-length have been achieved. Once the final femoral component size and position (e.g., anteversion) has been selected, a proximal centralizing jig is then utilized (V-line, Zimmer, Warsaw, IN). This jig creates two slots in the proximal femur that the proximal centralizing device seats into.

The femoral canal is then sized with sequentially larger sounds to choose the diameter of the distal centralizer to be utilized; the largest sized sound that passes down the canal easily is the appropriate size to be utilized. A cement restrictor is then placed into the femoral canal at an adequate depth to allow for a 2 cm cement mantle distal to the tip of the stem. The appropriately sized femoral component is then brought onto the field and the appropriately sized distal centralizer is applied along with the proximal centralizer. Two packages of Simplex-P cement (Howmedica, Rutherford, NJ) are then mixed under a vacuum, and placed into a cement gun.

As the cement is mixed, the femoral canal is then washed with pulsatile lavage to remove grossly loose cancellous bone, blood, and fat contents. The femoral canal is then packed with epinephrine-soaked gauze sponges to decrease local bleeding. This gauze sponge is inserted until the cement is ready to be inserted and then removed followed by the insertion of second dry gauze into the femoral canal for drying purposes.

At about 3.5 minutes after mixing, the bone cement is then carefully injected into the femoral canal in a retrograde manner, taking care to ensure that the tip of the cement gun does not fall below the level of the cement to avoid the introduction of voids in the cement mantle. At about four minutes, once the canal has been filled with cement, the cement is then slowly pressurized over one minute to ensure adequate interdigitation of the bone cement into the cancellous bone of the proximal femur. The femoral component is then inserted in the same anteversion as the broach (as guided by the V-fin proximal centralizer) taking care to ensure neural alignment of the femoral component within the canal. The stem should be inserted at a constant rate, slow enough to wet the surface without introducing air in the cement column. Firm pressure is maintained on the component while the cement is allowed to dry and excess cement is removed from the proximal femur.

CONCLUSIONS

Numerous studies have documented the importance of the cement mantle in total hip arthroplasty. Thin and less uniform cement mantles have been associated with higher rates of loosening and revision. Improved cement techniques have uniformly reduced the short term, intermediate term, and long-term femoral failure rate and surgeons should strive to reproducibly achieve optimum cement mantles. Proximal and distal centralizers improve the cement mantle in most surgeons hands; however, time will tell if this confers longevity. Lastly, the issue of stem geometry and finish is yet unsolved.

REFERENCES

1. Charnley J. Low friction arthroplasty of the hip. Theory and practice. New York: Springer-Verlag; 1979.
2. Callaghan JJ, Forest EE, Olejniczak JP, Goetz DD, Johnston RC. Charnley total hip arthroplasty in patients less than fifty years old. A twenty to twenty-five-year follow-up note. J Bone Joint Surg Am 1998; 80(5):704–714.
3. Schmalzried TP, Harris WH. Hybrid total hip replacement. A 6.5-year follow-up study. J Bone Joint Surg Br Jul 1993; 75(4):608–615.
4. Mulroy WF, Estok DM, Harris WH. Total hip arthroplasty with use of so-called second-generation cementing techniques. A fifteen-year-average follow-up study. J Bone Joint Surg Am 1995; 77(12):1845–1852.
5. Barrack RL, Mulroy RD Jr, Harris WH. Improved cementing techniques and femoral component loosening in young patients with hip arthroplasty. A 12-year radiographic review. J Bone Joint Surg Br May 1992; 74(3):385–389.
6. Smith SW, Estok DM 2nd, Harris WH. Total hip arthroplasty with use of second-generation cementing techniques. An eighteen-year-average follow-up study. J Bone Joint Surg Am 1998; 80(11):1632–1640.
7. Harvey EJ, Tanzer M, Bobyn JD. Femoral cement grading in total hip arthroplasty. J Arthroplasty Jun 1998; 13(4):396–401.
8. Berger RA, Kull LR, Rosenberg AG, Galante JO. Hybrid total hip arthroplasty: 7- to 10-year results. Clin Orthop Dec 1996(333):134–146.
9. Harris WH, McCarthy JC Jr, O'Neill DA. Loosening of the femoral component of total hip replacement after plugging the femoral canal. Hip 1982; 228–238.
10. Gruen TA, McNeice GM, AmstutzHC. "Modes of failure" of cemented stem-type femoral components: a radiographic analysis of loosening. Clin OrthopJun 1979(141):17–27.
11. Sutherland CJ, Wilde AH, Borden LS, Marks KE A ten-year follow-up of one hundred consecutive Muller curved-stem total hip-replacement arthroplasties. J Bone Joint Surg Am Sep 1982; 64(7):970–982.
12. Stauffer RN. Ten-year follow-up study of total hip replacement. J Bone Joint Surg Am Sep 1982; 64(7):983–990.
13. Callaghan JJ, Albright JC, Goetz DD, Olejniczak JP, Johnston RC. Charnley total hip arthroplasty with cement. Minimum twenty-five-year follow-up. J Bone Joint Surg Am 2000; 82(4):487–497.

14. Majkowski RS, Miles AW, Bannister GC, Perkins J, Taylor GJ. Bone surface preparation in cemented joint replacement. J Bone Joint Surg Br May 1993; 75(3):459–463.
15. Roberts DW, Poss R, Kelley K. Radiographic comparison of cementing techniques in total hip arthroplasty. J Arthroplasty 1986; 1(4):241–247.
16. Klapach AS, Callaghan JJ, Goetz DD, Olejniczak JP, Johnston RC. Charnley total hip arthroplasty with use of improved cementing techniques: a minimum twenty-year follow-up study. J Bone Joint Surg Am 2001; 83-A(12):1840–1848.
17. Askew MJ, Steege JW, Lewis JL, Ranieri JR, Wixson RL. Effect of cement pressure and bone strength on polymethylmethacrylate fixation. J Orthop Res 1984; 1(4):412–420.
18. Burke DW, Gates EI, Harris WH. Centrifugation as a method of improving tensile and fatigue properties of acrylic bone cement. J Bone Joint Surg Am Oct 1984; 66(8):1265–1273.
19. Wixson RL, Lautenschlager EP, Novak MA. Vacuum mixing of acrylic bone cement. J Arthroplasty 1987; 2(2):141–149.
20. Howie DW, Middleton RG, Costi K. Loosening of matt and polished cemented femoral stems. J Bone Joint Surg Br Jul 1998; 80(4):573–576.
21. Middleton RG, Howie DW, Costi K, Sharpe P. Effects of design changes on cemented tapered femoral stem fixation. Clin Orthop Oct 1998(355):47–56.
22. Collis DK, Mohler CG. Comparison of clinical outcomes in total hip arthroplasty using rough and polished cemented stems with essentially the same geometry. J Bone Joint Surg Am Apr 2002; 84-A(4):586–592.
23. Crowninshield RD, Jennings JD, Laurent ML, Maloney WJ. Cemented femoral component surface finish mechanics. Clin Orthop Oct 1998(355): 90–102.
24. Kale AA, Della Valle CJ, Frankel VH, Stuchin SA, Zuckerman JD, Di Cesare PE. Hip arthroplasty with a collared straight cobalt-chrome femoral stem using second-generation cementing technique: a 10-year-average follow-up study. J Arthroplasty Feb 2000; 15(2):187–193.
25. Sanchez-Sotelo J, Berry DJ, Harmsen S. Long-term results of use of a collared matte-finished femoral component fixed with second-generation cementing techniques. A fifteen-year-median follow-up study. J Bone Joint Surg Am Sep 2002; 84-A(9):1636–1641.
26. Dowd JE, Cha CW, Trakru S, Kim SY, Yang IH, Rubash HE. Failure of total hip arthroplasty with a precoated prosthesis. 4- to 11-year results. Clin Orthop Oct 1998(355):123–136.
27. Oishi CS, Walker RH, Colwell CW, Jr. The femoral component in total hip arthroplasty. Six to eight-year follow-up of one hundred consecutive patients after use of a third-generation cementing technique. J Bone Joint Surg Am Aug 1994; 76(8):1130–1136.
28. Ong A, Wong KL, Lai M, Garino JP, Steinberg ME. Early failure of precoated femoral components in primary total hip arthroplasty. J Bone Joint Surg Am May 2002; 84-A(5):786–792.
29. Berger RA, Seel MJ, Wood K, Evans R, D'Antonio J, Rubash HE. Effect of a centralizing device on cement mantle deficiencies and initial prosthetic alignment in total hip arthroplasty. J Arthroplasty Jun 1997; 12(4):434–443.

30. Hanson PB, Walker RH. Total hip arthroplasty cemented femoral component distal stem centralizer. Effect on stem centralization and cement mantle. J Arthroplasty Oct 1995; 10(5):683–688.

31. Breusch SJ, Lukoschek M, Kreutzer J, Brocai D, Gruen TA. Dependency of cement mantle thickness on femoral stem design and centralizer. J Arthroplasty Aug 2001; 16(5):648–657.

32. Noble PC, Collier MB, Maltry JA, Kamaric E, Tullos HS. Pressurization and centralization enhance the quality and reproducibility of cement mantles. Clin Orthop Oct 1998; (355):77–89.

33. Goldberg BA, al-Habbal G, Noble PC, Paravic M, Liebs TR, Tullos HS. Proximal and distal femoral centralizers in modern cemented hip arthroplasty. Clin OrthopApr 1998(349)(349):163–173.

34. Crowninshield RD, Brand RA, Johnston RC, Pedersen DR. An analysis of collar function and the use of titanium in femoral prostheses. Clin Orthop Jul-Aug 1981(158):270–277.

35. Oh I, Harris WH. Proximal strain distribution in the loaded femur. An in vitro comparison of the distributions in the intact femur and after insertion of different hip-replacement femoral components. J Bone Joint Surg Am Jan 1978; 60(1):75–85.

36. Ling RS. The use of a collar and precoating on cemented femoral stems is unnecessary and detrimental. Clin Orthop Dec 1992(285):73–83.

37. Meding JB, Ritter MA, Keating EM, Faris PM, Edmondson K. A comparison of collared and collarless femoral components in primary cemented total hip arthroplasty: a randomized clinical trial. J Arthroplasty Feb 1999; 14(2):123–130.

38. Settecerri JJ, Kelley SS, Rand JA, Fitzgerald RH, Jr. Collar versus collarless cemented HD-II femoral prostheses. Clin Orthop May 2002; (398):146–152.

39. Dall DM, Miles AW, Juby G. Accelerated polymerization of acrylic bone cement using preheated implants. Clin Orthop Oct 1986(211):148–150.

40. Iesaka K, Jaffe WL, Kummer FJ. Effects of preheating of hip prostheses on the stem-cement interface. J Bone Joint Surg Am Mar 2003; 85-A(3):421–427.

21

Treating Hip and Pelvic Osteolysis

Eric L. Martin, Stephen Burnett, and Wayne Paprosky
*Central Dupage Hospital, Winfield, and Department of
Orthopaedic Surgery, Rush University Medical Center, Chicago, Illinois, U.S.A.*

INTRODUCTION

Approximately 250,000 total hip arthroplasties are performed in the United States each year. The operation has noted uniform excellent long-term success rates. This has led to an expansion of the indications for hip arthroplasty. Younger patients, with more active lifestyles, are undergoing this surgery. Elderly patients are living longer and, continuing to be active longer. These factors place increased demand on the bearing surface of implants. They are forced to withstand more and more gait cycles. Wear is related to the number of gait cycles. More cycles equals more wear (1).

The vast majority of total hip arthroplasty surgeries performed in the United States use polyethylene as the part of the bearing surface. Small wear polyethylene particles created with every gait cycle have been shown to activate a cellular cascade leading to possible bone resorption. Different methods of polyethylene production have been associated with poor THA longevity. Bone resorption around prosthetic implants can lead to component loosening, prosthesis migration or fracture.

In the evolution of total hip arthroplasty multiple materials and different types and sizes of components have been used as bearing surfaces. Some of these different prostheses have been shown to increase the evolution of wear particles while some decrease particle production. Recognition of implants that are prone to increasing or decreasing wear is crucial to the adequate analysis of osteolysis.

This chapter will focus on the recognition and treatment of osteolytic defects around total hip arthroplasty components.

PARTICLE GENERATORS

Microscopic wear particles produced in normal and abnormal wear with total hip arthroplasty components can cause a spectrum of events that may lead to bony reabsorption or osteolysis. These particles can be produced from several sources labeled "Particle Generators." These "particles" may obtain access to the "effective joint space" or the immediate area around the implants that is continuous with the joint space. Particles can cause bone resorption in any area to which they have access.

Particle generators must be recognized so their mechanism of particle production can be blocked. If osteolytic lesions require surgical intervention, the generators can be addressed. Abnormal particle producers can be removed and increased amounts of normal wear can be inhibited. For example, oxidized, machined polyethylene can be exchanged for cross-linked polyethylene or metal-on-metal bearings if available.

Factors shown to promote increased particle production include: back side acetabular wear (2), 32 mm femoral heads (3), younger, more active patients (3–5), male gender (6), obese patients, polyethylene gamma irradiated in air (7), oxidized liners (i.e., long shelf life), machined polyethylene (8,9), poor cement mantles (6,10), thin polyethylene liners (<8 mm), femoral component modular head-neck corrosion (11–13), porous coating of either femoral or acetabular implants (Fig. 1), titanium femoral heads (13–15), cerclage cables, acetabular component orientation (16), cemented titanium femoral components (17), and poor congruity between the femoral heads and the acetabular shell (Table 1).

Osteolytic defects have been reported to be less prevalent when certain implants and prosthesis designs are used (Table 2). Ceramic bearings and metal-on-metal bearings, although not completely free of debris production (18–20), have shown decreased wear characteristics (21–25). Circumferential porous coating (26), thick cement mantles (10), 28 and 22 mm femoral heads, increased femoral offset (27) and cross-linked polyethylene (28), stable locking mechanisms (29), and smooth acetabular shell surfaces (29) are also associated with decreased wear and particle production.

CLINICAL PRESENTATION

Osteolysis has been labeled "the silent disease" by several authors. Its appearance and symptoms are variable. Most often its presence is unnoticed by the patient. Large lesions can often form without any clinical symptoms (30). If

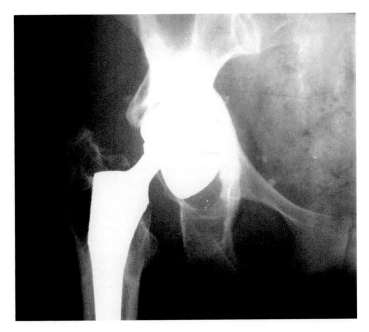

Figure 1 Metal particle shedding is evident from this loose acetabular component. The metal particles may lead directly to osteolysis or cause third body wear increasing the polyethylene load.

not followed radiographically, untreated lesions may progress to the point where prosthesis fracture, bony fracture (31), or prosthesis loosening occur.

DIFFERENTIAL DIAGNOSIS

The differential diagnosis of osteolysis differs slightly with the type of lesion that has developed. Lytic lesions around a total hip arthroplasty can be caused by infection metatstatic carcinoma (32), stress shielding, multiple myeloma, lymphoma (33), osteoporosis, Paget's disease (34,35), and fracture. Early failure of components, within two to four years, is not commonly due to osteolysis. Still, some cases of osteolysis have been reported in early follow-up. Poor surgical technique or component factors can cause these lesions. Regardless, the major differential is infection. Infection can give a similar clinical and radiologic appearance to osteolysis. Also, the two are not mutually exclusive and may coexist within the same patient.

HISTORY

A detailed history of the patient's prior surgeries and perioperative treatments should be obtained. Hospital records from previous operations may provide

Table 1 Possible Particle Generators Causing Osteolysis in Total Hip Arthroplasty

Particle generators

Components
   32 mm femoral heads
   Titanium femoral heads
   Modular acetabular components—backside wear
   Modular femoral components–fretting/corrosion
   Cemented titanium femoral components
   Unstable modular locking mechanism
   Rough inner acetabular surface
   Porous coating
   Design parameters (i.e., noncircumferential porous coating)
   Polyethylene
      Machined
      Long shelf life
      Gamma sterilized in air
      Thin polyethylene liners (<8 mm)
   Cerclage cables
Surgical factors
   Acetabular cup orientation
   Thin cement mantle
Third body wear
Patient factors
   Male gender
   Age
   Activity
   Weight

Table 2 Component Designs that Can Decrease Polyethylene Particle Production

Particle generator inhibitors

28/22 mm femoral heads
Stable polyethylene locking mechanism
Smooth concave acetabular shell surface
Cross-linked polyethylene
Metal-on-metal bearings
Ceramic bearings
Thick cement mantles
Fully circumferential porous coatings
No hole acetabular shells

clues to a patient's diagnosis. Records that list implanted components can be especially helpful.

Small osteolytic lesions are for the most part asymptomatic. Large lesions also commonly do not provoke symptoms. Maloney et al. (36) found 15 pelvic osteolyic lesions in acetabular shells placed without cement. Mean time to appearance of the osteolytic lesions was 65 months. All lesions were diagnosed on asymptomatic follow-up radiographs. Nine patients required acetabular revision.

Large lesions may cause pain in some patients. This may be due to abnormal, increased stresses placed on the remaining weight-bearing bone. This occurs because more force passes through the remaining bone that has not yet been resorbed. Microfractures or full stress fractures may result. Synovitis secondary to wear debris has been described as a source of pain. Inflammation of the iliopsoas tendon sheath secondary to particle debris has also been described (37).

Symptoms caused by osteolysis often appear abruptly. Patients have a history of a well-functioning implant that has become painful without any history of trauma. Symptoms can be due to prosthesis loosening, acute bony fracture, stress fracture, or component breakage. Symptoms are generally manifested as pain. Abrupt pain is likely caused by fracture of the implant or of bone. Patients are unable to bear weight on the affected extremity. Pain with weight bearing on the affected limb that is relieved by rest may be present. Gradual appearance of symptoms may indicate increasing loosening of a component or microstress fractures present in remaining weight-bearing bone. The location of the lesion affects the symptoms. Acetabular loosening or fracture can manifest with groin, lateral thigh, or buttock pain (38). Femoral loosening or fracture commonly appears with thigh pain (39). Patients may notice a gradual or acute change in leg length or in limb rotation.

PHYSICAL EXAMINATION

A full history and physical exam is essential. Neurovascular status of the affected and nonaffected extremity needs to be assessed. Signs of infection, such as draining sinuses or erythematous swelling should be looked for. Exam of the spine should be completed to evaluate if spinal pathology contributes to the patient's symptomatology.

Gross limb deformity, leg length discrepancy, or malrotation may be present. Pain associated with passive motion of the extremity and an antalgic limp may indicate a loose component or a fracture.

BLOOD TESTS

No commonly used laboratory test has been devised that can diagnosis osteolysis. Laboratory examination in cases with osteolytic lesions should be used to rule out infection (40). A complete white blood cell (WBC) count with differential, erythrocyte sedimentation rate (ESR) and C-reactive protein (CRP) are the laboratory tests most ordered. Together, these tests have a high likelihood of spotting an infected prosthesis. Underlying inflammatory conditions (i.e., collagen vascular diseases) may show evidence of inflammation on these tests. Patients taking corticosteroids will also have abnormal results.

An elevated WBC count is a relatively nonspecific test and requires additional data. Usually a WBC count greater than 10–11 is significant. A shift toward increased neutrophils points toward acute inflammation while increased macrophage numbers points to a more chronic inflammatory course. An ESR higher than 30–35 mm/hr indicates an increased amount of plasma proteins. It remains elevated for up to 10 months after surgery. The CRP is the most sensitive of these tests. It peaks 48 hours postoperatively. It remains elevated for only three weeks after surgery that is not complicated by infection. A level greater than 10 mg/L is significant. The significance of an elevated CRP is helped with an elevated WBC count and an elevated ESR.

These tests by themselves are moderately insensitive. Only together with the history, physical examination, and other investigative modalities do they become accurate in diagnosing infection.

RADIOGRAPHS

Because the majority of osteolysis cases are clinically silent, lesions can grow to a large size and not be detected by clinical examination. Radiographs are the most accessible and simple tests available to diagnosis and follow documented cases. Asymmetrical polyethylene wear and enlarging osteolytic lesions are best followed on serial X-ray exams. Routine radiographic evaluation after total hip arthroplasty has been advocated by several surgeons (41–43).

Standard films must be obtained so that accurate assessment of change can be reliably obtained. Anteroposterior hip and pelvis films along with a lateral hip film are the most common x-rays obtained. Unfortunately, pelvic osteolysis is commonly underestimated on standard radiographs (44). Judet films have been shown to assist in quantifying bone loss (45). Computerized tomography may also be helpful in quantifying bone loss. Many methods have been developed to accurately measure change in both polyethylene wear and osteolytic lesions. These include digital radiographs (46) and CT scans. No amount of radiographic pelvic or femoral lysis has, at this time, been labeled as the amount significant to require invasive treatment.

Polyethylene wear of the acetabular insert (Fig. 2) can be estimated on standard films. A rough estimate can be done by comparing the difference from the superior acetabular rim to the femoral head superior edge and subtracting this distance from the distance of the inferior femoral head

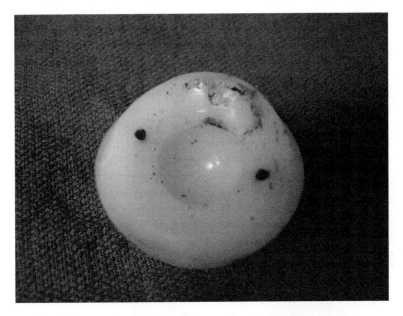

Figure 2 Retrieved polyethylene insert with grossly evident wear.

edge to the inferior acetabular rim (Fig. 3). With increasing wear superior femoral head migration is grossly evident (Fig. 4). Acetabular wear is related to the formation of osteolytic lesions. Polyethylene wear has been correlated with the frequency and size of osteolytic lesions (47). In one study, risk of acetabular revision was shown to increase with each millimeter of increased wear (48).

Total hip arthroplasty can be preformed using several fixation options. Press-fit components, cemented components, or a combination/hybrid can be used. Osteolytic lesions can have a different radiographic and clinical appearance depending on the component fixation method. The reliability of the peripheral interface depends on the seal obtained during fixation. Cemented components depend on a grout-like fixation to hold the components in place. Press-fit components rely on bony ingrowth for stable fixation. The ability of the "effective joint space" (49) to gain access to the prostheses–bone or cement–bone interfaces controls the manner in which osteolytic deficiencies form.

CEMENTED FEMORAL COMPONENTS

Cemented components have two interfaces to allow the passage of particles that can lead to osteolysis. One is the bone–implant interface and the second

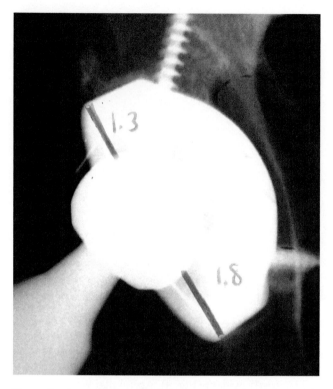

Figure 3 Asymmetric polyethylene wear can be measured by comparing polyethylene distance above and below the femoral head.

is the cement–bone interface. For bone resorption to occur some access to the bone must be present. Cemented femoral stems show early osteolysis in a linear fashion. Early osteolytic deficiencies appear as thin radiolucent lines that become apparent around the stem, commonly seen between the cement and the bone interface. A good cement mantle may prevent the joint space particles from reaching the metaphysis and diaphysis.

Radiographic signs of a loose femoral component include subsidence, cement mantle fracture, circumferential radiolucency, component fracture, and a stem that has progressively fallen into a varus or valgus position on serial radiographs. Implant loosening must be carefully considered as a cause of patient symptoms in the face of osteolysis. In cemented stems that are designed to subside, the criteria for loosening have been described (50) and the stem is considered definitely loose if there is any one of the following:

1. Subsidence or radiolucency at the stem–cement interface
2. Cement mantle fracture
3. Stem fracture

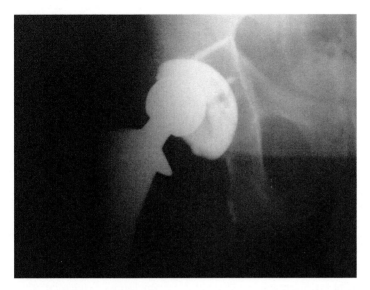

Figure 4 Severe asymmetric polyethylene wear with femoral head articulating with metal acetabular shell.

Probable loosening is present if there is a complete cement–bone radiolucent line, whereas if there is a cement–bone radiolucent line greater than 50% but less than 100%, the stem is possibly loose.

Deficiencies in the cement mantle are associated with early lysis (51). Osteolytic lesions seen in these cases may be isolated to the greater and trochanter and medial calcar region. Defects in the cement mantle allow access of wear particles. If access of particles more distally occurs, lesions can grow in size leading to the loosening of a component.

NONCEMENTED FEMORAL COMPONENTS

Proximal Porous Coated

Proximally porous coated femoral stems are designed for bone ingrowth in the metaphyseal area of the proximal femur. A tight press-fit is obtained at the time of surgery. Bone ingrowth is needed to retain implant stability. Two types of proximal porous coated stems have been designed, those with circumferential and noncircumferential porous coating. Noncircumferential porous coating stems showed early osteolysis when compared to cemented stems (52,53) and circumferentially porous coated. This occurred due to easier access of effective joint space to the femoral stem (54). The use of these stems has been abandoned. Circumferential proximally coated stems have excellent long-term survivorship (55,56). When bone ingrowth occurs, it serves as a good barrier to osteolytic particles. Femoral lysis in these cases is seen frequently around the greater and lesser trochanters. If joint fluid finds access distally, diaphyseal expansile osteolytic lesions can appear.

Signs of a stable proximally coated implant are present with or without osteolysis if the component is not grossly loose. Stability can be hard to define with x-rays. Signs of instability include migration, reactive lines surrounding the smooth implant surface, a distal pedestal, calcar hypertrophy, and implant migration (57). A stable component has spot welds indicating bone ingrowth and no change in component position with or without osteolytic lesions.

Fully Porous Coated

Fully coated ingrowth stems are designed to promote bone ingrowth primarily in the diaphyseal region. With an ingrown component, stresses placed though the hip joint bypass the proximal femur exiting through the distal stem. Bone hypertrophy is seen around the ingrowth diaphyseal region while bone resorption or "stress shielding" is noted proximally. In some cases, the bone resorption seen with stress shielding of ingrown stem may look like osteolysis. Stable fully coated femoral stems show distal spot welds and proximal bone hypertrophy (57). In stems that show fibrous-stable ingrowth, the fibrous tissue may provide a partial barrier to fluid and debris from the joint space. Osteolysis in these implants may develop and a common pattern of an expanding linear line around the component with progressive loss of diaphyseal bone is seen (Fig. 5).

In a study by Khalily and Whiteside (58) the presence of radiolucent lines around the porous coating of a femoral stem was 100% sensitive and 55% specific for predicting the need for future revision. The absence of radiolucent lines was 100% sensitive and 45% specific in predicting no need for revision in the first eight years after surgery.

Osteolytic lesions seen with fully coated stems are often seen in the proximal femur. Greater trochanteric or medial calacar lucencies are commonly seen. Diaphyseal lytic lesions have not been reported with an ingrown fully coated stem (59).

CEMENTED ACETABULAR COMPONENTS

The osteolysis that appears in association with cemented acetabular components occurs primarily along the interface between the cement and the pelvic bone. The cement blocks entrance of the osteolytic particles. Joint fluid must enter around the periphery of a component to gain access to periacetabular bone stock. Gaps in the cement mantle allow entry of joint fluid and wear particles. Cement covers any holes that may be present in the acetabular shell. Linear radiolucencies are most commonly seen between the cement and the metaphyseal bone (60). Larger expansile lesions although less

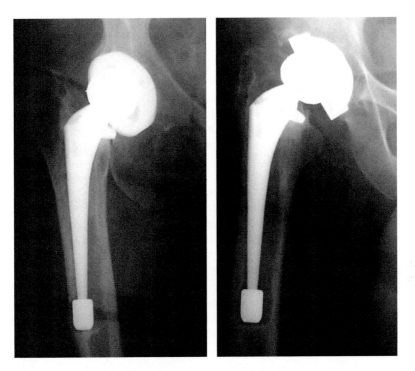

Figure 5 Noncemented femoral component with gross signs of loosening. AP and lateral views show circumferential osteolysis around the femoral stem. The stem subsided and fallen into a varus position. Note the asymmetric polyethylene wear and large femoral head size.

common, have been reported (61). DeLee and Charnley (62) described acetabular zones in terms of the osteolysis visualized on x-rays of cemented acetabular cups. Zone I is the lateral 1/3 of the acetabular shell. Zone II is the central 1/3 and zone III is the medial 1/3. Osteolysis, in a cemented acetabular component, is first seen in DeLee and Charnley zone I on the lateral edge of the component (63). Sockets without radiographic demarcation are firmly fixed but 94% of sockets with complete demarcation and all sockets that have migrated are loose (64).

Zicat et al. (71) followed 137 hips treated with total hip arthroplasty. Sixty-three patients had a cemented acetabular component inserted. The mean duration of follow-up was 105 months (54–142). Thirty-seven percent of acetabular shells inserted with cement demonstrated osteolysis. It appeared radiographically as a linear radiolucent line between the prosthesis and the pelvic bone. This finding correlated with a high prevalence of loose acetabular shells (30%).

NONCEMENTED ACETABULAR COMPONENTS

Press-fit, ingrowth, acetabular fixation has become the standard fixation used in primary hip arthroplasty. Excellent short to mid-term follow-up survivorship has been documented (65). Osteolysis lesions are seen less than with cemented acetabular fixation (66). Lytic lesions are seen more commonly at long-term follow-up (67,68). Early designs were nonmodular and the polyethylene could not be removed from the acetabular shell. Severe polyethylene wear, necessitating revision surgery, requires removal of the entire acetabular component. Modularity in acetabular arthroplasty allowed liner change only, with severe plastic wear, if the acetabular shell was intact and stable.

Acetabular shells destined for ingrowth require a tight press-fit at the time of implantation. This decreases any motion that might inhibit bone attachment to the prosthesis. Screws are commonly used as accessory fixation. Screw holes allow access of the joint particles into the central acetabular area. Osteolysis in press-fit acetabular components appears different clinically and radiographically than seen with cemented components. Linear osteolysis is less common. The modularity of the ingrowth acetabular component allows for backside wear between the plastic and the metal shell. Also, space between the metal shell and plastic allows the joint space access to the central acetabular bone. This is particularly true when screw holes are present. Osteolytic lesions, in these cases, appear as expansile, nonlinear lesions seen in the cancellous central bone of the acetabulum (69,70). They most commonly involve DeLee and Charnley zone II of the acetabulum (63). The periphery may or may not provide a barrier to the joint space. Large amounts of bone lysis can occur. Motion of the shell defines it as loose. If large osteolytic lesions are present and no motion of the cup is evident, surgery may be required to test the shell's integrity.

Zicat et al. (71) in their study of 137 hips treated with total hip arthroplasty all of which had a femoral reconstruction with an extensively porous coated stem. Seventy-four patients had a noncemented acetabular component inserted. Eighteen percent of acetabular shells inserted without cement demonstrated osteolysis. These osteolytic defects appeared localized and expansile. These lesions were not correlated with a loose acetabular component. More bone loss was produced from these lesions. Noncemented acetabular shells produced more femoral osteolysis.

RADIOGRAPHIC FOLLOW-UP

We recommend annual radiographic evaluation for total hip arthroplasty patients. Once radiographic osteolytic lesions have been identified, progression has been documented (72). Young, active, and obese patients should be closely evaluated. If a lesion is diagnosed radiographically and does not require surgical intervention it should be reevaluated within a three- to six-month period. If progression is documented intervention may be warranted (72). If no progression is seen, six to 12 month follow-up visits are appropriate.

ASPIRATION

If laboratory tests and diagnostic imaging gives an incomplete picture towards the presence or absence of infection, a hip aspiration is indicated. It is not considered to be a routine exam for all revision surgery. We perform all hip aspirations in a radiology suite with fluoroscopic guidance. Fluid obtained from the hip is sent for immediate Gram stain, cell count, and full cultures. Aspiration has been reported to demonstrate organisms in infected patients in about 90% of cases (73,74).

INTRAOPERATIVE TESTS

At the time of revision surgery, even if no signs of infection have been found, standard tests are completed. These include cell count of joint fluid, Gram stain, aerobic, anaerobic, fungal and tuberculosis cultures, acid-fast stains, and tissue frozen section for pathologic evaluation. Osteolytic lesions appear as granulation tissue with numerous macrophages and giant cells under pathologic examination (75).

CLASSIFICATION

Several defect classification systems exist to describe both femoral and acetabular osteolytic bone defects. These classification schemes have been developed to describe the clinical entity of osteolysis and point to possible treatments.

Acetabular osteolystic defects can be defined by radiographic examination and intraoperative findings. Preoperative physical exam can point to the location of the lesion and the stability of the components. Radiographs can hint at the amount of bone loss present, although this is commonly underestimated (76). Intraoperative examination is required to fully define the lesions in terms of the reconstruction needed.

Hozack et al. (77) have presented a staging system of acetabular lysis based on radiographic osteolysis, polyethylene wear, and patient symptoms (Table 3). Stage I are those patients with radiographic wear but no symptoms or lysis. Stage IIA patients have radiographic wear, no lysis or pain. Stage IIB patients have no pain but show wear and lysis on X-ray examination. Stage III patients present with pain as well as radiographic wear and lysis. The appearance of an osteolytic defect, Stage IIB and III, was described as a sentinel event after which surgical intervention must be considered. This staging system points toward when a reconstruction is needed but does not discuss treatment options.

Table 3 Staging System for Acetabular Osteolysis

	Polyethylene wear	Radiographic lysis	Pain
Stage I	Yes	No	No
Stage IIA	Yes	No	Yes
Stage IIB	Yes	Yes	No
Stage III	Yes	Yes	Yes

Source: From Ref. 77.

Acetabular osteolysis has recently been classified, by Rubash et al. (78) into three types relating to the stability of component and what if any surgical intervention will be required (Table 4). Type I describes defects where the acetabular component is completely stable. The acetabular shell is well ingrown, the mechanism for the polyethylene insert must be in full working order. The acetabular shell has a good track record for longevity and modular inserts must be available. Type II defects are those in which the acetabular cup is stable but it must still be removed. Reasons for this include: severe wear, a broken polyethylene locking mechanism, discontinued implants, or an acetabular shell with a poor longevity record. A caveat to the replacement of cups with a broken locking mechanism exists. In some cases, a polyethylene shell can be cemented into an acetabular shell obviating the need for an intact locking mechanism. The long-term results of this treatment and its indications have not as yet been clearly defined. Type III defects are those where the acetabular cup is unstable and revision of the component is mandatory.

Femoral osteolysis has been recently classified by Dunbar et al. (79) into four distinct types (Table 5). This classification relates to the type of revision implant that may be needed. It is based upon cancellous bone quality and the intactness of the cortical tube. The amount and location of bone loss is used to classify the defect type and to predict the type of reconstruction

Table 4 Classification of Acetabular Osteolysis

Type I	Stable/ingrown
	Undamaged locking mechanism
	Good long term track record
	Available implants
Type II	Stable/ingrown
	Damaged locking mechanism
	Poor long term track record
	Unavailable implants
Type III	Unstable component

Source: From Ref. 78.

Table 5 Femoral Osteolysis Classification

	Cancellous bone	Cortical bone
Type I	Intact	Intact
Type II	Deficient	Intact
Type III	Deficient	Deficient
Type IV	Absent	Absent

Source: From Ref. 79.

required. This classification system has been incorporated into a useful algorithm for the management of femoral osteolysis. Type I defects have both intact cancellous bone and an intact cortical tube. Primary femoral components can be utilized. Type II defects have deficient cancellous bone and an intact cortical tube. This is most commonly seen after linear osteolysis has caused the loosening of a cemented femoral component. A primary femoral component will not be adequately supported. Surgical options include a cemented component, a fully coated noncemented stem, and impaction allografting. Type III defects have both deficient cancellous bone and a deficient cortical tube. Distal bypass fixation is required with a fully porous coated femoral stem. Bone deficiencies may need to be restored with grafting techniques. Type IV defects include deficiencies with absent cancellous and cortical bone. Distal bypass fixation and the use of bulk allograft or tumor prostheses are used in these situations.

Femoral osteolytic defects can also be classified according to the stability of the implant and the reconstruction that may be required for the type of component already present (Table 6). Again preoperative physical exam and radiographs help to define the lesion. Intraoperative findings are used to fill in

Table 6 Classification of Femoral Components with Associated Osteolysis

Type I	Implant stable—ingrown or cement
	Intact/undamaged taper mechanism
	Acceptable implant longevity record
	Osteolytic lesion not compromising implant stability
Type II	Implant stable—ingrown or cement
	Damaged taper mechanism
	Unacceptable implant performance
	(i.e., noncircumferential coating)
	Component malposition (version, varus, offset)
	Osteolytic lesion(s) compromising implant stability with
	impending periprosthetic fracture
Type III	Implant loose + any osteolytic lesion
	Infection

the gaps. Type I defects are seen when the femoral component is stable. Treatment involves keeping the stem in situ. The component has good clinical longevity and modular components are available. Type II defects describe lesions where the stem is stable but the femoral trunion is damaged and cannot accept a new femoral head, nonmodular stems especially those with 32 mm heads, discontinued prosthetic lines, and femoral stems with poor long-term survivorship. Type III femoral osteolytic defects are those with an unstable femoral component that requires revision.

FEMORAL DEFECT CLASSIFICATION SYSTEMS

Assessment of osteolysis around femoral components in total hip arthroplasty has been classified in several different forms. The Committee on Hip and Knee Arthritis has outlined a classification which defines defects as Type I (segmental), Type II (cavitary), or Type III (combined) (80). These are subdivided into complete or partial deficiencies. Malalignment, stenosis, and discontinuity characterize Types IV, V, and VI, respectively. The level of the defect may then be localized as Level I (proximal to the inferior aspect of the lesser trochanter), Level II (lesser trochanter to 10 cm distal), and Level III (further distal). Defects are further graded by the severity of bone loss. Grade I defects demonstrate complete contact between the host bone and a revision prosthesis. Grade II lesions have areas with incomplete contact, which do not compromise stability, although bulk allografts are often used to augment initial stability. Grade III defects are those requiring structural allograft to stabilize the reconstruction. Despite being a concise descriptive defect classification, this system may be difficult to use in planning and predicting the type of surgical reconstruction required to predict the type of femoral reconstruction required in revision of femoral components in total hip arthroplasty.

The senior author has described a femoral defect classification that uses the bone loss present to point to the reconstruction that will be required (81). The type of defect predicted using this classification system is simple, easy to recall, and reproducible for communicating between surgeons. A brief overview of this defect classification system and the type of reconstruction options available to the surgeon follows (Table 7).

Paprosky Femoral Defect Classification

Type I Defects

These are minimal defects and the femur does not differ significantly from that encountered in the primary total hip. There is intact metaphyseal and diaphyseal bone stock, with only partial loss of the calcar and A-P bone. Examples include resurfacing and Moore-type prostheses. Type I defects are treated as in the primary arthroplasty, and may be managed with cemented, proximally porous coated, or extensively coated implants with successful outcome.

Table 7 Paprosky Acetabular Defect Classification

Defect type	Superior migration	Ischial lysis	Medial migration	Teardrop lysis
I	Insignificant	None	None	None
IIA	Insignificant	Mild	Grade I	Mild
IIB	Insignificant to Significant	Mild	Grade II	Mild
IIC	Significant	Mild	Grade III	Moderate to Severe
IIIA	Significant	Moderate	Grade II+ or III	Moderate
IIIB	Significant	Severe	Grade III+	Severe

Bradford M, Paprosky W. Acetabular defect classification: A detailed radiographic approach;

Type II Defects

These defects are isolated to the metaphysis, with intact diaphyseal bone. The calcar is completely deficient, and there is increased A-P loss of cancellous bone in the metaphysis. Examples include subsided prostheses, previous intertrochannteric fractures, and metaphyseal osteolysis surrounding an implant. Type II defects are not amenable to proximally porous coated implants or cementing. Canal filling, fully porous coated stems (6, 7, or 8 inches) are preferred for distal fixation. Calcar replacement may be required.

Type III Defects

These are divided into Types IIIA and IIIB defects. Type IIIA defects involve the metaphysis and the junction with the diaphysis; Type IIIB extend slightly further than type A into the diaphysis. The difference is based upon whether a minimum 4 cm scratch fit can be reliably obtained near the isthmus (IIIA) or requires diaphyseal fixation beyond the isthmus (IIIB). Examples include cemented and porous stems with metadiaphyseal osteolysis or aseptic loosening, proximal periprosthetic fractures, and femurs with varus remodeling. Type IIIA defects require the use of a fully porous coated stem with longer canal filling capacity (8 or 10 inch bowed stems, modular implants), and type IIIB defects are managed with similar stems, or impaction grafting if the "tube" is intact and the canal width exceeds 18 mm. Impaction grafting serves three purposes in this setting: (i) to reestablish bone stock to the proximal femur, (ii) provides a mechanically stable construct for cement fixation of the component, and (iii) to improve the quality of the bed into which cement is placed for fixation. Results of revisions with extensively porous coated stems for Type III defects are reported with a low 2.4% mechanical failure rate at eight years follow-up (82).

Type IV Defects

These defects represent extensive femoral metadiaphyseal damage, with thin cortices and widened canals that preclude reliable distal fixation, and a nonsupportive isthmus. Options include impaction allografting, or the use of an allograft prosthetic composite (APC). The surgeon must predict preoperatively if Type IIIB or IV defects are present, as allograft materials may be necessary for the reconstruction. Impaction grafting in the femur for massive osteolysis and loss of structural support has been described to restore bone stock. In this technique, cortical defects are strut grafted with cortical allografts secured with cerclage wires, and the authors note that strut grafting is especially important for defects that will not be bypassed by the short polished stem. Concerns related to high rate of femoral fracture, a steep learning curve, and the incidence of significant subsidence have made this technique challenging. However, it remains a useful addition to the list of surgical options for severe bone loss in the femur.

RESULTS

Osteolys is a relatively young clinical disease. Treatments specific to this disease do not all, as of yet, have long-term follow-up. The optimal treatment(s) for some aspects of the disease is still under investigation. Still, a significant amount of research data is available describing results of treatment of osteolytic lesions and results of component designs that may increase wear and lysis (Fig. 6).

Femoral Revision

Benson et al. (83) evaluated 17 hips requiring acetabular revision with incidental osteolytic defects around the proximal femur of a cementless component. The femoral components were all found to be stable. All were treated

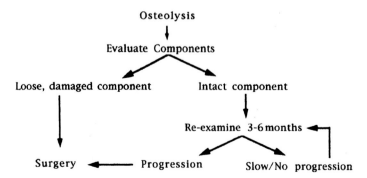

Figure 6 Flow diagram for decision making with osteolysis. *Source*: From Ref. 78.

with curettage and packing with cancellous allograft. At the minimum follow-up of 24 months, 15 of 17 lesions were decreased in size and no stems were radiographically or clinically loose.

Hozak et al. (84) found 154 osteolytic defects in 59 femoral components that were revised due to osteolysis. Clinical and radiographic evaluation was performed at two and five years. All patients were treated with cementless femoral revision stems. No failures to date. Of the 154 preoperative osteolytic defects, 27 stabilized, 65 regressed, and 62 healed.

Distal bypass fixation required in more advanced femoral osteolytic lesions can be obtained with fully porous coated stems or modular components. Wirtz et al. (85) reported on 142 revisions with modular components. Seventy of 142 cases had Paprosky Type 2C and Type 3 defects. At early follow-up five cases were re-revised for dislocation and two were re-revised for aseptic loosening. No further osteolytic defects were observed.

Acetabular Revision

Maloney et al. (86) studied the treatment of pelvic osteolysis with a stable noncemented acetabular component. Forty-six lesions were treated in 35 patients. All patients were treated with polyethylene insert exchange and synovectomy. Thirty-four of 46 lesions were bone grafted with allograft chips. At a minimum of two-year follow-up all grafts showed consolidation and there were no revisions.

Scmalzreid et al. (87) surgically treated 23 hips in 21 patients with pelvic osteolysis. Fifteen patients were treated with retention of the acetabular shell and eight were treated with acetabular revision. Eighteen of 23 hips were bone grafted with autograft or allograft. No lesions progressed regardless of treatment or bone grafting. Also, there was a significant decrease in operative and blood loss in the nonrevision group.

In a study of surgical treatment of pelvic osteolysis prepared by Maloney et al. (88) acetabular components were approached. Forty patients (Type I cases) were treated with polyethylene liner exchange and debridment of the lesion. Twenty-nine of 40 patients were grafted. At 3.5-year follow-up all the acetabular components were stable, no new lesions were identified, two-thirds of the lesions had decreased in size and one-third of the lesions had completely resolved. Twenty-eight patients (Type II cases) were treated with acetabular socket revision. Both treatment strategies were successful in stopping the osteolytic expansion. Removal of the acetabular component was associated with significantly increased bone loss.

Loss of cancellous bone can be treated with an impaction allografting technique (89). Satisfactory clinical and radiographic results at intermediate-term follow-up have reported by Leopold et al. (90). The reported complication rate in their series was high causing them to limit their indications. Mallory et al. (91) studied 51 hips with aseptic loosening and/or osteolytic lesions indicated for revision. All were treated with an impaction grafting. The defects were filled with fresh-frozen particulate allograft. The allograft was compressed and then a metal-backed, porous acetabular shell was cemented into the defect. Screw fixation was used prior to the cement curing. Polyethylene liners were inserted into the metal shell. At mid-term follow-up three hips have shown radiographic radiolucencies (one progressive requiring revision surgery, two nonprogressive). All other implants showed graft incorporation.

Component Design Factors

Several design factors invented to increase the longevity and stability of total hip components have proven to increase polyethylene wear and osteolysis in vivo. Implants that have a poor track record at long term follow-up must be considered for revision when osteolytic defects are being evaluated. Components are mentioned not to highlight failures, but to list some implants or fixation methods that may preclude long-term successful arthroplasty. These implants should be considered for exchange regardless of their stability at the time of revision (Table 8).

Screw Holes

Soto et al. (92) evaluated Harris–Galante acetabular cups for osteolysis at 7–9 year follow-up. One hundred twenty seven hips in 112 patients were assessed. X-rays showed 24% had acetabular osteolytic lesions. Seventy-three percent of these lesions were associated with screw holes.

Scmalzreid et al. (93) looked at 113 hips in 93 patients treated with acetabular components without cement. At mean follow-up of 64 months no component was radiographically loose or had been revised for loosening. The incidence of osteolytic lesions was 17% (19 hips). Most of the lesions were asymptomatic. Ten of 19 acetabular shells with osteolytic lesions had no screw holes. This showed elimination of screw holes decreased but did not stop the formation of osteolytic lesions. The effective joint space finds other routes to the acetabular bone interface. Porous ingrowth offers only some resistance to acetabular osteolysis.

Femoral Component Design

Cemented components precoated with polymethylmethacrylate have shown early osteolytic lesion form. Dowd et al. (94) reviewed 145 precoated femoral stems. Fifteen percent stem failure was seen at an average four-year follow-up. Debonding at the cement–bone interface was noted. It was thought that strengthening the cement–prosthesis interface predisposed to cement–bone interface failure, especially when a poor cement mantle was present.

Table 8 Components or Designs that Have an Increased Predispostion for Osteolysis

---

Components prone to increased/early osteolysis

Noncemented femoral
   Noncircumferentially porous coated stems
   Cementless femoral components without surface coating
   Small diameter stems (designs prone to fracture)
   Monoblock titanium stems
Cemented femoral
   Polymethylmethacrylate precoated stems
   Titanium cemented femoral stems
   Stems with a high surface roughness (Ra)
      Grit blasted Iowa stem
Acetabular shell
   Multiscrew holes cup
   Universal cup (Biomet)
   Harris–Galante I cup (Zimmer)
Acetabular liner
   AML PLUS acetabular shell ACS (acetabular cup system) liner (DePuy)
   Hylamer (DePuy) acetabular inserts
Femoral head
   Titanium femoral heads
   Large femoral heads

Cemented stems with a high Ra or surface roughness have shown a large number or early failures secondary to bone lysis. Collis reported that one of 12 original Iowa stems (Ra 30) and 12 of 22 (Ra 80) grit blasted stems required revision before five years (95).

Noncircumferential porous coating allows ingress of wear particles along the entire femoral stem. Emerson et al. (96) examined 126 hips with noncircumferential plasma-spray porous titanium coating compared with 90 patients with circumferential coating. Same design stem was used. Osteolysis in first group was 40% with noncircumferential coating versus 10% with circumferential coating.

Circumferentially porous coated components inhibit particle access to the metadiaphyseal region. Still osteolytic lesions are seen where the joint space comes in contact with bone. Rokkum et al. (97) reported on 94 consecutively implanted HA-coated implants. Ingrowth was seen in all cases. Sixty-six hips had osteolytic lesion, mostly in the greater trochanter and the acetabular regions.

Cementless femoral components without surface coating do not allow bone ingrowth. The failure rates with these stems are high. Failure rates between 23% and 37% at 10-year follow-up have been reported (98).

Titanium cemented femoral stems have shown early failure rates. Buly et al. (99) reported on 51 arthroplasties performed with a cemented titanium component at an average of 4.5 years. Both metallic and polyethylene particles were found at the time of revision. Femoral head burnishing was noted in 71% of revised cases. Increased metal particles were thought to increase third body wear.

Acetabular Component Design

Several acetabular components have been shown to have less than optimal wear characteristics. Bono et al. (100) reported on 94 AML PLUS components inserted with an ACS (Acetabular Cup System) polyethylene liner (DePuy) (100). The femoral component used 32 mm heads. The ACS design lacked a hemispherical geometry. The femoral head wore quickly and penetrated through the acetabular shell superior rim. Twenty-one percent clinical failures were reported. Puolakka et al. (101) reported on "alarming wear" of the first-generation liners of the Biomet Universal cup. Cylindrical design, thin polyethylene, and poor quality polyethylene were thought to be factors leading to early wear and subsequent osteolysis. Several authors have reported on Hylamer (DePuy) acetabular inserts that showed promising wear characteristics in vitro but, in vivo eccentric, early wear has been reported (102,103).

SURGICAL TREATMENT

The management of acetabular and femoral osteolysis associated with total hip arthroplasty continues to be a challenging problem and area of active investigation. Both cemented and cementless acetabular components may be associated with osteolysis.

ACETABULAR OSTEOLYSIS—MANAGEMENT

Noncemented Components

Revision for osteolysis of cementless components may involve either (i) removal of the well-fixed socket, with grafting and curettage of osteolytic defects and revision of the socket, or (ii) liner exchange with debridement and grafting of osteolytic lesions. The first option may be associated with significant bone loss if the component is well fixed and may require advanced reconstruction techniques, and the defect created by component removal is often much larger than the original lesion. The second option has developed as a result of difficulty with removal of these well-fixed components, and early results are promising.

We have followed a simple and effective algorithm for classifying lesions around the acetabulum, in order to manage these defects (104). This classification system directs the surgeon to assess not only the osteolytic lesion, but the defect associated with the lysis, and the implant itself, which is an important variable when considering surgical options. Similarly, patient age, symptoms, implant design, materials, "particle generators," and location of the lesion all play an important role in management of these lesions.

Type I Acetabular Components

The component is a stable, functional cup. There is progressive or symptomatic osteolysis, with an ingrown shell, asymmetric wear of the polyethylene and a focal osteolytic lesion may be present. In the preoperative planning phase X-rays, surgical approach, special equipment, modular exchange, trials (Low profile cups, lipped liners), a backup plan, bone graft, and special instruments needed for polyethylene and screw removal must be considered. In revision surgery, lack of preparation will inevitably lead to frustration, complications, and increased operative time.

The Type I component may often be asymptomatic, and first noted on radiographs at routine follow-up. Groin pain may be secondary to synovitis with associated soft tissue impingement, micromotion at the implant–bone interface, or secondary to small microfractures. The osteolysis is most commonly focal and located at the periarticular margins. Screws and screw holes may provide a conduit for particle flow, and osteolysis around these areas is not uncommon. Review of serial radiographs will allow the surgeon to establish whether the cup is stable and ingrown, or migrated. Judet views of the pelvis or CT scans may be useful to further assess the lesion extent. In Type I cups, the cup is stable by definition, has a locking mechanism which has an acceptable track record, and has asymmetric wear of the polyethylene. If the lesion is small and asymptomatic, follow-up with serial radiographs is warranted. Trials of oral bisphosphonate therapy are promising (105,106).

Patient age and general health must be considered. If the osteolytic lesion is symptomatic with pain, subluxation, dislocation, or increasing size on serial radiographs, surgical intervention may be warranted. A large asymptomatic lesion that may be at risk for fracture must also be carefully considered for operative treatment. Surgical treatment of these lesions is preferred with documented clinical or radiographic progression. Removal and identification of the particle generator must be assessed (Fig. 7).

Exposure for isolated acetabular modular polyethylene change may be performed through either the anterolateral or posterior approach. Adequate exposure requires complete visualization of the bony acetabular rim and interface between the modular polyethylene and the cup. This may require extensive excision of scar tissue, or capsule. If there is an indication to revise the femoral component, the order of revision may be used to facilitate exposure. Extended trochanteric osteotomy, trochanteric slide, or a standard trochanteric osteotomy may be necessary, and these procedures may facilitate acetabular exposure when indicated. Removal of modular femoral heads will

(A)   **(B)**

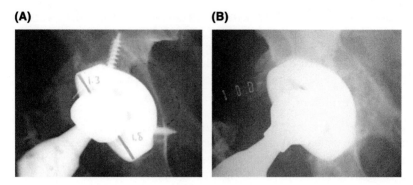

Figure 7 (**A**) Acetabular lysis evident in zone II with asymmetric polyethylene wear. No migration of the acetabular shell is evident. (**B**) Postoperative X-ray. Acetabular shell was found to be stable intraoperatively. Screws were removed, the lesion was bone grafted and a modular polyethylene exchange was conducted.

allow increased exposure, and exchange may be performed after the polyethylene has been exchanged. Excessive fretting and damage to the Morse taper must be identified as part of the process of assessment of the femoral component. If it has been significantly damaged or corroded, then revision of the femoral component is indicated. With the trochanteric slide, the slide may be retracted anteriorly and held with the Charnley retractor, and adequate exposure of the acetabulum is then facilitated. The posterior approach will maintain the abductor continuity. Regardless of approach, the femoral neck may be an obstacle to exposure. Nonmodular heads may be even more challenging to work around. The creation of an anterior-superior "pocket" for the femoral component may facilitate exposure in this instance. Significant capsular dissection may be required, and this must be considered if instability is present or anticipated to be a problem postoperatively. Removal of osteophytes or heterotopic bone around the acetabular rim may be necessary to visualize this interface. Currettes, small osteotomies, and high-speed burrs will aid the surgeon in exposure, and should be available.

Removal of polyethylene: The surgeon must plan preoperatively in order to remove the polyethylene, as specific instruments and equipment may be necessary. The operative report, along with the implant records from the original component packaging must be sought. In certain instances, it may be both useful and necessary to discuss the case preoperatively with the surgeon who performed the previous procedure, as the operative report may be lost or deficient. The company representative will often be able to provide useful literature, polyethylene extractor tools, and trial components to assess the reduction once the existing polyethylene has been removed. If a specific extractor is available, then the component may be removed simply. If there is difficulty in removing the component with standard extraction tools, then an alternate method must be used. The key principle at this point is to use a method that allows nontraumatic removal of the polyethylene with respect to the cup. Damage to the existing locking mechanism may be incurred during these alternate removal techniques, and new locking mechanisms must be available for insertion. Secondary damage to the cup or the need to revise the acetabular component must be anticipated and implants must be available to perform this at the time of revision. Tines on the locking mechanism may be retracted and the liner gently pried out of the cup with an osteotome. Polyethylene with locking rings or cold flow interference-fit liners may be difficult to extract. A 3.2 mm drill in the apex of the polyethylene may be used to create a hole to insert a 4.5 mm cancellous screw. The screw is screwed in, and upon contact with the metal shell, the liner is forced out of the locking mechanism. This technique will fail if the screw is inserted in a screw hole. The locking mechanism is often damaged with this technique, and exchange to a new ring must be anticipated preoperatively. If standard techniques fail, the surgeon may be required to section the polyethylene with a high-speed pencil burr into quadrants and remove the pieces separately. Careful attention to locking mechanism damage must be observed during this technique, and creation of undersurface metal defects must be carefully avoided.

Assessment of cup stability intraoperatively may be performed by several methods. Compression of the inside of the cup with a ball or blunt retractor may cause fluid to be expressed from the bone–implant interface if the cup has significant areas without ingrowth. Gentle pressure on the rim of the component with a Cobb elevator may demonstrate movement of the cup. Grasping the cup with a Kocher clamp and attempting to move it may also be tried.

Recognizing that simple liner change may not always be appropriate is an important part in the preoperative planning process. Contraindications to simple liner change include the malpositioned acetabular component, a damaged locking mechanism or damaged cup, poor cup design with known inadequate track record, and cups that have an ongrowth type surface, which are easily removed. In these instances the surgeon is dealing with Type II components.

Bone grafting of osteolytic defects associated with Type I components may be required at the time of revision. Lesions which are easily accessible to grafting (peri-articular lysis) and do not require violation of structural acetabular bone or creation of windows may be considered for grafting. The use of allograft or bone substitutes avoids the morbidity of autograft harvest, and radiographic incorporation of cancellous allograft has shown equal results to autograft. Complete debridement and cavitary curettage of the entire lesion is not necessary, and avoids creating large opening defects to access these lesions. Simple liner exchange without bone grafting of lesions has also shown acceptable results, and is performed routinely by many authors. Lesional currettage and bone grafting through acetabular screw holes may be performed in certain instances. This is a technically demanding technique, and newer instruments for delivery of graft into these defects have been developed to increase the volume and speed of delivery.

Modular polyethylene exchange is performed, and a new locking mechanism inserted, if necessary. The exchange of modular femoral heads is routine at our institution. The development of newer cross-linked polyethylene has created resurgence of interest in using larger femoral head diameters in these revision cases. The added stability and greater impingement-free range of motion may avoid the use of longer skirted head sizes and avoid using constrained components in these revision cases, which often are complicated by instability as a result of this "simple" surgery of polyethylene liner exchange. The results of larger femoral heads are in the early stages, however the early results seem to be promising. With the development of newer cross-linked polyethylene technology, the temptation to use a larger head for stability and sacrifice polyethylene thickness is experimental. The authors still recommend a minimum polyethylene thickness of 8 mm, as thin liners are more susceptible to fracture and accelerated polyethylene wear (107,108).

Type II Acetabular Components

These components have been defined as stable, with a damaged or nonfunctional shell due to excessive wear. Additionally, the locking mechanism may be broken (Fig. 8) or the acetabular component and polyethylene may be of a nonmodular design. These components require removal and revision.

The radiographic appearance of Type II cups may be similar to Type I, however, these cups are damaged or nonfunctional, and must be revised. The cup must be carefully assessed for a disrupted or a poor locking mechanism, and preoperative planning is essential to identify components with poor historical function. Backside wear of the shell must be sought, and is frequently encountered with catastrophic failure of the polyethylene liner. In the case of a well-fixed or ingrown socket that requires removal, the surgeon must again have the appropriate instruments available. With removal of such implants, reconstruction of the medial wall defect must be anticipated, and a defect larger than the existing osteolytic defect will be created. The principles of revision acetabular surgery guide the treatment for such cups. Adequate exposure of the rim of the cup, assessment of cup stability, and damage to the cup must be sought. Bone grafting of medial wall defects must be anticipated. The polyethylene liner is removed as described for Type I cups. Exposure of the circumferential rim of the implant may be aided with the use of osteotomes and high-speed burrs. Cup removal is then performed. The loose up is generally easy to remove. However, careful removal of the loose cup is advised, especially with medial defects, as neurovascular structures may be adherent to the soft tissue medial to the cup. If there is a significant

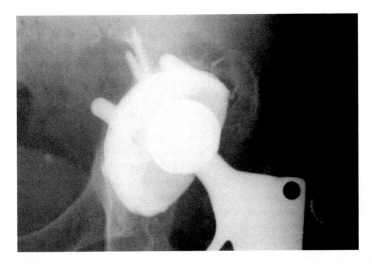

Figure 8 Asymmetric polyethylene wear with an acetabular shell with a broken locking ring. The broken tines are visable at the 3 o'clock position.

medial wall defect, the surgeon may wish to consider imaging the internal iliac vessels with contrast angiography or CT scanning, in order to predict proximity of vital neurovascular structures. The well-fixed Type II implant that must be removed provides the greatest challenge to the surgeon. Flexible curved sharp osteotomes may be useful, although they tend to remove a significant amount of acetabular bone despite meticulous technique and patience. Newer osteotome instruments that can rotate around the center of the cup axis and utilize sharp, flexible osteotomes (Zimmer Explant Cupout Extractor) with incremental sizes have shown promise. In our experience, however, the surgeon must not rely on the misguided osteotome or cutting instrument to remove all cups. The use of high-speed metal cutting burrs to section the acetabular component if it is well fixed and other methods have failed is also useful to have available, and may be used as an adjunctive tool. Cups that are medialized and approach the medial pelvic wall must not be blindly removed with osteotomes, as the pelvic vessels and viscera are at risk of damage. This is the ideal situation to section the cup into quadrants with high-speed metal cutting instruments under direct vision in order to directly visualize the removal. Circumferential disruption of the interface for 180°, and at the region of the quadrilateral plate is required before the implant may be able to be removed.

Material composition of components should be kept in mind, as some components will be easier to remove, knowing their history and biological characteristics. Cobalt–chrome sockets should be recognized preoperatively, as a number of metal cutting instruments and patience may be required in order to remove these implants, which are usually well fixed. Ongrowth cups, such those with a hydroxyapatite macrotextured surface may be easier to remove, and in certain instances (HA coated press fit—Osteonics) are removed routinely regardless of apparent implant stability because of its poor performance record (109). Titanium plasma sprayed components may also be simpler to remove, and recognition will aid in anticipating ease of extraction.

Nonmodular cups with excessive and eccentric wear of the polyethylene are also Type II cups. Newer cup materials have been developed which incorporate tantalum ingrowth surfaces (110) and utilize a nonmodular polyethylene monoblock design, in an attempt to eliminate backside motion and decrease concerns about polyethylene wear (111). Experience with removal of these implants is limited, but likely will require similar techniques as for removal of the well-fixed acetabular implant.

Removal of the well-fixed implant will likely incur the creation of a larger defect than on preoperative x-rays. It is our experience that removal of a well-fixed 52–54 mm cup will on average create a new rim defect, which requires a revision porous cup of approximately 66–68 mm outer diameter. Thus, a range of larger revision cups must be available to the surgeon when removal of a well-fixed cup is anticipated.

Currettage of membrane and bone grafting of osteolytic defects for Type II cups follows as in the assessment and classification of acetabular defects in revision surgery. Contained cavitary and medial wall defects are effectively managed with cancellous bone graft, and a porous revision cup with screws. Larger defects and those associated with segmental deficiencies of one or both columns are managed as described for revision of acetabular defects. Large porous cups with screws with available host bone coverage at least 50% is preferred. Rarely, femoral head allograft, distal femoral allograft, acetabular reconstruction cages, and acetabular hemi and total acetabular allograft reconstructions may be required. Preoperative classification and anticipation of these defects will allow the surgeon to prepare for the reconstruction, and often discussion with or referral to a surgeon familiar with these less commonly performed procedures may appropriate. The modular head exchange and polyethylene liner insertion then proceed as for revision acetabular surgery.

Type III Acetabular Components

These cups are unstable and the loose component may have collapsed into the osteolytic lesion (Fig. 9). All Type III cups require revision. The defect size may be underestimated on plain radiographs, and CT scanning may demonstrate the extent of the lesion more clearly. If the cup proceeds to migrate medially, the eventual outer acetabular diameter may decrease or become less than that of the component, making removal of this type of cup a challenging task. This will require removal of obstructing overhanging bone around the rim of the acetabulum prior to the removal of the cup. The cup that migrates into an osteolytic lesion will usually remain loose,

(A) **(B)**

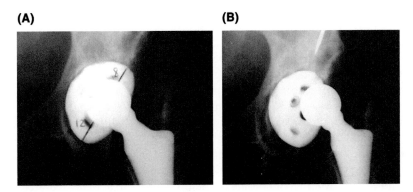

Figure 9 Type III acetabular component. (A) Radiograph shows a acetabular shell with linear lucency and some asymmetric polyethylene wear. Follow-up X-ray, just prior to surgery, shows component migration into the osteolytic lesion.

however on rare occasion, the cup may become partially ingrown in its new location, and removal more difficult than the surgeon had anticipated. Similarly, the loose, unstable acetabular component will create a defect that is significantly larger than that anticipated from preoperative radiographs, and the surgeon must recognize this and have available fixation options available. Porous cups with peripheral screw fixation or dome screw fixation provide different options to the surgeon. Inadequate host bone coverage may require acetabular antiprotrusio cages and/or supplemental structural allograft fixation for support. Reconstruction of osteolytic defects proceeds as for Type II defects, with curettage and grafting of the defect, which is easily accessible with cup removal.

FEMORAL OSTEOLYSIS—MANAGEMENT

The management of osteolysis of the femur in total hip arthroplasty is a challenging task. The complexity of revision surgery, along with patient factors, implant factors, and osteolysis often leads to confusion as to the appropriate route for management. Adherence to the basic principles of revision surgery for femoral arthroplasty, as well as understanding the mode of failure of the implant, the contributing factor(s) leading to the osteolysis, and the different reconstruction techniques available for femoral reconstruction will guide the surgeon to a solution that is tailored towards each patient. Although each patient and defect provides a challenging new problem, the basic management options for femoral osteolysis may be outlined as in Figure 6. A stable femoral reconstruction is the desired goal. The method(s) of reaching that goal are variable. Removing the source of wear and particle debris, curettage and grafting of accessible lesions, and a stable femoral reconstruction are the basic principles.

Defects with Associated Deformity

Proximal femoral deformity associated with femoral defects is most commonly seen as varus remodeling secondary to loosening of the femoral component and osteolysis of varying degrees. In these situations, we find that performing an extended proximal trochanteric osteotomy may serve several purposes. In cases associated with severe trochanteric osteolysis, the osteotomy is controlled, and avoids fracturing the trochanter during stem insertion. A straight entry for reaming is created, and the canal is directly visualized. The osteotomy allows for controlled removal of cement, under direct vision, avoiding cortical perforation and incomplete cement removal. Other indications for the osteotomy include removal of a well-fixed stem (cemented or cementless), and abductor tensioning. We have reported our results with extended trochanteric osteotomies (112), and found no nonunions and migration less than 2 mm in 87 cases over a two-year period. In Type II or III femurs with varus remodeling and one of the above indications, performing an osteotomy is a safe and efficient means of revising the femur with predictable healing rates and few complications.

Choice of implant fixation for femoral deficiency should follow a logical decision-making algorithm. Proximal bone quality, location and extent of femoral osteolysis, adequacy of cancellous bone, canal diameter, available isthmus fixation zone, and remodeling of the femur must all be considered before choosing the method of femoral revision. Patient factors must also be considered and used to choose the treatment option best for each patient's demands.

The location of osteolytic lesions and type of implant present will play an important role in management. With an extensively porous coated stem that is ingrown, osteolytic lesions frequently occur around the greater and lesser trochanters (Gruen zones 1 and 7) (113) and are not typically associated with implant loosening (71,114). The wear debris may gain access to these regions, and the circumferential ingrowth prevents distal debris migration, and osteolysis. These lesions may be bone grafted at the time of revision surgery, and with removal of the particle generator, reconstitution of the bone stock will occur. Fracture of the greater trochanter is known to occur in association with osteolysis (Fig. 10) (115) and may require operative fixation and grafting, or simple nonoperative treatment and later assessment along with the source of the osteolysis. As mentioned previously, plain radiographs frequently underestimate the severity of osteolysis, particularly in the greater trochanter. Also, metallic implants can obscure bone loss on routine radiographs. Therefore, when operative treatment is undertaken, the surgeon must be prepared for more severe bone loss than is visible on plain radiographs. In the cemented stem with stem tip osteolysis and regions of bubbly expansile lesions, stem loosening is likely, and the surgeon must be prepared to revise these components. Cavitary

(A) **(B)** **(C)**

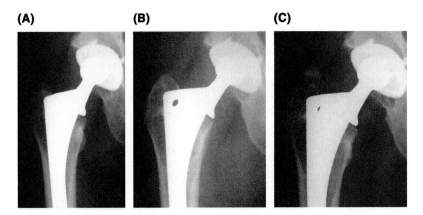

Figure 10 Trochanteric osteolytic fracture: (**A**) Postoperative radiograph. (**B**) Seven year follow-up with asymmetric polyethylene wear and greater trochanteric osteolytic lesion. The patient was asymptomatic. (**C**) Patient presented approximately seven and a half years postoperatively with hip pain. A trochanteric fracture was evident. The patient was treated nonoperatively and healed without residual problem.

lesions at and distal to the stem tip with progressive or destructive cortical erosions should be considered early for revision in order to avoid periprosthetic fracture in the future. Bypassing these lesions with fully porous coated stems or other methods must be the goal. When focal or large uncontained defects arise, consideration for the use of strut allografts to bridge the defects may be useful for structural support and to increase bone stock in the femur.

The challenge in managing osteolysis in the femur is in the ability to recognize when to operate, and what to do. The implant type, osteolytic defect, cement versus cementless, ingrown or loose, modular versus nonmodular, and implant performance record in the long term—all of these may be important factors in the decision making process. The senior author has used an acetabular implant classification system, which has been useful in preoperative planning and management of acetabular osteolysis in total hip arthroplasty. In order to address these similar concerns on the femoral side, we have proposed a new classification system that not only addresses osteolytic defects, but also the femoral implant itself (Table 6). This provides a useful outline for helping decide how to proceed in the presence of various forms of implants and osteolysis.

Type I Femoral Implant Osteolysis

Type I femoral implants are stable and do not require revision. The uncemented implant is ingrown or fibrous stable. The cemented implant is well fixed. Component positioning is satisfactory, and the overall performance of the implant has shown acceptable results in the literature. The taper mechanism is undamaged and intact, without signs of fretting. However, the associated osteolytic lesion may require surgical management (Fig. 11). The lesion is usually in the proximal regions of Gruen zones one or seven, and may be progressive. Typically involving the regions of the greater and lesser trochanter, these lesions are accessible at the time of revision surgery. The management of the particle generator is the primary focus, and curettage with bone grafting of lesions in the trochanteric regions may be undertaken at the same time. Patients may be symptomatic or asymptomatic, and osteolysis noted in addition to other findings on radiographs, such as polyethylene wear asymmetry or concomitant acetabular osteolysis. As noted above, the surgeon should beware that plain radiographs often underestimate the size and extent of these lesions, and careful management of the trochanter will avoid unwanted iatrogenic fracture or avulsion of the greater trochanter during revision. Attempted internal fixation of the osteolytic trochanter that has fractured is fraught with difficulty, and thus careful surgical technique is required to avoid this complication. Curettage of accessible lesions with bone grafting versus curettage alone, versus removal of the particle generator alone is currently practiced, and results may be similar for these methods. Currently, curettage of accessible lesions with or without bone grafting is commonly performed. Typically, a Type I femoral component is associated with asymmetric polyethylene wear and or acetabular osteolysis, and the femoral osteolysis may be managed at the time of polyethylene exchange or acetabular revision. With improved technology in porous coated implants and increased

(A)   **(B)**

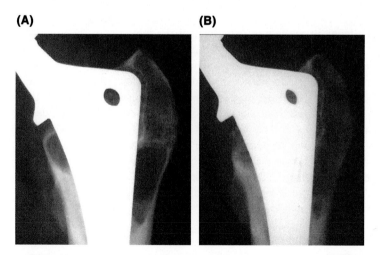

Figure 11 Trochanteric osteolysis. (**A**) Osteolysis evident at time of acetabular revision surgery was bone grafted. (**B**) Three year follow-up X-ray shows consolidation of the bone graft.

use of extensively porous coated stems in primary total hip arthroplasty, this type of implant and osteolysis is becoming one of the more commonly encountered by the orthopaedic surgeon following hip arthroplasty patients. Exchange of modular titanium heads for Co–Cr–Mo heads should be performed, and downsized to 28 or 26 mm diameter, to decrease volumetric wear.

Type II Femoral Implant Osteolysis

Type II femoral implants are stable, however revision is necessary, secondary to implant related factors or factors related to the extent or location of the osteolytic lesion.

The implant may again be either cemented or cementless, and is stable, without signs of loosening. However, surgeon threshold for revision of the femoral component is lowered as a result of several implant related factors. (i) If the modular taper mechanism shows excessive fretting or damage, modular head exchange may lead to a further source of particle debris and wear, propagating the osteolysis. (ii) Noncircumferential or "patch" porous coated implants have been shown to provide a poor barrier to distal wear debris flow, and are associated with progressive osteolysis of the femur. The removal of these implants is facilitated by their lack of circumferential coating. In the presence of osteolysis, these implants should be removed. These stems should be revised preferably before structural defects become so advanced that large allografts are needed or periprosthetic fracture occurs. However, a noncircumferentially coated component may be retained in elderly, sedentary patients, with grafting of the lesions and removal of the particle generators. This approach may be used occasionally in young, active patients if the stem is well fixed, and osteolysis is minimal, with close observation of the lysis. (iii) Monoblock titanium stems are associated with increased wear debris, and should be revised, except in the elderly patient with a well-fixed stem, where retaining the implant may be considered. (iv) Well-fixed stems that are small or designs which are prone to fracture should be revised before metal fatigue leads to breakage of the stem (116). (v) Femoral components that are stable but demonstrate varus malposition, poor offset, or poor version characteristics must be assessed at the time of surgery. If any of these factors is affecting the performance of the hip function, consideration must be given at the time of surgery to revise the component. Careful consideration must include patient age, hip stability, and type of implant, as the removal of a well-fixed cemented or cementless implant may create more complex or larger defects and advanced revision techniques will be required.

With Type II femoral implants, there is often an associated osteolytic lesion, which may be either expansile and focal, or linear, and which may lead to eventual failure of the implant or periprosthetic fracture. For small focal lesions or linear osteolysis, observation is recommended for elderly and less active patients. However, these types of osteolytic lesions are frequently progressive, and often require surgical intervention. If the defect is at the stem tip or distal, it is likely associated with an implant that has failed to provide a barrier to distal wear debris flow, and will likely require revision now or in the near future. Examples include cemented implants without definite signs of loosening, but probable or possible loosening, with incomplete bone cement radiolucencies. Similarly, the noncircumferentially porous coated implant is frequently associated with such lesions, and is a relative indication for femoral revision. The stable fibrous fully porous coated implant will rarely become unstable or loose, demonstrating the classic radiographic features of implant loosening. Expansile stem-tip lesions with associated diaphyseal expansile radiolucent lines indicate that the implant should be revised. Any lesion that is distal to the stem tip should be considered for revision with bypass fixation, using revision techniques as already discussed. If a cemented component is considered for the revision, it should bypass the most distal cortical defect by at least two to three cortical diameters (117). Curettage and grafting of accessible lesions is the gold standard of lesional treatment. Practically, however, removal of the particle generator, curettage of any accessible lesions, and femoral reconstruction that bypasses the defect are the principles. Advanced techniques to augment or restore bone stock such as strut allografts, structural allograft, or impaction allografting must be considered for structural cortical defects. The Type II implant without a bony defect is frequently encountered. The surgeon should be comfortable in removing both well-fixed cemented and cementless implants, and in revision femoral reconstruction. Early identification and treatment of impending fracture secondary to distal osteolytic lesions will hopefully prevent lesion propagation and periprosthetic fractures in this type of defect. The removal of well-fixed implants may be fraught with difficulty, and may increase the complexity of the revision. However, retaining such implants with the characteristics noted above may prove to be more detrimental in the long term. Controlled component removal during elective surgery provides a reasonable alternative to the wait and see method, and may prevent unnecessary emergency surgery for periprosthetic fractures.

The evolution of the extended proximal femoral osteotomy for removal of well-fixed cemented and cementless implants has been an important technique which has allowed controlled implant removal under direct vision. Cement removal instruments, including ultrasonic devices, have increased the surgeon's options for removal of well-fixed cemented implants. Availability of metal cutting instruments and trephine reamers is necessary in order to remove the well-fixed cementless component that must be revised.

Type III Femoral Implant Osteolysis

Type III femoral implants with associated osteolysis are loose implants, by definition, and require removal. We have included infected total hip arthroplasty in this category, as this will most often require removal of the stem, regardless of stem type or stability. The osteolytic defect that is encountered may range from the simple linear defects to expansile or focal lesions (Fig. 12). Loosening of the implant is determined by the criteria previously discussed, and is usually evident both clinically and radiographically. The important factors to consider in managing these defects are again in recognizing (i) the type of implant, and (ii) the nature of the osteolytic lesion. The type of implant is important to determine. Monoblock stems may be difficult to remove with challenges in exposing and dislocating the hip. Curved or bowed stems may be loose, however, bony remodeling or overgrowth in the proximal femur may make removal difficult, requiring an osteotomy. In this instance, the osteotomy serves a dual purpose—removal of the stem in the remodeled femur, and improved access to the femur for osteolytic lesions and femoral canal preparation. The osteotomy may also serve to tension the abductors as required for increased stability, by advancing the trochanteric fragment, as necessary. The surgeon must also recognize that the removal of curved stems from within a relatively straight proximal femur is not always straightforward. Loosening of the curved stem does not imply an easy

(A)   **(B)**

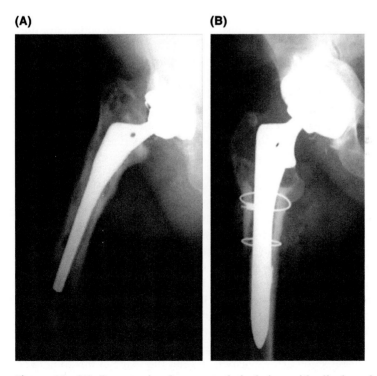

Figure 12 (**A**) Preoperative large osteolytic lesion with diaphyseal expansion. Femoral stem has subsided. (**B**) Postoperative X-ray showing placement of full porous coated stem with greater than 4 cm of diaphyseal press-fit.

removal, and the surgeon must be patient during exposure and in gentle extraction of the implant. Frequently, the implant has subsided or lateral bone has overgrown the edges of the prosthesis. Removal of all lateral bone which is impeding removal of the implant at the outset will not only expose the implant more adequately, but ensure an unimpeded, safer extraction. As noted previously, loss of proximal cancellous bone and osteolysis involving the trochanters is frequently encountered in association with these loose implants. Aggressive removal may lead to unwanted complications, such as fracture of the greater trochanter, or destruction of the remaining proximal femoral bone. Similarly, in removing these implants, the surgeon must pay close attention to the proximity of the abductor musculature, as forceful extraction techniques may inadvertently injure or avulse the already violated muscle, leading to loss of soft tissue balance and potential instability. Frequently this factor is overlooked, until the case has progressed without regard for the soft tissue quality.

The location and extent of the associated osteolytic lesions is the determining factor in how the femur will be reconstructed once the loose implant has been successfully removed, and follows from revision femoral reconstruction techniques. Often the extent and size of the lesions will be greater than on the preoperative radiographs. The surgeon should anticipate this, and have a primary reconstruction plan, a second option plan, and an unlikely but carefully thought out last resort plan if the first two methods are inadequate. As such, for every femoral revision, we always discuss at least two options for the femoral reconstruction, and ensure that the available instrumentation and materials are available (Fig. 13). Not infrequently, the surgeon may encounter difficulty with implant removal, larger than anticipated osteolytic defects, or other patient factors that alter the reconstruction. Thus, the backup plan is essential in the preoperative planning phase.

The infected total hip arthroplasty is included for two reasons in this group. Firstly, infection may mimic osteolysis, and all patients must be evaluated for infection, as previously discussed. Implants may be loose, well fixed, or show features on radiographs similar to those of osteolysis. Infection may also develop in the already loose implant with previous osteolysis, clouding the picture. Secondly, the infected total hip arthroplasty frequently requires removal and, two-staged reconstruction with antibiotic spacers have shown the most successful results. Both patient and organism factors are again considerations. Prior to stem removal for infection, the surgeon must consider whether other options are more appropriate for each particular patient. Discussion of single exchange reimplantation, chronic antibiotic suppression, or resection arthroplasty is beyond the scope of this topic. The loose infected stem is a somewhat easier decision for management than the solidly fixed implant, and should be removed at the time of irrigation and debridement.

(A) (B)

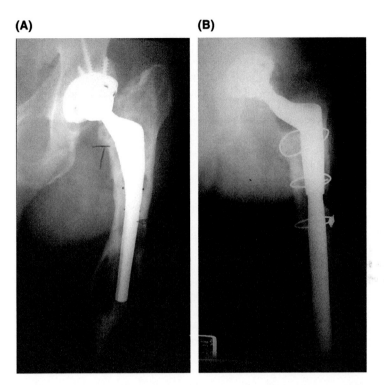

Figure 13 (A) Preoperative very large osteolytic diaphyseal lesion. (B) Postoperative X-ray. A modular femoral stem system was required to bypass the osteolytic defect.

CONCLUSION

Osteolysis is quickly becoming one of the prevalent diseases in total hip arthroplasty. Due to its silent nature, serial yearly examinations and X-ray follow-up are recommended. When lesions are discovered, close follow-up is warranted. Signs of progression of lesions or the appearance of new pain symptoms are indications for revision. The surgery required depends on many factors. Bone grafting around stable implants has been shown to be successful, but more research is required. Loose components should be revised so as to decrease particle generators and assess the bone defect that is present.

The recognition of implant related factors and patterns and locations of osteolytic lesions are important in order to select the appropriate form of management for each patient. In the process of planning the reconstruction, the surgeon must anticipate the technical difficulties that may be encountered, and have alternate plans as a backup. Finally, patient factors will play a role in the management of each defect, and must be considered as an important part of the planning for surgery or nonoperative treatment.

REFERENCES

1. Schmalzreid TP, Shepard EF, Dorey FJ, Jackson WO, dela Rosa M, Fa'vae F, McKellop HA, McClung CD, Martell J, Moreland JR, et al. Wear is a function of use, not time. Clin Orthop 2000; 381:36–46.
2. Chen PC, Mead EH, Pinto JG, Colwell CW. Polyethylene wear debris in modular acetabular prostheses. Clin Orthop 1995; 317:44–56.
3. Elfick A, Hall RM, Pinder IM, Unsworth A. Wear in retrieved acetabular components. Effect of femoral head radius and patient parameters. J Arthroplasty 1998; 13(3):291–295.
4. Xenos JS, Hopkinson WJ, Callaghan JJ, Heekin RD, Savory CG. Osteolysis around an uncemented cobalt chrome total hip arthroplasty. Clin Orthop 1995; 317:29–36.
5. Maloney WJ, Galante JO, Anderson M, Goldberg V, Harris WH, Jacobs J, Kraay M, Lachiewicz P, Rubash HE, Schutzer S, et al. Fixation, polyethylene wear, and pelvic osteolysis in primary total hip replacement. Clin Orthop 1999; 369:157–164.
6. Joshi RP, Eftekhar NS, McMahon DJ, Nercessian OA. Osteolysis after Charnley primary low-friction arthroplasty. A comparison of two matched paired groups. JBJS 1998; 80-B(4):585–590.
7. Sutula LC, Collier JP, Saum KA, Currier BH, Currier JH, Sanford WM, Mayor MB, Wodding RE, Sperling DK, Williams IR, et al. Impact of gamma sterilization on clinical performance of polyethylene in the hip. Clin Orthop 1995; 319:28–40.
8. Bankston AB, Keating M, Ranawat C, Faris PM, Ritter M. Comparison of polyethylene wear in machined versus molded polyethylene. Clin Orthop 1995; 317:37–43.
9. Bankston AB, Cates H, Ritter MA, Keating EM, Faris PM. Polyethylene wear in total hip arthroplasty. Clin Orthop 1995; 317:7–13.
10. Ranawat CS, Deshmukh RG, Peters LE, Umlas ME. Prediction of the long-term durability of all-polyethylene cemented sockets. Clin Orthop 1995; 317:89–105.
11. Urban RM, Jacobs JJ, Gilbert JL, Galante JO. Migration of corrosion products from modular hip prostheses. JBJS 1994; 76-A(9):1345–1359.
12. Bobyn JD, Tanzer M, Krygier JJ, Dujovne AR, Brooks CE. Concerns with modularity in total hip arthroplasty. Clin Orthop 1994; 298:27–36.
13. Bal BS, Vandelune D, Gurba DM, Jasty M, Harris WH. Polyethylene wear in cases using femoral stems of similar geometry, but different metals, porous layer, and modularity. J Arthroplasty 1998; 13(5):492–498.
14. Buly RL, Huo MH, Salvati E, Brien W, Bansal M. Titanium wear debris in failed cemented total hip arthroplasty. An analysis of 71 cases. J Arthroplasty 1992; 7(3):315–323.
15. Lombardi AV Jr, Mallory TH, Vaughn BK, Drouillard P. Aseptic loosening in total hip arthroplasty secondary to osteolysis induced by wear debris from titanium-alloy modular femoral heads. JBJS 1989; 71-A(9):1337–1342.
16. Kennedy JG, Rogers WB, Soffe KE, Sullivan RJ, Griffen DG, Sheehan LJ. Effect of acetabular component orientation on recurrent dislocation, pelvic

osteolysis, polyethylene wear and component migration. J Arthroplasty 1998; 13(5):530–534.

17. Scholl E, Eggli S, Ganz R. Osteolysis in cemented titanium alloy hip prothesis. J Arthroplasty 2000; 15(5):570–575.

18. Yoon TR, Rowe SM, Jung ST, Seon KJ, Maloney WJ. Osteolysis in association with a total hip arthroplasty with ceramic bearing surfaces. JBJS 1998; 80-A(10):1459–1467.

19. Klapperich C, Graham J, Pruitt L, Ries MD. Failure of a metal-on-metal total hip arthroplasty from progressive osteolysis. J Arthroplasty 1999; 14(7): 877–881.

20. Yoon TR, Rowe SM, Jung ST, Seon KJ, Maloney WJ. Osteolysis in association with a total hip arthroplasty with ceramic bearing surfaces. JBJS 1998; 80-A(10):1459–1468.

21. Cuckler JM, Bearcroft J, Asgian CM. Femoral head technologies to reduce polyethylene wear in total hip arthroplasty. Clin Orthop 1995; 317:57–63.

22. Dowson D. A comparative study of the performance of metallic and ceramic femoral head components in total hip replacement joints. Wear 1995; 190: 171–183.

23. Dorr LD, Zhinian W, Longjohn DB, Dubois B, Murken R. Total hip arthroplasty with use of the metasul metal-on-metal articulation. Four to seven-year results. JBJS 2000; 2-A(6):789–797.

24. Huo MH, Martin RP, Zatorski LE, Keggi KJ. Cementless total hip arthroplasties using ceramic-on-ceramic articulation in young patients. A minimum 5-year follw-up study. J Arthroplasty 1996; 11(6):673–678.

25. Higuchi F, Inoue A, Semlitsch M. Metal-on-metal McKee–Farrar total hip arthroplasty: characteristics from a long-term follow-up study. Arch Orthop Trauma Surg 1997; 116(3):121–124.

26. Emerson RH, Sanders SB, Head WC, Higgins L. Effect of circumferential plasma-spray porous coating on the rate of femoral osteolysis after total hip arthroplasty. JBJS 1999; 81-A(9):1291–1297.

27. Sakalkale DP, Sharkey PF, Eng K, Hozack WJ, Rothman RH. Effect of femoral component offset on polyethylene wear in total hip arthroplasty. Clin Orthop 2001; 388:125–134.

28. McKellop HA. Bearing surfaces in total hip replacements: State of the art and future developments. AAOS ICL 2001; 50, Chapter 17: 165–184.

29. Chen PC, Mead EH, Pinto JG, Colwell CW. Polyethylene wear debris in modular acetabular prostheses. Clin Orthop 1995; 317:44–56.

30. Maloney WJ, Jasty M, Rosenberg A, Harris WH. Bone lysis in well-fixed cemented femoral components. J Bone Joint Surg Br 1990; 72:966–970.

31. Chatoo M, Parfitt, Pearse MF. Periprosthetic acetabular fracture associated with extensive osteolysis. J Arthroplasty 1998; 13(7):843–845.

32. Schmidt AH, Walker G, Kyle RF, Thompson RC Jr. Periprosthetic metaastatic carcinoma: pitfalls in management of two cases initially diagnosed as osteolysis. J Arthroplasty 1996; 11:613–619.

33. Ito H, Shimizu A. Malignant lymphoma at the site of a total hip arthroplasty. Orthopedics 1999; 22(1):82–84.

34. Marr DS, Rosenthal DI, Cohen GL, Tomford WW. Rapid postoperative osteolysis in Paget disease: a case report. JBJS 1994; 76-A:274–277.
35. Anderson JT, Dehner LP. Osteolytic form of Pagets disease. Differential diagnosis and pathogenesis. JBJS 1976; 58(7):994–1000.
36. Maloney WJ, Paters P, Engh CA, Chandler H. Severe osteolysis of the pelvis in association with acetabular replacement without cement. JBJS 1993; 75-A(11): 1627–1635.
37. Berry DJ. UHMWPE: The good, bad & ugly. Management of osteolysis around total hip arthroplasty. Orthopedics 1999; 22(9):805–808.
38. Sanchez-Sotolo J, McGrory BJ, Berry DJ. Acute periprosthetic fracture of the acetabulum associated with osteolytic pelvic lesions: A report of 3 cases. J Arthroplasty 2000; 15(4):126–130.
39. Dunbar MJ, Blackley HR, Bournw RB. Osteolysis of the femur: Principles of management. AAOS ICL 2001; 50:197–209.
40. Spangehl MJ, Younger AS, Masri BA, Duncan CP. Diagnosis of infection following total hip arthroplasty. JBJS 1997; 79-A:1578–1588.
41. Schmalzreid TP, Fowble VA, Amstutz HC. The fate of pelvic osteolysis after reoperation. Clin Orthop 1998; 350:128–137.
42. Zicat B, Engh CA, Gokcen E. Patterns of osteolysis around total hip components inserted with and without cement. JBJS 1995; 77-A(3):432–439.
43. Maloney WJ, Herzwurm P, Paprosky W, Rubash HE, Engh CA. Treatment of pelvic osteolysis associated with a stable acetabular component inserted without cement as part of a total hip replacement. JBJS 1997; 79-A:1628–1634.
44. Maloney WJ, Paters P, Engh CA, Chandler H. Severe osteolysis of the pelvis in association with acetabular replacement without cement. JBJS 1993; 75-A(11): 1627–1635.
45. Zimlich RH, Fehring TK. Understimation of pelvic osteolysis. The value of the iliac oblique radiograph. J Arthroplasty 2000; 15(6):796–801.
46. Martell JM, Berdia S. Determination of polyethylene wear in total hip replacements with use of digital radiographs. JBJS 1997; 79-A(11):1635–1641.
47. Han CD, Choe WS, Yoo JH. Effect of polyethylene wear on osteolysis in cementless primary total hip arthroplasty. Minimal 5-year follow-up study. J Arthroplasty 1999; 14(6):714–723.
48. Sochart DH. Relationship of acetabular wear to osteolysis and loosening in total hip arthroplasty. Clin Orthop 1999; 363:135–150.
49. Schmalzreid TP, Callaghan JJ. Wear in total hip and knee replacements. JBJS 1999; 81-A(1):115–136.
50. Harris WH, Schiller AL, Scholler JM, et al. Extensive localized bone resorption in the femur following total hip replacement. JBJS-A 1976; 58:612–618.
51. Mulroy WF, Estok DM, Harris WH. Total hip arthroplasty with use of so-called second-generation cementing techniques. A fifteen-year-average follow-up study. JBJS 1995; 77-A:1845–1852.
52. Harris WH. The problem is osteolysis. Clin Orthop 1995; 311:46–53.
53. Tanzer M, Maloney WJ, Jasty M, Harris WH. The progression of femoral cortical osteolysis in association with total hip arthroplasty without cement. JBJS 1992; 74-A:404–410.

54. Urban RM, Jacobs JJ, Sumner DR, Peters CL, Voss FR, Galante JO. The bone–implant interface of femoral stems with non-circumferential porous coating. A study of specimens retrieved at autopsy. JBJS 1996; 78-A:1068–1081.
55. Dirksmeier P, Sinha RK. Double-tapered cementless stems for total hip arthroplasty. Oper Tech Orthop 2000; 10(2):120–122.
56. Head WC, Mallory TH, Emerson RH. The proximal porous coating alternative for primary total hip arthroplasty. Orthopedics 1999; 22:813–815.
57. Engh CA, Massin P, Suthers KE. Roentgenographic assessment of the biologic fixation of porous-surfaced femoral components. Clin Orthop 1990; 257: 107–128.
58. Khalily C, Whiteside LA. Predictive value of early radiographic findings in cementless total hip arthroplasty femoral components: an 8- to 12-year follow-up. J Arthroplasty 1998; 13(7):768–773.
59. Engh CA Jr, Culpepper WJ II, Engh CA. Long-term results of the use of anatomic medullary locking prosthesis in total hip arthroplasty. JBJS 1997; 79-A:177–194.
60. Wixon RL, Stulberg SD, Mehlhoff M. Total hip replacement with cemented, uncemented and hybrid protheses. A comparison of clinical and radiograpic results at two to four years. JBJS 1991; 73-A:257–270.
61. Pierson JL, Harris WH. Extensive osteolysis behind a acetabular component that was well fixed with cement. A case report. JBJS 1993; 75-A:268–271.
62. DeLee JG, Charnley J. Radiological demarcation of cemented sockets in total hip replacement. Clin Orthop 1976; 121:20–32.
63. Nayak NK, Mulliken B, Rorabeck CH, Bourne RB, Robinson EJ. Osteolysis in cemented versus cementless acetabular components. J Arthroplasty 1996; 11(2):135–140.
64. Hodgkinson JP, Shelly P, Wroblewski BM. The correlation between the roentgenographic appearance and operative findings at the bone–cement junction of the socket in Charnley low friction arthroplasties. Clin Orthop 1988; 228:105–109.
65. Callaghan JJ, Dysart SH, Savory CG. The uncemented porous-coated anatomic total hip prosthesis. JBJS 1988; 70-B:337–346.
66. Scmalzreid TP, Harris WH. The Harris–Galante porous-coated acetabular component with screw fixation. Radiographic analysis of eighty-three primary hip replacements at a minimum of five years. JBJS 1992; 74-A:1130–1139.
67. Kull LR, Jacobs JJ, Tompkins GS, Silverton CD, Galante JO. Primary cementless acetabular reconstruction: Osteolysis and interface changes at seven to ten year follow-up. Orthop Trans 1995; 19:401.
68. Owens TD, Moran CG, Smith SR, Pinder IM. Results of uncemented porous coated anatomic total hip replacement. JBJS 1994; 76-B:258–262.
69. Maloney WJ, Peters P, Engh CA, Chandler H. Severe osteolysis of the pelvis in association with acetabular replacement without cement. JBJS 1993; 75-A: 1627–1635.
70. Schmalzreid TP, Guttmann D, Grecula M, Amstutz HC. The relationship between the design, position and articular wear of acetabular components inserted without cement and the development of pelvic osteolysis. JBJS 1994; 76-A:677–688.

71. Zicat B, Engh CA, Gokcen E. Patterns of osteolysis around total hip components inserted with and without cement. JBJS 1995; 77-A(3):432–439.

72. Maloney WJ, Woolson ST. Increasing incidence of femoral osteolysis in association with uncemented Harris–Galante total hip arthroplasty. A follow-up report. J Arthroplasty 1996; 11(2):130–134.

73. Taylor T, Beggs I. Fine needle aspirates in infected hip replacements. Clin Radiol 1995; 50(3):149–152.

74. Manus TP, Berquist TH, Bender CE. Arthrographic study of painful total hip arthroplasty: refined criteria. Radiology 1987; 162:171.

75. Buechel FF, Drucker D, Jasty M, Jiranek, Harris WH. Osteolysis around uncemented components of cobalt–chrome surface replacement hip arthroplasty. Clin Orthop 1994; 298:202–211.

76. Maloney WJ, Peters P, Engh CA, Chandler H. Severe osteolysis of the pelvis in association with acetabular replacement without cement. JBJS 1993; 75-A(11):1627–1635.

77. Hozack WJ, Mesa JJ, Carey C, Rothman RH. Relationship between polyethylene wear, pelvic osteolysis and clinical symptomatology in patients with cementless acetabular components. A framework for decisionmaking. J Arthroplasty 1996; 11(7):769–772.

78. Rubash HE, Sinha RJ, Paprosky W, Engh CA, Maloney WJ. A new classification system for the management of acetabular osteolysis after total hip arthroplasty. AAOS ICL 1999; 48:37–42.

79. Dunbar MJ, Blackley HRL, Bourne RB. Osteolysis of the femur: Principles of management. AAOS ICL 2001; chapter 20, 50, 197–209.

80. D'Antonio J, McCarthy JC, Bargar WL, Borden LS, Cappelo WN, Collis DK, Steinberg ME, Wedge JH. Classification of femoral abnormalities in total hip arthroplasty. Clin Orthop 1993; 296:133–139.

81. Paprosky WG, Bradford MS, Younger TI. Classification of bone defects in failed prostheses. Chir Organi Mov 1994; 79(4):285–291.

82. Krishnamurthy AB, MacDonald SJ, Paprosky WG. 5–13 year follow up study on cementless femoral components in revision surgery. J Arthroplasty 1997; 12(8):839–847.

83. Benson ER, Christensen CP, Monesmith EA, Gomes SL, Bierbaum BE. Particulate bone grafting of osteolytic femoral lesions around stable cementless stems. Clin Orthop 2000; 381:58–67.

84. Hozak WJ, Bicalho PS, Eng K. Treatment of femoral osteolysis with cementless total hip revision. J Arthroplasty 1996; 11(6).

85. Wirtz DC, Heller KD, Holzwartth U, Siebert C, Pitto RP, Zeiler G, Blencke BA, Forst R. A modular femoral implant for uncemented stem revision in THR. Int Orthop 2000; 24(3):134–138.

86. Maloney WJ, Herzwurm P, Paprosky W, Rubash HE, Eng CA. Treatment of pelvic osteolysis associated with a stable acetabular component inserted without cement as part of a total hip replacement. JBJS 1997; 79-A(11).

87. Scmalzreid TP, Fowble VA, Amstutz HC. The fate of pelvic osteolysis after reoperation. Clin Orthop 1998; 350:128–137.

88. Maloney WJ, Paprosky W, Engh CA, Rubash H. Surgical treatment of pelvic osteolysis. Clin Orthop 2001; 393:78–84.

89. Flugsrud GB, Ovre S, Grogaard B, Nordsletten L. Cemented femoral impaction bone grafting for severe osteolysis in revision hip arthroplasty. Good results at 4-year follow-up of 10 patients. Arch Orthop Trauma Surg 2000; 120(7–8):386–389.

90. Leoplod SS, Berger RA, Rosenberg AG, Jacobs JJ, Quigley LR, Gaiante JO. Impaction allografting with cement for revision of the femoral component. A minimum four-year follow-up study with the use of a precoated femoral stem. JBJS 1999; 81-A(8):1080–1092.

91. Mallory TH, Lombardi AV, Fada RA, Adams JB, Kefauver CA, Eberle RW. Noncemented acetabular component removal in the presence of osteolysis. Clin Orthop 2000; 381:120–128.

92. Soto MO, Rodriguez JA, Ranawat CS. Clinical and radiographic evaluation of the Harris–Galante cup. Incidence of wear and osteolysis at 7 to 9 years follow-up. J Arthroplasty 2000; 15(2):139–145.

93. Scmalzreid TP, Guttmann D, Grecula M, Amstutz HC. The relationship between the design, position and articular wear of acetabular components inserted without cement and the development of pelvic osteolysis. JBJS 1994; 76-A(5):677–688.

94. Dowd JE, Cha CW, Trakru S, Kim SY, Yang IH, Ribash HE. Failure of total hip arthroplasty with a precoated prothesis. 4- to 11-year results. Clin Orthop 1998; 355:123–156.

95. Collies DK, Mohler CG. Loosening rates and bone lysis with rough finished and polished stems. Clin Orthop 1998; 355:113–122.

96. Emerson RH, Sanders SB, Head WC, Higgins L. Effect of circumferential plasma-spray porous coating on the rate of femoral osteolysis after total hip arthroplasty. JBJS 1999; 81-A(9):1291–1297.

97. Rokkum M, Brandt M, Bye K, Hetland KR, Waage S, Reigstad A. Polyethylene wear, osteolysis and acetabular loosening with an HA-coated hip prosthesis. A follow-up of 94 consecutive arthroplasties. JBJS 2000; 82-B(2): 305–306.

98. Kitamura S, Hasegawa Y, Iwasada S, Yamauchi K, Kawamoto K, Kanamono T, Iwata H. Catastrophic failure of cementless total hip arthroplasty using a femoral component without surface coating. J Arthroplasty 1999; 14(8):918–924.

99. Buly RL, Huo MH, Salvati E, Brien W, Bansal M. Titanium wear debris in failed cemented total hip arthroplasty. An analysis of 71 cases. J Arthroplasty 1992; 7(3):315–323.

100. Bono JV, Sanford L, Toussaint JT. Severe polyrthylene wear in total hip arthroplasty. Observation from retrieved AML PIUS hip implants with an ACS polyethylene liner. J Arthroplasty 1994; 9(2):117–118.

101. Puolakka TJ, Laine HJ, Moilanen TP, Koivisto AM, Pajamaki KJ. Alarming wear of the first-generation polyethylene liner of the cementless porpus-coated Biomet Universal cup: 107 hips followed for mean 6 years. Acta Orthop Scand 2001; 72(1):1–7.

102. Chmell MJ, Poss R, Thomas WH, Sledge CB. Early failure of Hylamer acetabular inserts due to eccentric wear. J Arthroplasty 1996; 11(3):351–353.

103. Vaughn BK, Dameron TB, Bauer TW, Mochida Y, Akisue T, Eberle RW. Early osteolysis following total hip arthroplasty with use of a Hylamer liner in combination with a modular ceramic femoral head. JBJS 1999; 81-A(10):1446–1449.

104. Rubash HE, Sinha RK, Paprosky WG, et al. AAOS Instr. Course Lect 1999; 48:37–42.

105. Jacobs JJ, Roebuck KA, Archibeck M, Hallab NJ, Glant TT. Osteolysis: basic science. Clin Orthop 2001; 393:71–77.

106. Shanbhag AS, Hasselman CT, Rubash HE. The John Charnley Award. Inhibition of wear debris mediated osteolysis in a canine total hip arthroplasty model. Clin Orthop 1997; 344:33–43.

107. Kawamura H, Dunbar MJ, Murray P, Bourne RB, Rorabeck CH. The porous coated anatomic total hip replacement. A ten to fourteen-year follow-up study of a cementless total hip arthroplasty. J Bone Joint Surg Am 2001; 83-A(9): 1333–1338.

108. Lee PC, Shih CH, Chen WJ, Tu YK, Tai CL. Early polyethylene wear and osteolysis in cementless total hip arthroplasty: the influence of femoral head size and polyethylene thickness. J Arthroplasty 1999; 14(8):976–981.

109. Massin P, Schmidt L, Engh CA. Evaluation of cementless acetabular component migration. An experimental study. J Arthroplasty 1989; 4(3):245–251.

110. Bobyn JD, Hacking SA, Chan SP, et al. Characteristics of a new porous tantalum biomaterial for reconstructive orthopedics. Scientific Exhibit, Proceedings of AAOS, Anaheim, CA, 1999.

111. Litsky AS. Elimination of cup-liner micromotion in acetabular components. Presented at the American Society for Biomaterials Annual Meeting, Anaheim CA, 1999.

112. Younger TI, Bradford MS, Magnus RE, Paprosky WG. Extended proximal femoral osteotomy. A new technique for femoral revision arthroplasty. J Arthroplasty 1995; 10(3):329–338.

113. Brown IW, Ring PA. Osteolytic changes in the upper femoral shaft following porous-coated hip replacement. J Bone Joint Surg Br 1985; 67(2):218–221.

114. Engh CA, Hooten JP Jr, Zettl-Schaffer KF, et al. Porous-coated total hip replacement. Clin Orthop 1994; 298:89–96.

115. Heekin RD, Engh CA, Herzwurm PJ. Fractures through cystic lesions of the greater trochanter: A cause of late pain after cementless total hip arthroplasty. J Arthroplasty 1996; 11:757–760.

116. Callaghan JJ, Salvati EA, Pellici PM, et al. Results of revision for mechanical failure after cemented total hip replacemt, 1979 to 1982: A two to five year follow up. JBJS 1985; 76A:1074–1085.

117. Panjabi MM, Trumble T, Hult JE, et al. Effect of femoral stem length on stress raisers associated with revision hip arthroplasty. J Orthop Res 1985; 3: 447–455.

22

Managing Knee Osteolysis

John Lyon and Aaron Rosenberg
Rush University Medical Center, Chicago, Illinois, U.S.A.

INTRODUCTION

Total knee arthroplasty has evolved into a reliable method of achieving pain relief and restoring essential knee functions. One of the current challenges is to maximize longevity of the total knee prosthesis. Bearing wear and osteolysis have emerged as significant problems jeopardizing the longevity of contemporary designs. Engh et al. (1) suggested that the most common reason for revision of modular-type total knee arthroplasty is polyethylene wear and osteolysis. This chapter briefly reviews the pathophysiology and natural history of osteolysis in total knee arthroplasty. These subjects are vital to proper diagnosis and management. The clinical presentation and work-up of patients with suspected osteolysis and polyethylene wear will be discussed. The principles of treatment are reviewed along with specific techniques necessary for surgical management. Finally, this chapter will review the results of these operative treatment methods.

PATHOPHYSIOLOGY AND NATURAL HISTORY

The treatment of advanced osteolysis of the knee can require technically difficult revision surgery. The key to management of established osteolysis lies in early recognition, before revision of fixed components becomes necessary. An understanding of the natural history of osteolysis facilitates the ability to recognize some of the clinical signs that herald future problems.

The problems of bearing wear and bone resorption essentially represent two steps in the continuum of the disease known as osteolysis. Wear and corrosion result in particulate debris production. Hydrostatic pressure within the joint is thought to pump the particulate debris into and around the periprosthetic interfaces, otherwise known as the effective joint space (2). Submicron particulate debris elicits a cellular immune response ultimately resulting in periprosthetic bone resorbtion known as osteolysis. Particles of metal, bone cement, and polyethylene have been implicated in the development of osteolysis. The most common location for osteolysis in total knee arthroplasty is the tibial metaphysis (3). Femoral and patellar lesions are less common. Ezzet et al. (4) found that the prevalence of osteolysis positively correlates with time in situ. The average time to radiographic appearance of osteolysis in total knees is approximately two and one half to three years [31 months Cadambi (5), and 35 months Peters (3)]. Once established, osteolysis is usually progressive (3). There is no clinical literature specifically examining the rate of lysis progression in total knee arthroplasty (6). As the periprosthetic bone resorbs, the bone stock supporting the implant is destroyed, jeopardizing the strength of the bone and the fixation of the prosthetic components. Prosthesis loosening, fracture, and or periprosthetic fracture can occur (7) These problems, when combined with severely compromised periprosthetic bone stock, can require extremely difficult revision procedures, even to a seasoned veteran of joint revision surgery.

THE CLINICAL PRESENTATION OF OSTEOLYSIS

The clinical problem of osteolysis generally manifests in one of two ways: (i) asymptomatic, radiographically apparent osteolytic lesions with or without advanced bearing wear (Fig. 1) or (ii) symptomatic disease. Recognition of symptoms potentially associated with wear should heighten the suspicion of existing wear and potential for osteolytic disease. There are a variety of symptoms associated with bearing wear and/or osteolysis. Usually, however, the symptoms are related to the presence of wear debris and bearing wear as opposed to the presence of osteolysis per se. The presence of wear debris in the joint can produce a reactive synovitis. Symptoms and signs include joint swelling, mild to moderate discomfort, and/or joint effusion. Rarely, the reaction to the wear debris is so extensive that a large swelling or pseudotumor can form adjacent to the knee (8). The pseudotumor typically contains wear debris, reactive synovium, and synovial fluid. Significant polyethylene wear can lead to pseudolaxity in the involved joint compartment, occasionally creating symptoms of joint instability. As bearing wear reaches the point of complete wear-through, the patello–femoral or femoral–tibial metal-on-metal contact can produce mechanical symptoms such as catching, grinding, and crepitus (8). The resulting metallic debris can manifest as a radiographically visible metal arthrogram. Once the lytic lesions have

(A)   **(B)**

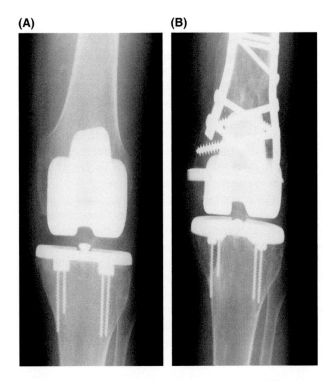

Figure 1 (A) AP view of the knee six weeks following a cementless total knee arthroplasty. (B) AP view of the knee 96 months postarthroplasty and 80 months post-open reduction and internal fixation of a periprosthetic supracondylar femoral fracture. Despite the fact that a large osteolytic lesion is noted in the medial tibial plateau, the patient is asymptomatic.

progressed to the point of significant bone stock loss, loosening and periprosthetic fractures can occur, causing acute pain.

Peters (3), Ezzet (4), and Cadambi have demonstrated that total knee arthroplasties with osteolysis do not have significantly different knee scores as compared to knees without osteolysis (5). In contrast, O'Rourke et al. (9) noted a statistically significant difference in knee society clinical scores when comparing knees with osteolysis to those without osteolysis. There may be an explanation for the difference between these studies. The development of symptoms may be associated with severity of the wear and osteolytic disease process. The following studies have demonstrated that knees with osteolysis are typically symptomatic at the time of revision. Knight et al. reviewed 18 cases with advanced polyethylene wear, with and without lysis, which underwent revision. All of these patients were symptomatic at the time of revision. Symptoms included swelling 89%, stiffness 72%, pain

67%, clicking 38%, and instability 22%. The onset of symptoms proceeded the revision procedure by an average of eight months. The authors did not, however, comment on symptoms in these patients during earlier stages of wear. In a study of knees which underwent revision for loosening and osteolysis, Mikulak et al. (10) noted that 15 of 16 knees were symptomatic with "synovitis" between one month and three years prior to the radiographic appearance of loosening or osteolysis. Lewonowski and Dorr (11) reported on a consecutive case series of 12 knees in 10 patients with osteolysis requiring revision. All but one of the patients were symptomatic with "recent pain." These studies suggest that patients tend to be symptomatic by the time the wear and osteolysis reaches advanced stages.

Routine clinical surveillance via radiographic examination is key to early recognition of asymptomatic bearing surface wear and osteolytic lesions. Wear and corrosion are inherently the first step in the development of osteolysis. One should have a high index of suspicion for the presence of osteolytic lesions if bearing wear is recognized. AP weightbearing (12), lateral, and merchant radiographic views orthogonal to the sagittal and coronal planes of the knee components are a prerequisite to visualization of periprosthetic bone and interfaces where osteolytic lesions manifest. Quantification of volumetric wear in vivo is difficult due to the geometry of the bearing surface and to our knowledge there currently are no precise methods to accomplish this (13). Hoshino et al. (14) described a method for objectively quantifying linear polyethylene wear in total knee arthroplasty based upon plain radiographs with markers. If standard x-rays are of insufficient quality, then selective views can be obtained via fluoroscopy.

A variety of nonradiographic methods have been used to detect the presence of polyethylene wear. Ultrasound has been clinically utilized as a means of detecting polyethylene wear (15). Aspiration and synovial fluid analysis by microscopy using polarized light can demonstrate polyethylene particles (16). This is, however, not necessarily a reliable method for quantifying polyethylene wear (12). Knight et al. (12) reported arthroscopy as a method of directly visualizing polyethylene wear related defects in symptomatic patients. They utilized arthroscopy only when other methods of detection had failed to establish a diagnosis.

Peters et al. (3) proposed criteria for the radiographic identification of osteolytic lesions: a lytic osseous defect that extends beyond the limits of that potentially caused by loosening of the implant alone, absent cancellous trabeculae, and geographically demarcated by a shell of bone. Several studies have determined that radiographic measurements on plain anteroposterior and lateral radiographs tend to underestimate the size of osteolytic defects as verified intra-operatively (11,12,17). Femoral components with boxes and tibial components with stems and/or fins are typically present with posterior-stabilzed prostheses. These prosthetic features can obstruct the visualization of peri-implant bone where osteolytic lesions tend to reside.

Oblique radiographs can facilitate the detection of lytic lesions in the setting of posterior-stabilized components (18). Computed axial tomography has been demonstrated to be more sensitive than plain radiographs for detection of osteolytic lesions associated with total knee arthroplasty. Reish et al. (19) compared plain radiographs to multidetector CT for the evaluation of periprosthetic knee osteolysis. They retrospectively reviewed radiographic studies of 26 knees with known osteolysis by CT scan. Twenty three of the knees in this study were posterior-stabilized designs with femoral boxes and tibial stems. Only 20% of the osteolytic lesions detected by CT scan were visible on plain radiographs. They suggested that CT scan can be useful in detecting osteolysis in the following cases: (i) where there is a strong index of suspicion but radiographs are negative, and (ii) when further definition of the morphology of the lesion could be useful for surgical planning and management.

Early detection of wear and osteolysis will allow for the implementation of a treatment plan before advanced osteolytic lesions have developed. The authors of this chapter advocate yearly clinical and radiographic examination of total knee arthroplasty. In cases where patients have symptoms suggestive of wear related problems (as detailed above) with negative plain radiographs, CT can be employed to evaluate further for osteolytic lesions.

PROPHYLAXIS: ANTICIPATING AND PREVENTING OSTEOLYSIS

The best treatment for osteolysis is prevention. The choice of implant design, material properties, manufacturing methods, and technique at index arthroplasty are all controllable factors that can affect the development of osteolysis in any given patient. The precise design and technical factors associated with development of osteolysis are expounded in the other chapters of this book. A solid knowledge of previous design failures and factors associated with the development of osteolysis is a prerequisite to decreasing the incidence of osteolysis in future patients. Selection of implant design for implantation should ideally involve investigation of the physical properties of that particular design and model knee implant. Some examples include the methods of processing, manufacture, and sterilization of polyethylene bearing surfaces. This technical information is available through company representatives. Physical implant properties do need to be considered in the context of other issues such as the kinematics, technical efficiency of implantation, mode of fixation, and, last but not least, in the context of any available in vivo survivorship studies. If one considers the fact that the vast majority of primary knee arthroplasties are performed by general orthopaedists, then this information is of importance to all orthopaedic surgeons, not just those with specialty training in arthroplasty.

Particular methods of fixation have been associated with a higher incidence of osteolysis. Ezzet et al. (4) examined 83 total knee arthroplasties to determine the effect on fixation method on osteolysis. At mean 51 month follow-up 20.5% of well-fixed knees had osteolysis. All of the osteolytic lesions were around the tibia with the exception of one patellar osteolysis. Knees with cementless femurs and cemented tibias with screw augmentation had a 30% osteolysis rate. Cemented femora with cemented tibiae and screw augmentation had a 13% osteolysis rate. Cementless femurs with cemented tibiae without screws had a 10% osteolysis rate. Knees with cemented femoral and tibial fixation without screws led to 0% osteolysis. Knees with cementless femurs and tibias were not included due to the small number of cases. They concluded that cemented femoral fixation may decrease the risk of osteolysis. Screw augmentation of cemented tibial components was not recommended due to the high osteolysis rate associated with this fixation mode.

Bearing surface wear is a function of the demand placed on the articulating surfaces. To our knowledge there are no clinical studies directly implicating specific activities as a causative factor of accelerated knee bearing wear. It has been demonstrated that osteolysis of the knee is more prevalent in heavy, young, active individuals (20). In a study on autopsy retrieved specimens, Lavernia et al. (21) found that the length of implantation was an important predictor of linear and volumetric wear in total knee arthroplasty. They downplayed the effect of activity level on wear. Clearly, younger patients with total knee arthroplasty are at greatest risk for wear and potential osteolysis. Prior to index arthroplasty, particularly with patients at risk, we recommend a realistic discussion of postarthroplasty activity modifications. The exact modifications imposed are up to the judgement of the surgeon based upon the clinical scenario. We recommend the avoidance of moderate to high impact activities and lifting of heavy objects combined with active knee range of motion. These modifications are reinforced and reviewed during yearly follow-up visits.

Prevention of osteolysis also occurs at the time of the index arthroplasty. Attention to surgical detail is imperative in minimizing the potential for osteolysis. Specific technique-related issues may contribute to development of wear and lysis. Engh (22) and Cadambi (5) addressed the issue of coronal plane malalignment and the presence of osteolysis. Although the results were not statistically significant to confirm a correlation, they did identify a trend. Saggital component orientation can effect the production of osteolysis in certain posterior-stabilized designs. Hyperextension, flexion of the femoral component, and excessive posterior tibial slope are associated with impingement of the anterior flange of the femoral box on the tibial post. This can result in accelerated polyethylene wear and lysis (20). Malrotation of posterior-stabilized components has also been suggested as a potential cause of postcam impingement, lysis, and loosening in posterior stabilized components (23). Another technique-related issue is the presence of retained bone and/or cement particles acting as third body wear debris

(24). Kloen et al. (25) reported third body bone cement particles entrapped in the bearing surface as the cause of polyethylene wear, osteolysis, and tibial loosening in a cemented posterior-stabilized knee design at just over two years postoperatively. Although this may be considered to be an uncommon problem, a separate study evaluating polyethylene wear demonstrated that 46% of 90 retrieved tibial surfaces contain embedded cement particles (26). Inspection and thorough irrigation of the knee joint prior to implantation of the final tibial bearing is one way to minimize the presence of retained cement debris which can act as third body wear particles.

MANAGEMENT OF ESTABLISHED OSTEOLYSIS

In considering the treatment options for this problem there are several issues to consider. First is the temporal relationship between index arthroplasty and onset of osteolysis/wear. Second is the age and activity of the patient. Third is the presence of a specific, identifiable source of wear.

The appearance of osteolysis or accelerated wear of knee components within the first two years of index arthroplasty is uncommon. Presentation of this problem should alert the physician to the possibility of a specific, correctable underlying etiology. Work-up should begin with an assessment of the patients vocational and leisure activities to determine if any consistent, untoward demand is being placed upon the implants. The brand and model of implant should be identified in an attempt to determine if the wear is related to known design or manufacturing issues. Technique-related problems such as gross component malalignment or third body debris particles should be ruled out. If lysis of bone is evident, then an attempt should be made to rule out infection. An erythrocyte sedimentation rate and C-reactive protein should be obtained. Synovial fluid should also be obtained for cell count, Gram stain, and culture.

After initial recognition of significant wear or osteolysis, close clinical monitoring is necessary. Radiographs obtained at 3–6 month intervals can determine the presence of rapid progression of osteolysis and possibly polyethylene wear, although the latter is much more difficult to quantify than in the hip. Objective criteria should be obtained about the rate of progression from radiographic studies. The polyethylene thickness on weight-bearing views can be measured compared to previous radiographs for an objective measurement of polyethylene wear; however, these measurements must be interpreted with caution given that slight changes in radiographic projections can result in substantial differences in apparent polyethylene thickness. McGovern et al. (27) defined accelerated wear as >1 mm/yr. Osteolytic lesions should be objectively measured and also evaluated for expansion/time. Surgical intervention needs to be strongly considered in patients with accelerated wear and osteolysis. Neglect of advanced wear and osteolysis only delays the inevitable need for more difficult surgery.

Patients without significant progression can continue to be observed. This latter group of patients should be counseled about activity modifications and precautions. Patients with symptoms related to debris synovitis can be started on NSAIDS.

Several recent in vitro and in vivo animal studies have shown promise for the use of pharmacological agents in the treatment and prevention of osteolysis. Shanbhag et al. (28) investigated the effect of alendronate on osteolysis in a canine hip arthroplasty model. Alendronate sucessfully inhibited periprosthetic bone loss in the presence of particulate wear debris. Millett et al. (29) examined the potential of bisphosphonates to prevent osteolysis and treat established osteolysis in a well-controlled study using a rat tibial implant model. A treatment group receiving concomitant alendronate and particulate debris experienced decreased bone loss as compared to controls. Alendronate did not completely block the osteolytic bone loss. Specimens with established particle-induced osteolysis were subsequently treated with alendronate. These specimens demonstrated large increases in trabecular bone volume. They concluded that alendronate can work in preventative and therapeutic modes in the treatment of osteolysis. In an in vitro study, administration of etidronate significantly reduced osteoclastic PMMA particle-induced resorption activity (30). Studies examining the effectiveness of bisphosphonates on osteolysis in human subjects are ongoing. Bisphosphonates are currently not FDA approved for the treatment of wear-related osteolysis.

SURGICAL TREATMENT OF OSTEOLYSIS AND WEAR

There are five factors which must be evaluated when considering operative intervention for osteolysis. First is the presence of factors potentially leading to particulate debris production. Examples include known prosthetic material and/or design flaws or technical error such as gross malalignment and retained cement debris. Second is the degree of bearing wear. Third is the amount of bone loss associated with the lysis. Fourth is the activity and age of the patient. Fifth is the rate of osteolysis progression. The rate of progression should be considered with respect to the timing of surgical intervention.

We propose the following indications for surgical intervention: (i) First-time presentation with advanced osteolysis in the presence of an identifiable cause of particle production. (ii) Progressive, radiographically documented osteolysis in an active individual. (iii) Advanced osteolytic lesions of any cause with impending failure of component fixation. (iv) Symptoms of wear-debris related synovitis which are refractory to conservative management. (v) Advanced polyethylene bearing wear in the presence of impending wear-through or related mechanical symptoms. Relative indications include elderly, sedentary individuals with moderate lysis.

The goals of surgery in osteolysis are to reduce particle debris load, restore bone stock where feasible, and revise loose components. Reduction of the particulate debris load involves removal of the sources of particle production. The findings from the preoperative evaluation should be considered in conjunction with intraoperative findings to determine the sources of wear. Exchange of damaged or worn modular polyethylene bearing surfaces is imperative. If evidence of backside wear is present, particularly in association with a poor quality locking mechanism, then revision of the tibial baseplate should be strongly considered. There is a paucity of clinical data on which to base indications for tibial bearing exchange versus revision of fixed components.

Surgical treatment should at the very least include removal of old worn polyethylene and exchange for new polyethylene along with debridement of inflammatory tissue from the joint and intraosseous lesions. Engh et al. (1) published one of the few clinical studies addressing this issue. They reviewed 48 isolated tibial bearing exchanges for advanced wear and/or osteolysis in the presence of otherwise stable components. A 15% failure rate occurred at an average 54 months postrevision as a result of accelerated wear of revised inserts. They concluded that revision total knee arthroplasty is necessary to correct design issues inherent to the fixed components. They recommended avoiding isolated polyethylene exchange if the following factors are present: (i) severe wear within 10 years of total knee arthroplasty, (ii) severe delamination, (iii) full thickness wear-through, or (iv) extensive back-sided polyethylene wear. The presence of metallosis associated with patellar wear-through did not seem to be a contraindication to retention of the femoral and tibial components as long as there was not advanced burnishing of the femoral component. They did acknowledge that the number of cases was small. Gamma irradiation in air was the method of polyethylene sterilization used in both the primary and revision cases in this study. The shelf life of the inserts was not indicated. Four of the revision inserts used were Hylamer-M which has been reported to have poor wear properties (31,32). It is certainly conceivable that inferior polyethylene material properties contributed to the early failure of the revised cases in this study. Two other reports (11,22) have advised revision of tibial and femoral components in symptomatic knees with osteolysis. The evidence on which this advice is based is not substantiated in the text of the articles.

Babis et al. (33) reviewed the outcome of 56 isolated tibial polyethylene insert exchanges for a variety of problems including wear and instability. Twenty-four knees underwent isolated tibial modular bearing exchange for wear. Sixteen of the knees survived at an average of 4.6 years with mean knee society scores of 87 points. Eight of these knees were determined to be failures at a mean of four year follow-up. Three knees developed recurrent wear of polyethylene. The other five knees that were considered failures due to problems, such as pain and stiffness, that were not directly related to tibial polyethylene wear. The authors concurred with Engh et al. and concluded that isolated tibial polyethylene exchange should not be performed within ten 10 years of index surgery.

In contrast, others have shown success with isolated tibial bearing exchange. Dehmukh and Scott (34) reviewed 2000 modular PCL-retaining arthroplasties at an average eight years postindex arthroplasty. Of these knees, 45 underwent isolated tibial insert exchange. These revised knees were the focus of their study. All implants had the same tibial baseplate design and were from the same manufacturer. Eighteen knees had isolated tibial polyethylene insert exchanges for polyethylene wear. Eight of these knees had synovitis and four of the knees had "osteolysis treatment." None of the 18 knees has a reoperation at 1–10 years follow-up. None of the total of 45 knees required re-revision at average five year (range 1–17 year) follow-up. Further details on the clinical knee scores is not readily available at this time. In contrast to the previous two studies, this review suggests that polyethylene bearing insert exchange, without exchange of the femoral and tibial components, can be successful at intermediate follow-up.

It is possible that design-specific differences between the prostheses in these studies can account for the differences in the outcomes with isolated tibial bearing exchange. More data is needed on isolated tibial bearing exchange to determine the efficacy of this procedure. Clearly, implant-related material and design problems need to be ruled out if one is planning retention of the tibial and femoral components. If the underlying problem is a material issue with the tibial polyethylene then bearing exchange with new polyethylene of adequate quality is a reasonable option. When deciding to perform a complete knee revision as opposed to isolated tibial polyethylene exchange one needs to consider the long-term results of total knee arthroplasty revision. The surgeon must also be prepared to manage potentially large bony defects. We recommend proceeding with revision of the tibial and femoral components if there are inherent design flaws in these components that place the bearing at risk for recurrent accelerated wear.

Before surgery, the processing method and shelf life of the in situ polyethylene can sometimes be determined in an effort to reveal wear-related material problems. Intraoperatively, the knee needs to be carefully evaluated for the source/etiology of wear. The tibial insert should be inspected for bearing side, and backside wear independently. The tibial baseplate surface should be evaluated to determine the surface characteristics. Is the baseplate titanium, cobalt–chrome, smooth, polished, or rough? (35). Are scratches or burishing present? What is the quality of the locking mechanism? The bearing and backside surfaces of the polyethylene should be evaluated for the presence and extent of wear. Extensive backside wear may be indicative of material and design flaws. Contraindications to isolated bearing exchange include ability to reinsert only very thin polyethylene, extensive burnishing of the femoral and/or tibial baseplate surfaces, severe backside wear in the absence of a third body cause, no quality polyethylene inserts available, and gross malalignment of components.

Regardless of what components are revised the particulate load in the joint should be reduced in an effort to halt the osteolytic process. An extensive synovectomy will aid in removing particles and active granulomatous inflammatory tissue. Synovectomy can be accomplished efficiently by identifying the plane between the synovium and capsule in the supra-patellar pouch area. A combination of blunt and bovie dissection then easily define the plane as one proceeds distally. Combining bovie cauterizer dissection and a rougeur and/or curettes may be utilized to resect synovium around the tibial baseplate and popliteal recesses if components are retained.

In their review of knees revised for advanced polyethylene wear, Knight et al. (12) noted that knees which did not undergo synovectomy tended to remain symptomatic after revision surgery. They concluded that residual symptoms resulted from failure to remove the particulate debris. Additional benefits noted in patients with debridement were facilitation of exposure and an implied debulking that facilitates recovery of motion postoperatively.

Osteolytic lesions should also be debrided. Simple debridement of periprosthetic osteolytic lesions has been demonstrated to halt the progression of further lysis provided that the particle generator has been removed (32,36). Revision of tibial or femoral components allows open access to osteolytic areas which are easily debrided with a curette. This debridement aids in defining the extent and characteristics of the bony defect. Defining these defects is crucial to planning and performing an appropriate reconstruction. Difficulty arises when there are osteolytic lesions behind well-fixed components. In this setting, the defect usually cannot be directly visualized. Definition of the extent of the defect in these cases may help in determining if adjacent components are at risk for failure or loosening. Lesions can be accessed with instruments such as curettes, probes, etc. Several techniques have been described to gain access to and debride these lesions (37). Cementless tibial components usually have screw holes through which the lesions can be debrided with a small curette. Saline can be used to irrigate the lesions via a large diameter angiocath and syringe. Modification of a standard femoral canal pulse irrigation tip will allow irrigation through larger screw holes. The granulomatous tissue can then be removed with a small kerrison rongeur or a frazier suction tip. Lesions behind well-fixed tibial or femoral components can also be accessed via a small bony window adjacent to the lesion. This is usually required in cemented implants. Access can sometimes be gained at the periphery of the well-fixed component where the lesion communicates with the joint space.

Provided that a thorough debridement of the lytic lesion is performed, bone grafting is not absolutely necessary in the presence of well-fixed components. We recommend grafting lesions associated with stable components where possible without jeopardizing crucial periarticular structures such as ligament and tendon insertions, and where areas of large bone stock loss is present. Studies on the treatment of osteolytic lesions around stable femoral and acetabular components in total hip replacement have demonstrated resolution or no progression of osteolytic lesions roughly three years after treatment with cancellous allograft bone grafting (36,38).

Engh et al. (22) reviewed 25 operations performed in knees for tibial osteolysis at a mean of 41 months follow-up. They classified knees into groups based upon surgical treatment. The decision to graft lesions was made based upon the size of the lesion and the ease of access to the lesion for grafting. In seven knees with tibial polyethylene change, removal of tibial screws, and curettage of lytic lesions, the lytic lesions remained unchanged in size and no new lesions developed. Two knees had polyethylene exchange without debridement of lysis or removal of screws. Lysis progressed in one requiring revision and remained unchanged in the other. Of knees with tibial component revision with curettage of tibial lesions and use of allografting in four patients and autograft in one, there was no new tibial lysis identified. Six of the knees treated with tibial revision had femoral osteolysis. The only femoral lesion treated with debridement progressed. Five femoral lesions were not curetted and remained stable without progression. Five knees underwent complete revision of the tibial and femoral components. 4/5 cases required a structural allograft for the femoral side and 3/5 on the tibial side. No loosening or lucencies developed in this latter group upon follow-up. They concluded that retaining stable components in the presence of osteolysis is effective only if multiple sources of particulate debris are removed. They also stated that incomplete removal of osteolytic debris was acceptable if the particle generators are removed. The study indicated that total knee arthroplasty revision in the setting of osteolysis requires the use of canal filling stems, frequently requires structural allograft use, and is complex and time consuming. Based upon the small numbers of patients in each of the treatment groups of this study, it is impossible to reach reliable conclusions about the efficacy of specific treatment methods for osteolytic lesions. There did, however, appear to be a trend: patients with lysis debridement and bone grafting were less likely to develop progression of bone defects.

Many bone graft options are currently available including allograft, autograft, and bone graft substitutes. To our knowledge, there is no literature addressing optimal graft type in this setting. Currently we are using particulate allograft cancellous bone, which can be packed into the bony defect with a footed impactor and mallet. This graft provides osteoinductive as well as osteoconductive properties, which may aid in consolidation of the defect. In areas where bone graft may dislodge from a cavitary space, the use of a thin bone cement cap or incorporation of bone graft substitutes which provide some cohesive properties has been suggested in the setting of hip osteolysis. These techniques may be useful in areas such as the posterior femoral condyles. We caution against the use of a cement cap, particularly in areas where dependant migration of the cement could result in third body bearing wear.

Stable components can be retained. The decision to retain components that have evidence of scoring/burnishing is one which needs to be made on a case-by-case basis depending on the extent and location of associated bearing wear, and ability to rectify the problem which caused the burnishing in the first place. To our knowledge, there is no outcome data specifically examining the results of revisions in the setting of retained, but damaged bearing or backside surfaces. Engh (37) recommends revision of the femoral components if there is visible damage or scoring palpable with a probe.

When osteolysis accompanies loose components, there are generally large bony deficiencies, which must be addressed at revision surgery. A stable base must be present, onto which revised components can be seated. The classification system proposed by Engh (39) is useful for guiding reconstruction when faced with tibial or femoral bony deficiency. In this classification, there are three basic types of defects. Type I defects involve intact metaphyseal bone with small cavitary defects. Type II defects involve damaged metaphyseal bone requiring prosthesis augmentation with cement, metal, or structural allograft. Type III defects involve segmental loss of metaphyseal areas, which compromise a large area of plateau or condyle and can involve detachment of ligament insertions.

There are a number of methods for managing bony defects associated with osteolysis. The morphology and location of the defect influences the reconstruction options available. Cavitary defects with a stable rim of bone can be managed by impacting cancellous particulate graft into the defect. Bulk allograft can be used to fill cavitary defects. Uncontained defects require the use of prosthetic augmentation with modular metal augments (Fig. 2), or bulk structural allograft. An uncontained defect can be converted to a contained defect with wire mesh. The defect is then filled using impaction grafting. Use of structural allograft should be considered when modular metallic augments available with standard revision knee instrumentation do not provide at least 50% prosthesis–host bone contact.

The most efficient methods of reconstruction with allograft employ techniques where the graft and host bone are contoured to complementary geometric or cylindrical shapes while removing the least amount of viable native bone. The allograft is then secured to the host bone using either k-wires or 3.5 mm screws if the defect is uncontained. The reconstructed bone stock is then cut in situ to match the contour of the fixation side of the implant. Modular stem augments transfer stress from the metaphseal construct to diaphyseal bone. Cemented implants are indicated as biologic in-growth does not occur at the site of allografting. Allograft prosthetic composites can be utilized in reconstruction of massive segmental bone loss

(A)   **(B)**   **(C)**

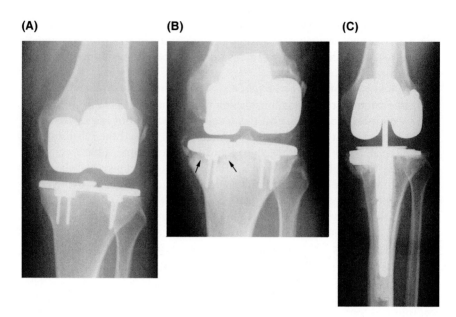

Figure 2 (A) AP view of the knee six months following a cementless total knee arthroplasty. (B) AP view of the knee 127 months postoperatively demonstrating a large area of osteolysis subjacent to the medial aspect of the tibial component (*arrows*) and progressing distally along the fixation screw tracks. Due to the fact that the medial portion of the tibial component was unsupported by the remaining bone, the tibial component sustained a fatigue fracture. (C) AP of the knee two months following revision surgery. The medial tibial defect was addressed by placing a modular medial block augment on the undersurface of the tibial component.

where less than 50% host bone contact is anticipated. This type of reconstruction is preferred in younger individuals. Modular oncology-type prostheses can be used in lieu of allograft prosthetic composites in elderly individuals with large areas of segmental bone loss.

Robinson et al. (17) reviewed the technical challenges involved in 17 total knee arthroplasty revisions performed for severe osteolysis and catastrophic failure. Exposure was difficult and required a rectus snip, v–y quadricepsplasty, tibial tubercle osteotomy, or lateral release in over half of the cases. Both cavitary and noncavitary osteolytic defects were present. Sizes of the bony defects were consistently underestimated by the preoperative radiographs. Bone loss was managed with cement only in 47%, allograft in 30%, and metallic augments in 35%. Thirty percent of the cases required constrained condylar-type devices. They concluded that revision in the setting of advanced osteolysis is technically challenging. Further, they indicated that surgeons attempting this type of surgery should be armed with the knowledge of a variety of revision reconstructive techniques and should have allograft and revision components available.

Lewonowski and Dorr (11) reviewed their pre- and intra-operative experience of 12 consecutive knee revisions in the setting of osteolysis. In this brief technical procedure review they indicated that removal of components always resulted in more bone loss than expected preoperatively. Use of a metal pin was suggested as one method of locating potential areas of lysis. Demineralized cancellous chips and hydroxyapetite granules were used to fill the identified lytic defects. The outcomes of these methods were not discussed in this report.

CONCLUSION

Osteolysis has been only recently recognized in association with total knee arthroplasty. Recognition of symptom patterns associated with osteolysis and new techniques of radiographic evaluation have improved detection of this disease. Early recognition of wear and osteolysis as well as close clinical follow-up is necessary to identify patients who need treatment. New pharmacological modalities hold the potential for prophylaxis or retarding osteolysis progression in its early stages. When lysis has progressed to the point of component failure and/or loosening, then surgical revision offers considerable technical challenges, but is noncontroversial. Management of the patient with osteolysis in modular TKAs without fixed component failure is controversial. There is a relative paucity of literature on the outcome of surgical management in this setting. Numbers of patients tend to be small in individual studies, making statistically valid conclusions about treatment methods difficult to reach. In addition, our knowledge about the design and manufacturing issues associated with osteolysis has brought new factors into consideration which may not have been fully recognized or generally accepted at the time that some of the earlier studies were published. Clearly, more studies on the outcome of various treatment methods of osteolysis are needed to more concretely define indications for selective component revision versus total knee revision.

The answer to the problem of knee related osteolysis truly lies in prevention. The future holds the promise of improved components and bearing surfaces with a low propensity for particulate debris production. In the meantime, careful surgeon selection of implant designs and materials will help to reduce the future incidence of osteolytic and wear-related disease.

REFERENCES

1. Engh GA, Koralewicz LM, Pereles TR. Clinical results of modular polyethylene insert exchange with retention of total knee arthroplasty components. JBJS Am 2000; 82:516–523.

2. Schmalzried TP, Jasty M, Harris WH. Periprosthetic bone loss in total hip arthroplasty: the role of polyethylene wear debris and the concept of the effective joint space. JBJS Am 1992; 74:849.
3. Peters PC Jr, Engh GA, Dwyer KA, Vinh TN. Osteolysis after total knee arthroplasty witout cement. JBJS Am 1992; 74:864–876.
4. Ezzet KA, Garcia R, Barrack RL. Effect of component fixation method on osteolysis in total knee arthroplasty. Clin Orthop 1995; 321:86–91.
5. Cadambi A, Engh GA, Dwyer KA, Vinh TN. Osateolysis of the distal femur after total knee arthroplasty. J Arthroplasty 1994; 9:579–594.
6. Wright TM, Goodman SB. What is the clinical scope of implant wear in the knee and how has it changed since 1995? In: Implant Wear in Total Joint Replacement: Clinical and Biological Issues, Material and Design Considerations. 2001, AAOS.
7. Huang CH, Yang CY, Cheng CK. Case report: Fracture of the femoral component associated with polyethylene wear and osteolysis and after total knee arthroplasty. J Arthroplasty 1999; 14:375–379.
8. Chavda DV, Garvin KL. Failure of a polyethylene total knee component presenting as at high mass. Clin Orthop 1994; 303:211–216.
9. O'Rourke MR, Callaghan JJ, Goetz DD, Sullivan PM, Johnston RC. Osteolysis associated with a cemented modular posterior-cruciate-substituting total knee design. JBJS Am 2002; 84:1362–1371.
10. Mikulak SA, Ormonde MM, Dela Rosa MA, Schmalzried TP. Loosening and osteolysis with the press-fit condular posterior-cruciate-subtituting total knee replacement. JBJS Am 2001; 83:398–403.
11. Lewonowski K, Dorr LD. Revision of cementless total knee arthroplasty with massive osteolytic lesions. J Arthroplasty 1994; 9:6661–6663.
12. Knight JL, Ggorai PA, Atwater RD, Grothaus L. Tibial polyethylene failure after primary porous coated anatomic total knee arthroplasty: Aids to diagnosis and revision. J Arthroplasty 1995; 10(6):748–757.
13. Wright TM, Goodman SB, How should wear-related implant surveillance be carried out and what methods are indicated to diagnose wear-related problems? In: Implant Wear in Total Joint Replacement: Clinical and Biological Issues, Material and Design Considerations. 2001, AAOS.
14. Hoshino A, Fukuoka Y, Ishida A. Accurate in-vivo measurement of polyethylene wear in total knee arthroplasty. J Arthroplasty 2002; 17:490–496.
15. Yashar AA, Adler RS, Grady-Benson JC, Matthews LS, Freiberg AA. An alternative method to evaluate polyethylene component wear in total knee replacement arthroplasty. Am J Orthop 1996; 25:702–704.
16. Kovacik, Osteolytic indicators found in total knee arthroplasty synovial fluid aspirates. CORR 2000; 379;186–194.
17. Robinson EJ, Mulliken BD, Bourne RB, Rorabeck CH, Alvarez C. Catastrophic osteolysis in total knee replacement: A report of 17 cases. Clin Orthop 1995; 321:96–105.
18. Nadaud M, Fehring TK, Fehring K. Use of oblique radiographs in detection of osteolysis in posterior stabilized components. Poster Presentation. AAHKS, Dallas, 2002.

19. Reish TG, Scott WN, Cushner FD, Math K. Osteolysis around total knee arthroplasty diagnosed by multi-detector computed tomography. Presented at AAOS, San Francisco, 2004.

20. O'Rourke MR, Callaghan JJ, Goetz DD, Sullivan PM, Johnston RC. Osteolysis associated with a cemented modular posterior-cruciate-substituting total knee design. JBJS Am 2002; 84:1362–1371.

21. Lavernia CJ, Sierra RJ, Hungerford DS, Krackow K. Activity level and wear in total knee arthroplasty: a study of autopsy retrieved specimens. J Arthroplasty 2001; 16:446–453.

22. Engh GA, Parks NL, Ammeen DJ. Tibial osteolysis in cementless total knee arthroplasty: a review of 25 cases treated with and without tibial revision. CORR 1994; 309:33–43.

23. Mikulak SA, Ormonde MM, Dela Rosa MA, Schmalzried TP. Loosening and osteolysis with the press–fit condular posterior-cruciate-subtituting total knee replacement. JBJS Am 2001; 83:398–403.

24. Helmers S, Sharkey PF, McGuigan FX. Efficacy of irrigation for removal of particulate debris after cemented total knee arthroplasty. J Arthroplasty 1999; 14:549–552.

25. Kloen P, Burke DW, Chew FS, Mildrum R. Radiographic pseudochondrocalcinosis in early failure of a cemented total knee replacement. J Arthroplasty 1998; 13:8.

26. Landy MM, Walker PS. Wear of ultra high mollecular weight polyethylene components of 90 retrieved knee prostheses. J Arthroplasty 1998; 76(suppl):73.

27. McGovern, Ammeen DJ, Collier JP, Currier BH, Engh GA. Rapid polyethylene failure of unicondylar tibial components sterilized with gamma irradiation in air and implanted after long shelf life. JBJS 901–906, 2002:84-A1.

28. Shanbhag AS, Hasselman CT, Rubash HE. Inhibition of wear debris mediated osteolysis in a canine total hip arthroplasty model. Clin Orthop 1997; 344: 33–43.

29. Millett PJ, Allen MJ, Bostrom MP. Effects of alendronate on particle-induced osteolysis in a rat model. JBJS Am 2002; 84:236–249.

30. Sabokbar A, Fujikawa Y, Murray DW, Athanasou NA. Bisphosphonates in bone cement inhibit particle induced bone resorbtion. Ann Rheum Dis 1998; 57:614–618.

31. Ahn NU, Nallamshetty L, Ahn UM, Buchowski JM, Rose PS, Lemma MA, Wenz JF. Case report: early failure associated with the use of hylamer-M spacers in three primary AMK total knee arthroplasties. J Arthroplasty 2001; 16:136–139.

32. Reis MD, Bellare A, Livingston BJ, Cohen RE, Spector M. Early delamination of a hylamer-M tibial insert. J Arthroplasty 1996; 11:974.

33. Babis GC, Trousdale RT, Morrey BF. The effectiveness of isolated tibial insert exchange in revision total knee arthroplasty. JBJS AM 2002; 84:64–68.

34. Dehmukh RV, Scott RD. The incidence and outcome of modular tibial insert exchange in 2000 consecutive primary PCL-retaining knee arthroplasties. Presented at AAOS, New Orleans, 2003.

35. Wasielewski RC, Parks N, Williams I, Surprenant H, Collier JP, Engh GA. Tibial insert undersurface as a contributing source of polyethylene wear debris. Clin Orthop 1997; 345:53–59.

36. Maloney WJ, Herzwurm P, Paprosky W, Rubash HE, Engh CA. Treatment of pelvic osteolysis associated with a stable acetabular component inserted without cement as a part of total hip replacement. JBJS Am 1997; 79:1628–1634.

37. Engh GA, Ammeen DJ. Periprosthetic osteolysis with total knee arthroplasty. AAOS Instr Course Lect 2001; 50:391–398.

38. Benson ER, Christensen CP, Monesmith EA, Gomes SL, Bierbaum BE. Particulate bone grafting of osteolytic lesions around stable cementless stems. Clin Orthop 2000; 381:58–67.

39. Engh GA. Bone defect classification. In: Engh GA, Rorabeck CH, eds. Revision Total Knee Arthroplasty. Baltimore: Williams and Wilkins, 1997:63–120.

23

Advances in Metals

Cheryl R. Blanchard, Dana J. Medlin, and Ravi Shetty

Corporate Research and Clinical Affairs, Zimmer, Inc., Warsaw, Indiana, U.S.A.

INTRODUCTION

Metals have found successful application in the field of orthopaedics as prosthetic and fracture fixation devices because of their biocompatibility, good mechanical properties, sufficient corrosion resistance, and manufacturability at a reasonable cost. The earliest written record of a metal being used as a surgical fixation device was in 1565 when Petronius recommended repairing cleft palates with gold plates (1). In 1666, Fabricius described the use of gold, bronze, and iron wires in studies of tissue tolerance of metals and concluded that platinum was the best tolerated metal (2). Bell tried a variety of materials such as gold, silver, and platinum alloys in dental applications in the early 1800s (2). In 1829, Levert studied the tissue tolerance of a variety of metals and also concluded that platinum was the best tissue compatible metal (1).

Three major developments in the 19th century significantly changed the field of orthopaedic surgery by facilitating surgery, improving patient recovery, and improving surgical techniques (3–6). In 1846, ether was used for the first time to induce anesthesia for the surgical removal of a tumor. In the 1880s, Lister developed antiseptic surgical techniques that reduced postoperative infections. Then, in 1895, Roentgen discovered X-rays that allowed surgeons to use X-ray techniques to view fractures before and after surgery.

In 1912, Sherman, the head of U.S. Steel's Medical Application Department, directed landmark research that resulted in an improved material for bone plates and screws called vanadium steel. This research project was the first biomedical partnership between surgeons and engineers and set a precedent for future medical materials research collaborations (1). Even though the resulting vanadium steel was only utilized for a short period of time because of insufficient corrosion resistance, this pioneering research led to the understanding of corrosion resistance and biocompatibility of metal in the saline environment of the human body. It also revealed that both of these material characteristics can be mutually exclusive. Just because a material is corrosion resistant does not mean that it is biocompatible. For example, copper is a corrosion resistant metal in the saline environment, but it vigorously reacts with tissues and provokes negative reactions in vivo (7).

In 1926, a new metal developed in Germany called 18-8 stainless steel was introduced in the United States. The expeditious and successful application of this material for orthopaedic use was due to its higher strength and improved biocompatibility when compared to vanadium steel. Even though 18-8 stainless steel had improved characteristics compared to vanadium steel, it was still susceptible to pitting corrosion in saline environments. The addition of a small amount of molybdenum to the stainless steel reduced this problem (8), and the resulting 18-8 SMO alloy became a standard implant material for many years (2). During the 1930s and 1940s, American researchers made slight modifications to the 18-8 stainless steel alloy and developed a three number alloy identification system established under the American Iron and Steel Institute as AISI-302, AISI-304, and AISI-316. These alloys are now usually referred to simply as 302, 304, and 316 stainless steel. The work that C.R. Murry and C.G. Fink did found that 302 and 316 stainless steels were the most desirable metals for internal fixation devices (2). Subsequent supporting research from other institutions persuaded the American College of Surgeons in 1946 to endorse 316 stainless steel for surgical implant applications (1).

In the 1930s cast cobalt–chromium–molybdenum alloys (Co–Cr–Mo) were used in dental applications. Their success in the dental field resulted in their eventual use in orthopaedic implants. Cobalt-based alloys are still successfully used for numerous orthopaedic implant components, designs, and applications today.

In 1964, Jergensen (9) discussed research from the 1950s explaining that titanium could be used as a suitable implant material and subsequent research has shown that titanium and titanium alloys are some of the most versatile metals for surgical implants. During the last half of the 20th century, a wide variety of metals and alloys have been developed and used for a variety of orthopaedic implant applications. Table 1 lists the chronology of the clinical use of some of these metals. Except for the vanadium steel developed in 1912 and the nickel-free stainless steel introduced in 2000, none of the other metals listed in Table 1 were developed specifically for medical use. The alloys were initially developed for other industrial applications and later found to be suitable for medical implant use.

Table 1 Chronology of Metal Alloys in Orthopaedic Implant Applications

Alloy	Year	Application	Performance
Vanadium steel	1912	Bone plates	Corrosion problems
18-8 stainless steel	1926	Implant material	Minor pitting issues
18-8 SMO stainless steel	1937	Implant material	Well accepted
Cast Co–Cr–Mo	1927	Dental devices	Well accepted
Cast Co–Cr–Mo	1938	Orthopaedic implants	Well tolerated, adequate strength
302 stainless steel	1938	Bone plates/screws	Corrosion resistant
316 stainless steel	1946	Trauma implants	Improved corrosion resistance and strength
Titanium	1965	Hip implants (England)	Corrosion resistant, osteoconductive
316L stainless steel	1968	Trauma implants	Further improvements in corrosion resistance, strength
MP35N	1972	European hip prostheses	High strength
Ti–6Al–4V	1974	Trauma implants	High strength, biocompatible
Ti–6Al–4V	1976	Hip prostheses	High strength, low modulus
Forged Co–Cr–Mo	1978	Hip prostheses	High fatigue strength
22-13-5 stainless steel REX 734 stainless steel	1981	Hip implants, trauma	High strength, forgeable
Ti–6Al–7Nb	1982	Hip implants	High strength, biocompatible
Cold-forged 316L	1983	Compression hip screw	High strength
Ni-free stainless steel	2000	Implants	Reduced nickel sensitivity
Zirconium (oxidized zirconium)	2001	Joint prostheses	Abrasion resistance

Abbreviation: Co–Cr–Mo, cobalt chromium molybdenum.
Source: From Refs. 3,4.

Today, the most common metals used in orthopaedic implants are Co–Cr–Mo alloys, titanium alloys, and stainless steel alloys. Examples of implants made from each of these materials are shown in Figure 1. The subtle differences in corrosion resistance, biocompatibility, mechanical properties, and manufacturability of each alloy result in the more advantageous utilization of one alloy group over another for specific implant

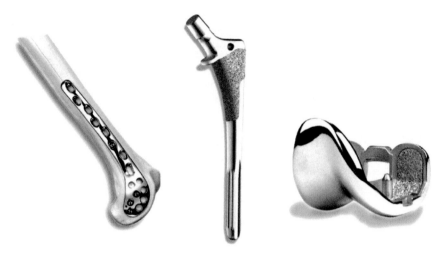

Figure 1   Examples of orthopaedic implants made from stainless steel (distal medial femoral periarticular bone plate), titanium (porous hip stem) and Co–Cr–Mo (knee prosthesis). *Abbreviation*: Co–Cr–Mo, cobalt chromium molybdenum. *Source*: Courtesy of Zimmer Inc., Warsaw, IN.

applications. In addition, the enhancements and improvements proposed with surface coatings and surface treatments of implant materials, as well as the development and application of porous coatings and new implant materials, have increased the need for a more fundamental understanding of materials and processing techniques available and the resulting biomaterial property changes.

METAL MANUFACTURING PROCESSES

Cast Metals

Co–Cr–Mo alloy castings made for orthopaedic implants are manufactured using the investment casting process. Figure 2 shows the sequence of steps required to investment cast implants. Step 1 involves making a wax mold of the engineered implant to be cast, such as a femoral knee component. Usually, hot wax is injected into a mold of the implant and then the mold is chilled to solidify the wax replica into the final shape of the component being cast. The next step is removing the wax replica from the mold and inspecting it for surface defects such as seams and voids (step 2). Next, several of the wax replicas are attached to a wax assembly post or tree by carefully surface melting and welding the replicas onto the tree (step 3). Several wax replicas are attached to one tree so that several cast components can be poured simultaneously. Usually, additional gates and runners are added

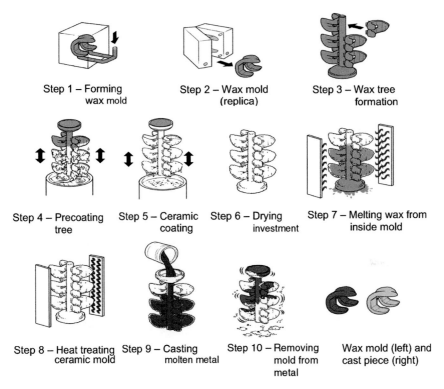

Step 1 – Forming wax mold

Step 2 – Wax mold (replica)

Step 3 – Wax tree formation

Step 4 – Precoating tree

Step 5 – Ceramic coating

Step 6 – Drying investment

Step 7 – Melting wax from inside mold

Step 8 – Heat treating ceramic mold

Step 9 – Casting molten metal

Step 10 – Removing mold from metal

Wax mold (left) and cast piece (right)

Figure 2 Schematic diagram illustrating the investment casting process used to manufacture some orthopaedic implants. The casting of femoral knee components is shown here.

between the wax components and the post to assist with liquid metal flow and gas evacuation during casting. Steps 4 and 5 involve coating the entire wax tree with a wet ceramic slurry layer and then a dry ceramic powder. This process is repeated several times in order to build a thick ceramic mold or investment around the wax tree. The completed ceramic mold is dried (step 6) and then heated to melt the wax from the inside of the ceramic mold (step 7), leaving a hollow shell. The hollow shell is heat treated to high temperatures to cure the ceramic shell, thereby giving it the strength needed for handling and pouring (step 8). Next, the investment mold is preheated to near the melting point of the Co–Cr–Mo alloy, the mold is filled with molten metal (step 9) and then the metal-filled mold is allowed to cool. Finally, the solidified tree is shaken to break the ceramic mold material from the cast metal tree and the parts are cut from the post (step 10). Because the metal components can be cast to a geometry close to the final shape, relatively little machining, grinding, or polishing is required to complete the process. The assembly post, gates, and runners are often recycled during subsequent

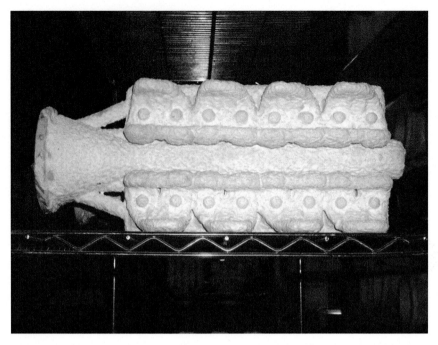

Figure 3 Photograph of an investment mold prepared to cast femoral knee components. *Source*: Courtesy of Zimmer Inc., Warsaw, IN.

casting operations. A photograph of an investment mold of eight femoral knee components is shown in Figure 3.

The microstructures of cast components contain relatively large grains, large interdendritic primary carbides, and metallurgical imperfections that result in lower mechanical properties relative to wrought and forged components. However, properly cast components exhibit the required strength, corrosion properties, and wear resistance for many orthopaedic implant applications including knee implants, endo-prostheses, and low demand hip stems. Figure 4 shows the microstructure of a cast Co–Cr–Mo alloy.

Metallurgical imperfections that remain after casting, such as voids, can be reduced by hot isostatic pressing (HIPing) cast components thus slightly improving some of the mechanical properties. HIPing involves heating the cast components to 900–1200°C and pressurizing the parts in an inert gas environment to 15,000–25,000 psi for several hours to close pores in the parts. Using an inert gas prevents oxidation and hydrostatic gas pressurization provides a uniform surface pressure that will not permanently alter the dimensions of the parts.

Like Co–Cr–Mo alloys, titanium alloys can also be cast using either a rammed graphite mold process or an investment casting process (10).

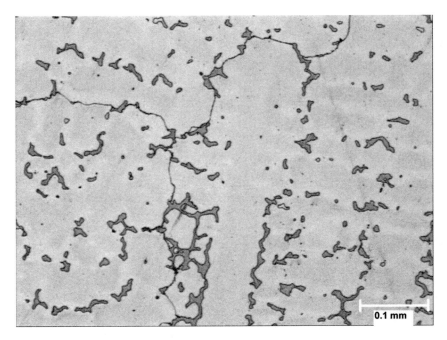

Figure 4 Example of a cast Co–Cr–Mo alloy microstructure. Note the relatively large grains and large interdentritic primary carbides. *Abbreviation*: Co–Cr–Mo, cobalt chromium molybdenum.

The rammed graphite mold process uses graphite powder mixed with suitable organic binders. The mold material is rammed around the pattern and the mold is cured at high temperatures in a reducing atmosphere to convert the organic binders to carbon. The mold that is formed takes the shape of the object, and is used to pour the molten metal into the required shape. The pouring of titanium is usually done in a vacuum to prevent oxidation. Figure 5 shows the cast microstructure of a Ti–6Al–4V alloy.

The titanium investment casting process, on the other hand, uses a method very similar to the investment casting process described for Co–Cr–Mo alloys. The ceramic slurry materials used to make molds for titanium casting must not react with the molten titanium metal. Cast titanium alloys are also HIPed to improve the mechanical properties of the implant. The mechanical properties of cast and HIPed titanium alloys are comparable to wrought and forged titanium alloys.

Wrought Metals

"Wrought" is a metallurgical term that refers generally to thermomechanically processing a metal after casting to improve its mechanical properties by making the microstructure finer and more uniform throughout the cross

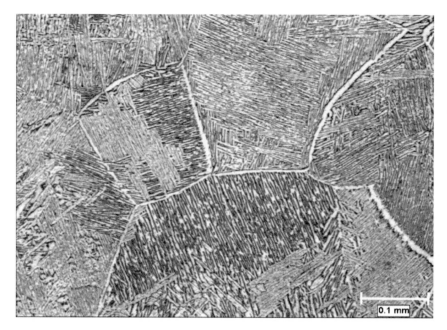

Figure 5   The cast microstructure of a Ti–6Al–4V alloy.

section of a part. As mentioned previously, cast metals have large dendritic microstructures and exhibit alloy segregations that result in relatively lower strength and ductility. Reheating a metal and hot working by repeated rolling or forging, or by using other mechanical means to achieve progressively smaller thicknesses, homogenizes chemical and microstructural segregations and refines the microstructure. This results in metal alloys with improved strength and ductility when compared to cast metals.

When large-scale heats or batches of metal are melted (up to 10,000 pounds), they are cast into rectangular molds called ingots. The ingots are reheated to homogenize the solidification segregation and then hot rolled to reduce the diameter. Round and square bars of various diameters can be produced in a rolling mill. The repeated rolling operations sequentially reduce the bar thickness, reduce chemical segregation, and refine the grain size of the bar stock, as shown in Figure 6. When the rolling operations are performed at temperatures above the recrystallization temperature of the alloy, the process is called hot rolling and when the rolling reductions are performed below the recrystallization temperature of the alloy, the process is called cold rolling.

Wrought metal alloys are machined into final shapes using a variety of machining processes. An example of an implant being machined on a high speed, five-axis mill is shown in Figure 7.

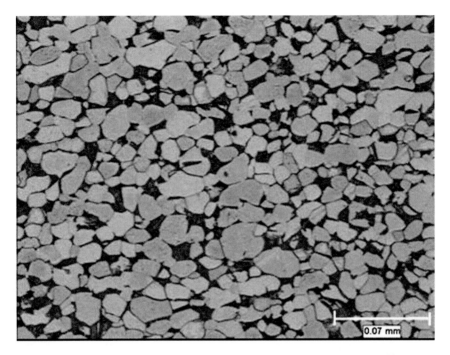

Figure 6 The microstructure of a wrought Ti–6Al–4V alloy. Note the smaller, more uniform grain size and chemistry.

Forged Metals

Forging involves the gradual (sequential) shaping of a cast or wrought blank into a final shape by successive dynamic compression impacts between mating dies in a press. A series of three or more die sets may be used, with the first die set being of a rough shape and the last die set being of a final component shape. Figure 8 shows a schematic diagram of the sequential steps used in forging a hip stem. The metal used for forging is usually a wrought blank. It is heated to a temperature high enough to make the metal flow under dynamic load. This improves the microstructure, and extends the forging die life. With proper temperature and strain control during forging, the grain size and chemical segregation may be further reduced when compared to the original wrought metal. In most manufacturing environments, machining a component from wrought bar stock is usually more economical than forging a component. However, when large volumes of parts are forged and the processes are carefully controlled, forging can be more economical. In designs where relatively high mechanical properties are required, implant performance issues usually dictate the need for forging.

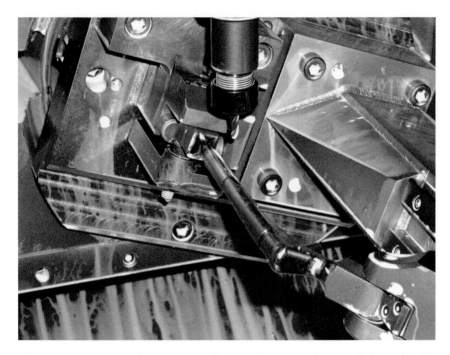

Figure 7 Photograph of a hip stem being machined on a high speed, five-axis mill. *Source*: Courtesy of Zimmer Inc., Warsaw, IN.

Ambient temperature forging can also be used to form metal components. This is referred to as cold working. Cold working can substantially increase the yield and ultimate tensile strengths of a metal, but it will decrease the ductility of the metal. With careful process control, cold working will also increase the fatigue performance of a cold forged component; however, there are limitations to this benefit that must be clearly understood when utilizing this processing technique.

COBALT–CHROMIUM ALLOYS

Many of the present-day commercial cobalt-based alloys were derived from cobalt–chromium–tungsten and cobalt–chromium–molybdenum ternary systems first investigated by Elwood Haynes in the early 1900s (11). Haynes named them Stellite alloys after the Latin word *stella*, for star, because of their star-like luster. He discovered that these alloys had outstanding wear resistance, corrosion resistance, and high temperature mechanical properties (of little use in medical devices). These alloys have been widely used in harsh industrial applications such as drill bits, trimming dies, oil drilling

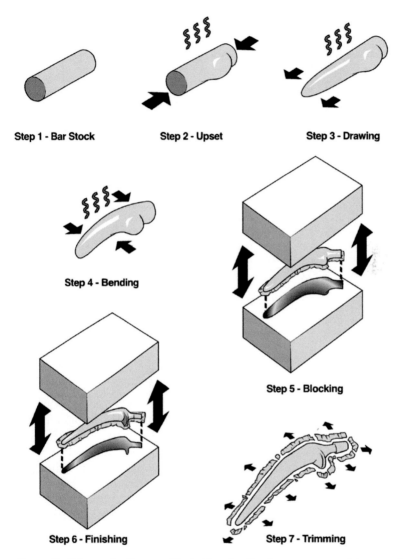

Figure 8 Schematic diagram illustrating the forging process used to manufacture some hip stems.

equipment, engine valves and seats, and industrial turbines. Some of these alloys were used for dental implants due to their high strength, corrosion resistance, wear resistance, and biocompatibility. Their success in the dental field eventually led to their use in orthopaedic implants (11).

The beneficial properties of these alloys arise from the crystallographic nature of cobalt, the solid solution strengthening effects of chromium,

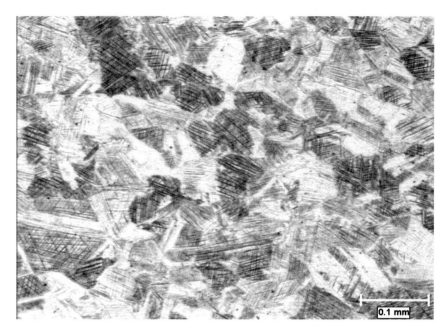

Figure 9 The microstructure of a forged Co–Cr–Mo alloy.

tungsten, and molybdenum, the formation of hard alloy carbides in the microstructure, and the corrosion resistance imparted by chromium and molybdenum. Figure 9 shows a typical microstructure of a forged, high-carbon, Co–Cr–Mo alloy. Chromium forms a passive surface oxide (Cr_2O_3) film that is chemically resistant to a variety of environments, including the saline environment of the human body. The crystal structure of these alloys allows significant strain hardening to occur during some fabrication techniques, such as machining. Interestingly, this very property initially made machining and other fabrication techniques difficult and inefficient on these alloys. However, over the years, specialized machining techniques have been developed that have greatly simplified the manufacture of cobalt-based alloys.

Table 2 lists the typical compositions of some present-day cobalt-based alloys used for medical implant applications. The most popular cobalt alloys for orthopaedic implant use are F-75 (castings), F-799 (forgings), and F-1537 (wrought). All three of these cobalt-based alloys are derived from the same basic chemistry family with slight alloy modifications that are chosen depending upon the final application. However, some of the other cobalt alloys with higher nickel contents, such as MP35N, have not been widely used as implants due to potential nickel sensitivity or toxicity concerns.

Table 2 Nominal Compositions of Cobalt-Based Alloys for Orthopaedic Implant Applications[a]

Designation	ASTM F-75	ASTM F-799	ASTM F-1537	ASTM F-90	ASTM F-562	ASTM F-563
Designation	ISO 5832-4		ISO 1532-12	ISO 5832-5	ISO 5832-6	ISO 5832-8
Trade names	Haynes Stellite-21	Haynes Stellite-21	Haynes Stellite-21	Haynes Stellite-25 L605	MP35N	—
Alloy group and condition	Co–Cr–Mo Castings	Co–Cr–Mo Forgings	Co–Cr–Mo Wrought	Co–Cr–W–Ni Wrought	Co–Ni–Cr–Mo Wrought	Co–Ni–Cr–Mo–W–Fe Wrought
Cobalt	Balance	Balance	Balance	Balance	Balance	Balance
Chromium	27.00–30.00	26.00–30.00	26.00–30.00	19.00–21.00	19.00–21.00	18.00–22.00
Molybdenum	5.00–7.00	5.00–7.00	5.00–7.00	—	9.00–10.50	3.00–4.00
Tungsten	0.20 max	—	—	14.00–16.00	—	3.00–4.00
Carbon	0.35 max	0.35 max	0.35 max	0.05–0.15	0.025 max	0.05 max
Nickel	1.00 max	1.00 max	1.00 max	9.00–11.00	33.00–37.00	15.00–25.00
Iron	0.75 max	0.75 max	0.75 max	3.00 max	1.00 max	4.00–6.00
Silicon	1.00 max	1.00 max	1.00 max	0.40 max	0.15 max	0.5 max
Manganese	1.00 max	1.00 max	1.00 max	1.00–2.00	0.15 max	1.00 max
Nitrogen	0.25 max	0.25 max	0.25 max	—	—	—
Sulfur	0.01 max	—	—	0.03 max	0.01 max	0.01 max
Titanium	—	—	—	—	1.00 max	0.50–3.50
Phosphorus	0.02 max	—	—	0.04 max	0.015 max	—

[a]Values in weight percent.
Source: From Ref. 38.

TITANIUM AND TITANIUM ALLOYS

Commercially pure (CP) titanium and titanium alloys are relatively new materials for orthopaedic applications compared to stainless steels and cobalt-based alloys. Titanium was discovered in 1791 by William Gregor, but was considered mostly a laboratory curiosity until W.J. Kroll invented a process to extract titanium from titanium ore in 1932 (12). During the 1950s, the use of titanium alloys grew substantially in the developing aerospace industry due to their attractive physical, mechanical, and chemical properties. A tremendous amount of government funded research for military aerospace applications developed a large database of mechanical properties on many titanium alloys, including Ti–6Al–4V. In the 1970s, to address the desire for a lower stiffness alloy and improved fatigue strength over cast Co–Cr, the large-scale use of titanium alloys in orthopaedics began in the United Kingdom in hip stems (13).

Ti–6Al–4V has predominately a hexagonal close-packed (HCP) crystal structure at room temperature and transforms to a body-centered cubic (BCC) crystal structure when heated above the phase transformation temperature of 883°C. Upon cooling, the titanium returns to an HCP crystal structure below the transformation temperature. The HCP structure is called the alpha (α) titanium phase and the BCC structure is called the beta (β) titanium phase.

Alloying elements change the transformation temperature depending upon their ability to be alpha stabilizers or beta stabilizers. Alpha stabilizers, such as aluminum, oxygen, carbon, and nitrogen, increase the temperature range at which the alpha phase is stable. Alternatively, beta stabilizers, such as vanadium, molybdenum, chromium, tantalum, hydrogen, and copper, result in stability of the beta phase at lower temperatures. The amount and type of alloying elements determine the phase structure retained at ambient temperatures. Ti–6Al–4V is the most widely used titanium alloy in the aerospace industry due to its combination of properties, manufacturability, and processing costs. Because aluminum and vanadium are the primary alloying elements, this alloy is referred to as an alpha/beta alloy. With most heat treatments, this alloy is predominantly alpha phase with small amounts of beta phase at ambient temperatures. By adding more beta stabilizing elements to the alloy, the microstructure can be beta phase at ambient temperatures. These titanium alloys are referred to as beta (β) alloys.

Because of the successful application of Ti–6Al–4V in aerospace applications, a large amount of research data was available for engineers in the orthopaedic industry to use for considering this alloy as an implant material. Initially, the strength-to-weight ratio made this material very appealing. However, their outstanding corrosion resistance, biocompatibility, and lower modulus of elasticity compared to other metals quickly made titanium alloys one of the primary implant metals. The outstanding corrosion

Table 3 Nominal Compositions of Titanium-Based Alloys for Orthopaedic Implant Applications[a]

Designation	ASTM F-67	ASTM F-136	ASTM F-1108	ASTM F-1295	ASTM F-1713
Designation Alloy group and condition	ISO 5832-2 CP titanium Wrought, Grade 1	ISO 5832-3 Ti-6Al-4V ELI Wrought	– Ti-6Al-4V Casting	ISO 5832-11 Ti-6Al-7Nb	– Ti-13Nb-13Zr Wrought
Titanium	Balance	Balance	Balance	Balance	Balance
Aluminum	–	5.50–6.50	5.50–6.75	5.50–6.50	–
Vanadium	–	3.50–4.50	3.50–4.50	–	–
Niobium	–	–	–	6.50–7.50	12.50–14.00
Oxygen	0.18 max	0.13 max	0.20 max	0.20 max	0.15 max
Nitrogen	0.03 max	0.05 max	0.05 max	0.05 max	0.05 max
Carbon	0.08 max	0.08 max	0.10 max	0.08 max	0.08 max
Hydrogen	0.015 max	0.012 max	0.015 max	0.009 max	0.012 max
Iron	0.20 max	0.25 max	0.30 max	0.25 max	0.25 max
Tantalum	–	–	–	0.50 max	–
Zirconium	–	–	–	–	12.50–14.00

[a]Values in weight percent.
Source: From Ref. 38.

resistance of titanium alloys is attributed to the formation, under ambient conditions, of a thin, adherent, surface oxide film (TiO_2) that is chemically resistant, especially to saline environments. This is often referred to as a passive oxide film or passive layer.

Table 3 lists the compositions of some common titanium-based alloys used in medical implant applications. Commercially pure titanium (ASTM F-67) has the highest corrosion resistance when compared to other titanium alloys. Commercially pure titanium is available in four grades (grades 1–4) representing varying levels of oxygen, iron, and nitrogen. Small increases in the oxygen, iron, and nitrogen content increase the strength and decrease the ductility, respectively. Ti–6Al–4V-ELI (ASTM F-136) is another common titanium alloy used for implant applications in which the interstitial elements (hydrogen, carbon, nitrogen, and oxygen) are reduced to improve stress corrosion properties when compared to standard Ti–6Al–4V. Commercially pure titanium and the Ti–6Al–4V alloys can be used in the cast, wrought, or forged process condition. However, maintaining the extra low interstitial contents in Ti–6Al–4V–ELI makes this particular alloy difficult to cast. More recently, beta-titanium alloys have been successfully used as implant materials (14). Two examples of beta-titanium alloys are Ti–15Mo (ASTM F-2066) and Ti–13Nb–13Zr (ASTM F-1713).

STAINLESS STEEL ALLOYS

Stainless steel alloys are classified into three general groups: ferritic, martensitic, and austenitic. Ferritic and martensitic stainless steels have magnetic properties that make them unsuitable as implantable materials due to the use of magnetic imaging techniques. However, adding high amounts of nickel (>10%) stabilizes the face-centered cubic (FCC) microstructure of austenite at ambient temperatures, resulting in a nonmagnetic alloy. Manganese, carbon, and nitrogen also stabilize the austenite phase, but to a lesser degree than nickel. Molybdenum is also added to enhance the pitting corrosion resistance in acidic and saline environments. The addition of more than 12% chromium gives the alloy corrosion resistance due to the formation of a thin, chromium oxide layer on the surface of the metal, similar to the passive layer formed on cobalt-based alloys. Maintaining chromium as a solid solution in the alloy matrix and not forming chromium carbides or nitrides is important for proper corrosion resistance. Improper heat treating or welding can cause the formation of detrimental carbides and nitrides and decrease the free chromium available for chromium oxide formation to passivate the surface of the steel.

Table 4 lists the chemical compositions of several common stainless steels used in orthopaedic implant applications. One of the more historical implant alloys is 316L stainless steel, where the "L" signifies an extra low carbon content in the alloy to prevent the formation of detrimental

Table 4 Nominal Compositions of Stainless Steels for Orthopaedic Implant Applications[a]

Designation	ASTM F-138	ASTM F-621	ASTM F-1314	ASTM F-1314	ASTM F-1586	ASTM F-621
Designation	ISO 5832-2	ISO 5832-3	—	ISO 5832-11	ISO 5832-9	—
Alloy group and condition	316L S.S Wrought	316L S.S. Forging	22–13–5 S.S. Wrought	22–13–5 S.S. Forging	REX 734 Wrought	REX 734 Forging
Iron	Balance	Balance	Balance	Balance	Balance	Balance
Chromium	17.00–19.00	17.00–19.00	20.50–23.50	20.50–23.50	19.50–22.00	19.50–22.00
Nickel	13.00–15.00	13.00–15.00	11.50–13.50	11.50–13.50	9.00–11.00	9.00–11.00
Molybdenum	2.25–3.00	2.25–3.00	2.00–3.00	2.00–3.00	2.00–3.00	2.00–3.00
Manganese	2.00 max	2.00 max	4.00–6.00	4.00–6.00	2.00–4.25	2.00–4.25
Silicon	0.75 max	0.75 max	0.75 max	0.75 max	0.75 max	0.75 max
Copper	0.50 max	0.50 max	0.50 max	0.50 max	0.25 max	0.25 max
Carbon	0.030 max	0.030 max	0.030 max	0.030 max	0.08 max	0.08 max
Nitrogen	0.10 max	0.10 max	0.20–0.40	0.20–0.40	0.25–0.50	0.25–0.50
Sulfur	0.010 max	0.010 max	0.010 max	0.010 max	0.010 max	0.010 max
Phosphorous	0.025 max	0.025 max	0.025 max	0.025 max	0.025 max	0.025 max
Niobium	—	—	0.10–0.30	0.10–0.30	0.25–0.80	0.25–0.80
Vanadium	—	—	0.10–0.30	0.10–0.30	—	—

[a]Values in weight percent.
Source: From Ref. 38.

chromium carbides during processing. This alloy has an excellent history as an implant material and is inexpensive when compared to the other implantable alloys. Another common stainless steel developed more recently is 22Cr–13Ni–5Mn, which has higher strengths while maintaining good ductility when compared to 316L. The higher strengths are attributed to higher alloy contents of chromium and manganese and additional elements like nitrogen, niobium, and vanadium. This alloy has lower nickel contents, but the austenite phase stability is maintained by increased nitrogen and manganese contents. Another stainless steel developed in Europe is REX-734, which has alloy contents and mechanical properties very similar to 22Cr–13Ni–5Mn.

Stainless steels are generally used in the wrought or forged condition. Wrought processed stainless steel has a uniform microstructure with fine grains, as shown in Figure 10. In the annealed condition, stainless steel has relatively low-mechanical strength and high ductility; however, the strength can be increased by cold working. The FCC structure of austenite work hardens easily and results in substantial increases in strength and fatigue performance with moderate decreases in ductility. Austenitic stainless steels can be hot forged into appropriate shapes rather easily due to the high ductility in the annealed condition. They can also be formed by cold

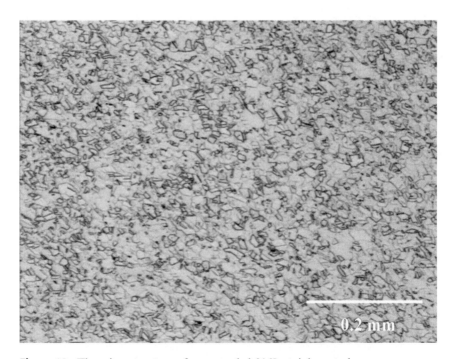

Figure 10 The microstructure of an annealed 316L stainless steel.

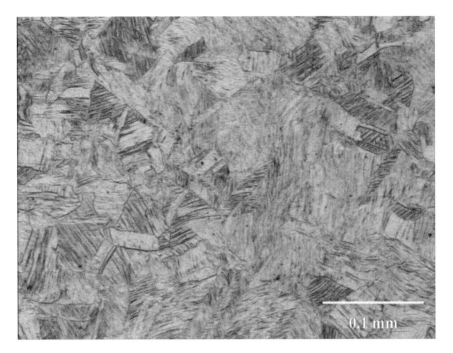

Figure 11   The microstructure of a cold worked 22-13-5 stainless steel.

working (forging) into appropriate shapes, which results in improved mechanical properties. Figure 11 shows a typical microstructure of a cold worked 22Cr–13Ni–5Mn stainless steel alloy.

In the United States and in many Asian markets, the use of stainless steel for joint replacement applications (primarily hip and knee joint prostheses) has decreased to a very low level. The reasons for this are primarily based on business and cost factors and clinical philosophies. The use of stainless steel, especially for hip implants, in Europe and particularly in the United Kingdom, has remained a popular option for surgeons in the more cost sensitive markets. The less cost sensitive markets have tended to shift towards more modern titanium and cobalt-based alloys as technologies and clinical philosophies have developed over the years.

MECHANICAL PROPERTIES

Some of the material properties of a cobalt-based (F-799) alloy are compared with a titanium alloy (Ti–6Al–4V–ELI) and a common implantable stainless steel (316L) in Table 5. The modulus of elasticity (Young's modulus) and the density of the three alloys are of interest. The density of titanium is almost half the density of Co–Cr–Mo and stainless steel.

Table 5 Material Properties for Typical Orthopaedic Implant Metals

Property	Stainless steel (316L)	Titanium (Ti–6Al–4V–ELI)	Co–Cr–Mo (F-1537)
Density (g/cc)	8.00	4.40	8.34
Young's modulus (GPa)	205	110	240
Shear modulus (GPa)	80	43	93
Poisson's ratio	0.27	0.31	0.30
Thermal exp. coeff. (1/°C)	16.8×10^{-6}	8.5×10^{-6}	14.0×10^{-6}

Source: From Ref. 38.

Also, the modulus of elasticity of Co–Cr–Mo and stainless steel are both over 200 GPa, while the elastic modulus of titanium is almost half, at 110 GPa. This means that under the same applied load, titanium will elastically deflect twice as much as Co–Cr–Mo alloys and stainless steel alloys. This could be significant in implant applications that require very rigid fixation or in applications where stress shielding or bone remodeling is a concern.

The mechanical properties of several cobalt-based alloys are shown in Table 6. It is important to compare the properties between the cast (ASTM F-75) alloy and the forged (ASTM F-799) alloy, specifically noting the increase in both strength and ductility of the forged alloy. These properties clearly show the advantage of forging a component when compared to casting. The wrought alloys (ASTM F-90 and F-562) in the annealed condition have relatively low strength and fatigue properties, but ductilities of over 50%. Cold working these alloys will substantially improve their strength and fatigue properties, but decrease the ductility to levels similar to the cast and forged alloys. The ability to obtain a variety of strength and fatigue levels by cold working makes these alloys suitable for numerous implant applications and processing techniques.

The mechanical properties of commercially pure titanium and several titanium alloys are shown in Table 7. As a group, the strength and fatigue properties of the titanium alloys are lower when compared to the cobalt-based alloys. Commercially pure titanium (ASTM F-67) has four grades depending upon the interstitial purity. Grade 1 has the lowest interstitial content (particularly oxygen) and has the lowest mechanical properties when compared to Grade 4. The most commonly used titanium alloy for implants is wrought Ti–6Al–4V-ELI (ASTM F-136) due to its extensive use in the aerospace industry and thus availability. The designation of "ELI" refers to "extra low interstitials" and by controlling the amounts of carbon, oxygen, and hydrogen to low levels, improvements in properties can be achieved. The extensive use of this alloy is due to its outstanding

Table 6 Mechanical Properties of Cobalt-Based Alloys for Orthopaedic Implant Applications

Alloy condition	Hardness	Fatigue limit[a] (MPa)	Tensile properties[b]		
			YS (MPa)	UTS (MPa)	% Elongation
ASTM F-75 (cast)	R_C 25-35	275	515	725	10
ASTM F-799 (forged)	R_C 37-44	760	895	1240	14
ASTM F-90 (wrought/ annealed)	R_C 20-25[c]	205	455	960	60
Annealed + 10% CW	–	315	710	1015	44
Annealed + 15% CW	–	380	840	1090	28
Annealed + 20% CW	–	425	950	1200	18
ASTM F-562 (wrought/ annealed)	R_B 90-100	185	415	930	70
Annealed + 40% CW + aged	R_C 40-45	745	1655	1860	10

[a]Typical experimental values (MPa) determined at 10^7 cycles and $R = -1$.
[b]Typical experimental values.
[c]Higher values may be obtained by cold working.
Source: From Refs. 38,39.

combination of mechanical properties, manufacturability, biocompatibility, corrosion resistance, and availability. Ti–6Al–4V can also be used in the cast condition (ASTM F-1108); however, the ductility, strength, and fatigue properties are lower compared to its wrought counterpart.

The last three alloys listed in Table 7 are considered beta-titanium alloys. The mechanical properties of these three alloys are similar to the wrought Ti–6Al–4V alloys; however, the elastic modulus of the beta alloys is slightly lower than the modulus of the alpha and alpha–beta alloys.

The mechanical properties of stainless steel alloys are shown in Table 8. As a group, the properties are between the titanium and cobalt alloys. As discussed earlier, the stainless steel alloy 316L (ASTM F-138 and F-139) has successfully been used as an implant alloy for decades. Similar to the cobalt alloys, this alloy can be cold worked to substantially increase the strength and fatigue performance, however, the ductility decreases dramatically. Another stainless steel alloy with an excellent history as an implant

Table 7 Mechanical Properties of Titanium Alloys for Orthopaedic Implant Applications

Alloy condition	Hardness	Fatigue limit[a] (MPa)	Tensile properties[b]		
			YS (MPa)	UTS (MPa)	% Elongation
ASTM F-67 grade-1 (CP-Titanium)	R_B 70–85	125	170	240	10
ASTM F-67 grade-4 (CP-Titanium)	R_C 20–28	340	480	550	14
ASTM F-136 (Ti–6Al–4V–ELI) wrought	R_C 30–35	550	825	895	15
ASTM F-1108 (Ti–6Al–4V) cast	R_C 30–35	485	760	825	10
ASTM F-1295 (Ti–6Al–7Nb) wrought	R_C 30–35	550	825	895	15
ASTM F-2066 (Ti–15Mo) wrought	R_C 25–30	–	480	690	20
ASTM F-1713 (Ti–13Nb–13Zr) wrought aged	R_C 30–35	–	725	860	10

[a]Typical experimental values (MPa) determined at 10^7 cycles and $R = -1$.
[b]Typical experimental values.
Source: From Refs. 38,39.

material is 22Cr–13Ni–5Mn (ASTM F-1314). This alloy exhibits slightly improved corrosion resistance when compared to 316L and higher strength and fatigue performance. Just like 316L, this alloy can also be strengthened by cold working to relatively high values. The REX-734 alloy (ASTM F-1586) has mechanical properties and corrosion resistance very similar to 22Cr–13Ni–5Mn.

MECHANICAL INTEGRITY OF IMPLANTS—MATERIALS AND DESIGN ELEMENTS

Orthopaedic implants are engineered components that are subjected to repetitive loading and sometimes high loading scenarios in vivo. In order to

Table 8 Mechanical Properties of Stainless Steel Alloys for Orthopaedic Implant Applications

Alloy condition	Hardness	Fatigue limit[a] (MPa)	Tensile properties[b]		
			YS (MPa)	UTS (MPa)	% Elongation
ASTM F-138, F-139 (316L annealed) wrought	R_B 75-100	180	240	550	50
ASTM F-138, F-139 (316L 60% CW) wrought	R_C 30-5	450	1000	1240	12
ASTM F-1314 (Fe–22Cr–13Ni–5Mn) annealed–wrought	R_C 25-30z	380	760	965	35
ASTM F-1314 (Fe–22Cr–13Ni–5Mn) 60% CW–wrought	R_C 35-40	670	1480	1585	9
ASTM F-1586 (REX 734 annealed) wrought	R_C 25-30	380	760	965	35

[a]Typical experimental values (MPa) determined at 10^7 cycles and $R = -1$.
[b]Typical experimental values.
Source: From Refs. 38,39.

design implants that can provide useful lifetimes, engineers must consider both material and design elements. The design of a new orthopaedic implant involves the use of a number of engineering tools and processes including finite element analysis, kinematic analysis, and extensive biomechanical, wear and fatigue testing of both materials and implants. As the clinical and engineering science of orthopaedics has evolved over the last few decades, both materials and designs have improved, along with better operative techniques, to provide implants with improved mechanical integrity and clinical outcomes (15,16).

Historically, in the 1960s cast or annealed stainless steel or cast Co–Cr–Mo alloy was used for hip hemi-arthroplasty (17). The most common implants included the Thompson and Austin–Moore prostheses. Over time, many of these hip stems loosened because of inadequate fixation of the stem to the bone. In order to overcome this problem, Charnley, in 1970, used acrylic cement to fix the hip stem into the bone (18). Since then, the clinical practice of total hip arthroplasty has been revolutionized and become what is considered to be a very successful surgery for most patients. In the 1970s cast Co–Cr–Mo alloy and cold worked 316L stainless steel were primarily used for hip stem applications. These materials possess higher fatigue strengths when compared to the cast or annealed stainless steels used previously. The incidence of fatigue fracture of hip stems has been significantly reduced because of the use of these materials. In the 1980s the high-strength Ti–6Al–4V alloy and Co–Cr–Mo alloy forgings appeared in the market. These materials possess higher fatigue strengths than the cold worked 316L stainless steel and cast Co–Cr–Mo alloy. These alloy developments provided engineers and surgeons an enabling tool to design hip stems with increased mechanical integrity. Because of these material developments, hip stem fractures are very rarely seen in modern hip implants. Similar developments have also been taking place in the material selection and design of other implants such as femoral heads, acetabular components, knee prostheses, and fracture fixation devices.

POROUS COATINGS FOR BONE INGROWTH

Total joint arthroplasty devices have traditionally been implanted using bone cement (polymethylmethacrylate or PMMA) for fixation. This type of fixation is primarily mechanical in nature. Specifically, the bone cement is pressurized into the interstices of the cancellous bone and subsequently interdigitated into small surface irregularities on the implant. The cement acts as a grout to fix the implant and provide mechanical stability. The failure of the implant–bone cement interface resulting in loosening is a potential issue in some cemented implants. Therefore, porous coated implants (19) offer the promise for mitigating bone–cement interface loosening issues. Porous coated devices provide implant fixation via bone in-growth into or on-growth onto the implant surface (20). Four types of porous coatings have been used commercially for the last two decades: diffusion bonded titanium or Co–Cr–Mo fiber metal, sintered titanium, plasma sprayed titanium, and titanium or Co–Cr–Mo beads.

Fiber Metal Coatings

Fiber metal porous coatings are made by compacting and diffusion bonding randomly oriented CP titanium or Co–Cr–Mo wires. The porous fiber metal pad formed is placed in intimate contact with the surface of the device to be coated. The combination of pressure, elevated temperature, and time at temperature allows solid-state diffusion to occur and form strong metallurgical bonds between the wires both in the fiber metal pad and between the pad

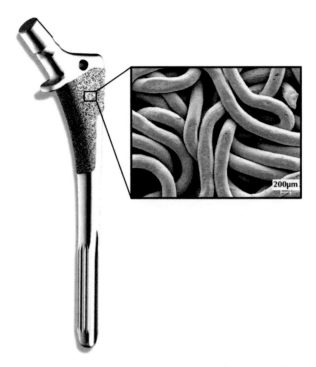

Figure 12 Porous titanium hip stem with a titanium fiber metal coating. Inset shows the microstructure of the fiber metal coating. *Source*: Courtesy of Zimmer Inc., Warsaw, IN.

and the implant surface. The fiber metal coating contains interconnected, randomly oriented pores and is approximately 40–50% porous with a mean pore size of approximately 300 μm. The fiber metal porous coated devices may be either titanium alloy or cobalt alloy. A typical titanium fiber metal coating is shown in Figure 12 on a porous coated titanium hip stem.

Bead Coatings

Porous bead coatings of titanium and Co–Cr–Mo alloys are manufactured by attaching multiple layers of beads to a metallic substrate using a suitable binder and subjecting this composite structure to temperatures that are 90–95% of the melting point of the substrate alloy. At these temperatures, the binder is vaporized and the beads become sintered to each other and to the substrate. CP titanium beads are generally used for bead coated titanium alloy implants while Co–Cr–Mo beads are used for beaded Co–Cr–Mo alloy implants. The highly interconnected pores created during the process are engineered to produce a pore size ranging from 100 to 1000 μm, a pore volume of approximately 40–50% of the total coating

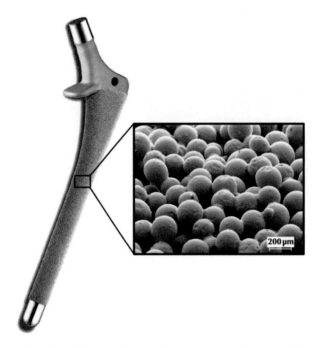

Figure 13 Porous Co–Cr–Mo hip stem with a Co–Cr–Mo beaded metal coating. Inset shows the microstructure of the bead coating. *Abbreviation*: Co–Cr–Mo, cobalt chromium molybdenum. *Source*: Courtesy of Zimmer Inc., Warsaw, IN.

volume and a thickness ranging from 500 to 1,500 μm depending on the device and the manufacturer. A typical Co–Cr–Mo bead coating is shown in Figure 13 on a porous coated Co–Cr–Mo hip stem.

Plasma Spray Coatings

Plasma spray coatings are created by ionizing a gas using an electric arc and transforming that gas into a high temperature plasma. When a metallic powder is blown through the gas plasma at high velocity, the powder is melted. The molten metal stream strikes the device to be coated and immediately solidifies to form the porous coating. By controlling the processing parameters, the porosity of the coating and the coating thickness can be varied. Plasma spray coatings generally have a rough surface containing a variable degree of porosity averaging approximately 35% with a pore size ranging from 20 to 200 μm. CP titanium and Ti–6Al–4V alloy plasma spray coatings are generally used in the manufacture of orthopaedic implants. A typical CP titanium plasma spray coating is shown in Figure 14 on a hip stem.

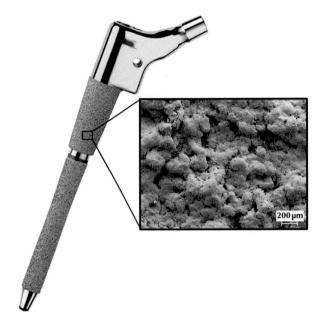

Figure 14 Titanium plasma spray-coated hip stem. Inset shows the microstructure of the plasma spray coating. *Source*: Courtesy of Zimmer Inc., Warsaw, IN.

Porous Coating Issues

The use of porous coatings on orthopaedic implants has provided clinicians with a noncemented fixation option which has received widespread clinical use. However, the application of any porous coating raises engineering and manufacturing issues that must be carefully considered when designing a porous coated implant. Specifically, when any type of porous coating is applied or attached to an implant surface, it produces effective "notches" at the coating/substrate interface. The shape and size of these notches depend upon the geometry of the bond sites formed at the interface. These notches act as stress concentrators and have the overall effect of lowering fatigue strength relative to the uncoated alloy. This phenomenon is not problematic per se as long as it is taken into consideration when designing an implant. In general, titanium and titanium alloys are more sensitive to notches than Co–Cr–Mo alloys. As a result, the fatigue strength of porous coated Ti–6Al–4V, for example, is approximately 40% lower than the fatigue strength of porous coated Co–Cr–Mo alloy. For higher fatigue strength applications of porous coated devices, plasma sprayed Ti–6Al–4V alloy or plasma sprayed Co–Cr–Mo alloy implants generally are used in the design of porous implants. Other issues that are relevant to porous coated implants include coating bond strength and coating integrity.

SURFACE TREATMENTS FOR IMPROVED WEAR RESISTANCE

Ion Implantation

Ion implantation is a specialized surface treatment process by which metal alloys can be hardened using high energy ion beams (21,22). Several ion species have been evaluated in an attempt to modify implant surfaces for improved abrasion resistance and to improve polyethylene wear. Among them, the nitrogen ion implantation process has emerged as the most successful process to harden orthopaedic implants. The nitrogen ions impinge onto the surface of the alloy producing a hardened surface layer approximately 0.2 µm thick. This process does not alter the bulk properties of the alloy.

The nitrogen ion implantation process has been used since the mid-1980s to harden Ti–6Al–4V alloy implants, reduce polyethylene wear, and increase the implant's resistance to scratching (23). This process was also applied to Co–Cr–Mo implants in the 1990s (24). Again, the hardness and the scratch resistance of Co–Cr–Mo implants are increased due to nitrogen ion implantation. There is, however, no measurable reduction in polyethylene wear when articulated against an ion-implanted Co–Cr–Mo alloy relative to an untreated Co–Cr–Mo alloy when evaluated in a hip simulator (25).

Nitriding

Ti–6Al–4V alloy implants are also hardened using a low-temperature nitrogen diffusion hardening process called nitriding (26). The process produces a nitrogen-rich region on the prosthesis surface. Nitrogen reacts with titanium on the implant surface to form titanium nitrides and a solid solution of nitrogen in the titanium matrix. Hardening is also somewhat enhanced by coincidental diffusion of oxygen into the surface of the alloy. As a result, the prosthesis surface hardness and abrasive wear resistance are increased without compromising the bulk properties of the alloy. This process produces hardened layers up to 2 µm in depth compared to the nitrogen ion implantation process, which produces only a 0.2 µm hardened layer.

The nitrogen diffusion hardening process has been used to harden polished Ti–6Al–4V alloy hip and knee implants since the 1990s with good clinical results (27). Studies have demonstrated a significant increase in hardness, decrease in polyethylene wear, and increase in abrasion resistance in joint simulator studies of nitrogen diffusion hardened implants (26).

Surface Treatment Issues

Integral hardened layers are produced on Ti–6Al–4V alloy implants from nitrogen ion implantation and nitrogen diffusion hardening processes. The hardened layer produced from these processes is a part of the alloy and there is an alloy gradient formed at the hardened layer and substrate interface. These hardened layers are metallurgically sound and difficult to delaminate.

Hard coatings such as TiN, CrN, and diamond-like carbon (DLC) deposited on implants exhibit a sharp demarkation at the coating/substrate interface. These coatings may be prone to delamination because of manufacturing issues and the modulus mismatch between the coating and the substrate material. This type of coating failure may lead to third body wear and increased corrosion at the implant–coating interface. Moreover, there are no reliable non destructive test methods available to date to assure the quality of these coatings. As a result, hard coatings have not been widely used on implants, but instead have found utility on cutting instruments.

RECENT ADVANCES IN METALS

Recently, a number of advances in metals have been implemented in orthopaedic devices and are being used clinically. An example of a new porous coating/porous metal and a new surface treatment are given.

Porous Tantalum (Trabecular Metal™)

Trabecular Metal (Implex Corp., Allendale, NJ) is an open-cell, porous tantalum (Ta) structure that has the microstructural appearance of trabecular bone (28). This porous metal structural material has a relatively high porosity of 75–85% (compared to 35–50% for conventional porous coatings) and is characterized by continuous interconnecting pores that have the shape of a dodecahedron cell structure with a nominal pore diameter of 550 μm. Trabecular Metal is manufactured using a chemical vapor deposition (CVD) process in which pure tantalum metal is precipitated onto a reticulated vitreous carbon (RVC) foam, or skeleton. The CVD process completely encases the RVC skeleton with tantalum metal, as shown in Figure 15. The nominal composition of Trabecular Metal is approximately 99% Ta and 1% vitreous carbon, by weight. Elemental tantalum is useful as an implant material due to its biocompatibility and relatively high-corrosion resistance compared to other metals (29).

Unlike other porous coatings, Trabecular Metal is also a stand-alone structural material. The compressive strength and modulus of elasticity are typically 65 MPa and 3 GPa, respectively, for an 80% porous material (28,30,31). These values are between the compressive strength and modulus values of trabecular and cortical bone. The Trabecular Metal torsional strength is approximately 50 MPa and the bending fatigue strength is about 35 MPa at 1.0×10^6 cycles (31). Due to its high porosity, Trabecular Metal has been reported to have excellent bone ingrowth characteristics resulting in improved mechanical properties of the bone–implant interface relative to other porous coatings (32). It has also been shown to have favorable soft

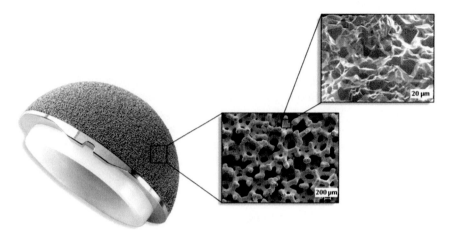

Figure 15 Trabecular metal monoblock acetabular cup. Inset shows the microstructure of trabecular metal. *Source*: Courtesy of Zimmer Inc., Warsaw, IN.

tissue ingrowth characteristics, which has prompted its use for soft tissue attachment onto orthopaedic implants (33).

Trabecular Metal has been in use clinically since 1995 (30). Since then, a number of orthopaedic devices have used Trabecular Metal as a porous bone and soft tissue ingrowth surface in applications including acetabular cups, tibial knee components, and patella components. It is also in use clinically for bone ingrowth applications as a stand-alone implant in spinal fusion devices and an avascular necrosis device. Figure 15 shows a photo of an acetabular cup application using Trabecular Metal.

Oxidized Zirconium (Oxinium™)

Zirconium (Zr) is a biocompatible metal, like titanium, but has not been used widely as an orthopaedic implant material, primarily due to its inferior mechanical properties compared to titanium. However, as with other metals, the strength of zirconium can be increased by alloying with other elements. Zirconium–2.5 niobium (Nb) is one such alloy that was originally developed for commercial applications. Its mechanical properties were improved over Zr by alloying with Nb and oxygen. To date, there are no known applications of zirconium, or more specifically the Zr–2.5 Nb alloy, in orthopaedics other than Smith and Nephew Orthopaedic's (Memphis, TN) oxidized zirconium, or Oxinium, femoral knee and femoral head products (34–37).

Oxinium is the Zr–2.5 Nb alloy that has been oxidized at an elevated temperature to grow a zirconium oxide ceramic layer on the surface of the implant. The proposed benefit of this technology is to offer an implant that is resistant to abrasion while avoiding the risk of fracture associated with an all-ceramic component. Oxinium is manufactured by heating the Zr–2.5 Nb alloy in an air or oxygen atmosphere at 535°C for three to four hours. The implant surface is then polished. This process produces a 5 µm thick blue-black or black zirconium oxide layer. This layer has a hardness close to that of a monolithic zirconium oxide ceramic. Wear studies performed in joint simulators on oxidized zirconium knees and hips have demonstrated an increase in the abrasion resistance of oxidized zirconium relative to Co–Cr parts (35). The material has been in use clinically in femoral knee components for two years, and was introduced in femoral heads in 2003.

SUMMARY

Total hip and knee arthroplasty procedures have been performed for more than three decades with great success. During this period, a number of metals have been used in a variety of orthopaedic implant designs. The mechanical properties, particularly the fatigue strength of metals, have steadily increased over the years as a result of new alloy developments and improved processing and manufacturing techniques. Today's higher strength metals are effectively used to design implants that provide excellent clinical results. However, there remains ample opportunity to continue to improve the mechanical properties and wear resistance of current alloys even further. Continuous advances in metallurgy will remain important as implants are used in younger and more active patients.

REFERENCES

1. Mears DC. Materials and Orthopaedic Surgery. Baltimore: Williams and Wilkens, 1979:1–28.
2. Encyclopedic Handbook of Biomaterials and Bioengineering, Part B: Applications. Wise DJ, Trantolo DJ, Altobelli DE, ed. New York: Marcel Dekker 1995:509–539.
3. Park JB. Biomaterials Science and Engineering. New York: Plenum Press, 1984:6–9.
4. Park JB, Lakes RS. Biomaterials—An Introduction. 2nd ed. New York: Plenum Press, 1992:3–6.
5. Park JB, Bronzino JD. Biomaterials—Principles and Applications. New York: CRC Press, 2002:1–10.
6. Cullity BD. Elements of X-ray Diffraction. 3rd ed. New York: Prentice Hall, 2001:1–15.
7. Bothe RT, Beaton KE, Davenport HA. Reaction of bone to multiple metallic implants. Surg Gynecol Obstet 1940; 71:589.
8. Smith WF. Structure and Properties of Engineering Alloys. 2nd ed. New York: McGraw-Hill, 1993:312–322.
9. Jergensen FD. Metallic surgical implants. J Bone Joint Surg Am 1993; 46(2): 401–408.

10. Eylon DJ, Newman JR, Thorne JK. Titanium and Titanium Alloy Casting. ASM Metals Handbook. ASM International, Materials Park, OH, Vol. 2, 10th ed, 1990:635–646.
11. Crook P. Cobalt and Cobalt Alloys. ASM Metals Handbook. ASM International, Materials Park, OH, Vol. 2, 10th ed, 1990:446–454.
12. Smith WF. Structure and Properties of Engineering Alloys. 2nd ed. New York: McGraw-Hill, 1993:433–438.
13. Windler M, Klabunde R. Titanium for hip and knee prosthesis. In: Brunette D, Tengvell P, Textor M, Thomsen P, eds. Titanium in Medicine: Material Science, Surface Science, Engineering, Biological Responses and Medical Applications. New york: Springer, 2001:703–746.
14. Freese HL, Volas MG, Wood JR. Metallurgy and Technological Properties of Titanium and Titanium Alloy. In: Brunette D, Tengvell P, Textor M, Thomsen P, eds. Titanium in Medicine: Material Science, Surface Science, Engineering, Biological Responses and Medical Applications. New york: Springer, 2001:25–52.
15. Dall DM, Learmonth ID, Solomon MI, Davenport JM. Fracture and loosening of Charnley femoral stems: comparison between first-generation and subsequent designs. J Bone Joint Surg Br 1993; 75(2):259–265.
16. Heck DA, Partridge CM, Reuten JD, Lanzer WL, Lewis CG, Keating EM. Prosthetic component failures in hip arthroplasty surgery. J Arthroplasty 1995; 10(5):575–580.
17. Roaf R. Implants in orthopaedic surgery. In: Williams DF, Roaf R, eds. Implants in Surgery. Philadelphia: W.B. Saunders, 1973:437–480.
18. Charnley J. Total hip replacement by low friction arthroplasty. Clin Orthop 1970; (72):7–21.
19. Andersen PJ. Medical and dental applications. Metals Handbook. 19th ed. Vol 7. Metals Park, OH: American Society for Metals, 1984:657–663.
20. Galante J, Rostoker W, Lueck R, Ray RD. Sintered fiber metal composites as a basis for attachment of implants to bone. J Bone Joint Surg Am 1971; 53(1):101–114.
21. Higham PA. Ion implantation as a tool for improving the properties of orthopaedic alloys. In: Biomedical Materials. Pittsburgh: Materials Research Society, 1986:253–261.
22. Sioshansi P, Oliver RW. Improvements in the hardness of surgical titanium alloys by ion implantation. In: Biomedical Materials. Pittsburgh: Materials Research Society, 1986:237–241.
23. Sioshansi P. Improving the properties of titanium alloys by ion implantation. JOM 1990; 42(3):30–31.
24. Sioshansi P. Ion implantation of cobalt-chromium prosthetic components to reduce polyethylene wear. Orthop Today 1991; 11(8):24–25.
25. Schmidt MB, Lin M, Greer KW. Wear performance of UHMWPE articulated against ion implanted CoCr. Transactions of 21st Annual Meeting of the Society for Biomaterials, 1995, 230.
26. Shetty RH. Mechanical and Corrosion Properties of Nitrogen Diffusion Hardened Ti–6Al–4V Alloy. Medical Applications of Titanium and Its Alloys: The Material and Biological Issues, ASTM STP 1272, 1996:240–251.

27. Bobyn JD, Galante JO, Jordan LR, Rosenberg AG, Rubash HE, White RE. A radiographic assessment of bone resorption and biological fixation with the Multilock® hip prosthesis—A multi-center study. 61st Annual Meeting of the AAOS, 1994.

28. Zardiackas LD, Parsell DE, Dillon LD, Mitchell DW, Nunnery LA, Poggie R. Structure metallurgy, and mechanical properties of a porous tantalum foam. J Biomed Mater Res 2001; 58(2):180–187.

29. Black J. Biological performance of tantalum. Clin Mater (Engl) 1994; 16(3): 167–173.

30. Rapp SM. Bone-building implant used for segmental replacement. Orthop Today (Int Ed) 2000; 3(3):26–28.

31. Bobyn JD, Hacking SA, Chan SP, Toh K, Krygier JJ, Tanzer M. Characterization of a new porous tantalum biomaterial for reconstructive surgery. Transactions of AAOS, 66th Annual Meeting, 1999, 250.

32. Bobyn JD, Stackpool GJ, Hacking SA, Tanzer M, Krygier JJ. Characteristics of bone ingrowth and interface mechanics of a new porous tantalum biomaterial. J Bone Joint Surg Br, 1999; 81(5):907–914.

33. Hacking SA, Bobyn JD, Toh K, Tanzer M, Krygier JJ, Miller JO. Fibrous tissue ingrowth and attachment to porous tantalum. J Biomed Mater Res, 2000; 52(4):631–638.

34. Davidson JA, U.S. Patent 5,370,694, 1994.

35. Mishra AK, Davidson JA. Zirconia/zirconium: a new abrasion resistant material for orthopaedic applications. Mat Tech, 1993; (8):16–21.

36. White SE, Whiteside LA, McCarthy DS, Anthony M, Poggie RA. Simulated knee wear with cobalt chromium and oxidized zirconium knee femoral components. Clin Orthop 1994; (309):176–184.

37. Spector BM, Ries MD, Bourne RB, Sauer WA, Long M, Hunter G. Wear performance of ultra-high molecular weight polyethylene on oxidized zirconium total knee femoral components. J Bone Joint Surg Am 2001; 83(suppl 2 Pt 2): 80–86.

38. American Society for Testing Materials, Annual Book of Standards 2002, Vol 13.01, Medical Devices and Emergency Medical Services, ASTM International, 2002.

39. Black J. Orthopaedic Biomaterials in Research and Practice. New York: Churchill Livingstone, 1988:163–190.

24

Advances in Polyethylene

Anuj Bellare

Department of Orthopaedic Surgery, Brigham & Women's Hospital, Harvard Medical School, Boston, Massachusetts, U.S.A.

Lisa A. Pruitt

Department of Mechanical Engineering, University of California at Berkeley, Berkeley, California, U.S.A.

Ultra high molecular weight polyethylene (UHMWPE) is a tough, wear resistant, biocompatible polymer that has been used for over four decades as a bearing material in total joint replacement prostheses. Despite its superior wear properties, osteolysis associated with particulate wear debris of UHMWPE released during in vivo use has been a major factor determining the longevity of hip replacements utilizing UHMWPE components. In the case of knee components, fatigue damage wear mechanisms, such as delamination wear have led to loosening of the implants leading to premature revision surgery. Aging of γ-irradiated components is the primary factor promoting delamination wear of UHMWPE tibial components. In this chapter, various aspects of UHMWPE synthesis, morphology, processing, and their effects of mechanical and wear properties of clinical relevance have been outlined. The role of chain entanglements, radiation sterilization, radiation cross-linking, and crystallinity in controlling wear resistance and mechanical properties are also discussed. Currently, processing techniques and methods of chemical modification by radiation are being developed and optimized to maximize the mechanical and tribological performance of UHMWPE, as it varies for each joint. We have identified that chemical factors, such as the number of chain entanglements and degree of cross-linking, are beneficial for wear resistance while physical factors such as density or degree of crystallinity lead to an increase in several clinically relevant mechanical properties such as resistance to creep deformation and resistance to fatigue crack propagation. All of these factors may be affected in the long term if free radicals associated with γ-sterilization or radiation cross-linking remain in the UHMWPE component after processing and packaging. Long-term oxidative degradation can be decreased by packaging of UHMWPE components in reduced-oxygen environments but it remains to be seen whether in vivo oxidation will affect their mechanical and wear performance in the long term.

INTRODUCTION

During 1958–1960, John Charnley designed total hip replacement prostheses based on the low friction polymer, polytetrafluoroethylene (PTFE) (1–3). The early results of Charnley's low friction arthroplasty (LFA) were encouraging with negligible wear of PTFE (4). However, over 99% of prostheses needed revision within two to three years due to excessive wear of PTFE and inflammatory response associated with PTFE wear debris. The failure of PTFE prompted Charnley to examine other bearing materials for joint arthroplasty. In 1962, a bearing salesman provided Charnley's technician, H. Craven, with ultra high molecular weight polyethylene (UHMWPE) samples, which were marketed using the trade name RCH-1000, manufactured by the German company, Ruhrchemie (currently Ticona). Although initially dismissed by Charnley, Craven conducted a three week long wear test on the samples during Charnley's absence, which showed less wear after three weeks than PTFE tested for a period of a day under similar wear test conditions (5). These remarkable results convinced Charnley to conduct a biocompatibility study comparing UHMWPE and PTFE (by implanting bulk and particulate samples in his own thigh!) which showed that UHMWPE was biocompatible (6). Charnley began implanting UHMWPE acetabular cups in patients in November 1962. Thus, UHMWPE was introduced into joint arthroplasty due to the combined efforts of an engineer and a surgeon. Four decades later, after considering several other polymers for joint arthroplasty, UHMWPE remains the gold standard as a bearing material for total joint replacement prostheses since it combines superior wear resistance along with high fracture toughness compared to other polymers. Despite the excellent resistance of UHMWPE to wear, numerous studies have shown that UHMWPE components also have significant wear rates and generate particulate debris as they articulate against a metal or ceramic counterface (2,7–18). In the 1994 NIH Consensus statement it was stated that particulate wear debris can result in tissue inflammation, bone resorption (referred to as osteolysis), and implant loosening (7). Osteolysis due to

UHMWPE wear can cause complications during revision surgery. In recent years, orthopaedic implant wear has been recognized to be the leading problem in orthopaedic surgery. Osteolysis can occur in the periprosthetic tissue surrounding the hip, but can also occur in other joints such as the knee joint (8–13).

UHMWPE WEAR: HIP VS. KNEE COMPONENTS

In the case of total hip replacements (THRs), the motion of the metallic or ceramic femoral component relative to the motion of the UHMWPE acetabular component follows a quasi-elliptical path during a patient's gait cycle (19). Thus, wear in the acetabular component is dominated by particulate wear mechanisms, which results in penetration of the femoral component into the acetabular component during the wear process. The resulting UHMWPE submicrometer wear debris has been associated with osteolysis, which is generally more prevalent in the hip than in the knee (14). In addition, third body wear particles (bone chips, hydroxyapatite, cement particles) and scratches on the metallic counterface can lead to accelerated wear of UHMWPE in hip replacements (20–24). The load distribution across the surface area of the cup varies with the location on the cup and determines the direction and extent of wear (25). Other complications can also occur due to surgical misalignment, which can lead to impingement of the femoral neck on to the rim of acetabular cups, thereby imposing cyclic loads on the rim. This fatigue related loading history can lead to eccentric wear, fatigue damage mechanisms, and catastrophic failure (such as rim cracking), or can lead to dislocation and socket loosening (26–30).

The contact area between the bearing components remains largely constant in the hip, compared to the knee components, where sliding and rolling of the counterface leads to the imposition of cyclic loads on knee components. In the case of total knee replacement (TKR) prostheses, the UHMWPE components comprise the tibial and patellar components. These components are subjected to a large variety of damage modes such as catastrophic failure, fatigue damage, delamination wear, as well as scratching, pitting, and burnishing (15,16,31–33). Particulate wear also occurs in TKR components, although the particle size distribution differs from that of THR wear particles, and TKR particles have been shown to be generally larger than THR wear particles (18). These mechanisms of wear occur due to the vastly different design of the TKR components that result in larger contact stresses in the patellofemoral and tibial components compared to the acetabular component (34–41). In the case of metal backed patellar components with low conformity, the contact stresses often exceed the yield stress of UHMWPE, leading to cold flow (permanent deformation) of the implant eventually leading to catastrophic failure. Permanent deformation can also occur without exceeding the yield stress due to creep deformation associated with viscoelasticity. More contemporary designs of UHMWPE knee components utilize higher conformity of the femoral component against the UHMWPE component to increase the contact area, thereby decreasing the contact stresses.

POLYETHYLENE: SYNTHESIS AND MOLECULAR STRUCTURE

Liquid forms of low molecular weight polyethylene were known since 1869. Solid polyethylene was first invented almost by chance in March, 1933 at the Imperial Chemical Industries Ltd, U.K. when researchers E.W. Fawcett and R.O. Gibson were investigating the effects of high pressures on several chemical reactions, one of which involved ethylene and toluene (42). But the vast technological and commercial impact of polyethylene over the course of the 20th century was driven by the invention of an inexpensive, low-pressure polymerization process using new coordination catalysts by Karl Ziegler for which he shares the 1963 Nobel Prize in chemistry with Giulio Natta. The free radical polymerization of ethylene gas into solid polyethylene can be simply depicted by the following equation:

$$CH_2{=}CH_2 \xrightarrow{\text{catalyst}} \text{-}(CH_2\text{-}CH_2)_{n-} \tag{1}$$

where "n" refers to the number of monomers that make up the linear polymer. Currently, there are several types of polyethylene resins available, which are categorized based primarily on their density (specific gravity), which is usually controlled by the amount of small or large branches on an otherwise linear macromolecule. Some examples of commercial polyethylene are high density polyethylene (HDPE), low density polyethylene (LDPE), linear low density polyethylene (LLDPE), ultra low density polyethylene (ULDPE), very low density polyethylene (VLDPE), and UHMWPE. The density of UHMWPE, which generally falls within a range of 0.93–0.95 g/cc, is similar to that of LDPE. The reason for the low density of UHMWPE is the high degree of chain entanglement of the linear macromolecule. Commercial LDPE has low density due to a large number of chain branches. The molecular weight of UHMWPE is usually 500,000–5,000,000 g/mole. Thus, the number of monomers that make up the polymer is at approximately 20,000–200,000.

Over the last few decades, there have been various grades of UHMWPE resins available, primarily from Ruhrchemie AG, which later changed its name to Hoechst, and is currently called Ticona (Bayport, Texas, U.S.A). Their earlier UHMWPE resin trade name, used by Charnley, was called RCH-1000 or (R)uhr(CH)emie (similar resin to the current GUR 1020 UHMWPE resin) and was classified as a form of HDPE, which is why earlier papers refer to UHMWPE as HDPE (43). Later the orthopaedic grade of UHMWPE was called CHIRULEN followed by GUR or (G)ranular (U)HMWPE

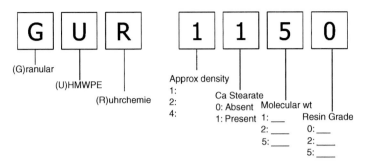

Figure 1 A schematic explaining the numbers or grade associated with GUR UHMWPE resins. *Abbreviation*: UHMWPE, ultra high molecular weight polyethylene.

(R)uhrchemie in the 1990s. The most common grades used today are GUR 1050 and GUR 1020. The numbers following GUR currently refer to the following: first digit refers to approximate density (1), second digit refers to presence (1) or absence (0) of calcium stearate which is a lubricant that assists in processing, third digit refers to molecular weight (2 = 2 million g/mole and 5 = 5 million g/mole) and the fourth digit (0) refers to the resin grade (numbering schematic in Fig. 1). There were some reports of increased levels of oxidation and fusion defects associated with calcium stearate (44–47). This not an issue for new joint replacement devices since orthopaedic grade resins, GUR 1050 and GUR 1020, do not contain calcium stearate. Another source of UHMWPE was Montell [Formerly Himont (Wilmington, Delaware, U.S.A.)], which produced the Hi-Fax 1900H resin, which has a different structure and properties compared to the Hoechst resins (48). Montell no longer manufactures UHMWPE after a new merger involving Shell and BASF.

UHMWPE: A HIERARCHY OF STRUCTURES

The nanostructure of UHMWPE is qualitatively similar to other semicrystalline polymers. In order to understand the macromolecular organization of polyethylene at the nanometer scale, it is necessary to know its transition temperatures and processing history. There are two primary transition temperatures in semicrystalline polymers that greatly affect their structure and properties, which are: (i) glass transition temperature or T_g, and (ii) melting temperature of crystals or T_m. The T_m for atmospheric pressure crystallized UHMWPE is approximately 133°C whereas the T_g is approximately −120°C. If a sample of polyethylene is raised to a temperature above its T_m, the macromolecules form long randomly coiled, entangled linear chains, just like entangled balls of wool or entangled spaghetti. Most medium molecular weight polyethylenes (less than approximately 250,000 g/mole) form a viscous melt that can flow upon melting. In the case of UHMWPE, the chain molecules are extremely long and their entanglement density is high. Therefore, UHMWPE remains undeformed in the melt state, remaining stationary like a gel. (It must be noted, however, that final machined components of UHMWPE should not be melted since residual stresses from machining can lead to some deformation and loss of tolerances.) When the temperature is reduced to a temperature below its T_m, crystallization occurs. The rate of crystallization, the nucleation density of crystals, crystalline lamella thickness and overall degree of crystallinity can be controlled by the temperature and time of crystallization (49). The applied pressure during crystallization can also have a large effect on the thickness of the crystals and overall degree of crystallinity. For a comprehensive review of various aspects of polyethylene crystallization kinetics, structure, mechanisms and theories, see Hoffman and Miller (50).

The crystals of UHMWPE are in the form of ribbon-like lamellae, which sandwich amorphous layers, as depicted in Figure 2. The polyethylene chains are held in fixed positions in the crystals to form a lattice of orthorhombic unit cells. In the case of dilute solution crystallized polyethylene, the macromolecules exit the crystalline lamellae and fold back into the adjacent unit cell. Thus, the amorphous regions comprise chain folds and chain ends. However, when the crystallization occurs from the entangled melt, the chains cannot fully reptate (snake-like motion) and form an ordered structure. Thus, as shown in Figure 2, the chains in the amorphous region comprise loose loops, adjacent folds, chain ends or randomly coiled chains before they re-enter a neighboring lamella. This depiction has been referred to as a telephone "switchboard" model. When the crystallization occurs from a melt state under pressures higher than 3.6 kbar and temperatures higher than 230°C, polyethylene crystallizes into a hexagonal unit cell, which is a more open structure capable of thickening to a much larger extent than crystallization below 3.6 kbar (51). Upon removal of the pressure, the original orthorhombic crystal is restored but the thick crystalline lamellae remain. This strategy can be used to increase the overall crystallinity of UHMWPE from approximately 45–55% up to 80%. A similar process was employed in the case of Hylamer^{TM} (Depuy Orthopaedics, Warsaw, Indiana, U.S.A.), which was used for the manufacture of acetabular cups in the 1990s, and had a degree of crystallinity of 68–75%. Crystalline lamellae present in bulk UHMWPE are approximately 10–50 nm in thickness whereas high pressure processing can increase the crystalline lamellae to a thickness of approximately 200 nm (0.2 μm). A similar high pressure process was used to manufacture Hylamer-M^{TM}, which had a degree of crystallinity of approximately 65% and was used to manufacture tibial plateaus for TKR prostheses.

Polyethylene lamellae have a high modulus of elasticity (stiffness) whereas the amorphous regions in between the lamellae are liquid like at room temperature. If the temperature of polyethylene is decreased to a temperature below T_g (−120°C), then the amorphous regions vitrify and

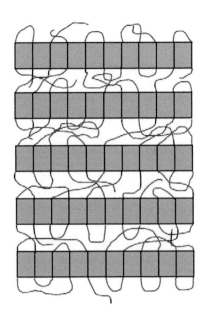 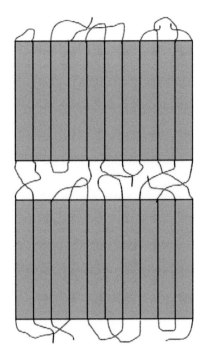

Figure 2 Semicrystalline structure of UHMWPE: The gray regions are crystalline lamellae with amorphous regions in between. The left figure shows thin lamellae, which can be thickened by a factor of up to 40 (*right figure*) using high pressure crystallization. *Abbreviation*: UHMWPE, ultra high molecular weight polyethylene.

form a glass, thereby transforming polyethylene into an extremely brittle, glassy, semicrystalline polymer. Thus at room or body temperatures, polyethylene is a nanocomposite comprising thin layers of crystals and melt of nanometer thickness. This imparts superior toughness to polyethylene combined with its light weight, which has resulted in its vast commercial impact on a variety of consumer applications, such as packaging films and bottles.

At the micrometer scale, medium molecular weight polyethylenes form a ball-like structure called "spherulites" which are of the order of 10–100 μm in diameter. As crystallization progresses from a nucleus of a bundle of lamellae, the lamellae grow until the growing spherulites impinge upon each other, forming three-dimensional polygonal shapes, as shown by the low voltage scanning electron micrograph in Figure 3. In the case of UHMWPE, a high concentration of nuclei precludes the formation of spherulites, and the structure of UHMWPE is simply space filling, 10–50 nm thick lamellae that are tortuous and meander through the bulk material (52). Figure 4 is a freeze fractured UHMWPE specimen of a rod stock that was etched using a standard permanganic acid etching technique to reveal the

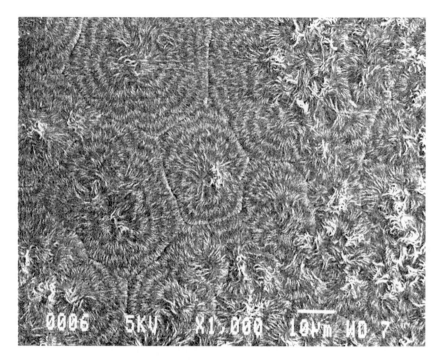

Figure 3 Low voltage scanning electron micrograph of spherulitic morphology in polyethylene.

lamellar morphology (53). Under high pressure crystallization, the lamellae of UHMWPE can be considerably thickened to approximately 0.2 μm (Fig. 5).

UHMWPE: THE ROLE OF DEGREE OF CRYSTALLINITY OR DENSITY

The total degree of crystallinity or density of UHMWPE is a very important morphological parameter. Higher crystallinity UHMWPEs generally have a larger modulus of elasticity, superior yield strength, improved resistance to creep deformation, and enhanced fatigue strength. All of these are desirable properties for joint components. Also, a study comparing Hylamer™ (approximate crystallinity of 68–75%) sterilized using gas plasma sterilization with unsterile, conventional UHMWPE (approximate crystallinity of 50–55%) showed that the degree of crystallinity did not affect wear rates substantially within this range of crystallinity (54). The resistance to creep deformation is an important mechanical property for joint arthroplasty since orthopaedic surgeons quantify UHMWPE wear in patients by monitoring the degree of femoral head penetration into the acetabular component, estimated using X-ray radiographs. It is important to distinguish the

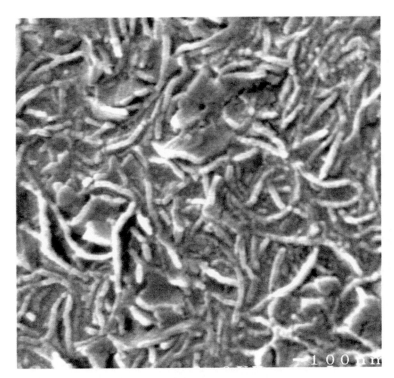

Figure 4 LVSEM of a permanganic acid etched freeze fracture cross section of bulk UHMWPE showing 20–50 nm thick lamellae (white regions are crystalline lamellae). *Abbreviations*: UHMWPE, ultra high molecular weight polyethylene; LVSEM, low voltage scanning electron micrograph.

relative contribution of UHMWPE creep deformation and wear to femoral head penetration. Obviously, a low amount of creep deformation is desirable. The fatigue strength is also very important since it relates to the ability of UHMWPE to resist cyclic damage modes, which are prevalent in knee components and also in the rims of malpositioned acetabular cups.

The density of UHMWPE samples may be measured using a density gradient column. The degree of crystallinity can be estimated from the density of the UHMWPE sample since the density of the crystal is 1.0 g/cc and that of the amorphous phase is 0.855 g/cc. Alternatively, a common method of measurement of crystallinity is using a differential scanning calorimeter (DSC). In this method, an approximately 5 mg sample of UHMWPE is heated from room temperature at a heating rate of 10°C/min until 170°C. An endothermic reaction occurs as the sample absorbs heat to melt the crystals. Sample DSC thermographs for a rod stock UHMWPE sample and a high pressure crystallized UHMWPE are presented in Figure 6. The peak of the melting curve represents the melting temperature of the samples. As

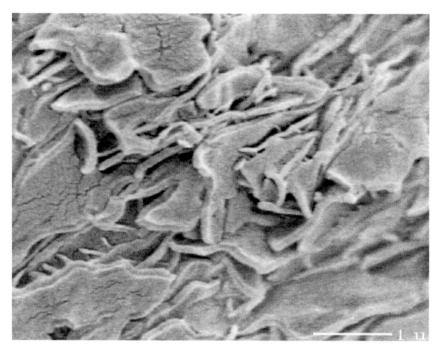

Figure 5 LVSEM micrograph of permanganic acid etched high pressure crystallized UHMWPE showing 0.2 μm thick lamellae. *Abbreviations*: LVSEM, low voltage scanning electron micrograph; UHMWPE, ultra high molecular weight polyethylene.

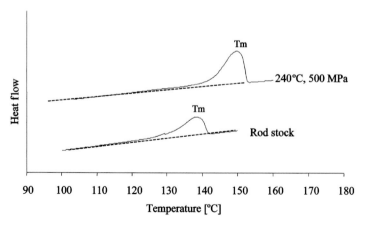

Figure 6 Differential scanning calorimeter thermograph showing heating and melting of UHMWPE rod stock and UHMWPE crystallized under 240°C and 500 MPa pressure. Dashed lines represent baseline. *Abbreviation*: UHMWPE, ultra high molecular weight polyethylene.

can be observed, the thicker crystalline lamellae of the high pressure crystallized sample (Fig. 5) melt at a higher temperature (146°C) compared to the melting temperature (138°C) of the relatively thinner crystalline lamellae of the rod stock (Fig. 4), both of which are higher than the melting temperature (133°C) of atmospheric pressure crystallized UHMWPE. The broad melting curves are due to the presence of a broad distribution of thickness of the lamellae in UHMWPE. Melting curves can also be affected by defects in lamellae, constrained chains in amorphous regions, and other factors. The degree of crystallinity is equal to the ratio of the area under the thermographs and the heat of fusion of 100% polyethylene crystal ($= 293 \, J/g$). The degree of crystallinity and density are related by the following equation:

$$\rho = \rho a x + \rho c (1 - x) \tag{2}$$

where ρ is the overall density, ρa is density of amorphous region ($0.855 \, g/cc$), ρc is density of PE crystal ($1.0 \, g/cc$), and x is the degree of crystallinity. Thus, these quantities can be estimated by one of the two aforementioned methods. It must be noted, however, that the density can also be affected by porosity (apparent density). Thus, the density estimated using the degree of crystallinity often differs in value from the density measured using a density gradient column.

UHMWPE: POWDER MORPHOLOGY

The as-synthesized or nascent UHMWPE powder contains particles that are approximately 100 μm in size (Fig. 7A). The broad size distribution of GUR 4150 powder particles have been measured by Pienkowski et al. (55). Each powder particle contains 10–30 μm size aggregates (Fig. 7B) comprising approximately 1 μm size nodules connected to each other by fibrils (Fig. 7C). It has been shown by Olley et al. (56) that the consolidation of UHMWPE powder can lead to voids or defects on two length scales since fusion of powder during ram extrusion or compression molding must occur on the 100 μm as well as the 1 μm length scales. Figure 8 shows that even well-consolidated UHMWPE shows the presence of powder boundaries using light microscope examination of thin sections of bulk UHMWPE. While it has been suggested that incomplete consolidation of powder particles of UHMWPE may contribute to wear, Gul et al. (57) showed that there was no correlation between the degree of consolidation of UHMWPE powder particles and the rate of generation of particulate wear debris under the processing conditions examined by the authors.

The nanostructure of the nascent UHMWPE powder contains a combination of extended chain crystals as well as thin lamellae (58). The melting temperature (141°C) observed using DSC suggests that the powder contains mostly extended chain crystals, as present in high pressure crystallized

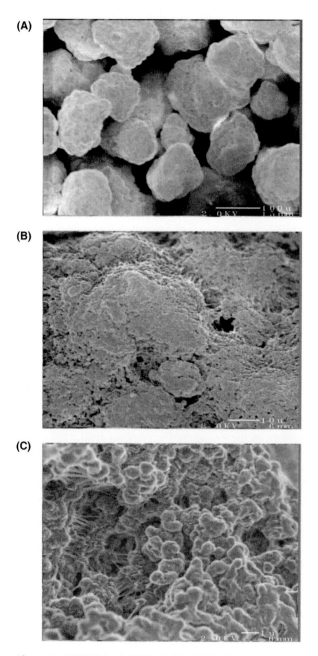

Figure 7   LVSEM of GUR 1050 UHMWPE powder showing (**A**) a base resin particle size of approximately 100 μm; (**B**) 10–30 μm size aggregates of UHMWPE
within the nascent powder; and (**C**) fibrils and nodules of approximately 1 μm size.
Abbreviations: LVSEM, low voltage scanning electron micrograph; UHMWPE, ultra
high molecular weight polyethylene.

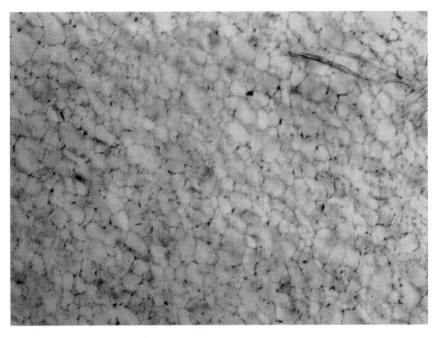

Figure 8 Low magnification (4x) polarized light micrograph showing resin-particle boundaries present in a bulk GUR 4150 UHMWPE component. *Abbreviation*: UHMWPE, ultra high molecular weight polythylene.

UHMWPE. However, a combination of several morphological, chemical, and molecular techniques indicated that a dual lamellar structure existed. It has been suggested that the fibrils (Fig. 7C) of the powder contain thick, extended chain crystalline lamellae while 20 nm thick lamellae exist in the spherical domains (58). The presence of fibrils in the powder also suggests that the as-synthesized powder has UHMWPE chains trapped in an aligned state of low entanglement, compared to the melt crystallized UHMWPE. This must be beneficial for the molding or ram extrusion processes used to consolidate the powder into bulk components. A highly entangled state would make it much more difficult to consolidate the powder since it would require the chains from powder particles to disentangle, reptate, and then entangle with the chains of the adjacent powder particles.

UHMWPE: PROCESSING TECHNIQUES

In most cases, UHMWPE powder particles are consolidated into bulk stock using either compression molding into thick sheets or by ram extrusion process. The final implant is usually machined from these UHMWPE stocks. Both of these processes involve compaction of UHMWPE nascent powder at elevated temperatures and pressures for an extended duration. The resulting bulk components are usually annealed. Compression molded sheets of one to three inch thickness of GUR 1020 and GUR 1050 UHMWPE resins are commercially produced by two companies: Perplas Medical (U.K.) and Poly Hi Solidur (U.S.A). Another common process, ram extrusion, is employed to sinter nascent UHMWPE powder into 1–12 inch diameter rod stock of UHMWPE that are several feet in length (Fig. 9). Ram extruded, UHMWPE rods are manufactured by Perplas Medical, Poly Hi Solidur, and West Lake plastics (U.S.A.). The proprietary, extrusion processes are also usually followed by annealing. The resulting bulk UHMWPE stock is generally uniform except for small spatial variations in anisotropy due to spatially nonuniform crystallization occurring due to low thermal conductivity of polyethylene (59). The final implant is machined from these bulk consolidated UHMWPE stocks and sheets. In some cases, direct compression molding of tibial and acetabular components has been carried out. The advantage of direct compression molding is that the articular surfaces of the joint components are smooth, lacking machine marks or grooves. However, due to processing control issues, the common choice for implant manufacture is machining of compression molded sheets and ram extruded, rod stock of UHMWPE.

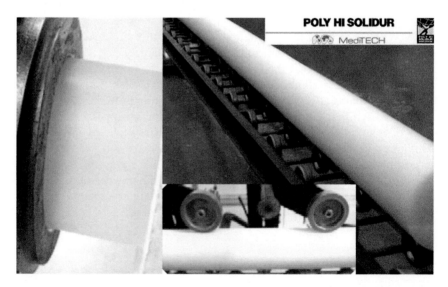

Figure 9 Ram extrusion of UHMWPE rod stock. *Abbreviation*: UHMWPE, ultra high molecular weight polythylene.

UHMWPE: THE STERILIZATION ISSUE

Sterilization of UHMWPE components deserves special mention since it is known to degrade the mechanical and wear properties of UHMWPE (43,60–78).Until recently, UHMWPE components of total joint replacements were packaged in air and thereafter sterilized using a 25–37 kGy dose of gamma radiation. It is well known that radiation causes cross-linking, chain scission, and long-term oxidative degradation of polyethylene. The effects of ionizing radiation on postirradiation aging of several types of polyethylene, including pressure crystallized UHMWPE (62) was studied in detail by Bhateja et al. (61–66). More recently, Costa et al. (67–69,79,80) demonstrated the detailed mechanism of oxidation, and have shown that oxidation can also occur in ethylene oxide sterilized UHMWPE, albeit to a much smaller extent than gamma radiation sterilized UHMWPE. It is now well established that long-term postirradiation aging can have detrimental effects on the morphology and mechanical properties of UHMWPE (72–75). The effects of postirradiation aging on TKRs have been well documented (77) in analyses of TKR retrievals. Recent reviews summarize various issues related to sterilization, its chemistry and effects on UHMWPE for TJR prostheses (43,60,80).

The major issue associated with oxidative degradation was that, in many cases, gamma-air sterilized UHMWPE components were stored on the shelf for long durations prior to implantation. These components, especially when stored over a period of six months or longer, exhibited oxidative degradation to the extent that their wear performance was compromised. It was originally believed that oxidation was associated primarily with fatigue damage mechanisms, such as delamination wear, that occurs in TKRs. However, it is now well known that the rate of particulate wear debris generation can also increase due to the molecular weight reduction and embrittlement in both tibial components (reciprocating motion) as well as in acetabular cups (multidirectional motion) (54,81). Initially, gamma radiation increases resistance to wear debris generation due to the low level of cross-linking that accompanies gamma radiation. However, with aging, oxidative effects begin to dominate and negate any initial benefits of gamma radiation, leading to higher wear rates.

Orthopaedic manufacturers have now recognized the deleterious effects of long-term oxidation. In response, some manufacturers sterilize UHMWPE using nonradiation methods, such as ethylene oxide or gas plasma sterilization. Some orthopaedic manufacturers have resorted to packaging of components in low oxygen environments, such as vacuum-foil packaging, packaging in nitrogen or argon gas. These methods would slow down the rate of oxidation during storage. However, it is not yet known whether in vivo oxidation rates would eventually affect the clinical performance of conventional UHMWPE, packaged in low oxygen environments and then sterilized using 25–37 kGy dose of gamma radiation.

UHMWPE: ALTERNATE FORMS

Contact stresses of UHMWPE components in TKRs can be reduced by a design approach that increases the conformity of the metal and UHMWPE components. However, this can limit the range of motion for a patient. Also, more constraint imparts greater stresses on fixation interfaces. A preferable approach would be to improve the material and tribological properties of UHMWPE that would allow for greater flexibility in implant design. One approach that was attempted more than two decades ago was to blend UHMWPE with carbon fibers to fabricate total joint replacement components (82,83). However, while the devices manufactured using carbon-fiber reinforced polyethylene showed excellent resistance to creep and improved compressive strength in in vitro tests, there was a large decrease in fatigue resistance. More importantly, no improvement in resistance to wear resistance was observed, and black colored debris due to the presence of carbon fibers was present surrounding worn implants. In fact, the material faired poorly in a clinical setting, and within a short time after implantation many devices failed due to elevated wear.

In the early 1990s, proprietary high pressure crystallization was employed to produce UHMWPE components. High crystallinity in UHMWPE results in an increase in mechanical properties such as yield stress, Young's modulus, resistance to creep deformation, and resistance to fatigue crack propagation (84–86). This bulk material obtained from the GUR 4150 resin was known as Hylamer^{TM} (Depuy Orthopaedics, Warsaw, U.S.A) for THRs and Hylamer-M for TKRs. Thus, it would seem that this form of UHMWPE would be advantageous for use in joint replacement applications. However, early clinical results showed that some acetabular cups of Hylamer failed early due to excessive wear rates (87,88). It is now well recognized that Hylamer was more susceptible to oxidative degradation associated with gamma radiation sterilization, leading to early failure due to high wear rates (89–91). Hylamer is no longer manufactured, although a significant number of Hylamer acetabular cups are in use today.

UHMWPE: CROSS-LINKING

In the 1980s, cross-linking was shown to improve the wear performance of UHMWPE (92–94). In recent years, cross-linking of the otherwise linear macromolecules of UHMWPE has been revisited by several groups (95–97). Laboratory wear tests have shown that there is a decrease in wear rate with an increase in degree of cross-linking of UHMWPE (98). However, a concern associated with cross-linking of UHMWPE is that there is a reduction in the fatigue crack propagation resistance upon cross-linking of UHMWPE (99,100), as well as a decrease in the fracture toughness (101). Since these are important mechanical properties for UHMWPE for application in TKR components, it is not yet clear that the benefits of resistance to particulate wear due to cross-linking would outweigh the risk of fatigue failure of UHMWPE components in TKRs. However, the potential benefits of reduced particulate wear of cross-linked UHMWPE in acetabular cups are well documented, and consequently has led to a large number of commercially available radiation cross-linked polyethylenes such as Durasul™ (95 kGy electron beam radiation, ethylene oxide sterilized), Longevity™ (100 kGy electron beam radiation, gas plasma sterilized), Crossfire™ (75 kGy gamma radiation, 25 kGy gamma radiation sterilized), XLPE™ (100 kGy gamma radiation, ethylene oxide sterilized), and Marathon™ (50 kGy gamma radiation, gas plasma sterilized). With the exception of Crossfire, these products are all melted after being subjected to radiation to quench the free radicals and initiate crosslinking. Crossfire is also heated, but to a temperature below the melting temperature of UHMWPE. The reason for this is to maintain some of the processing history and morphology induced by ram extrusion or compression molding and still gain the advantage of cross-linking, which is promoted by the elevated annealing temperature. One potential concern for Crossfire is that it contains residual free radicals, which could lead to oxidative degradation. However, it is not known whether the extent of in vivo oxidation would outweigh the benefit of a high degree of cross-linking and lead to excessive wear. Regardless, all of these commercially available, radiation crosslinked UHMWPE acetabular cups are now in clinical use, and it is to be determined whether they will lead to a higher survivorship compared to conventional, uncrosslinked UHMWPE.

UHMWPE: FUTURE DIRECTIONS

In the future, the application of polyethylene in joint replacements may involve the use of new polyethylenes synthesized using metallocene catalysts. The "holy grail" of manufacturing of implant components is to be able to injection mold components of polyethylene that are wear resistant. This is, however, not possible under current processing technology. UHMWPE required for high resistance to wear cannot be injection molded due to extremely high viscosity. Until new forms of polyethylene and processing technology are developed, components will be manufactured from ram extruded rod stock and compression molded sheets of UHMWPE, along with the intermediate radiation processing treatment. Both ram extrusion and compression molding involve the application of heat and pressure to compact UHMWPE powder. If a new injectable polyethylene resin were to be developed, issues of consolidation could be avoided and manufacturing costs would be much lower than the costs associated with current manufacturing methods.

In the near future, we can expect radiation cross-linking processes to be optimized to improve the resistance to particulate wear without a large decrease in mechanical properties such as resistance to fatigue crack propagation, tensile work of fracture, and J integral fracture toughness. One problem with most of the radiation cross-linking methods that employ complete melting to initiate cross-linking is that melting of UHMWPE erases the thermal history induced by ram extrusion and compression molding. Since cooling or recrystallization after melting is carried out without any application of pressure, it generally decreases the overall degree of crystallinity of radiation crosslinked UHMWPE. This in turn leads to a low Young's modulus in radiation cross-linked UHMWPE, which is generally associated with a lower resistance to creep deformation. In fact, the imperfect crystals present in radiation cross-linked UHMWPE leads to a decrease in modulus compared to the uncros-slinked UHMWPE even when their overall degree of crystallinity, measured by differential scanning calorimeter, is identical (101). One possible method to restore crystallinity in cross-linked UHMWPE is to utilize high pressure crystallization on the crosslinked UHMWPE to increase crystallinity (102). In fact, the high pressures used in the Hylamer process, could also be used to substantially increase the crystallinity of radiation crosslinked UHMWPE, with the potential for a high resistance to fatigue crack propagation and a high

Table 1 Summary of Fatigue Crack Inception Measurements for UHMWPE Resins with Four Process Conditions: Conventional UHMWPE (PE), UHMWPE Cross-Linked with 50 kGy Gamma Irradiation and Subsequently Melted and Annealed (XPE), Conventional UHMWPE Subjected to 180°C and 300 MPa Pressure (HP-PE), and Cross-Linked UHMWPE Subjected to 240°C and 500 MPa Pressure (HP-XPE). Cross-Linking and Enhanced Crystallinity via High-Pressure Methods to Improve the Mechanical Properties of UHMWPE

Material/Property	PE	HP-PE	X-linked	HP-X-linked
Processing conditions	0 kGy	0 kGy, 180°C, 300 MPa	50 kGy	50 kGy, 240°C, 500 MPa
Crystallinity (%)	50.2	70.9	46.2	67.5
Lamellae thickness (nm)	28.1	131.2	23.1	50.6
Ultimate true tensile strength (MPa) (SD)	231.1 (10.1)	78.8 (10.0)	157.7 (11.2)	167.8 (20.8)
Ultimate strain (%) (SD)	375 (7.1)	230 (21.6)	317 (31.5)	325 (23.8)
Yield strength (MPa) (SD)	21.3 (0.19)	23.4 (0.28)	19.0 (0.17)	20.6 (0.42)
Elastic Modulus (MPa) (SD)	495 (14.0)	675 (19.8)	334 (7.8)	695 (5.1)
ΔKth^* (MPa$\sqrt{m}$) (SD)	1.14 (0.22)	1.57 (0.23)	0.82 (0.25)	1.03 (0.25)

Abbreviations: UHMWPE, ultra high molecular weight polyethylene; HP-PE, high pressure polyethylene.
Source: From Ref. 100.

resistance to creep deformation associated with Hylamer. A recent study by Simis et al. (102) investigated the coupled effects of cross-linking and enhanced crystallinity via high-pressure methods to improve the mechanical properties of UHMWPE. This tailored microstructure provided a material with good wear resistance due to the cross-linking and improved fatigue resistance due to higher crystallinity and larger lamellae. Table 1 provides a summary of the fatigue crack inception values for a range of processing conditions. It is clear that high-pressure processes improve fatigue crack propagation resistance for both conventional and highly cross-linked UHMWPE. Figure 10 shows the corresponding wear factors measured for the same material groups. These material developments are especially important for TKRs where high cyclic stresses can lead to fatigue wear mechanisms. Such a process followed by nonionizing sterilization methods (gas plasma, ethylene oxide) would induce the beneficial properties of Hylamer in radiation cross-linked UHMWPE without the problem of high susceptibility to oxidative degradation.

Another method that is currently being explored is to infiltrate UHMWPE with Vitamin E, which is a radical scavenger (103). This has two advantages: (i) Vitamin E would prevent long-term oxidation associated

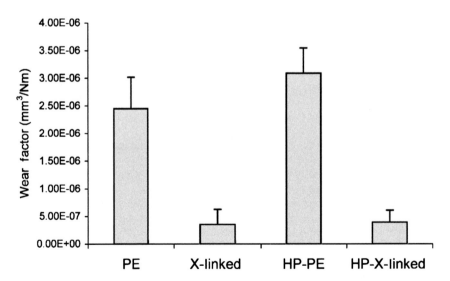

Figure 10 Wear factors for UHMWPE resins with 4 process conditions: conventional UHMWPE (PE), UHMWPE cross-linked with 50 kGy gamma irradiation and subsequently melted and annealed (X-linked), conventional UHMWPE subjected to 180°C and 300 MPa pressure (HP-PE), and cross-linked UHMWPE subjected to 240°C and 500 MPa pressure (HP-X-linked), cross-linking and enhanced crystallinity via high-pressure methods to improve the mechanical properties of UHMWPE (100). *Abbreviations*: UHMWPE, ultra high molecular weight polyethylene; HP-PE, high pressure polyethylene. *Source*: From Ref. 100.

with the presence of free radicals, and (ii) the presence of Vitamin E has shown to increase fatigue crack resistance of cross-linked UHMWPEs. However, biocompatibility studies of Vitamin E and the degradation products of Vitamin E after radical scavenging must be conducted prior to its implementation in TJR prostheses. Other approaches are currently under investigation to increase the fatigue crack growth resistance of radiation cross-linked UHMWPE so that its superior resistance to wear can also be accompanied by superior mechanical properties.

ACKNOWLEDGMENT

The LVSEM images of Figures 4 and 5, and DSC data presented in Figure 6 were collected and provided by Mary Beth Turell. Figure 11 was provided by Lou Matrisciano, Poly Hi Solidur Inc.

REFERENCES

1. Charnley J, Low Friction Arthroplasty of the Hip: Theory and Practice. Berlin: Springer, 1979.
2. Li S, Burstein AH. Current concepts review: ultra-high molecular weight polyethylene. J Bone Joint Surg 1994; 76-A:1080–1090.
3. Kurtz SM. The UHMWPE Handbook: Principles and Clinical Applications in Total Joint Replacement. Amsterdam: Elsevier Academic Press, 2004.
4. Charnley J. Arthroplasty of the hip: a new operation. Lancet 1961; I:1129–1132.
5. Waugh W, John Charnley. The Man and the Hip. London: Springer, 1990.
6. Charnley J. Tissue reaction to the polytetrafuoroethylene. Lancet 1963; II:1379.
7. Total Hip Replacement. NIH Consensus Statement 1994; 12(5):1–31.
8. Willert HG. Reactions of the articular capsule to wear products of artificial joint prostheses. J Biomed Mater Res 1977; 11(2):157–164.
9. Dannenmaier WC, Haynes DW, Nelson CL. Granulomatous reaction and cystic bony destruction associated with high wear rate in a total knee prosthesis. Clin Orthop 1985; 198:224–230.
10. Howie DW. Tissue response in relation to type of wear particles around failed hip arthroplasties. J Arthroplasty 1990; 5(4):337–348.
11. Peters PC Jr, Engh GA, Dwyer KA, Vinh TN. Osteolysis after total knee arthroplasty without cement. J Bone Joint Surg Am 1992; 74(6):864–876.
12. Maguire JKJ, Coscia MF, Lynch MH. Foreign body reaction to polymeric debris following total hip arthroplasty. Clin Orthop 1987; 216:213–223.
13. Santavirta S, Konttinen YT, Hoikka V, Eskola A. Immunopathological response to loose cementless acetabular components. J Bone Joint Surg Br. 1991; 73(1):38–42.
14. McKellop HA, Campbell P, Park SH, Schmalzried TP, Grigoris P, Amstutz HC, Sarmiento A. The origin of submicron polyethylene wear debris in total hip arthroplasty. Clin Orthop 1995; 311:3–20.
15. Wright TM, Rimnac CM, Stulberg SD, Mintz L, Tsao AK, Klein RW, McCrae C. Wear of polyethylene in total joint replacements. Observations from retrieved PCA knee implants. Clin Orthop 1992; (276):126–134.

16. Landy MM, Walker PS. Wear of ultra-high-molecular-weight polyethylene components of 90 retrieved knee prostheses. J Arthroplasty 1988(suppl 3): S73–S85.

17. Hirakawa K, Bauer TW, Stulberg BN, Wilde AH. Comparison and quantitation of wear debris of failed total hip and total knee arthroplasty. J Biomed Mater Res 1996; 31(2):257–263.

18. Shanbhag AS, Bailey HO, Hwang DS, Cha CW, Eror NG, Rubash HE. Quantitative analysis of ultrahigh molecular weight polyethylene (UHMWPE) wear debris associated with total knee replacements. J Biomed Mater Res 2000; 53(1):100–110.

19. Ramamurti BS, Bragdon CR, O'Connor DO, Lowenstein JD, Jasty M, Estok DM, Harris WH. Loci of movement of selected points on the femoral head during normal gait. Three-dimensional computer simulation. J Arthroplasty 1996; 11(7):845–852.

20. Morscher EW, Hefti A, Aebi U. Severe osteolysis after third-body wear due to hydroxyapatite particles from acetabular cup coating. J Bone Joint Surg Br 1998; 80(2):267–272.

21. McKellop H, Shen FW, DiMaio W, Lancaster JG. Wear of gamma-cross-linked polyethylene acetabular cups against roughened femoral balls. Clin Orthop 1999; 369:73–82.

22. Minakawa H, Stone MH, Wroblewski BM, Lancaster JG, Ingham E, Fisher J. Quantification of third-body damage and its effect on UHMWPE wear with different types of femoral head. J Bone Joint Surg Br 1998; 80(5):894–899.

23. Que L, Topoleski LD. Third-body wear of cobalt–chromium–molybdenum implant alloys initiated by bone and poly(methyl methacrylate) particles. J Biomed Mater Res 2000; 50(3):322–330.

24. Affatato S, Bersaglia G, Foltran I, Taddei P, Fini G, Toni A. The performance of gamma- and EtO-sterilised UHWMPE acetabular cups tested under severe simulator conditions. Part 1: role of the third-body wear process. Biomaterials 2002; 23(24):4839–4846.

25. Yamaguchi M, Bauer TW, Hashimoto Y. Three-dimensional analysis of multiple wear vectors in retrieved acetabular cups. J Bone Joint Surg Am 1997; 79(10):1539–1544.

26. Wroblewski BM. Direction and rate of socket wear in Charnley low-friction arthroplasty. J Bone Joint Surg Br 1985; 67(5):757–761.

27. Wroblewski BM, Lynch M, Atkinson JR, Dowson D, Isaac GH. External wear of the polyethylene socket in cemented total hip arthroplasty. J Bone Joint Surg Br 1987; 69(1):61–63.

28. Scifert CF, Brown TD, Pedersen DR, Heiner AD, Callaghan JJ. Development and Physical Validation of a Finite Element Model of Total Hip Dislocation. Comput Methods Biomech Biomed Engin 1999; 2(2):139–147.

29. Callaghan JJ, Brown TD, Pedersen DR, Johnston RC. Choices and compromises in the use of small head sizes in total hip arthroplasty. Clin Orthop 2002; 405:144–149.

30. Barrack RL, Burke DW, Cook SD, Skinner HB, Harris WH. Complications related to modularity of total hip components. J Bone Joint Surg Br 1993; 75(5):688–692.

31. Collier JP, Mayor MB, McNamara JL, Surprenant VA, Jensen RE. Analysis of the failure of 122 polyethylene inserts from uncemented tibial knee components. Clin Orthop 1991; 273:232–242.

32. Mintz L, Tsao AK, McCrae CR, Stulberg SD, Wright T. The arthroscopic evaluation and characteristics of severe polyethylene wear in total knee arthroplasty. Clin Orthop 1991; 273:215–222.

33. Kilgus DJ, Moreland JR, Finerman GA, Funahashi TT, Tipton JS. Catastrophic wear of tibial polyethylene inserts. Clin Orthop 1991; 273:223–231.

34. Bartel DL, Bicknell VL, Wright TM. The effect of conformity, thickness, and material on stresses in ultra-high molecular weight components for total joint replacement. J Bone Joint Surg Am 1986; 68(7):1041–1051.

35. Bartel DL, Burstein AH, Toda MD, Edwards DL. The effect of conformity and plastic thickness on contact stresses in metal-backed plastic implants. J Biomech Eng 1985; 107(3):193–199.

36. Bartel DL, Rawlinson JJ, Burstein AH, Ranawat CS, Flynn WF, Jr. Stresses in polyethylene components of contemporary total knee replacements. Clin Orthop 1995; 317:76–82.

37. Jin ZM, Dowson D, Fisher J. A parametric analysis of the contact stress in ultra-high molecular weight polyethylene acetabular cups. Med Eng Phys 1994; 16(5):398–405.

38. McNamara JL, Collier JP, Mayor MB, Jensen RE. A comparison of contact pressures in tibial and patellar total knee components before and after service in vivo. Clin Orthop 1994; 299:104–113.

39. Takeuchi T, Lathi VK, Khan AM, Hayes WC. Patellofemoral contact pressures exceed the compressive yield strength of UHMWPE in total knee arthroplasties. J Arthroplasty 1995; 10(3):363–368.

40. Star MJ, Kaufman KR, Irby SE, Colwell CWJ. The effects of patellar thickness on patellofemoral forces after resurfacing. Clin Orthop 1996; 322:279–284.

41. Buechel FF, Pappas MJ, Makris G. Evaluation of contact stress in metal-backed patellar replacements. A predictor of survivorship. Clin Orthop 1991; (273):190–197.

42. Trossarelli L, Brunella V. Polyethylene: Discovery and growth. In: Costa L, Brach del Prever EM, Bracco P, eds. In: UHMWPE for arthroplasty: from synthesis to implant. Turin, Italy: University of Turin, 2003:6–18.

43. Kurtz SM, Muratoglu OK, Evans M, Edidin AA. Advances in the processing, sterilization, and crosslinking of ultra-high molecular weight polyethylene for total joint arthroplasty. Biomaterials 1999; 20(18):1659–1688.

44. Wrona M, Mayor MB, Collier JP, Jensen RE. The correlation between fusion defects and damage in tibial polyethylene bearings. Clin Orthop 1994; 299: 92–103.

45. Hamilton JV, Wang HC, Sung C. The effect of fusion defects on the mechanical properties of UHMWPE. Transactions of the 5th World Biomaterials Congress, 1996; 511.

46. Schmidt MB, Hamilton JV. The effects of calcium stearate on the properties of UHMWPE. Transactions of the 42nd Annual Meeting of the Orthopaedic Research Society, 1996; 22.

47. Swarts D, Gsell R, King R, Devanathan D, Wallace S, Lin S. Aging of calcium stearate—free polyethylene. Transaction of the 5th World Biomaterials Congress, 1996; 196.

48. Weightman B, Light D. A comparison of RCH 1000 and Hi-Fax 1900 ultra-high molecular weight polyethylenes. Biomaterials 1985; 6(3):177–183.

49. Turell MB, Bellare A. A study of the nanostructure and tensile properties of ultra-high molecular weight polyethylene. Biomaterials 2004; 25(17):3389–3398.

50. Hoffman JD, Miller RL. Kinetics of crystallization from the melt and chain folding in polyethylene fractions revisited: theory and experiment. Polymer 1997; 38(13):3151–3212.

51. Rastogi S, Kurelec L, Lemstra PJ. Chain mobility in polymer systems: on the borderline between solid and melt. 2. Crystal size influence in phase transition and sintering of ultrahigh molecular weight polyethylene via the mobile hexagonal phase. Macromolecules 1998; 31:5022–5031.

52. Bellare A, Schnablegger H, Cohen RE. A small-angle x-ray scattering study of high-density polyethylene and ultra-high molecular weight polyethylene. Macromolecules 1995; 17:2325–2333.

53. Olley RH, Hodge AH, Bassett DC. A permanganic etchant for polyolefins. J Polym Sci Polym Phys Ed 1979; 17:627–643.

54. McKellop H, Shen FW, Lu B, Campbell P, Salovey R. Effect of sterilization method and other modifications on the wear resistance of acetabular cups made of ultra-high molecular weight polyethylene. A hip-simulator study. J Bone Joint Surg Am 2000; 82-A(12):1708–1725.

55. Pienkowski D, Jacob R, Hoglin D, Saum K, Kaufer H, Nicholls PJ. Low-voltage scanning electron microscopic imaging of ultrahigh-molecular-weight polyethylene. J Biomed Mater Res 1995; 29(10):1167–1174.

56. Olley RH, Hosier IL, Bassett DC, Smith NG. On morphology of consolidated UHMWPE resin in hip cups. Biomaterials 1999; 20(21):2037–2046.

57. Gul RM, McGarry FJ, Bragdon CR, Muratoglu OK, Harris WH. Effect of consolidation on adhesive and abrasive wear of ultra high molecular weight polyethylene. Biomaterials 2003; 24(19):3193–3199.

58. Cook JTE, Klein PG, Ward IM, Brain AA, Farrar DF, Rose J. The morphology of nascent and moulded ultra-high molecular weight polyethylene. Insights from solid-state NMR, nitric acid etching, GPC and DSC. Polymer 2000; 41:8615–8623.

59. Bellare A, Cohen RE. Morphology of rod stock and compression-moulded sheets of ultra-high-molecular-weight polyethylene used in orthopaedic implants. Biomaterials 1996; 17(24):2325–2333.

60. Premnath V, Harris WH, Jasty M, Merrill EW. Gamma sterilization of UHMWPE articular implants: an analysis of the oxidation problem. Ultra High Molecular Weight Poly Ethylene. Biomaterials 1996; 17(18):1741–1753.

61. Bhateja SK. Changes in the crystalline content of irradiated linear polyethylenes upon ageing. Polymer 1982; 23:654–655.

62. Bhateja SK. Radiation-induced crystallinity changes in pressure-crystallized ultra high molecular weight polyethylene. J Macromol Sci—Phys 1983; B22(1):159–168.

63. Bhateja SK. Radiation-induced crystallinity changes in linear polyethylene: influence of aging. J Appl Polym Sci 1983; 28:861–872.
64. Bhateja SK, Andrews EH, Young RJ. Radiation-induced crystallinity changes in linear polyethylene. J Polym Sci Polym Phys Ed 1983; 21:523–536.
65. Bhateja SK, Andrews EH. Radiation-induced crystallinity changes in polyethylene blends. J Mater Sci 1985; 20:2839–2845.
66. Bhateja SK, Andrews EH, Yarbrough SM. Radiation induced crystallinity changes in linear polyethylenes: long term aging effects. Polym J 1989; 21(9):739–750.
67. Costa L, Luda MP, Trossarelli L, Brach del Prever EM, Crova M, Gallinaro P. In vivo UHMWPE biodegradation of retrieved prosthesis. Biomaterials 1998; 19(15):1371–1385.
68. Costa L, Luda MP, Trossarelli L, Brach del Prever EM, Crova M, Gallinaro P. Oxidation in orthopaedic UHMWPE sterilized by gamma-radiation and ethylene oxide. Biomaterials 1998; 19(7–9):659–668.
69. Costa L, Jacobson K, Bracco P, Brach del Prever EM. Oxidation of orthopaedic UHMWPE. Biomaterials 2002; 23(7):1613–1624.
70. Nusbaum HJ, Rose RM. The effects of radiation sterilization on the properties of ultra high molecular weight polyethylene. J Biomed Mater Res 1979; 13:557–576.
71. Shinde A, Salovey R. Irradiation of ultra-high-molecular-weight polyethylene. J Polym Sci Polym Phys Ed 1985; 23:1681–1689.
72. Roe R-J, Grood ES, Shastri R, Gosselin CA, Noyes FR. Effect of radiation sterilization and aging on ultrahigh molecular weight polyethylene. Journal of Biomedical Materials Research 1981; 15:209–230.
73. Birkinshaw C, Buggy M, Daly S, O'Neill M. Mechanism of ageing in irradiated polymers. Polymer Degradation and Stability 1988; 22:285–294.
74. Birkinshaw C, Buggy M, Daly S, O'Neill M. The effect of gamma radiation on the physical structure and mechanical properties of ultrahigh molecular weight polyethylene. Journal of Applied Polymer Science 1989; 38:1967–1973.
75. Pruitt L, Ranganathan R. Effect of sterilization on the structure and fatigue resistance of medical grade UHMWPE. Mater Sci Eng c-biomimet Mater Sensors Sys 1995; c3:91–93.
76. Bostrom MP, Bennett AP, Rimnac CM, Wright TM. The natural history of ultra high molecular weight polyethylene. Clin Orthop 1994; 309:20–28.
77. Sutula LC, Collier JP, Saum KA, Currier BH, Currier JH, Sanford WM, Mayor MB, Wooding RE, Sperling DK, Williams IR, et al. The Otto Aufranc Award. Impact of gamma sterilization on clinical performance of polyethylene in the hip. Clin Orthop 1995; 319:28–40.
78. Pruitt L, Ranganathan R. Effect of sterilization on the structure and fatigue resistance of medical grade UHMWPE. Mater Sci Eng c-Biomimet Mater Sensors Syst 1995; c3(2):91–93.
79. Brach del Prever E, Crova M, Costa L, Dallera A, Camino G, Gallinaro P. Unacceptable biodegradation of polyethylene in vivo. Biomaterials 1996; 17(9):873–878.
80. Costa L, Brach del Prever E, eds. UHMWPE for Arthroplasty: Characterisation, sterilisation and degradation. Torino: Edizioni Minerva Medica; 2000.

81. Besong AA, Tipper JL, Ingham E, Stone MH, Wroblewski BM, Fisher J. Quantitative comparison of wear debris from UHMWPE that has and has not been sterilised by gamma irradiation. J Bone Joint Surg Br 1998; 80(2):340–344.

82. Wright TM, Fukubayashi T, Burstein AH. The effect of carbon fiber reinforcement on contact area, contact pressure, and time-dependent deformation in polyethylene tibial components. J Biomed Mater Res 1981; 15(5):719–730.

83. McKellop H, Clarke I, Markolf K, Amstutz H. Friction and wear properties of polymer, metal, and ceramic prosthetic joint materials evaluated on a multi-channel screening device. J Biomed Mater Res 1981; 15(5):619–653.

84. Li S, Howard EGJ; DuPont De Nemours & Co., assignee. Process of manufacturing ultra high molecular weight polyethylene shaped articles. US patent # 5037928. DuPont De Nemours, Wilmington, DE 1991.

85. Baker DA, Hastings RS, Pruitt L. Study of fatigue resistance of chemical and radiation crosslinked medical grade ultra high molecular weight polyethylene. J Biomed Mater Res 1999; 46(4):573–581.

86. Champion AR, Li S, Saum K, Howard E, Simmons W. The effect of crystallinity on the physical properties of UHMWPE. 1994; 585.

87. Chmell MJ, Poss R, Thomas WH, Sledge CB. Early failure of Hylamer acetabular inserts due to eccentric wear. J Arthroplasty 1996; 11(3):351–353.

88. Livingston BJ, Chmell MJ, Spector M, Poss R. Complications of total hip arthroplasty associated with the use of an acetabular component with a Hylamer liner. J Bone Joint Surg Am 1997; 79(10):1529–1538.

89. King R, Kirkpatrick L, Devanathan D, Lin S, Krebs S, Rohr W. Long-term aging of implant grades of polyethylene. 1996; 196.

90. Yamauchi K, Hasegawa Y, Iwasada S, Sakano S, Kitamura S, Warashina H, Iwata H. Head penetration into Hylamer acetabular liner sterilized by gamma irradiation in air and in a nitrogen atmosphere. J Arthroplasty 2001; 16(4):463–470.

91. Collier JP, Bargmann LS, Currier BH, Mayor MB, Currier JH, Bargmann BC. An analysis of hylamer and polyethylene bearings from retrieved acetabular components. Orthopedics 1998; 21(8):865–871.

92. Grobbelaar CJ, Du Plessis TA, Marais F. The radiation improvement of polyethylene prostheses: a preliminary study. J Bone Joint Surg 1978; 60:370–374.

93. Oonishi H, Ishimaru H, Kato A. Effect of cross-linkage by gamma radiation in heavy doses to low wear polyethylene in total hip prostheses. J Mater Sci Mater Med 1996; 7:753–763.

94. Oonishi H, Kadoya Y. Wear of high-dose gamma-irradiated polyethylene in total hip replacements. J Orthop Sci 2000; 5(3):223–228.

95. McKellop H, Shen FW, Lu B, Campbell P, Salovey R. Development of an extremely wear-resistant ultra high molecular weight polyethylene for total hip replacements. J Orthop Res 1999; 17(2):157–167.

96. Muratoglu OK, Bragdon CR, O'Connor DO, Jasty M, Harris WH. A novel method of cross-linking ultra-high-molecular-weight polyethylene to improve wear, reduce oxidation, and retain mechanical properties. Recipient of the 1999 HAP Paul Award. J Arthroplasty 2001; 16(2):149–160.

97. Wang A, Essner A, Polineni VK, Stark C, Dumbleton JH. Lubrication and wear of ultra-high molecular weight polyethylene in total joint replacements. Tribology International 1998; 31(1–3):17–33.
98. Muratoglu OK, Bragdon CR, O'Connor DO, Jasty M, Harris WH, Gul R, McGarry F. Unified wear model for highly crosslinked ultra-high molecular weight polyethylenes (UHMWPE). Biomaterials 1999; 20(16):1463–1470.
99. Baker DA, Bellare A, Pruitt L. The effects of degree of cross-linking on the fatigue crack initiation and propagation resistance of orthopedic-grade polyethylene. J Biomed Mater Res 2003; 66A(1):146–154.
100. Krzypow D, Bensusan J, Sevo K, Haggard W, Parr J, Goldberg V, Rimnac C. The fatigue crack propagation resistance of gamma radiation or peroxide crosslinked UHMW polyethylene. 2000; 382.
101. Gomoll A, Wanich T, Bellare A. J-integral fracture toughness and tearing modulus measurement of radiation cross-linked UHMWPE. J Orthop Res 2002; 20(6):1152–1156.
102. Simis KS, Pruitt LA, Bistolfi A, Bellare A. Fatigue behavior of crosslinked UHMWPE with high crystallinity. 2003; 1471.
103. Oral E, Wannomae KK, Hawkins N, Harris WH, Muratoglu OK. Alpha-tocopherol-doped irradiated UHMWPE for high fatigue resistance and low wear. Biomaterials 2004; 25(24):5515–5522.

25

Improving UHMWPE Using Electron Beam Irradiation

Orhun K. Muratoglu and William H. Harris

Department of Orthopaedic Surgery, Orthopaedic Biomechanics and Biomaterials Laboratory, Massachusetts General Hospital, Harvard Medical School, Boston, Massachusetts, U.S.A.

INTRODUCTION

Ultra high molecular weight polyethylene[a] has been the material of choice for bearing surfaces used in total hip and knee arthroplasty for 40 years and polyethylene has been successfully used in acetabular components, tibial inserts, and patella buttons. Yet there are certain in vivo damage mechanisms associated with this material that can compromise device performance.

In total hip replacements (THR), the primary failure mechanism is the periprosthetic osteolysis secondary to particulate debris, which often results in loosening, massive bone loss, or pathologic fractures. Particulate debris is primarily generated by the adhesive and abrasive wear of polyethylene acetabular components. Recently, periprosthetic osteolysis secondary to particulate debris has been recognized as an important factor contributing to clinical failure in total knee replacement (TKR) as well (5,12). The amount

---

[a] In the remainder of this chapter ultra high molecular weight polyethylene (polyethylene) will be referred to as polyethylene.

of bone loss in some circumstances in TKR is extensive, leading to component loosening or fracture (43). Unfortunately, revision surgery in these cases is made particularly difficult, often necessitating the use of special augments to the components and bone allografts (44).

Adhesive wear of polyethylene, the main mechanism of particulate debris generation, is initiated by the orientation and strain hardening of the polyethylene surface. With implant motion, adhesive wear results in the removal of small wear debris, usually on the order of a few micrometers or less in size. There is a higher frequency of somewhat larger size debris (>1 μm) in total knee patients (18,46,48). This increase in size and irregularity of the shape of the particles is thought to decrease the biological activity of the particles and result in a reduced rate of osteolysis in the total knee compared with total hip.

Another mechanism of particulate debris generation is abrasive wear, which occurs through the rubbing action of the hard asperities on the surface of the femoral component. It is also enhanced by hard third body particles, such as bone chips or bone cement particles, entering the articulation. Abrasive wear progresses by the cutting and removal of the soft polyethylene articular surface.

Delamination is another polyethylene failure mechanism, which primarily occurs in polyethylene tibial inserts and patella components of TKR. Delamination is initiated by reduction in the mechanical properties of polyethylene that results from oxidation secondary to gamma sterilization. Oxidation leads to the embrittlement of the components, which act as a precursor to subsurface cracks. These cracks propagate to the articulating surface, leading to the removal of relatively large (>0.5 mm) flake-like debris. Delamination can rapidly lead to a loss of geometric conformity at the articulation, disrupting the intended load distribution in the total joint, and eventually resulting in implant failure through disengagement, fracture, or complete wear-through of the polyethylene component.

Therefore, improvements in adhesive/abrasive wear, delamination, and oxidation resistance of polyethylene would enhance device performance in vivo in both THR and TKR.

SOLUTIONS TO POLYETHYLENE OXIDATION AND WEAR

There are a number of solutions that address the traditional gamma sterilization induced oxidation of polyethylene. Material factors such as resin type and consolidation methods have been reported to affect the oxidation resistance of polyethylene (13,25,55). The use of Himont 1900 resin in combination with direct compression molding has been shown to have superior resistance to delamination when compared to other resin and manufacturing methods. Direct compression molded Himont 1900 polyethylene resin has been used in the conforming posterior-stabilized Insall-Burstein I (IB-I)[b] (13), anatomic graduated component (AGC)[c] with a less conforming flat-on-flat design (11), as well as in the less conforming Miller–Galante I (MG-I)[b] knee prostheses (55).

The delamination in the surgically retrieved polyethylene tibial inserts with the IB-I, AGC, and MG-I designs was near to absent over the first 10 years of in vivo use (11,13,42,50,55). With a wide variation in articular surface conformity, these designs all exhibited a high resistance to delamination in vivo because of the increased oxidation resistance of direct compression molded Himont 1900 resin.

Other solutions to reduce long-term oxidation and thus the incidence of delamination in tibial inserts in vivo include both the sterilization with gamma radiation and storage in an inert environment or alternatively sterilization with ethylene oxide gas. The former sterilization method leads to the formation of residual free radicals but prevents oxidation during irradiation and subsequent storage by keeping the implant free of exposure to oxygen. As a result, oxidation is delayed until the polyethylene component is implanted. While the rate and extent of in vivo oxidation is not known, this sterilization method is expected to delay oxidation and related damage mechanisms, such as delamination, of the polyethylene components.

Ethylene oxide sterilization does not alter the molecular structure of polyethylene and does not produce free radicals. As a result, in the long-term oxidation is not expected to occur in polyethylene components sterilized with this method. This effect was demonstrated by Williams et al. (54), who reported on 1603 tibial knee inserts that had been gamma sterilized in air with an average in vivo duration of 57 months and 32 inserts that had been sterilized with ethylene oxide gas with an average in vivo duration of 115 months. Fifty-five percent of the former group showed evidence of delamination, while none of the latter group appeared to have delamination type damage. The absence of delamination is anticipated to correlate with low levels of oxidation. However, while ethylene oxide gas sterilization prevents long-term oxidation in polyethylene components, its wear resistance is less than the same material after gamma sterilization.

The key method to improve polyethylene wear resistance is to generate a highly crosslinked network structure. There are three long-term reports by various investigators who studied the effect of increased crosslink density on the in vivo performance of polyethylene acetabular components. The methods used included crosslinking polyethylene with high dose (100 Mrad) gamma radiation in air (37,49) with gamma radiation (10 Mrad) in the presence of acetylene gas (10,14,15), and with silane chemistry (56).

---

[b] Zimmer, Warsaw, Indiana, U.S.A.

[c] Biomet, Warsaw, Indiana, U.S.A.

Retrospective clinical studies of these three series demonstrated marked improvement in wear behavior of these highly crosslinked polyethylenes. The radiographic wear measurements of Oonishi et al. (37) showed a decreased average rate of femoral head penetration (0.072–0.076 mm/yr) for the 100 Mrad-irradiated polyethylene, in comparison with the control polyethylene (0.098–0.25 mm/yr) that had been gamma sterilized in air. Grobbelaar et al. (15) reported on two different clinical follow-up series with polyethylene that had been gamma irradiated (10 Mrad) in the presence of acetylene gas. The first is a 14–22 year follow-up (average 15.5 years) of 62 patients showing no measurable wear in 56 cases and a total of 1.0–4.0 mm linear penetration in eight cases. The average wear rate of this series was about 0.011 mm/yr. The second series was a 13–22 year follow-up (average 15.5 years) of 39 patients with no measurable wear in 30 cases and a total of 0.7–1.5 mm linear penetration in nine cases. Among these 103 hips (one bilateral case) combined no wear was detectable in 83% at an average of 15.5 years. Wroblewski et al. (56) reported on the wear behavior of 22-mm diameter, silane crosslinked high-density polyethylene acetabular components. The clinical and joint simulator studies of Wroblewski and colleagues showed remarkable agreement in the wear rates of the crosslinked polymer. After an initial "bedding-in" penetration of 0.2–0.4 mm with an average penetration rate of 0.29 mm/yr, presumably representing creep, the subsequent average penetration rate (or wear rate) decreased by an order of magnitude to 0.02 mm/yr, presumably representing wear. Mean clinical follow-up was 10 years and 6 months, with a total of 14 patients.

There are several contemporary approaches to crosslink polyethylene for improved wear resistance. These differ in some ways from the aforementioned historical examples. Today radiation chemistry is the preferred method of crosslinking and silane chemistry is not used. In addition, postirradiation thermal treatment steps are used in an effort to reduce the residual free radicals and improve the long-term oxidative stability.

A contemporary solution to polyethylene wear and oxidation is electron beam irradiation and melting. Irradiation crosslinks the polyethylene molecules and leads to the formation of residual free radicals. Subsequent melting quenches the residual free radicals to prevent their long-term oxidative effects. Crosslink density of polyethylene increases with increasing radiation dose level used in the electron beam irradiation process (34). The absence of detectable residual free radicals achieved through the postirradiation melting greatly diminishes the long-term oxidation of polyethylene and is expected to improve the delamination resistance especially in TKRs.

BASICS OF RADIATION CHEMISTRY OF POLYETHYLENE

The exposure of polyethylene to ionizing radiation leads to chain scission and crosslinking. Chain scission is a result of carbon–hydrogen bond cleavage.

Crosslinking is the product of the recombination of two free radicals, which are formed by carbon–carbon or carbon–hydrogen bond cleavage as shown in Figure 1. Chain scission reduces the molecular weight and leads to the degradation of the polymer. Crosslinking is the primary reaction that competes with chain scission. The number of the crosslinking reactions is about three times larger than that of chain scission in polyethylene (3,16). As a result, the net effect of ionizing radiation on polyethylene is predominantly crosslinking.

Crosslinking reactions, i.e., free radical recombination, take place mainly in the amorphous phase of the polymer, where the molecules are in close enough proximity to allow the formation of the interchain carbon–carbon bond that constitutes the crosslink (9,26). In the crystalline phase, because of the increased distance between the molecules, crosslinking is not favored. Therefore, free radicals generated in the crystalline regions

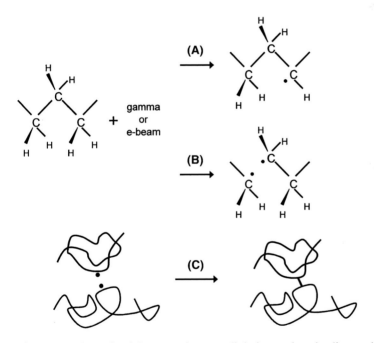

Figure 1 Schematic of the two primary radiolytic reactions leading to the formation of (**A**) primary free radicals and (**B**) chain scission. The primary free radicals are formed by the cleavage of a carbon–hydrogen bond, which also liberates a hydrogen free radical. The hydrogen-free radicals readily recombine with each other, form hydrogen gas, and diffuse out of the polymer. Chain scission is the consequence of the cleavage of the carbon–carbon bond along the backbone of the molecule. The majority of primary free radicals shown in (**A**) react with each other to form crosslinks as shown in (**C**).

are postulated not to take part in the crosslinking reactions (19,23,41). Instead these free radicals migrate along the backbone of the chain and become trapped, primarily in the crystalline/amorphous interfaces. These are the *residual* free radicals and are known to initiate oxidation-induced embrittlement in polyethylene.

A cascade of events involving the residual free radicals leads to the oxidation and eventual embrittlement of polyethylene. Residual free radicals generated by the ionizing radiation react with oxygen and form peroxy free radicals, which readily form hydroperoxides by abstracting a hydrogen atom from a nearby chain. The abstraction of hydrogen produces a new free radical, which, in turn, takes part in the oxidation cascade. The hydroperoxides are unstable and decay into carbonyl species, mainly ketones and acids. The formation of acids reduces the molecular weight of the polymer leading to recrystallization, increase in stiffness, and embrittlement of the component.

The necessity of the elimination of residual free radical subsequent to irradiation to avoid the significant adverse effects of the residual free radicals on polyethylene is now widely recognized (28,33,34). The most effective method is to raise the temperature of polyethylene above its peak melting transition (about 137°C) to eliminate the crystalline domains and liberate the trapped, residual free radicals. This allows the rapid removal of the residual free radicals through recombination reactions. Another method for reducing the residual free radical concentration of irradiated polyethylene is to anneal below its peak melting transition. But because the polyethylene will only be partially molten at the annealing temperature, this method only leads to a partial reduction of the residual free radicals through a series of recombination reactions.

While the cascade of events that leads to the formation of crosslinks and residual free radicals is identical for both gamma irradiation and electron beam irradiation, there are still important differences between the two irradiation methods, specifically in terms of penetration of the effects of radiation and radiation dose rate achieved. Gamma irradiation sources are commonly based on the artificial isotope of cobalt [^{60}Co] that generates gamma photons. While the penetration of gamma radiation into polyethylene has no practical limitations, the activity level of the gamma source limits the radiation dose rate. With an electron beam irradiator, the radiation is in the form of accelerated, charged particles. The penetration of the effects of electron beam radiation is limited by the kinetic energy of the electron beam, measured in million electron volts (MeV). With a 10 MeV electron beam incident on a polyethylene surface radiation penetrates about 4–4.5 cm depending on temperature. The radiation dose rate that a commercial electron beam accelerator provides is about two orders of magnitude larger than that from a commercial gamma source.

Electron Beam Cross-linked and Melted Polyethylene

There are three types of electron beam irradiated and melted polyethylenes available to the practicing clinician today (Table 1): Durasul™ (Sulzer Orthopaedics, Inc., Austin, TX) used in the fabrication of acetabular liners, tibial inserts, and patella components; Longevity™ (Zimmer, Inc., Warsaw, IN) used in the fabrication of acetabular liners; and Prolong™ (Zimrner, Inc., Warsaw, IN) used in the fabrication of tibial inserts. In all three cases, a polyethylene block is heated to a temperature below the melting point of polyethylene (<137°C) and irradiated at that temperature with a 10 MeV electron beam source. Radiation dose levels used vary between 65 and 100 kGy (6.5 and 10 Mrad) as indicated in Table 1. Subsequent to irradiation, the polyethylene block is melted at around 150°C to eliminate the residual free radicals. The hip and knee implant components are then machined and packaged for sterilization. In all three cases, gas sterilization methods, namely ethylene oxide gas or gas plasma, are used. Unlike gamma sterilization, gas sterilization methods are not known to have long-term adverse effects on the properties of polyethylene. As a result, all three electron beam crosslinked and melted polyethylenes have a crosslinked network structure with no detectable residual free radicals. The former is essential for improved wear resistance and the latter for long-term oxidative stability.

OPTIMUM RADIATION DOSE

Radiation crosslinking not only influences the wear and oxidation resistance but also the mechanical properties of polyethylene. Increasing radiation dose level increases the crosslink density, which results in a decrease in large-strain mechanical properties of polyethylene, namely elongation at break, toughness, and ultimate tensile strength (34). The low strain mechanical properties such as yield strength and elastic modulus of polyethylene depend on the level of crystallinity, which decreases as a result of the post-irradiation melting. The decrease in crystallinity and concomitant decrease in yield strength and elastic modulus are independent of the radiation dose (34). Therefore, the optimization of the radiation dose level involves the maximization of increase in wear resistance and minimization of the changes in the large-strain mechanical properties of polyethylene.

The effect of radiation dose level on the wear rate of two types of electron beam crosslinked and melted polyethylenes is shown in Figure 2. Wear rate decreases with increasing radiation dose level and begins to level off at around 10 Mrad. Above 10 Mrad of radiation dose, the improvement in wear behavior with increasing dose is minimal. Therefore, the benefits of reduction in wear through radiation crosslinking are maximized at a dose level of around 10 Mrad. At 10 Mrad of radiation dose, highly crosslinked

Table 1 The Details of the Processing Steps Used in the Fabrication of the Three Electron Beam Cross-linked and Melted Polyethylenes

Polyethylenes	Manufacturer	Radiation temperature (°C)	Radiation (kGy*)	Radiation type	Postirradiation thermal treatment	Sterilization method	Application
Prolong™	Zimmer	~125	65	E-beam	Melted at 150°C	Gas plasma	Tibial inserts
Durasul™	Sulzer	~120–125	95			EtO	Acetabular liners
							Tibial inserts
							Patellar components
Longevity	Zimmer	~40	100			Gas plasma	Acetabular liners

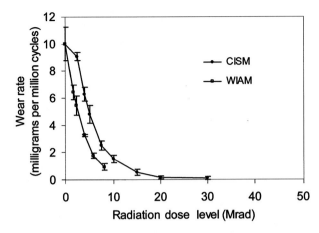

Figure 2 The wear rate of two types of electron beam cross-linked and melted polyethylenes as a function of radiation dose on the bi-directional knee simulator is shown here. One was cold irradiated (room temperature) and subsequently melted (CISM) and the other was warm (125°C) irradiated and subsequently melted (WIAM). In both cases, the wear rate decreased with increasing radiation dose level.

polyethylene still maintains its properties within the ranges that are typical of surgical grade polyethylene. The mechanical properties of polyethylene at this radiation dose level are listed in Table 2 along with the standard ranges of properties required for surgical grade polyethylene resins.

Table 2 Mechanical Properties of the Three Electron Beam Cross-linked and Melted Polyethylenes Along with Typical Minimums Required by National Standards. Note that the Properties of Conventional Polyethylene, when Gamma Sterilized in Air, Decay to Levels Considered Not Suitable for Surgical Grade Polyethylene

	Ultimate tensile strength (MPa)	Yield strength (MPa)	Elongation at break (%)	Izod toughness (kJ/m²)	Tensile modulus (MPa)
Durasul™	30 ± 1	20 ± 0.5	330 ± 25	62 ± 3	660 ± 40
Longevity™	38 ± 3	19 ± 0	262 ± 9	64 ± 2	689 ± 110
Conventional polyethylene	47 ± 4	20 ± 0.5	420 ± 50	100 ± 15	890 ± 100
ASTM F-648 (minimums)	27	19	250	30	NA
ISO 5834–2 (minimums)	27	19	250	25	NA
FDA (range)	27–60	19–26	200–400	NA	600

Abbreviation: NA, not available.

IN VITRO EVIDENCE IN TOTAL HIP

There are numerous in vitro studies comparing the wear behavior of radiation crosslinked and melted polyethylene versus conventional polyethylene (27,29,33–35). The in vitro wear models used in such studies have been developed to closely simulate the in vivo environment in terms of motion, loading profile, lubrication, and polyethylene wear mechanisms. These wear models are built on pin-on-disk wear testers or hip simulators.

Historically, pin-on-disk wear testing has been carried out by rubbing of a pin against a counterface in a unidirectional path. This method of wear testing is adequate for a number of wear couples where the mechanism of wear is independent of the changes in the directionality of the wear path. Pooley and Tabor (39) have shown that with polymers articulating against a hard counterface the frictional force changes with changes in the wear path direction. Their observation indicated that for bearing surface applications where direction of motion varies, wear testing with a unidirectional path may be inadequate. The studies of Jasty et al. (21) on 128 surgically and autopsy-retrieved acetabular liners showed that the surface of the polyethylene undergoes large-strain plastic deformation during in vivo use. In their study, the polyethylene articulating surfaces showed numerous elongated fibrils, primarily oriented in the longitudinal direction of flexion–extension direction. This orientation is expected to result in strain hardening of the surface in the sliding direction, and weakening of the surface in the transverse direction. As a result, wear of polyethylene surface is anticipated to depend on the changes in the directionality of motion, so-called crossing motions, at the articulating interface as was evident from the studies of Pooley and Tabor (39). Ramamurti et al. (40) have shown that crossing motions are present in the human hip and are mostly induced by the abduction/adduction and rotation.

Contemporary pin-on-disk wear models for the study of polyethylene wear as it occurs in the human hip now incorporate a crossing motion pattern. Bragdon et al. (2) have reported on the development of a bi-directional pin-on-disk model where the pin articulates against a counterface following a rectangular wear path. In their study, the wear rate of polyethylene pin articulating against an implant finish cobalt–chrome disk increased by two orders of magnitude (from 0.1 to 10 mg/million cycles) when the wear path was modified from a unidirectional to a bi-directional rectangular one, demonstrating the importance of crossing path in the wear of polyethylene. Using this bi-directional pin-on-disk wear tester, Muratoglu et al. (34) studied the effect of electron beam radiation dose on the wear rate of polyethylene and demonstrated a linear correlation between wear rate and crosslink density of the polyethylene (Fig. 2). Another pin-on-disk model used by Saikko et al. (45) generated the crossing path by translating the pin without rotation against a counterface in a circular path. Wear behavior of one type of electron beam crosslinked and melted polyethylene was studied by Saikko et al. (45) using the bi-circular pin-on-disk machine. That study also showed a marked reduction in the wear rate of polyethylene upon crosslinking even when it was articulating against roughened counterfaces.

Hip simulators, like the new generation pin-on-disk machines, incorporated the essential element of crossing motion. The Boston Hip Simulator (AMTI, Watertown, Massachusetts, U.S.A.) adopted the human hip kinematics to achieve the level and nature of crossing path as it occurs in vivo (Fig. 3). The kinematics is synchronized with a physiologic load profile to better simulate the in vivo conditions. Typically the physiologic load profile is derived from instrumented hip prosthesis studies of Bergmann et al. (1) and Paul (38) with a peak load of 750 pounds. The motions used are usually ±23° of flexion/extension, ±10° of external/internal rotation, and ±8.5° of abduction/adduction adopted from Johnston and Schmidt (22).

A number of investigators reported on the wear behavior of electron beam crosslinked and melted polyethylene using the Boston Hip Simulator (33,35). Figure 4 is an example showing the stark difference between the weight change of acetabular components as a function of simulated gait cycles of conventional versus electron beam crosslinked and melted polyethylene (33,35). The rate of weight loss in these components ranged from 14 ± 2 to 48 ± 5 mg/million cycles with conventional polyethylene articulating against varying femoral head sizes. In contrast, the highly crosslinked polyethylene components initially showed an increase in weight associated by the fluid absorption followed by a near zero steady rate of weight change, regardless of the femoral head size used. Figure 5 shows representative

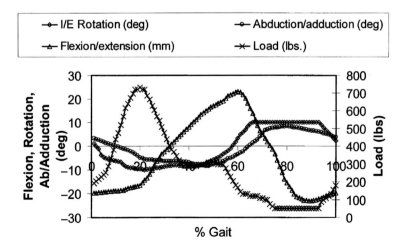

Figure 3 The normal gait kinematics and load profile typically used in the Boston hip simulator.

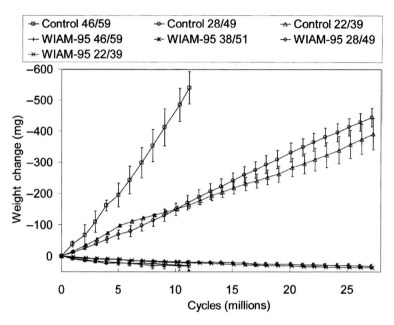

Figure 4 Weight change of polyethylene acetabular liners as a function of simulated gait are shown here. The tests were performed on a 6-station Boston hip simulator. The control liners were manufactured from GUR 1050 polyethylene stock and sterilized with gamma irradiation. Two electron-beam cross-linked and melted polyethylenes were cold irradiated (room temperature) and subsequently melted (CISM) or warm (125°C) irradiated and subsequently melted (WIAM). Control liners exhibited a steady wear rate, which increased with increasing head size while the wear with the WIAM and CISM liners were not measurable.

micrographs of the articulating surfaces at the dome of the acetabular components at different stages of the hip simulator test. The machining marks present on the surfaces of the highly crosslinked polyethylene liners (Fig. 5A) persisted even after 27 million cycles of simulated gait while the machining marks on the surfaces of conventional liners were polished away in less than 0.5 million cycles.

Today, electron beam crosslinked and melted polyethylene acetabular components are widely used in total hip arthroplasty. Components are available to be used with conventional femoral head sizes of 22, 28, and 32 mm as well as larger femoral head sizes of 36, 38, and 44 mm (35). The use of larger femoral head sizes is made possible by the advance of the electron beam crosslinked and melted polyethylene, which addressed the adhesive wear problem. The advantages of larger head sizes are improved stability, reduced rate of dislocations, and improved range of motion (4,36). Furthermore, the greater range of motion available is more forgiving

(A) **(C)**

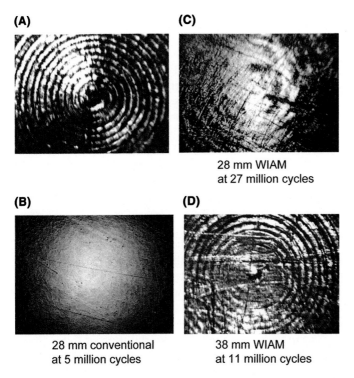

28 mm WIAM
at 27 million cycles

(B) **(D)**

28 mm conventional   38 mm WIAM
at 5 million cycles   at 11 million cycles

Figure 5 Representative optical micrographs of articulating surfaces of polyethylene acetabular liners tested on the Boston hip simulator. The original articular surface contains undulated machining marks (**A**), which are polished away in the conventional polyethylene liners with a femoral head diameter of 28 mm (**B**) as a result of adhesive wear during hip simulator testing. In contrast, the machining marks on the articular surface of warm (125°C) irradiated and subsequently melted (WIAM) liners persisted with a femoral head diameter of 28 mm (**C**) and 38 mm (**D**) even after 27 million cycles of simulated gait indicating a marked improvement on wear resistance.

to the inherent errors in acetabular placement providing an increased margin of safety (20).

IN VIVO EVIDENCE

Thus far, early clinical experience with electron beam crosslinked and melted polyethylene in the total hip has shown no adverse effects on device performance. There have been no reported instances of early increased wear or fatigue failure. Muratoglu et al. (32) reported on a number of revision surgeries performed for sepsis, recurrent dislocation secondary to implant malpositioning, or acetabular shell loosening with various types of highly crosslinked polyethylenes. Preliminary observations of the articulating surfaces of these explants showed the unexpected finding of numerous scratches. Such scratching may be attributed to one of two factors: wear resulting in loss of material or plastic deformation of the surface without loss of material.

Experiments devised by Muratoglu et al. (32) tested the hypothesis that the primary mechanism of scratching was surface reconfiguration through plastic deformation induced through abrasive third body particles. Their analyses showed that the in vivo surface scratching is indeed dominated by surface plastic deformation which leads to only minimal material removal. They investigated 16 highly crosslinked and 19 conventional polyethylene components with comparable in vivo durations ranging from 5 days to 18 months. Visual analysis of all the implants showed no delaminations or cracks on any of the surfaces. Scratching of the articulating surfaces was apparent in both groups of explants with more polishing through adhesive wear in the conventional polyethylene group. When present, this fine and heavy scratching induced a slightly dull, opaque appearance on the articulating surfaces unlike the polished appearance that is commonly observed on the articulating surfaces of highly worn long-term retrievals of conventional polyethylene acetabular liners (21). Polishing was not common in the highly crosslinked implants, with only three of them showing evidence of polishing after an average in vivo duration of 14 months. Polishing was more common in the conventional group with an average in vivo duration of five months. Most of the highly crosslinked polyethylene explants also exhibited the persistence of machining marks juxtaposed with surface scuffing (Fig. 6).

Muratoglu et al. (32) used the shape memory property of high molecular weight polymers to study the root cause of the surface scratching. Shape memory is retained in the molecular structure of the high-molecular-weight polymer and can be activated by melting. For instance, machining of acetabular components operates through the principle of cutting the surface at a microscopic level, leaving behind an undulated surface structure, representing surface memory. If this surface is scratched through plastic deformation, melting can be used to restore the original undulated machining marks. On the other hand, if scratching is a result of material removal, that is wear, the melt recovery of the original surface topography is no longer possible. This shape memory phenomenon is demonstrated in Figure 7.

A region in the superior aspect of a typical, highly crosslinked retrieval with an in vivo duration of three months, before and after the melt recovery experiment is shown in Figure 8. Before melting, the surface contained multidirectional scratches and the machining marks were not visible (Fig. 8A). After melting, the surface scratches were no longer visible and the original machining marks which had been generated during fabrication reappeared (Fig. 8B). This example demonstrates the restoration of the original machining marks on a heavily scratched surface even though no machining marks were visible before melting. Out of seven highly crosslinked explants included in the melt-recovery experiments, five showed full recovery and two partial

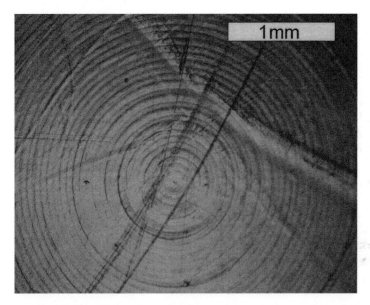

Figure 6 Typical surface morphology observed on the articulating surface of a highly cross-linked acetabular liner after 18 months in vivo, showing presence of machining marks with superimposed surface scratches at the dome of the liner. Recorded with optical microscopy. The scale bar indicates 1 mm.

recovery of the original surface machining marks. The latter two with partial recovery had been in vivo for about 15 months, indicating that there was some material removal during this period. Still, the extent of removal was less than the typical height of machining marks (less than 10 μm) in 15 months, which amounts to a linear wear rate of less than 0.008 mm/yr.

Among the 12 conventional retrievals that were subjected to the melt-recovery experiments, three showed near-full recovery upon melting, four partial recovery, and five almost no recovery. With the advance of the wear front, enough of the surface material that retained the surface shape memory had been worn away in vivo from the conventional polyethylene explants, preventing recovery of original surface topography.

Future investigations on retrieved highly cross-linked polyethylene acetabular liners with longer term in vivo durations will be essential in further understanding the evolution of the surface features described by Muratoglu et al. (32). Such investigations will complement the on-going radiographic follow-up studies with contemporary highly cross-linked polyethylenes.

IN VITRO EVIDENCE IN TOTAL KNEE

The use of radiation crosslinked and melted polyethylene in TKRs to address both the delamination type polyethylene damage and adhesive/abrasive

(A-1)   **(B-1)**   **(C-1)**

(A-2)   **(B-2)**   **(C-2)**

(A-3)   **(B-3)**   **(C-3)**

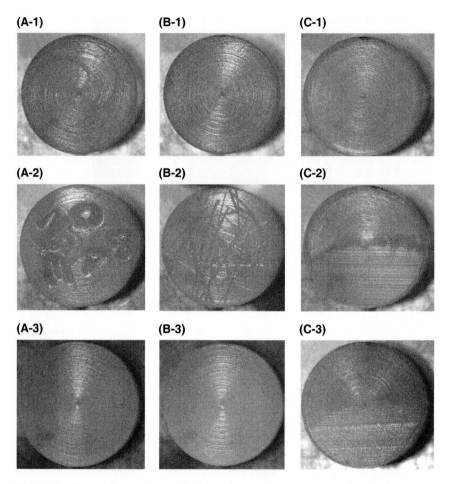

Figure 7 The results of the controlled melt recovery experiments on surfaces that were intentionally altered with plastic deformation or material removal are shown here. The surfaces of three pins made out of warm (125°C) irradiated and subsequently melted (WIAM) polyethylene as shown in (**A**-1) and (**B**-1) were subjected to damage modes without material removal, namely indentation with metal letter dies (**A**-2) and scribing with a blunt metal tool (**B**-2). The damaged surfaces of the same cylinders are shown following melting in (**A**-3) and (**B**-3) demonstrating near full recovery of the original surface with the machining marks, demonstrating the shape memory property of polyethylene. Another cylindrical pin (**D**-1) was microtomed to remove a wedge shaped 50 μm thin section from the lower half of the surface (**D**-2). Following microtoming, the upper half of the surface displayed machining marks and the lower half showed complete removal of the machining marks. After melting, no recovery of the initial machining marks occurred in the lower half (**D**-3) because the material containing the machining marks had been removed by the microtome and shape memory had been lost.

(A) **(B)**

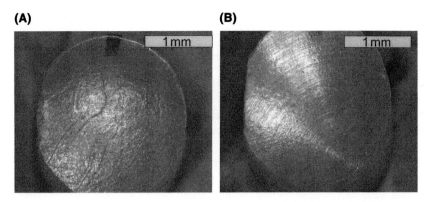

Figure 8 Typical surface morphology of one of the explanted highly cross-linked polyethylene (Longevity™, Ziminer Inc., Warsaw, IN) liners after three months in vivo before melting (**A**) showing extensive scratching in the dome aspect of the articulating surface where machining marks are no longer obvious. After melting (**B**) there is nearly full recovery of the original machining marks, indicating that very little if any material had been removed. Scale bars indicate 1 mm.

wear is a new concept. It is widely accepted that delamination is often the result of oxidation-induced embrittlement secondary to gamma sterilization and storage in air (6,54). Electron beam crosslinked and melted polyethylene components have no detectable residual free radicals and are sterilized with either ethylene oxide gas or gas plasma. Their oxidation resistance is far superior to the gamma sterilized conventional polyethylene components. Consequently, radiation crosslinked and melted polyethylene components are expected to have excellent oxidative stability both on the shelf and in vivo, which will result in superior resistance to delamination as well. The in vitro and in vivo experiences with THRs have demonstrated a marked increase in adhesive/abrasive wear resistance with highly crosslinked poly-ethylenes (31,47,52). Even though the contact mechanics at the tibiofemoral articulation differs somewhat from that of the total hip, one would expect increased crosslink density to improve the wear resistance of polyethylene in total knees as well.

Several investigators tested the hypothesis that radiation crosslinking and thermal treatment would both reduce delamination and decrease adhesive/abrasive wear of polyethylene tibial inserts (17,31,47,52). These studies used contemporary in vitro knee wear simulators capable of producing in vivo damage mechanisms of delamination and adhesive/abrasive wear to critically assess the benefits of this technology.

Recently developed knee simulators use physiologic kinematics and provide the aforementioned crossing motion, which is one prerequisite for the adhesive/abrasive wear to occur. Among these are force- and displacement-driven knee simulators. The Stanmore simulator, developed by Walker et al. (51), is a force-driven knee wear simulator where a physiologic flexion motion along with axial load and simulated soft tissue constraint are applied to the implants. The specific articular surface geometry and design of the implant being tested dictates the internal/external rotation and anterior/posterior translation of the tibial insert (51). This simulator has been shown to generate adhesive–abrasive wear of polyethylene tibial inserts with typical wear rates of 15 and 25 mg/million cycles with the Kinematic[d] and IB-II[b] designs, respectively (51).

Contemporary displacement-driven knee simulators control the complete kinematics of the knee and axial load to simulate the in vivo conditions. Typical wear rates achieved with displacement-driven simulators depend on the type of kinematics and knee design used (24,30,53). With a common range of tibial rotation of 10°, the wear rate of conventional polyethylene was reported to be 14 mg/million cycles on a flat-on-flat cruciate-retaining design (30).

The crossing motion that dominates hip articulation is also present in the knee as a result of tibial rotation, the extent of which highly depends on the articular surface design. The effect of tibial rotation on the wear behavior of conventional polyethylene has been studied on contemporary knee simulators by Muratoglu et al. (30), Wang et al. (53), and Kawanabe et al. (24). Muratoglu et al. (30) showed that with a cruciate retaining total knee design the wear rate of conventional polyethylene (gamma sterilized in nitrogen) increased by about 60-fold from 0.4 to 23 mg/million cycles when the tibial rotation range was increased by 9° (from 5 to 14°). The study by Wang et al. (53) showed a decrease in the rate of weight loss from 14.4 mm^3/million cycles with a 13.5° internal–external rotation to 3.9 mm^3/million cycles with no rotation of the tibia. Similarly, Kawanabe et al. (24) demonstrated that the addition of a $\pm 5°$ tibial rotation increased the wear rate from 1.7 mg/million cycles to 10.6 mg/million cycles on a cruciate retaining design.[e] Therefore, knee simulator testing has to be tailored for each design based on known or expected in vivo kinematics.

Reproduction of delamination type polyethylene damage is also essential for the validation of an in vitro knee simulator. Only when conventional polyethylene is oxidized either on the shelf or through accelerated aging have researchers been able to generate delamination type damage in knee simulators (7,8). For example, Currier et al. (7) observed delaminations on aged conventional polyethylene components, the extent of which increased with severity of the subsurface oxidation. Therefore, it is necessary to simulate clinically relevant oxidation levels in polyethylene components through

---

[d] Howmedica, Rutherford, New Jersey, U.S.A.
[e] Anatomic Graduated Component, AGC, Biomet, Warsaw, Indiana, U.S.A.

accelerated aging prior to knee simulator testing to better study the delamination behavior of different designs and candidate bearing materials.

Several groups used the above described in vitro tools to simulate delamination and adhesive/abrasive wear of highly cross-linked and conventional polyethylenes (17,31,47,52). Wang et al. (52) used gamma irradiation to cross-link polyethylene with subsequent annealing at 50°C and investigated the wear behavior with a maximum of 22° of flexion motion. The wear rate was about $20 \, mm^3$/million cycles in the conventional polyethylene inserts that had been sterilized with ethylene oxide gas. The crosslinked inserts exhibited no change in wear rate between 2.5 and 5 Mrad of radiation dose. When compared to the wear rate measured at 2.5 Mrad, there was 40% decrease in wear rate at 7.5 Mrad and 50% decrease at 10 Mrad. In another study, Schimidig et al. (47) showed a reduction in adhesive/abrasive wear rate of polyethylene tibial inserts following 10 Mrad gamma irradiation with subsequent annealing at 135°C. The wear rate of conventional inserts, which had been gamma sterilized, was about 12 mg/million cycles on a force-driven knee simulator. The wear rate of the crosslinked inserts (10 Mrad) was 1.3 mg/million cycles. In neither of the above noted studies (47,52) were the tibial inserts subjected to accelerated aging, therefore the effect of the respective crosslinking methods used on delamination resistance of polyethylene was not revealed.

Recently, Muratoglu et al. (31) combined the methods of accelerated aging and a displacement-driven knee simulator to compare the wear behavior of conventional versus crosslinked and melted polyethylene. In their study polyethylene was crosslinked to a dose level of 9.5 Mrad at an elevated temperature (125°C) using electron beam irradiation with subsequent melting. The knee simulator test was done using normal gait kinematics with a peak load of 750 pound and motions consisting of 55° of flexion/extension, 10 mm of anterior/posterior translation, and ±10° of internal/external rotation. The wear rate of unaged conventional inserts that had been gamma sterilized in an inert gas environment was ~8 mg/million cycles. The highly crosslinked inserts were subjected to accelerated aging and showed both a significant decrease in the adhesive/abrasive wear rate and no detectable subsurface cracking or delamination on the articular surfaces after 10 million cycles of simulated gait. In contrast, the aged conventional polyethylene inserts showed delaminations in less than five million cycles.

Collective observations from these studies indicate that irradiation and melting significantly increases the delamination and adhesive/abrasive wear resistance of polyethylene. Currently, the application of cross-linking technology in total knees consists of electron beam irradiation and melting[f]

---

[f] Durasul used in Natural Knee II, Sulzer Orthopaedics and Prolong used in NexGen, Zimmer.

and its use is a first entry into a very broad field. The in vivo benefits of increased crosslinking will become more evident with long-term clinical studies, which will rely on the analysis of explanted components.

SUMMARY

The contemporary polyethylene technology of electron beam cross-linking and melting offers a highly cross-linked network structure with no detectable residual free radicals and will likely have significant impact on the performance of total hip and total knee arthroplasty by reducing adhesive/abrasive wear and preventing long-term oxidation, thus decreasing incidence of delamination.

REFERENCES

1. Bello A, Barrales-Rienda JM. Fractionation of Polymers. In: Brandrup J, Immergut EH, eds. Polymer Handbook. New York: John Wiley & Sons, 1989:233–377.
2. Bergmann G, Graichen F, Rohlmann A. Hip joint loading during walking and running, measured in two patients. J Biomech 1993; 26:969–990.
3. Bragdon CR, O'Connor DO, Lowenstein ID, Jasty M, Biggs SA, Harris WH. A new pin-on-disk wear testing method for simulating wear of polyethylene on cobalt–chrome alloy in total hip arthroplasty. J Arthroplasty 2001; 16:658–665.
4. Burroughs BR, Golladay GJ, Hallstrom B, Harris WH. A novel constrained acetabular liner design with increased range of motion. J Arthroplasty 2001; 16(suppl 1):31–36.
5. Cadambi A, Engh GA, Dwyer KA, Vinh TN. Osteolysis of the distal femur after total knee arthroplasty. J Arthroplasty 1994; 9:579–594.
6. Collier JP, Sperling DK, Currier JH, Sutula LC, Saum KA, Mayor MB. Impact of gamma sterilization on clinical performance of polyethylene in the knee. J Arthroplasty 1996; 11:377–389.
7. Currier JH, Duda JL, Sperling DK, Collier JP, Currier BH, Kennedy FE. In vitro simulation of contact fatigue damage found in ultra-high molecular weight polyethylene components of knee prostheses. Proc Inst Mech Eng Part H—J Eng Med 1998; 212:293–302.
8. Deluzio KJ, O'Connor DO, Bragdon CR, Muratoglu OK, O'Flynn H, Rubash H, Jasty M, Wyss UP, Harris WH. Development of an in vitro knee delamination model in a knee simulator with physiologic load and motion. Annual Meeting of Orthopaedic Research Society, Orlando, Florida, 2000.
9. Dole M. Crosslinking an crystallinity in irradiated polyethylene. Polym Plast Technol Eng 1979; 13:41–64.
10. DuPlessis T, Grobbelaar C, Marais F. The improvement of polyethylene prostheses through radiation crosslinking. Radiat Phys Chem 1977; 9:647–652.
11. Emerson RH Jr, Higgins LL, Head WC. The age total knee prosthesis at average 11 years. J Arthroplasty 2000; 15:418–423.

12. Engh GA, Koralewicz LM, Pereles TR. Clinical results of modular polyethylene insert exchange with retention of total knee arthroplasty components. J Bone Joint Surg Am 2000; 82:516–523.
13. Furman B, Awad J, Chastain K, Li S. Material and performance differences between retrieved machined and molded insall/burstein type total knee arthroplasties. Trans Orthop Res Soc 1997; 643.
14. Grobbelaar CJ, DuPlessis TA, Marais F. The radiation improvement of polyethylene prostheses. J Bone Joint Surg 1978; 60-B:370–374.
15. Grobbelaar CJ, Weber FA, Spirakis A, DuPlessis TA, Cappaert G, Cakic JN. Clinical experience with gamma irradiation-crosslinked polyethylene—a 14 to 20 year follow-up report. South African Bone Joint Surg 1999; XI:140–147.
16. Guven OE. Crosslinking and scission in polymers. In: Guven O, ed. NATO ASI series, Mathematical and Physical Sciences. Boston: Kluwer, 1988.
17. Hastings R, Huston D, Reber E, DiMaio W. Knee wear testing of a radiation crosslinked and remelted uhmwpe. 1999 Society for Biomaterials 25th Annual Meeting Transactions, Providence, RI, 328, 1999.
18. Hirakawa K, Bauer TW, Stulberg BN, Wilde AH, Borden L. Characterization of debris adjacent to failed knee implants of 3 different designs. Clin Orthop Rel Res 1996; 331:151–158.
19. Jahan MS, Wang C, Schwartz G, Davidson JA. Combined chemical and mechanical effects on free radicals in uhmwpe joints during implantation. J Biomed Mater Res 1991; 25:1005–1017.
20. Jaramaz B, Nikou C, DiGioia AM. Effect of combined acetabular/femoral implant version on hip range of motion. Trans of 45th Annu Meet ORS, 926, 1999.
21. Jasty MJ, Goetz DD, Lee KR, Hanson AE, Elder JR, Harris WH. Wear of polyethylene acetabular components in total hip arthroplasty. An analysis of 128 components retrieved at autopsy or revision operation. JBJS 1997; 79(A):349–358.
22. Johnston RC, Schmidt GL. Measurement of hip-joint motion during walking. J Bone Joint Surg Am 1969; 51(A):1083.
23. Kashiwabara H, Shimada S, Hori Y. Free radicals and crosslinking in irradiated polyethylene. Radiat Phys Chem 1991; 37:43–46.
24. Kawanabe K, Clarke IC, Tamura J, Akagi M, Good VD, Williams PA, Yamamoto K. Effects of a–p translation and rotation on the wear of uhmwpe in a total knee joint simulator. J Biomed Mater Res 2001; 54:400–406.
25. Lewis G. Polyethylene wear in total hip and knee arthroplasties. J Biomed Mater Res 1997; 38:55–75.
26. McGinniss V. Crosslinking with radiation. In: Brandrup J, Immergut EH, eds. Polymer Handbook. New York: Wiley 1989:418–449.
27. McKellop H, Shen F-W, DiMaio W, Lancaster JG. Wear of gamma- crosslinked polyethylene acetabular cups against roughened femoral balls. Clin Orthop Rel Res 1999; 369:73–82.
28. McKellop H, Shen FW, Lu B, Campbell P, Salovey R. Effect of sterilization method and other modifications on the wear resistance of acetabular cups made of ultra-high molecular weight polyethylene. A hip-simulator study. J Bone Joint Surg Am 2000; 82A:1708–1725.

29. McKellop H, Shen F-W, Lu B, Campbell P, Salovey R. Development of an extremely wear resistant ultra-high molecular weight polyethylene for total hip replacements. J Orthop Res 1999; 17:157–167.
30. Muratoglu O, Bragdon C, O'Connor D, Jasty M, Harris W. A highly cross-linked, melted uhmwpe: expanded potential for total joint arthroplasty. In: Rieker C, Oberholzer S, Wyss U, eds. World Tribology Forum in Arthroplasty. Bern: Hans Huber 2001:245–262. In: Rieker C, Oberholzer S, Wyss U, eds. World Tribology Forum in Arthroplasty. Bern: Hans Huber, 2001:245–262.
31. Muratoglu OK, Bragdon CR, Jasty M, O'Connor DO, Von Knoch R, Harris WH. Knee simulator testing of conventional and crosslinked polyethylene tibial inserts. J Arthroplasty 2004; 19:887–897.
32. Muratoglu OK, Bragdon CR, O'Connor DO, Jasty M, Harris WH. 1999 HAP Paul Award. A novel method of crosslinking UHMWPE to improve wear, reduce oxidation and retain mechanical properties. J Arthroplasty 2001; 16:149–160.
33. Muratoglu OK, Bragdon CR, O'Connor DO, Jasty M, Harris WH, Gul R, McGarry F. Unified wear model for highly crosslinked ultra-high molecular weight polyethylenes (uhmwpe). Biomaterials 1999; 20:1463–1470.
34. Muratoglu OK, Bragdon CR, O'Connor DO, Perinchief RS, Estok DM, Jasty M, Harris WH. Larger diameter femoral heads used in conjunction with a highly cross-linked ultra-high molecular weight polyethylene. A new concept. J Arthroplasty 2001; 16:24–30.
35. Muratoglu OK, Greenbaum E, Bragdon C, Jasty M, Freiberg A, Harris WH. Surface analysis of early retrieved acetabular polyethylene liners. A comparison of standard and highly crosslinked polyethylenes. J Arthroplasty 2004; 19:68–77.
36. Noble PC, Paravic V, Ismaily S. Are big heads the solution to dislocation after total hip replacement? 48th Annual Meeting of the Orthopaedic Research Society, Dallas TX, 2002.
37. Oonishi H, Takayama Y, Tsuji E. The low wear of cross-linked polyethylene socket in total hip prostheses. In: Wise DL, Trantolo DJ, Altobelli DE, Yaszemski MJ, Gresser JD, Schwartz ER, eds. Encyclopedic Handbook of Biomaterials and Bioengineering. Part A: Materials. New York: Marcel Dekker, 1995:1853–1868.
38. Paul JP. Forces transmitted by joints in the human body. Proc Inst Mech Eng 1966; (Pt 3F8):181.
39. Pooley CM, Tabor D. Friction and molecular structure: the behavior of some thermoplastics. Proc R Soc Lond 1972; 329A:251–274.
40. Ramamurti B, Bragdon C, O'Connor D, Lowenstein J, Jasty M, Estok D, Harris W. Loci of movement of selected points on the femoral head during normal gait. Three-dimensional computer simulation. J Arthroplasty 1996; 11: 845–852.
41. Randall JC, Zoepfl FJ, Silverman J. High-resolution solution carbon 13 nmr measurements of irradiated polyethylene. Radiat Phys Chem 1983; 22:183–192.
42. Ritter MA, Worland R, Saliski J, Helphenstine JV, Edmondson KL, Keating EM, Faris PM, Meding JB. Flat-on-flat, nonconstrained, compression molded polyethylene total knee replacement. Clin Orthop Rel Res 1995:79–85.

43. Robinson EJ, Mulliken BD, Bourne RB, Rorabeck CH, Alvarez C. Catastrophic osteolysis in total knee replacement—a report of 17 cases. Clin Orthop Rel Res 1995:98–105.

44. Rorabeck CH, Smith PN. Results of revision total knee arthroplasty in the face of significant bone deficiency. Orthop Clin North Am 1998; 29:361–371.

45. Saikko V, Calonius O, Keranen J. Effect of counterface roughness on the wear of conventional and crosslinked ultra high molecular weight polyethlene studied with a multi-directional motion pin-on-pin device. J Biomed Mater Res 2001; 57:504–512.

46. Schmalzried TP, Campbell P, Schmitt AK, Brown IC, Amstutz HC. Shapes and dimensional characteristics of polyethylene wear particles generated in vivo by total knee replacements compared to total hip replacements. J Biomed Mater Res 1997; 38:203–210.

47. Schmidig G, Essner A, Wang A. Knee simulator wear of cross-linked uhmwpe. 46th Annual Meeting, ORS, Orlando, Florida, 2000.

48. Shanbhag AS, Bailey HO, Hwang DS, Cha CW, Eror NG, Rubash HE. Quantitative analysis of ultra high molecular weight polyethylene (uhmwpe) wear debris associated with total knee replacements. J Biomed Mater Res 2000; 53: 100–110.

49. Shikata T, Oonishi H, Hashimato Y, Al E. Wear resistance of irradiated uhmw polyethylenes to Al_2O_3 ceramics in total hip prostheses. Transactions of the 3rd Annual Meeting of the Society for Biomaterials 1977:118.

50. Thadani PJ, Vince KG, Ortaaslan SG, Blackburn DC, Cudiamat CV. Ten- to 12-year followup of the insall-burstein i total knee prosthesis. Clin Orthop Rel Res 2000:17–29.

51. Walker PS, Blunn GW, Perry JP, Bell CJ, Sathasivam S, Andriacchi TP, Paul JP, Haider H, Campbell PA. Methodology for long-term wear testing of total knee replacements. Clin Orthop Rel Res 2000:290–301.

52. Wang A, Polineni VK, Essner A, Sun DC, Stark C, Dumbleton JH. Effect of radiation dosage on the wear of stabilized uhmwpe evaluated by hip and knee joint simulators. 23rd Annual Meeting of the Society for Biomaterials, New Orleans, LA, 1997.

53. Wang A, Sun DC, Stark C, Dumbleton JH. Wear mechanisms of uhmwpe in total joint replacements. Wear 1995; 181–183:241–249.

54. Williams IR, Mayor MB, Collier JP. The impact of sterilization method on wear in knee arthroplasty. Clin Orthop Rel Res 1998; 356:170–180.

55. Won CH, Rohatgi S, Kraay MJ, et al. Effect of resin type and manufacturing method on wear of polyethylene tibial components. Clin Orthop Rel Res 2000; 161–171.

56. Wroblewski B, Siney P, Fleming P. Low-friction arthroplasty of the hip using alumina ceramic and cross-linked polyethylene. A ten-year follow-up report. J Bone Joint Surg 1999; 8l-B:54–55.

26

Alternate Bearing Materials: Metal-on-Metal

Mauricio Silva and Thomas P. Schmalzried

Joint Replacement Institute at Orthopaedic Hospital, Los Angeles, California, and Harbor-UCLA Medical Center, Torrance, California, U.S.A.

INTRODUCTION

Despite generally inferior clinical results with metal-on-metal total hip replacements, many metal-on-metal implants lasted over two decades or are still functioning in patients who received the implant at a young age (1,2). Acetabular component wear and loosening limit the survival of Charnley hips (3–7). Because of this, long-term survival rates of the Charnley hip and the McKee-Farrar are similar (8). Consequently, there is renewed interest in metal-on-metal bearings.

Aseptic loosening of early implants with a metal-on-metal bearing was multi-factorial and not uniformly due to the metal-on-metal bearings. There is evidence indicating that some metal-on-metal bearing couples were poorly designed and/or manufactured leading to high frictional torque and/or excessive wear which could have been the cause of failure. However, as has been seen with hips which have metal-on-polyethylene bearings, loosening of hips with metal-on-metal bearings occurred due to other factors such as suboptimal stem and/or cup design, manufacturing, or implantation technique (1,2,9–11). There is now more than a decade of experience with second-generation metal-on-metal bearings adding further definition to the benefits and risks of this alternate bearing technology.

FRICTIONAL TORQUE

The coefficient of friction for the metal-on-metal bearing of the McKee-Farrar hip is roughly two to three times greater than that for a metal-on-polyethylene hip bearing. The larger diameter of the McKee-Farrar (about 40 mm) amplifies this difference and the result is a frictional torque that is up to ten times greater than that in the Charnley (2). This value is still an order of magnitude less than the static torque-to-failure of an acutely implanted cemented acetabular component and lower than that reported for metal-on-polyethylene surface replacement components (12–18).

Contrary to theoretical considerations, frictional torque has not been demonstrated to be important in the initiation of aseptic loosening of either femoral or acetabular components. Accumulating evidence indicates that periprosthetic inflammation from polyethylene (PE) wear particles has a greater effect on the durability of implant fixation than frictional torque (14,16–18). From this perspective, the success of the Charnley low friction arthroplasty is primarily a function of the low volumetric wear of the 22-mm-diameter bearing, not low frictional torque. Within the range of frictional torques generated by implants used to date, wear is a more important factor in survivorship than frictional torque. Large diameter bearings can be successful if the wear rate is sufficiently low (19).

MATERIALS AND DESIGN CONSIDERATIONS

The interplay of material(s), macrogeometry (diameter and clearance), microgeometry (surface topography), and lubrication influences the wear of metal-on-metal bearing total hip replacements to a far greater degree than with metal-on-polyethylene bearing. Insight into optimizing the performance of metal-on-metal bearings can be obtained from several sources including theoretical models (20), wear simulator studies (21), and analysis of metal-on-metal bearings retrieved after in vivo cycling (2,22–26).

Because of their harness, alloys of cobalt (Co) and chromium (Cr) have traditionally been preferred for metal-on-metal bearings in total hip replacement. High chromium content provides good corrosion resistance. During manufacturing, carbon-rich compounds of chromium (Cr), cobalt (Co) and molybdenum (Mo) are formed. These carbides, which are firmly adherent to the surrounding matrix, are approximately five times harder than the austenitic metallic phase of the matrix and are relatively brittle (25). The size and distribution of the carbides depends on the manufacturing process. Cast cobalt–chromium–molybdenum alloy (ASTM, F-75), which was used to manufacture the majority of first generation metal-on-metal hips, has a relatively high carbon content of 0.2–0.3% and contains primarily Cr and Mo carbides which result in asperities on the polished surface. The importance of dispersed carbides for wear resistance has been generally acknowledged (25).

The macrogeometry of a metal-on-metal bearing can be described in terms of the diameter(s) of the ball and the socket and the clearance of the resultant bearing couple. Clearance is the size of the gap between the surfaces at the equator of the bearing. For hemispherical bearings, clearance is a function of the difference in the diameters of the surfaces of the ball and socket. A ball and socket of exactly equal diameter mated together would have zero clearance and have maximal contact area for that size bearing. Contact area can be increased by increasing the size (diameter) of the bearing surfaces and/or by decreasing the clearance. Conversely, for a given diameter, increase in clearance decreases contact area. Contact stresses are a function of material properties and are inversely proportional to contact area. Clearance also influences lubrication, as the size of the gap has implications for the amount and type of lubrication. Smaller clearances encourage fluid film lubrication. Large clearances lead to a reduced contact area, loss of effective lubrication, and more rapid wear. However, too little clearance may lead to equatorial contact, very high frictional forces, high torque, and loosening of the implant (20). The limitations of current mass production manufacturing sets the lower limit of clearance at about 20 μm. Wear rate, particularly during the initial run-in, increases rapidly with clearances above about 150 μm (21,24,27).

For a given material or combination of materials with known mechanical properties, implant diameter and clearance can be combined into a single parameter called the effective radius. The effective radius of a hemispherical bearing is the radius of another sphere which, if it were in contact with a flat surface, gives the same contact area as that of the actual ball and socket geometry. For example, for a 28-mm-diameter cobalt–chromium on cobalt–chromium hemispherical bearing (14 mm radius) with a clearance of 100 μm , the effective radius is about 3.9 m (20).

In addition to the contact area, another important variable is where the contact occurs. Given bearings of equivalent diameters, equatorial contact is associated with higher frictional torques than the same contact area in a more polar location. Equatorial bearing may have been a factor associated with failure of some early metal-on-metal total hip replacements and this is supported by retrieval studies (22). Consequently, relatively polar contact is preferred (2,22,24,28). Retrieval analyses of McKee-Farrar hips demonstrate variability in these parameters and likely represent an evolution of bearing surface design and manufacturing (2,22).

LUBRICATION

The lubricating fluid and conditions are important variables which influence friction and wear. The synovial fluid of normal, osteoarthrotic and rheumatoid joints has been characterized to some degree. The fluid is thixotropic; viscosity if a function of the shear strain rate, or velocity of motion for practical purposes (20). Less is known about the fluid formed around total joint arthroplasties, but the composition and rheology are likely variable. Full-film lubrication completely separates the surfaces of a bearing. In this situation, the load is carried by the fluid and wear of the bearings is minimal. Mixed-film lubrication partially separates the surfaces.

Mixed-film lubrication appears to be the operative mechanism in most metal-on-metal hip joints. For a given load and surface velocity, fluid film thickness is dependent on the properties of the fluid but can be influenced by the properties of the bearing materials, the macrogeometry of the bearing (which is a function of diameter and clearance), and the surface microtopography (surface finish) (20). Within the apparent contact area, the surfaces make actual contact only at the tips of asperities and a lubricant film can influence wear significantly. As wear proceeds, the contact area at the asperity tips increases and such "running-in" can produce a more favorable microgeometry for lubricant films to separate the surfaces and reduce wear (21).

Fluid-film lubrication is encouraged by making the femoral head as large as practically possible and the clearance as small as practically possible. For metal-on-metal bearings, in distinction from PE bearings, larger diameters can actually produce lower wear rates for similar manufacturing parameters (29,30).

HIP SIMULATOR TESTS

Medley et al. (21) compared the wear rates of different metal-on-metal bearings in a hip simulator. The bearing couples were made from one of three alloys, had either small (28 mm) or large (45 mm) diameter, and clearances ranging from 10 to 630 μm, with calculated effective radii ranging from 1.6 to 11.4 m. The mass loss per million cycles ranged from 0.7 mg to over 500 mg but 14 of the 17 pairs tested were between 2.5 and 40 mg. This translates to calculated wear volumes ranging from 0.09 to 61 mm^3 per million cycles and linear wear rates ranging from 1.3 to 100 μm per million cycles. In most tests, the wear rate decreased substantially after the first 0.1 to 0.5 million cycles. The greatest variability was seen in this initial "run in" period after which 14 of 17 pairs demonstrated low wear rates ranging from a total mass loss of less than 1 mg per million cycles to about 6 mg per million cycles (0.12–0.72 mm^3 per million cycles).

No definitive statements could be made regarding the choice of alloy or size of the bearing. The authors suggest that lower wear was associated with larger effective radius (6–11 m) but there was a fair amount of scatter in the data. The poorest performance, however, was associated with a very high clearance of 630 μm (smallest effective radius, 1.6 m).

Chan et al. (27) also evaluated the wear of metal-on-metal bearings using a hip simulator. The implants were made from CoCrMo alloy, either wrought or cast, with average surface roughness (R_a) ranging from 2 to

20 nm and clearances ranging from 10 to 107 µm. Higher wear occurred within the first million cycles, followed by a marked decrease in wear rate to lower, steady-state values. The volumetric wear at three million cycles was small, ranging from 0.15 to 2.56 mm³. An average wear rate of 0.40 mm³ per million cycles (range: 0.02–1.9) was observed during the run-in period (first million cycles). Once the steady state was reached, an average wear rate of 0.08 mm³ per million cycles (range: 0.03–0.21) was observed. With roughness held relatively constant, wear increased with increasing clearance ($R^2 = 0.65$, $p = 0.001$). Mass manufacturing control of tolerances below 20 µm is difficult and the probability to match parts with an excessively tight fit would increase. The authors conclude that slightly larger clearances are necessary to increase the margin of safety.

RETRIEVAL STUDIES

Twenty-year performance has been reported of metal-on-metal hip articulations obtained at revision surgery after a mean implantation time of 21.3 years (2). The amount of wear was too small to be measured radiographically or by the so-called shadowgraph technique. A computerized coordinate measuring machine (CMM) was used to quantify the amount of wear by assessing the sphericity of bearing surfaces and comparing the measured dimensions in multiple planes to the best-fit circle (Fig. 1). The worst-case estimate of combined femoral and acetabular linear wear was 4.2 µm per year, about twenty-five times less than that typically seen with PE.

Table 1 summarizes linear and volumetric wear rates obtained from retrieval analyses of first generation metal-on-metal prosthesis (22,24–26). A comparison with linear and volumetric wear rates for metal-on-polyethylene joints is provided (6,31–35). The average linear wear rate on the retrieved heads was about 0.004 mm/year, with an average volumetric wear rate of 1.5 mm³/year (22,24–26). The average linear wear rates on the cups were about 0.003 mm/year. No data on the average volumetric wear rates for the cups were provided. The mean wear rate of the smaller diameter McKee-Farrar balls was about twice that of the larger diameter balls (1.4 vs. 0.7 mm³ per year). This could be due to associated factors such as differences in clearance and/or effective radius, lubrication, or patient activity (24).

The wear rate of the metal-on-metal bearings decreases with time in situ. This is consistent with an initial "conditioning phase" or "running-in"; more rapid wear over the first 1–2 years, which is then followed by a lower steady-state wear rate. Thus, the overall wear rate decreases with time in situ (23–25,36).

In a retrieval study, McKellop et al. (24) observed that wear rate tended to increase as clearance increased. A McKee-Farrar prosthesis with an unusually large clearance of 1.7 mm had a volumetric wear rate of 11.2 mm³/year, which was about 16 times the rate of the other large diameter

Metal-on-metal-Wear Patterns: Retrievals

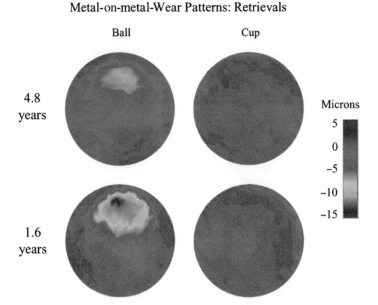

Ball   Cup

4.8
years

1.6
years

Microns

5

0

-5

-10

-15

Figure 1 Coordinate measuring machine quantitative analysis of wear. Wear is determined by assessing the deviation from sphericity of the bearing surfaces. The color coding (shown here in gray scale) indicates the deviation from sphericity in that location.

McKee-Farrars. However, a relationship between clearance and time to revision could not be established. Kothari et al. (22) observed several bearings with small clearances that would theoretically allow hydrodynamic lubrication, but no correlation was found between clearance and measured wear. There are numerous clinical variables, including those related to the patient and to surgical technique, that could explain the lack of a correlation between clearance and wear in retrieval studies.

McCalden et al. (23) described a fine abrasive wear involving the superior or polar portion of the head and corresponding portion of the cup as the most common type of surface wear. McKellop et al. (24) suggested that the bearing surfaces could be divided in three distinct zones: 1. *The non-contact zone,* which exhibited the original surface as polished by the manufacturer, typically containing residual polishing scratches, 2. *The transition zone,* which exhibited mild to severe surface damage, such as third-body scratches, and 3. *The main wear zone,* from which the most material had been removed. This region is often more polished than the original, non-contact zone. Scratches in the main wear zone were observed to fade or "polish out" with continued use. This "self-healing" property of metal-on-metal bearings makes them relatively tolerant of hard third bodies. These authors have not observed a case of run-away wear with a metal-on-metal bearing.

Table 1 Wear of Total Hips In Vivo

Study	Acetabular bearing	Femoral head	Diameter (mm)	Number of hips	Average linear wear rates[a]	Range linear wear rates[a]	Average volumetric wear rate (mm³/year)	Range volumetric wear rate (mm³/year)	Comments
Wrobleski, 1985	PE	SS	22	22	0.21	0–0.41	42.4	0–83	Radiographic
Isaac et al., 1992	PE	SS	22	22	0.19	0.017–0.52	38.0	3.4–104.8	Direct
	PE	SS	22	87	0.21	<0.005–0.6	42.3	<1–120.9	Direct
Schmalzried et al., 1992	PE	SS, CoCr	22	2	0.15	0.11–0.18	29.6	23.4–35.9	Autopsy
	PE	—	26	5	0.16	0.05–0.3	48.8	14.2–101.5	Autopsy
Kabo et al., 1993	PE	—	32	5	0.06	0.04–0.07	25.0	16.5–30.7	Autopsy
	PE	SS	22	5	0.13	—	25.9	—	Direct
	PE	CoCr	26	3	0.23	—	63.4	—	Direct
	PE		28	23	0.23	—	75.6	—	Direct
	PE	CoCr	32	9	0.21	—	88.7	—	Direct
	PE		36–54	20	0.38	—	313.5	—	Direct
Sychters et al., 1996	PE	CoCr	32	21	0.07	0.02–0.18	36.7	1–131.3	Autopsy
	PE	AlO₂	32	5	0.08	0.03–0.17	52.9	24.5–124.7	Autopsy
Jasty et al., 1997	PE	—	—	22	—	—	35	8–116	Autopsy
	PE	—	—	84	—	—	62	8–256	Revision, Cemented
	PE	—	—	22	—	—	94	12–284	Revision,

(*Continued*)

Table 1 Wear of Total Hips In Vivo (*Continued*)

Study	Acetabular bearing	Femoral head	Diameter (mm)	Number of hips	Average linear wear rates[a]	Range linear wear rates[a]	Average volumetric wear rate (mm³/year)	Range volumetric wear rate (mm³/year)	Comments
McKellop et al., 1996	CoCr	CoCr	34.9	8	4.1	0.4–8.0	1.4	0.12–3.1	Cemented, MB
	CoCr	CoCr	41.3	3	1.6	0.7–2.5	0.7	0.21–1.3	McKee-Farrar Heads Only
	CoCr	CoCr	34.9	7	3.6	0.0–4.9	—	—	McKee-Farrar Heads Only
	CoCr	CoCr	41.3	2	0.9	0.0–1.8	—	—	McKee-Farrar Cup Only
	CoCr	CoCr	37	1	3.1	—	0.9	—	McKee-Farrar Cup Only
	CoCr	CoCr	42	5	6.9	4.1–11.0	3.4	2–5.5	Muller Heads Only
	CoCr	CoCr	40–40.8	2	5.2	1.7–8.7	2.3	1.6–3	Muller Heads Only
									Ring Heads Only

Study									
Kothari et al., 1996	CoCr	CoCr	34.9–41.3	22	—	—	2.2	0.15–4.9	McKee-Farrar Heads Only
Schmidt et al., 1996	CoCr	CoCr	—	17	6.6	0.1–28.0	—	—	McKee-Farrar Heads
	CoCr	CoCr	—	13	4.9	0.2–30.0	—	—	McKee-Farrar Cups
	CoCr	CoCr	—	10	2.0	0.7–6.2	—	—	Muller Heads
	CoCr	CoCr	—	14	2.0	0.0–3.9	—	—	Muller Cups
Willert et al., 1996	CoCr	CoCr	—	3	9.9	1.6–24.0	8.6	0.66–22.36	McKee-Farrar Cups and Heads
	CoCr	CoCr	—	3	8.3	5.7–10.0	2.6	0.22–5.98	Muller Cups and Heads

[a] mm/year for metal-polyethylene and microns/year for metal-metal.

For the McKee-Farrar prosthesis, evidence of neck-socket impingement is present in 33–43% of cases (23,24). Substantial amounts of third bodies can be generated by this mode of wear. Such abrasives create scratches, primarily in the transition zone, where the local clearance between the ball and the cup is comparable with the largest dimension of the abrasive particles.

Calcium phosphate surface deposits have been seen adjacent to or in the periphery of the main contact zone (23,24). This location suggests that the precipitation was induced by elevated bearing surface temperatures. Any deposits formed in the main contact zone were probably quickly worn away. Proteins, phosphates, and other constituents of joint fluid in vivo may influence lubrication and wear but the effect(s) of these constituents and associated precipitates and/or deposits are currently unknown.

SECOND-GENERATION METAL-ON-METAL BEARINGS

The Metasul (Sulzer Medical Technology, Winterthur, and Switzerland) total hip bearing utilizes a carbide-containing, forged, cobalt–chromium–molybdenum alloy (Protasul-21WF), which reportedly has a clearance of 150 µm for the 28 mm articulation (37). In 1988, Weber implanted the first Metasul bearing couple. Well over 100,000 Metasul bearings have subsequently been implanted with a variety of Sulzer hip systems. This metal-on-metal bearing technology has also been extended to large diameter surface replacement components (38).

Clinical results of total hip systems with these bearings have generally been good (38–41). There are no reports of reoperations for a problem directly attributable to the metal-on-metal articulation. There has been no evidence of run-away wear, and few metal particles are seen in histologic sections (38,40,41). There have, however, been reoperations for infection, heterotopic ossification, instability, impingement, and aseptic loosening.

Impingement wear can be a source of metallosis, especially if a titanium alloy neck impinges on the CoCr acetabular articulation (42). For this reason, metal-on-metal articulations are more position sensitive than metal–polyethylene joints. Larger diameter bearings have a greater arc of motion, which decreases impingement risk.

Sieber et al. (36) reported on 118 Metasul components (65 heads and 53 cups) retrieved for dislocation (24%), loosening of the stem (17%), loosening of the cup (28%), and other reasons such as heterotopic ossification or infection (31%). None were revised for osteolysis. The mean time of implantation was 22 months (range: 2–98 months). The mean annual linear wear rate was found to decrease with the time from insertion, being 25 µm/year for the first year and about 5 µm/year after the third year. The volumetric wear after the run-in period was estimated to be 0.3 mm^3/year, concluding that these metal-on-metal bearings have a volumetric wear rate about 60 times lower than that of conventional PE bearings.

In clinical reports of hips with second-generation metal-on-metal bearings, with follow-up between 2.2 and 5 years, osteolysis is rare (38–41). Beaule at al. (43), however, have reported a case of a well-fixed, cementless total hip replacement with a Metasul bearing with progressive diaphyseal osteolysis occurring within two years. There was minimal bearing surface wear and only small numbers of inflammatory cells in the tissues. Absent evidence of a foreign-body reaction, it was hypothesized that this was a case of osteolysis secondary to transmission of joint fluid pressure, rather than particulate-induced osteolysis (44).

Between 1991 and 1994, 74 Metasul bearings in the Weber cemented cup were implanted with a variety of femoral components. With up to four years follow-up (average 2.2), the clinical results were good to excellent and no hips had loosened. Twenty-seven of these patients had a contralateral metal on plastic bearing hip of similar design and none of these patients could detect a difference between the two hips (39). Complete clinical and radiographic data on 56 of these patients (56 hips), with follow-ups between 4 and 6.8 years (average 5.2 years) has also been reported (45). Good to excellent clinical results were found in 99% of cases. One patient required acetabular revision for loosening secondary to sub-optimal cement technique. There were no loose or revised femoral components. There was no apparent osteolysis (45).

METAL-ON-METAL WEAR PARTICLES

Wear particles from metal-on-metal bearings are nanometers in linear dimension, substantially smaller than PE wear particles (46,47). Light microscopic analysis of tissue obtained from around metal-on-metal joints showed particles with variable and irregular shape (47). The size of metal particles reported by scanning electron microscopy (SEM) studies ranges from 0.1 to 5 μm. SEM studies have suggested that large metallic particles observed with light microscopy were agglomerates of the smaller particles (47,48).

Transmission electron microscopy (TEM) has demonstrated wear particles from cobalt–chromium–molybdenum bearings (CoCrMo) to be round to oval in shape with irregular boundaries. Most of the particles are smaller than 50 nm [range: 6 nm to 1 μm (47,49)]. Additional analysis of these retrieved wear particles indicates that the particles have several different elemental compositions. There are CoCrMo particles, but there is an even greater number of chromium oxides particles (Fig. 2) (50). It has been hypothesized that the CoCrMo particles are produced by the wear of the carbides on the bearing surfaces and the prosthesis matrix, and that the chromium oxide particles come from the passivation layer on the implant surface and possibly from oxidized chromium carbides (50).

There is little known about the rates of metallic particle production in vivo, lymphatic transport of metallic particles from the joint, and systemic

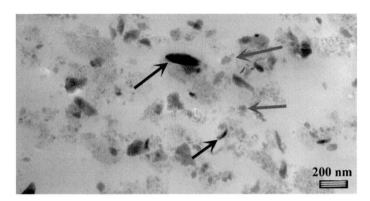

Figure 2 Transmission electron microscopy image of particles retrieved from a metal-on-metal joint. Most of the particles are smaller than 50 nm. Although there are some CoCrMo particles (*black arrows*), there is an even greater number of chromium oxide particles (*gray arrows*).

dissemination (51,52). Utilizing information on volumetric wear rate and average particle size, it has been estimated that $6.7 \times 10^{12} - 2.5 \times 10^{14}$ metal particles are produced per year, which is 13–500 times the number of PE particles produced per year by a typical metal-on-polyethylene joint (47). The aggregate surface area of these metal wear particles is substantial.

BIOLOGICAL CONSIDERATIONS

The large aggregate surface area of metal wear particles may have both local and systemic effects. Surface area has been identified as a variable affecting the macrophage response to particles (53). However, the local tissue reaction around metal-on-metal prosthesis, indicated by the number of histiocytes, is about one grade lower than that around metal-on-polyethylene prosthesis (47,51). A number of hypotheses have been proposed to explain this discrepancy (47). As metal particles are considerably smaller than PE particles, histiocytes are able to store a larger number of metal particles and, therefore, the total number of histiocytes required to store the metal particles is lower. Very small particles may enter macrophages by pinocytosis instead of phagocytosis, which may alter the cellular response to the particles. It is also recognized that CoCr particles have greater potential for cytotoxicity than PE and the cell may be incapable of the same inflammatory response. There may be a difference in the relative proportion of metal wear particles that are retained locally versus systemically distributed compared to PE wear particles. Dissolution of metal particles result in elevation of serum and urine cobalt and chromium ions.

    In vitro studies have shown a dose–response effect with metal particles (54). Low to moderate concentrations of metal particles stimulate the release of cytokines, such as interleukin-1 (IL-1), interleukin-6 (IL-6), tumor necrosis factor-α, and prostaglandin E^2, that can lead to periprosthetic osteolysis and aseptic loosening (54–60). At higher concentrations, however, CoCr particles have been found to be cytotoxic (54–57,61,62), altering the phagocytic activity of macrophages and leading to cell death (54,57 60,63).

Although the volume of reactive periprosthetic inflammatory tissue associated with metal-on-metal bearings is less than with metal-on-polyethylene, osteolysis can occur in hips with metal-on-metal bearings (1,2,43). The incidence of osteolysis associated with metal-on-metal bearings has not been well established, but appears to be comparatively low (10,11).

SERUM AND URINE IONS

It is important to recognize that in modern total hip replacement prostheses there may be several sources of metal particle and ion generation. Systemic dissemination of soluble and particulate corrosion products from modular junctions has been described, including the presence of metallic particles in the lymph nodes, liver, and spleen (59,64–67). In control subjects (no metallic implants) the levels of serum and urine cobalt and chromium are undetectable, or nearly undetectable (64).

For patients with clinically well-functioning hips with a metal-on-polyethylene bearing, 36 months following surgery, the average serum cobalt level was 0.27 ng/mL (range: 0.15–1.59). The average serum chromium level was 0.18 ng/mL (range: 0.015–1.46) and the average urine chromium level was 0.28 ng/mL (range: 0.008–1.77). In these apparently well-functioning hips, the ion levels were 1–5 times higher than controls.

In modular total hips with a metal-on-polyethylene bearing, with no or mild corrosion at the modular head and neck junction, serum and urine levels of cobalt averaged 0.94 ng/mL (range: <0.54–1.65) and 0.92 ng/mL (range: <0.3–1.14), respectively, and urine chromium levels averaged 1.0 ng/mL (range: 0.54–1.92). With moderate or severe corrosion at the modular head and neck junction, the serum and urine levels of cobalt averaged 1.06 ng/mL (range: 0.8–1.4) and 0.87 ng/mL (range: <0.3–1.3), respectively, and the average urine chromium levels was 1.59 ng/mL (range: 0.6–3.0) (64).

The levels of metal ions in serum and urine are further elevated in patients with metal-on-metal bearings. In some reports, the ion levels are higher in the short-term and decrease over time. This is consistent with a conditioning phase or running-in of the bearing. In resurfacing prostheses with an average bearing diameter of 45 mm (38–52 mm) and average follow-up of 12.4 months (2–19 months), the average serum cobalt level was 3.77 ng/mL (range: 1.0–9.6) and the average serum and urine chromium levels were 3.86 ng/mL (range: 2.65–5.72) and 5.10 ng/mL (range: 1.33–11.0), respectively (68).

Jacobs et al. (68) have also measured ion levels in subjects with cobalt–chromium alloy metal-on-metal total hip replacements that had been in situ for an average of 24 years. The average serum cobalt level was 0.9 ng/mL (range: <0.3–2.0). The average serum chromium level was 1.28 ng/mL (range: 0.21–2.56) and the average urine chromium level was 1.22 ng/mL (range: 0.26–2.59) (68).

The longer-term serum and urine ion levels produced by metal-on-metal bearings are not much higher than those produced by the modular junctions of femoral components which demonstrated moderate to severe corrosion at revision surgery. Unfortunately, the toxicological importance of these trace metal elevations has not been established and available data do not answer questions regarding the risks of ion hypersensitivity, toxicity, and carcinogenesis (52,68–70). Since wear of a metal-on-metal bearing cannot generally be measured on a radiograph, serum and urine metal ion concentrations may be useful indicators of patient activity and the tribological performance of these bearings.

HYPERSENSITIVITY

Due to the fact that all metals in a biological environment corrode (71,72), the ions released can combine with proteins and activate the immune system as antigens and elicit hypersensitivity responses (73). Nickel is the most common metal sensitizer in humans, followed by cobalt and chromium (73–77). Because of the elevated level of cobalt and chromium ions in patients with a metal-on-metal bearing, there may be an increased risk of developing hypersensitivity.

Implant-related hypersensitivity reactions are generally delayed cell-mediated responses (73,78,79). Delayed-type hypersensitivity (DTH) is characterized by antigen activation of sensitized T lymphocytes that releases cytokines, resulting in a recruitment and activation of macrophages (73). Several case reports have associated the use of orthopaedic implants with the appearance of immunogenic reactions (80–85).

Historically, testing for DTH has been done in vivo by skin testing and in vitro by lymphocyte transformation testing and leukocyte migration inhibition testing. There are, however, many concerns about the applicability of skin test to the study of immune responses to implants. Unlike the typical acute dermal exposure to the antigen that occurs with the patch testing, it takes weeks to months of constant exposure prior to reports of dermal reactions to orthopaedic implants (73). Moreover, the diagnostic utility of patch testing could be affected by immunological tolerance, which could suppress dermal response to implants, or by impaired host immune response (73). In vitro DTH testing remains an unpopular means of assessing metal hypersensitivity, mainly because of its labor-intensive characteristics and limited clinical results (73).

In patients with well-functioning implants, the prevalence of metal sensitivity is approximately 25%, which is roughly twice of that of the general population (73). The prevalence is approximately 60% among patients with a failed or poorly functioning implant. Because a malfunctioning or loose implant can generate metal particles, it is unclear whether metal hypersensitivity causes implant failure or vice versa (73). In either event, DTH should be considered when a patient with a well-fixed implant experiences chronic, aching pain with evidence of synovitis (an irritable range of motion), but has no objective evidence of infection.

CANCER RISK

Cobalt and chromium wear particles have been shown to induce carcinoma in animal models (86,87), giving rise to the concern that such alloys could have the same effect in human tissues if present in sufficient amounts for a sufficient length of time.

The first well-documented case of cancer associated with total joint replacement was in a patient who developed a malignant fibrous histiocytoma three and half years after a metal-on-metal total hip replacement performed in December 1969 (88). There have been at least 24 additional cases reported in the English literature of malignancy occurring in association with a total hip or knee prostheses (89). Of the 25 reported cases of cancer following a total joint replacement, 21 involved sarcomas (89).

The risk of cancer after metal-on-metal total hip replacement has been assessed specifically in only one epidemiological study (70). In that study, the relative risk of cancer was reported to be 0.95 (95% confidence interval, 0.8–1.1), suggesting that there is no apparent increased risk of cancer development after metal-on-metal total hip arthroplasty. In addition, the risk of sarcoma after metal-on-metal total hip replacement was found to be 0.00 (95% confidence interval, 0.0–6.6) (70). However, the same study found the relative risk of hematopoietic cancer to be 1.59 (95% confidence interval, 0.8–2.8) following metal-on-metal total hip replacement and 3.77 (95% confidence interval, 0.9–17.6) for leukemia when metal-on-metal implants were compared with metal-on-polyethylene implants. The confidence intervals are very broad for these data and encompass unity, indicating that the risk is statistically neither increased nor decreased. From an epidemiological perspective, these data are limited because of the small number of patients (579) who underwent metal-on-metal total hip replacement. Rigorous long-term studies are needed.

SUMMARY

Metal-on-metal bearings have wear rates that are 20–100 times lower than conventional PE. The amount of wear is generally the same order of magnitude for the head and the cup. There is an initial run-in period of higher wear followed by lower, steady-state wear. Wear rate is a function of the interplay of material(s), macrogeometry, microgeometry, and the resultant type and amount of lubrication. The wear resistance and clinical performance of a metal-on-metal bearing are more sensitive to macrogeometry and lubrication than a metal-on-polyethylene bearing.

Metal wear particles are nanometers in linear dimension. They are much smaller and more numerous than the submicron PE wear particles, but the volume of periprosthetic inflammatory tissue is less. Osteolysis appears to be relatively rare. Little is known about the systemic distribution of metal particles and ions. The significance of systemic distribution is also not known. The levels of serum and urine cobalt and chromium ions are elevated in patients with metal-on-metal bearings, but the long-term, steady state levels are not much higher than those associated with moderate to severe corrosion of modular femoral components.

Because of the elevated levels of cobalt and chromium ions, theoretically there is a greater risk of DTH. There is also concern about the potential for malignant degeneration secondary to exposure to these elements. The available data are insufficient to address this concern. Rigorous long-term studies are needed. It will take decades of close clinical observation to determine if the wear resistance of metal-on-metal bearings outweigh the associated risks.

ACKNOWLEDGMENTS

The authors would like to acknowledge Isabelle Catelas B. Eng. (Ph.D. candidate) and Harry McKellop Ph.D. for their contribution to this chapter.

REFERENCES

1. Schmalzried TP, Szuszczewicz ES, Akizuki KH, Petersen TD, Amstutz HC. Factors correlating with long term survival of McKee-Farrar total hip prostheses. Clin Orthop 1996; 329(suppl):S48–S59.
2. Schmalzried TP, Peters PC, Maurer BT, Bragdon CR, Harris WH. Long-duration metal-on-metal total hip arthroplasties with low wear of the articulating surfaces. J Arthroplasty 1996; 11:322–331.
3. Garcia-Cimbrelo E, Diez-Vazquez V, Madero R, Munuera L. Progression of radiolucent lines adjacent to the acetabular component and factors influencing migration after Charnley low-friction total hip arthroplasty. J Bone Joint Surg Am 1997; 79-A:1373–1380.
4. Kobayashi S, Takaoka K, Saito N, Hisa K. Factors affecting aseptic failure of fixation after primary Charnley total hip arthroplasty. Multivariate survival analysis. J Bone Joint Surg Am 1997; 79-A:1618–1627.

5. Wroblewski BM. Charnley low friction arthroplasty in patients under the age of 40 years. In: Sevastik J, Goldie I, eds. The Young Patient with Degenerative Hip Disease. Stockholm: Almquvist and Wiksell, 1985:197–201.
6. Wroblewski BM. Direction and rate of socket wear in Charnley low-friction arthroplasty. J Bone Joint Surg Br 1985; 67-B:757–761.
7. Wroblewski BM. 15–21-year results of the Charnley low-friction arthroplasty. Clin Orthop 1986; 211:30–35.
8. Jacobsson SA, Djerf K, Wahlstrom O. Twenty-year results of McKee-Farrar versus Charnley prosthesis. Clin Orthop 1996; S60-S68.
9. Amstutz HC, Campbell PA, McKellop H, Schmalzried TP, Gillespie WJ, Howie D, Jacobs J, Medley J, Merritt K. Metal on metal total hip replacement workshop consensus document. Clin Orthop 1996; 329S:297–303.
10. Szuszczewicz ES, Schmalzried TP, Petersen TD. Progressive bilateral pelvic osteolysis in a patient with McKee-Farrar metal-on-metal total hip prostheses. J Arthroplasty 1997; 12:819–824.
11. Zahiri CA, Schmalzried TP, Ebramzadeh E, Szuszczewicz ES, Salib D, Kim C, Amstutz HC. Lessons learned from loosening of the McKee-Farrar metal-on-metal total hip replacement. J Arthroplasty 1999; 14:326–332.
12. Charnley J, Kamangar A, Longfield MD. The optimum size of prosthetic heads in relation to the wear of plastic sockets in total replacement of the hip. Med Biol Eng 1969; 7:31–39.
13. Charnley J. Low Friction Arthroplasty of the Hip: Theory and Practice. Berlin: Springer-Verlag, 1979.
14. Andersson GBJ, Freeman MAR, Swanson SAV. Loosening of the cemented acetabular cup in total hip replacement. J Bone Joint Surg Br 1972; 54-B: 590–599.
15. Wilson JN, Scales JT. Loosening of total hip replacements with cement fixation. Clinical findings and laboratory studies. Clin Orthop 1970; 72:145–160.
16. Ma SM, Kabo JM, Amstutz HC. Frictional torque in surface and conventional hip replacement. J Bone Joint Surg Am 1983; 65-A:366–370.
17. Eftekhar NS, Pawluk RJ. Role of surgical preparation in acetabular cup fixation. In: Anonymous the Hip. Proceedings of the Eighth Open Scientific Meeting of the Hip Society. St. Louis: C.V. Mosby, 1980:308–328.
18. Volz RG, Wilson RJ. Factors affecting the mechanical stability of the cemented acetabular component in total hip replacement. J Bone Joint Surg Am 1977; 59-A:501–504.
19. Mai MT, Schmalzried TP, Dorey FJ, Campbell PA, Amstutz HC. The contribution of frictional torque to loosening at the cement-bone interface in Tharies hip replacements. J Bone Joint Surg Am 1996; 78-A:505–511.
20. Schey JA. Systems view of optimizing metal on metal bearings. Clin Orthop 1996; 329(suppl):S115–S127.
21. Medley JB, Chan FW, Krygier JJ, Bobyn JD. Comparison of alloys and designs in a hip simulator study of metal on metal implants. Clin Orthop 1996; 329(suppl):S148–S159.
22. Kothari M, Bartel DL, Booker JF. Surface geometry of retrieved McKee-Farrar total hip replacements. Clin Orthop 1996; 329(suppl):S141–S147.

23. McCalden RW, Howie DW, Ward L, Subramanian C, Nawana N, Pearcy MJ. Observation on the long-term wear behaviour of retrieved McKee-Farrar total hip replacement implants. Trans Orthop Res Soc 1995; 20:242.

24. McKellop H, Park SH, Chiesa R, Doorn P, Lu B, Normand P, Grigoris P, Amstutz H. In vivo wear of three types of metal on metal hip prostheses during two decades of use. Clin Orthop 1996; 329S:128–140.

25. Schmidt M, Weber H, Schon R. Cobalt chromium molybdenum metal combination for modular hip prostheses. Clin Orthop 1996; 329(suppl):S35–S47.

26. Willert HG, Buchhorn GH, Gobel D, Koster G, Schaffner S, Schenk R, Semlitsch M. Wear behavior and histopathology of classic cemented metal on metal hip endoprostheses. Clin Orthop 1996; 329(suppl):S160–S186.

27. Chan FW, Bobyn JD, Medley JB, Krygier JJ, Tanzer M. Wear and lubrication of metal-on-metal hip implants. Clin Orthop 1999; 369:10–24.

28. Walker PS, Gold BL. The tribology (friction, lubrication and wear) of all-metal artificial hip joints. Wear 1971; 17:285–299.

29. Dowson D. New joints for the millennium: wear control in total replacement hip joints. Proc Inst Mech Eng [H] 2001; 215:335–358.

30. Smith SL, Dowson D, Goldsmith AAJ. The effect of diametral clearances, motion and loading cycles upon lubrication of metal-on-metal hip replacements. Proc Inst Mech Eng [C] 2001; 215:1–5.

31. Isaac GH, Wroblewski BM, Atkinson JR, Dowson D. A tribological study of retrieved hip prostheses. Clin Orthop 1992; 276:115–125.

32. Jasty M, Goetz DD, Bragdon CR, Lee KR, Hanson AE, Elder JR, Harris WH. Wear of polyethylene acetabular components in total hip arthroplasty. An analysis of one hundred and twenty-eight components retrieved at autopsy or revision operations. J Bone Joint Surg Am 1997; 79-A:349–358.

33. Kabo JM, Gebhard JS, Loren G, Amstutz HC. In vivo wear of polyethylene acetabular components. J Bone Joint Surg Br 1993; 75-B:254–258.

34. Schmalzried TP, Kwong LM, Jasty M, Sedlacek RC, Haire TC, O'Connor DO, Bragdon CR, Kabo JM, Malcolm AJ, Harris WH. The mechanism of loosening of cemented acetabular components in total hip arthroplasty. Analysis of specimens retrieved at autopsy. Clin Orthop 1992; 274:60–78.

35. Sychterz CJ, Moon KH, Hashimoto Y, Terefenko KM, Engh CA Jr, Bauer TW. Wear of polyethylene cups in total hip arthroplasty. A study of specimens retrieved post mortem. J Bone Joint Surg Am 1996; 78-A:1193–1200.

36. Sieber HP, Rieker CB, Kottig P. Analysis of 118 second-generation metal-on-metal retrieved hip implants. J Bone Joint Surg Br 1999; 81-B:46–50.

37. Müller ME. The benefits of metal-on-metal total hip replacements. Clin Orthop 1995; 311:54–59.

38. Wagner M, Wagner H. Preliminary results of uncemented metal on metal stemmed and resurfacing hip replacement arthroplasty. Clin Orthop 1996; 329(suppl):S78–S88.

39. Hilton KR, Dorr LD, Wan Z, McPherson EJ. Contemporary total hip replacement with metal on metal articulation. Clin Orthop 1996; 329(suppl):S99–S105.

40. Weber BG. Experience with the Metasul total hip bearing system. Clin Orthop 1996; 329(suppl):S69–S77.

41. Wagner M, Wagner H. Medium-term results of a modern metal-on-metal system in total hip replacement. Clin Orthop 2000; 379:123–133.

42. Iida H, Kaneda E, Takada H, Uchida K, Kawanabe K, Nakamura T. Metallosis due to impingement between the socket and the femoral neck in a metal-on-metal bearing total hip prosthesis. A case report. J Bone Joint Surg Am 1999; 81-A:400–403.

43. Beaule PE, Campbell P, Mirra J, Hooper JC, Schmalzried TP. Osteolysis in a cementless, second generation metal-on-metal hip replacement. Clin Orthop 2001; 386:159–165.

44. Schmalzried TP, Akizuki KH, Fedenko AN, Mirra J. The role of access of joint fluid to bone in periarticular osteolysis. A report of four cases. J Bone Joint Surg Am 1997; 79-A:447–452.

45. Dorr LD, Wan Z, Longjohn DB, Dubois B, Murken R. Total hip arthroplasty with use of the Metasul metal-on-metal articulation. Four to seven-year results. J Bone Joint Surg Am 2000; 82-A:789–798.

46. Doorn PF, Campbell PA, Amstutz HC. Metal versus polyethylene wear particles in total hip replacements. A review. Clin Orthop 1996; 329(suppl): S206–S216.

47. Doorn PF, Campbell PA, Worrall J, Benya PD, McKellop HA, Amstutz HC. Metal wear particle characterization from metal on metal total hip replacements: transmission electron microscopy study of periprosthetic tissues and isolated particles. J Biomed Mater Res 1998; 42:103–111.

48. Hanlon J, Ozuna R, Shortkroff S, Sledge CB, Thornhill TS, Spector M. Analysis of metallic wear debris retrieved at revision arthroplasty. Implant Retrieval Symposium of the Society for Biomaterials, St. Charles, Il, 1992.

49. Soh EW, Blunn GW, Wait ME, Walker PS. Size and shape of metal particles from metal-on-metal total hip replacements. Trans Orthop Res Soc 1996; 21:462.

50. Catelas I, Campbell P, Medley JB, Zukor DJ, Huk OL, Bobyn JD. Quantitative and compositional analysis of particles from metal-metal THRs. European Society for Biomaterials 25th Anniversary Conference, 2001:T46.

51. Doorn PF, Mirra JM, Campbell PA, Amstutz HC. Tissue reaction to metal on metal total hip prostheses. Clin Orthop 1996; 329(suppl):S187–S205.

52. Merritt K, Brown SA. Distribution of cobalt chromium wear and corrosion products and biologic reactions. Clin Orthop 1996; 329(suppl):S233–S243.

53. Shanbhag AS, Jacobs JJ, Black J, Galante JO, Glant TT. Macrophage/particle interactions: effect of size, composition and surface area. J Biomed Mater Res 1994; 28:81–90.

54. Haynes DR, Boyle SJ, Rogers SD, Howie DW, Vernon-Roberts B. Variation in cytokines induced by particles from different prosthetic materials. Clin Orthop 1998; 352:223–230.

55. Howie DW, Rogers SD, McGee MA, Haynes DR. Biologic effects of cobalt chrome in cell and animal models. Clin Orthop 1996; 329(suppl):S217–S232.

56. Nakashima Y, Sun DH, Trindade MC, Chun LE, Song Y, Goodman SB, Schurman DJ, Maloney WJ, Smith RL. Induction of macrophage C-C chemokine expression by titanium alloy and bone cement particles. J Bone Joint Surg Br 1999; 81-B:155–162.

57. Shanbhag AS, Jacobs JJ, Black J, Galante JO, Glant TT. Human monocyte response to particulate biomaterials generated in vivo and in vitro. J Orthop Res 1995; 13:792–801.
58. Lee SH, Brennan FR, Jacobs JJ, Urban RM, Ragasa DR, Glant TT. Human monocyte/macrophage response to cobalt-chromium corrosion products and titanium particles in patients with total joint replacements. J Orthop Res 1997; 15:40–49.
59. Archibeck MJ, Jacobs JJ, Black J. Alternate bearing surfaces in total joint arthroplasty: biologic considerations. Clin Orthop 2000; 379:12–21.
60. Catelas I, Campbell P, Dorey F, Frausto A, Mills B, Amstutz HC. Relationship between cytokines and metal particles in metal-metal THA's. Combined ORS, Rhodes, 2001:123.
61. Maloney WJ, Smith RL, Castro F, Schurman DJ. Fibroblast response to metallic debris in vitro. Enzyme induction cell proliferation, and toxicity [see comments]. J Bone Joint Surg Am 1993; 75-A:835–844.
62. Shanbhag AS, Jacobs JJ, Black J, Galante JO, Glant TT. Effects of particles on fibroblast proliferation and bone resorption in vitro. Clin Orthop 1997; 342: 205–217.
63. Rae T. A study on the effects of particulate metals of orthopaedic interest on murine macrophages in vitro. J Bone Joint Surg Br 1975; 57-B:444–450.
64. Jacobs JJ, Urban RM, Gilbert JL, Skipor AK, Black J, Jasty M, Galante JO. Local and distant products from modularity. Clin Orthop 1995; 319:94–105.
65. Shea KG, Lundeen GA, Bloebaum RD, Bachus KN, Zou L. Lymphoreticular dissemination of metal particles after primary joint replacements. Clin Orthop 1997; 338:219–226.
66. Urban RM, Jacobs JJ, Tomlinson MJ, Black J, Turner TM, Galante JO. Particles of metal alloys and their corrosion products in the liver, spleen and para-aortic lymph nodes of patients with total hip replacement prostheses. Trans Orthop Res Soc 1995; 20:241.
67. Urban RM, Jacobs JJ, Tomlinson MJ, Gavrilovic J, Black J, Peoc'h M. Dissemination of wear particles to the liver, spleen, and abdominal lymph nodes of patients with hip or knee replacement. J Bone Joint Surg Am 2000; 82-A: 457–476.
68. Jacobs JJ, Skipor AK, Doorn PF, Campbell P, Schmalzried TP, Black J, Amstutz HC. Cobalt and chromium concentrations in patients with metal on metal total hip replacements. Clin Orthop 1996; 329(suppl):S256–S263.
69. Gillespie WJ, Henry DA, O'Connell DL, Kendrick S, Juszczak E, McInneny K, Derby L. Development of hematopoietic cancers after implantation of total joint replacement. Clin Orthop 1996; 329(suppl):S290–S296.
70. Visuri T, Pukkala E, Paavolainen P, Pulkkinen P, Riska EB. Cancer risk after metal on metal and polyethylene on metal total hip arthroplasty. Clin Orthop 1996; 329(suppl):S280–S289.
71. Black J. Systemic effects of biomaterials. Biomaterials 1984; 5:11–18.
72. Jacobs JJ, Gilbert JL, Urban RM. Corrosion of metallic implants. In: Stauffer RN, ed. Advances in Operative Orthopaedics. St. Louis: CV Mosby, 1994: 279–319.

73. Hallab N, Merritt K, Jacobs JJ. Metal sensitivity in patients with orthopaedic implants. J Bone Joint Surg Am 2001; 83-A:428–436.

74. Basketter DA, Briatico-Vangosa G, Kaestner W, Lally C, Bontinck WJ. Nickel, cobalt and chromium in consumer products: a role in allergic contact dermatitis? Contact Dermatitis 1993; 28:15–25.

75. Gawkrodger DJ. Nickel sensitivity and the implantation of orthopaedic prostheses. Contact Dermatitis 1993; 28:257–259.

76. Haudrechy P, Foussereau J, Mantout B, Baroux B. Nickel release from nickel-plated metals and stainless steels. Contact Dermatitis 1994; 31:249–255.

77. Kanerva L, Sipilainen-Malm T, Estlander T, Zitting A, Jolanki R, Tarvainen K. Nickel release from metals, and a case of allergic contact dermatitis from stainless steel. Contact Dermatitis 1994; 31:299–303.

78. Hensten-Pettersen A. Allergy and hypersensitivity. In: Morrey BF, ed. Biological, Material, and Mechanical Considerations of Joint Replacements. New York: Raven Press, 1993:353–360.

79. Kuby J. Immunology. 2nd ed. New York: WH Freeman, 1994.

80. Barranco VP, Soloman H. Eczematous dermatitis from nickel. JAMA 1972; 220:1244.

81. Cramers M, Lucht U. Metal sensitivity in patients treated for tibial fractures with plates of stainless steel. Acta Orthop Scand 1977; 48:245–249.

82. Halpin DS. An unusual reaction in muscle in association with Vitallium plate: a report of possible metal hypersensitivity. J Bone Joint Surg Br 1975; 57-B: 451–453.

83. Merle C, Vigan M, Devred D, Girardin P, Adessi B, Laurent R. Generalized eczema from vitallium osteosynthesis material. Contact Dermatitis 1992; 27: 257–258.

84. Rostoker G, Robin J, Binet O, Blamoutier J, Paupe J, Lessana-Leibowitch M, Bedouelle J, Sonneck JM, Garrel JB, Millet P. Dermatitis due to orthopaedic implants. A review of the literature and report of three cases. J Bone Joint Surg Am 1987; 69-A:1408–1412.

85. Thomas RH, Rademaker M, Goddard NJ, Munro DD. Severe eczema of the hands due to an orthopaedic plate made of Vitallium. Br Med J (Clin Res Ed) 1987; 294:106–107.

86. Heath JC, Freeman MA, Swanson SA. Carcinogenic properties of wear particles from prostheses made in cobalt-chromium alloy. Lancet 1971; 1:564–566.

87. Freeman MA, Swanson SA, Heath JC. Study of the wear particles produced from cobalt-chromium-molybdenum-manganese total joint replacement prostheses. Ann Rheum Dis 1969; 28(suppl):29.

88. Swann M. Malignant soft-tissue tumour at the site of a total hip replacement. J Bone Joint Surg Br 1984; 66-B:629–631.

89. Tharani R, Dorey FJ, Schmalzried TP. The risk of cancer following total hip or knee arthroplasty. J Bone Joint Surg Am 2001; 83-A:774–780.

27

Alternate Bearing Materials: Ceramic-on-Ceramic

Justin P. Hawes and Jonathan P. Garino
Department of Orthopaedic Surgery, Hospital of the University of Pennsylvania, Philadelphia, Pennsylvania, U.S.A.

HISTORY

The introduction and subsequent refinement of total hip replacement principles and techniques have enabled orthopaedic surgeons to provide relief to millions of patients worldwide. Several series have verified the long-term durability of this operation (1–4) with the original concept of a metal head and polyethylene liner as proposed by Chamley (5) currently accepted as the "gold standard." These results, however, have also been accompanied by reports of both late and catastrophic, early failures related to localized bone loss and component loosening (Fig. 1). Initially felt to be due to "cement disease" (6), research into the etiology of aseptic failure has identified particulate wear debris as the primary cause of osteolysis (7,8). The generation of particulate debris, particularly ultra high molecular weight polyethylene (UHMWPE), is the common weak link among early hip implants and the majority of prostheses currently in use throughout the world. The ensuing inflammatory destruction of bone support and eventual implant loosening represent one of the major limitations to the long-term survival of total hip replacements (9). As hip arthroplasty is now being performed in a younger population of patients, alternatives to the conventional metal/polyethylene articulation are being sought that would minimize the creation of particulate debris.

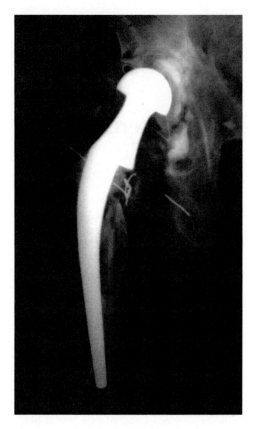

Figure 1 Hip prosthesis with osteolysis.

In an effort to eliminate the complications associated with the catastrophic wear seen in early prosthetic designs, investigation into the use of other bearing materials in total hip surgery began in Europe in the 1960s. Memories of polytetrafluoroethylene (PTFE), the initial bearing surface used by Charnley (10,11) which had disastrous results, fueled an anticipation of polyethylene having a similar fate. This led other investigators to seek hard-on-hard solutions. Metal on metal was the first of the alternative bearings employing a hard-on-hard articulation. In 1970, Pierre Boutin was the first to introduce a ceramic-on-ceramic hip arthroplasty (Fig. 2) (12). He postulated that die wear characteristics of aluminum oxide (alumina) would create a better articulating surface and lead to decreased wear of the implant. A matched pair of alumina (aluminum oxide) bearings (acetabulum and ball) was developed for this purpose by the Ceraver Company. Acetabular fixation of these early designs proved to be the Achilles heel of this innovative design, with early loosening of the sockets occurring with high frequency. The

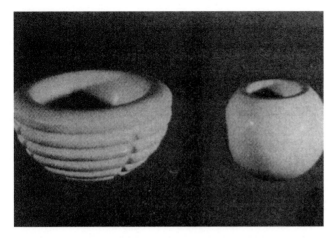

Figure 2 Original ceramic-on-ceramic hip prostheses.

mid-term results (10 year) revealed a loosening rate of the acetabular components of approximately 15% (13). Interestingly, unlike the early failures of Charnley's PTFE, bone stock was minimally affected and osteolysis was rarely seen. This led to straightforward revisions. The very marked difference between the modulus of elasticity of the ceramic and the cement is believed to be the cause of this early loosening. The femoral side was treated with a polished titanium stem that was cemented into the femoral canal. This stem has enjoyed a great deal of long-term success with a 25-year survivorship reported at over 90% (14). The initial ball heads in this series were fixated to the stem with additional cement.

In Germany, the government noted the difficulties experienced by Boutin in mating ceramic ball heads to metal stems and in the fixation of ceramic cups to bone, and funded research into ceramic technology. This led to the introduction of medical grade alumina and the use of the Morse Taper with ceramic balls on the femoral stem. The application of taper technology to hip replacement surgery allows for the coupling of different materials so as to maximize the biomechanical properties of the individual components; ceramic can be used as a bearing surface with cemented or cementless femoral fixation (15). The medical grade ceramics also allowed for manufacturing of components in an "unmatched" fashion. This enabled any femoral head to be successfully coupled with any acetabular cup from the manufacturer. Employment of these advances in Europe has led to the use of ceramic-on-ceramic articulations in hip replacement surgery with over 20 years of follow-up (16).

Mittelmeier was considered the other real pioneer in the use of ceramic–ceramic bearings and was successful in marketing his design throughout the world. The all-cementless total hip replacement that bears his name had a single, monoblock piece of alumina ceramic that was threaded. It was screwed into the patient's acetabulum after appropriate reaming. The cementless stem, which was fashioned after an Austin–Moore design, had dimples and hollow areas for "macro" interlocking. Neither the cup nor the stem had any porous coating or other biologically active coatings to enhance fixation (Fig. 3).

The early experience with ceramic-on-ceramic coupling in the United States did not meet with the same success as in Europe, with several factors contributing to the rejection of ceramics as a potential bearing surface. The early 1980s were a time for innovation with cementless designs in the United States. As such, the Mittelmeier design, with its cementless ceramic–ceramic articulation was quite intriguing. By this time, however, the polyethylene–metal articulation of Charnley was far exceeding initial expectations for success, and the need for a hard-on-hard bearing, particularly ceramics, was questioned. The early European ceramic-on-ceramic studies demonstrated no advantage over the obvious success of the Charnley design, which had now emerged as the gold standard.

Nonetheless, the Autophor, as the Mittelmeier design became known as (Smith & Nephew Richards, Memphis, Tennessee, U.S.A.), was introduced into the United States in 1984. The crude instrumentation and lack of forgiveness of the screw in socket placement did not meet with much acceptance within the American marketplace. That, coupled with reports of early loosening (17), led to the device being pulled from the market.

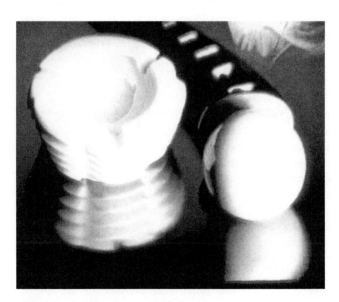

Figure 3 Mittelmeier cementless ceramic–ceramic hip prosthesis. *Source*: Photo courtesy of Ceram Tec.

The device had numerous design shortcomings with respect to obtaining consistent long-term fixation of the components and would have probably seen a similar fate with standard metal–plastic bearings as well. The American surgeon did not see through these design flaws and laid the blame of the sub optimal outcomes directly on the shoulders of the ceramic bearings. In addition, early ceramic quality technology and a lack of appreciation of the precision required in taper technology led to reports of excessive wear and ball head fractures, and further reduced enthusiasm at this time. These incidents led the Food and Drug Administration to classify ceramic-on-ceramic hip implants as class III, an experimental device that requires thorough investigation and premarket approval. In spite of the ups and downs of the past, the ceramic–ceramic bearing total hip replacement (THR) has once again moved back toward the spot light. The problems of wear, osteolysis, and need for THR in a growing segment of younger patients have elevated the enthusiasm for a more durable hip replacement. With our understanding of the basic designs and materials required for consistent long-term fixation reasonably well appreciated, manufacturers have directed more of their focus on the bearing, with most companies developing a ceramic–ceramic alternative. Once a technology ahead of its time, the recent advances in ceramics manufacturing and taper technology have inspired a renaissance of the ceramic bearings in THR with potential opportunities to improve other prosthetic replacements as well.

At the time of this writing, FDA approved Investigational Device Exemptions have been completed for two manufacturers and await final FDA approval for general marketing and sale in the United States. Several other companies are in various stages of completion of additional Investigation Device Exemption (IDE) studies.

BIOMECHANICS AND MATERIAL PROPERTIES

With the focus of this chapter being on the ceramic–ceramic articulation in THR, it should be noted that alumina is the only ceramic presently used in this manner. Zirconia, with its potential for phase change, has not yet been adopted for this application, although testing of the zirconia–zirconia couple continues at this time. Comparisons of these two ceramic materials commonly used in orthopaedic applications will be made.

The rationale behind the choice of ceramics, alumina in particular, as a bearing material is based on their mechanical properties and inert nature when implanted. Ceramics can be highly polished, making them an ideal bearing surface from that perspective alone. In addition, the hardness of ceramics makes them exceptionally wear resistant. Since first being used in the late 1960s, medical grade alumina has undergone technological advances that have enhanced its inherent characteristics. Improvements in density, grain size, and hardness, coupled with superior methods of manufacturing, processing, and testing have resulted in ceramic implants of significantly higher quality. These improvements have had only a small impact on the wear resistance of ceramic bearings, but profound effects in the reduction of fractures. With this in mind, the focus of future improvements will revolve around a further strengthening and toughening of ceramic bearing materials to increase their safety and to expand their applications.

Hardness

Ceramics, in general, are very hard materials, with alumina being the hardest, second only to diamond. The hardness of ceramics has long been appreciated by industry where they have been adapted and successfully utilized as cutting tools. Hardness refers to a material's ability to resist plastic deformation at its surface and gives an indication of its capacity to resist wear. Pressing an indenter into the material and measuring any resultant surface depressions measures hardness in orthopaedic implants (18). As with all hardness scales, the scale used to measure implant-grade ceramics is relative, higher values being indicative of a harder material. The early ceramic-on-ceramic designs used alumina with a hardness value of 1700 HV. This compares with other materials used in orthopaedic surgery, such as cobalt–chrome and titanium, which have values below 500 HV, and UHMWPE, which has a value between 60 and 70. Technological advances have subsequently led to the production of alumina with values around 2000 HV. Modern zirconia, by comparison, has a hardness rating of approximately 1,200 HV (Fig. 4). It is this superior hardness that makes alumina the current choice of ceramic in ceramic–ceramic bearing systems. This superior hardness also imparts significant protection from third body wear in the form of tremendous scratch resistance.

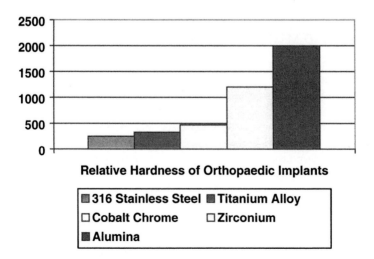

Figure 4   Relative hardness values of orthopaedic materials.

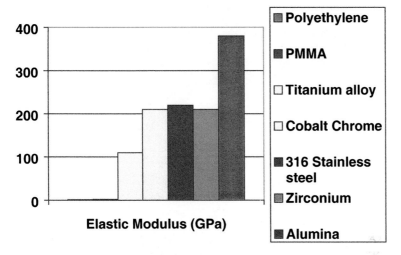

Figure 5 Comparison of stiffness of materials in orthopaedic surgery. *Abbreviation:* PMMA, polymethylmethacrylate.

Stiffness

Stiffness, or modulus of elasticity, is an indication of the amount of deformation a given material undergoes per unit force applied (stress/strain), regardless of geometry. The crystalline structure and strong ionic bonds found in alumina make it a very stiff material, much more so than the metals and alloys used in hip implants (Fig. 5). Because of its high stiffness, alumina resists deformation, even under high compressive loads. This quality, however, is only present during compression as alumina is weak in tension. Additionally, when used as either a screw-in or cemented acetabular liner, the mismatch in elastic modularity between alumina, bone, and cement can lead to an increased risk of fatigue failure at the material interfaces (19). This, however, can be overcome with proper implant design.

Brittleness

The crystalline structure of alumina also makes it a very brittle material. Brittle compounds are those that have little or no potential for plastic deformation; they fracture before undergoing any permanent change in shape (Fig. 6). Therefore, deformations seen in metals and plastics when the yield strength is exceeded are not possible with ceramics. However, modem manufacturing of these materials has provided ceramics with significant strength when combined with a proper loading environment. An improvement in the understanding of the manner in which the performance of these materials is optimized has contributed greatly. Taper technology has

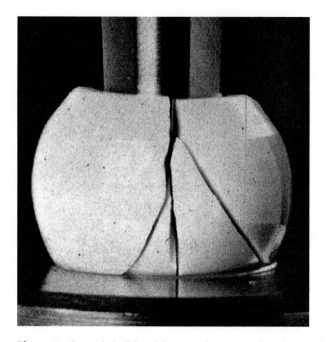

Figure 6 Ceramic ball head fracture demonstrating the brittle nature of these materials. However, when engaged on a properly designed taper, axial loads in excess of 15,000 pounds are needed to create this failure.

probably contributed the most to enhancing ceramic performance (further discussed in "design and manufacturing" section below). Like alumina, zirconia also is quite brittle and will fail catastrophically when its ultimate yield strength is exceeded.

Fracture Toughness

It is a common misconception that ceramic materials will fracture under light impact loads. This is not the case for modern ceramic components. A catastrophic failure will take place when the stress intensity exceeds a critical level for the material in question. This parameter is the fracture toughness of the material. It is usually determined by the ability of a crack to propagate under strict laboratory conditions. Alumina has a fracture toughness of about 5 MPa/m while that of zirconia approaches 9 MPa/m. It is the grain size of the ceramic material that has the largest effect on the fracture toughness, with the toughness increasing inversely with the grain size. Some additives are also used in ceramic manufacturing and are designed to enhance the fracture toughness by making it more difficult to propagate a crack. Furthermore, purification steps in the manufacturing process impart homogeneity to the ceramic and significantly reduce the potential for internal stress risers. Modem alumina ceramics have a grain size of $1.8\,\mu m$ and a density of $3.98\,g/cm^3$ while zirconia has respective values of $0.5\,\mu m$ and $6.0\,g/cm^3$. The lower grain size and higher density structurally explains the increased strength of zirconia. Ceramics have demonstrated improved wear characteristics over metal ball heads when articulating with polyethylene (20). With similar wear characteristics to alumina when articulating against polyethylene, the higher fracture toughness has made zirconia the favored choice for ceramic-poly articulation. In addition, this higher fracture toughness has allowed the safe manufacturing and implantation of 22 mm ball heads directly onto metal tapers.

BIOCOMPATIBILITY

Alumina is composed of aluminum in its most oxidized state (Al_2O_3). Generated particles are unreactive, remaining insoluble and resistant to corrosion, even in an aqueous environment. The lattice structure of pure alumina has six atoms of oxygen arranged in a hexagonal arrangement that completely surrounds the smaller aluminum atom. Alumina is a covalent molecular compound that is thermodynamically stable. Localized and systemic effects, therefore, are due to the size and number of particles generated. There is also some evidence that the cellular response to particles may be dependant on the total surface area of the debris (21). This may prove to be an important consideration in ceramic-on-ceramic arthroplasty as hard-on-hard articulations have been shown to generate not only fewer, but smaller particles (22), making the available surface area, in some circumstances, similar to that produced in bearings with polyethylene in combination with either ceramic or metal (23). This is much more of a problem with metal–metal articulations as the particles generated are in the nanometer size range, but the number of particles generated in these designs is usually several orders of magnitude higher. With the small and numerous particles, elevated levels of the ionized forms of cobalt and chromium can be easily detected. The potential systemic hazards of this phenomenon are not clear and are dealt with in greater detail in other chapters in this text.

Although it is non reactive with its surroundings, in bulk form, alumina's ionic bonds make it very hydrophilic and give it a low wetting angle ($\approx 45°$). In an aqueous solution, water is adsorbed on to the surface, allowing for increased lubrication by this thin film of fluid and further enhancing the wear characteristics (24).

Alumina has also been shown to be biologically inert in both bulk and particulate forms (24,25). In vitro animal studies have demonstrated that unloaded bone responds to implanted bulk alumina with the initial formation of woven bone that quickly matures over the next few months. Unlike other bioactive ceramics, however, alumina does not bond to the advancing bone. The two interfaces do come in very close contact with each other but remain separated by an interposed proteoglycan layer (24).

Under loaded conditions, animal studies have also shown that alumina demonstrates some structural biocompatibility. Porous, bulk alumina is able to undergo bony ingrowth, which improves with increasing stress at the bone–implant interface; in addition, implants with geometric irregularities that are placed under compression show more osseointegration than those with a smooth surface. This possibility for ingrowth is being considered in various applications. The porosity, however, does have a negative impact on the density and therefore the strength of the component.

Like other wear-generated particles, alumina exists in equilibrium between particle generation and host phagocytosis. When this balance tips toward excessive production, it induces a foreign-body response, with the production and release of numerous cellular mediators that have been implicated in the osteolytic process (26).

The tissue response to particulate alumina has been studied in both in vivo animal experiments (24) and in cell culture studies. Using flow cytometry, Catelas et al. (27) demonstrated that the release of tumor necrosis factor-α (TNF-α) by macrophages was significantly higher in the presence of polyethylene particles compared with either alumina or zirconia. Using a rabbit model, Kubo et al. (28) demonstrated that particle composition, rather than size or calculated total surface area, was the strongest factor in inducing a histiocytic response, with the reaction to UHMWPE being the most severe and that due to titanium and alumina being significantly more mild.

There is one case report of an aggressive soft tissue sarcoma detected 15 months following alumina ceramic-on-ceramic total hip arthroplasty (29). This finding must be viewed with the understanding that implant associated neoplasms generally arise following prolonged periods of implantation (24) and that the referenced patient had previously undergone internal fixation with metallic screws for a posterior fracture dislocation of the hip 13 years earlier.

Design and Manufacturing

The initial ceramic ball heads employed by Boutin were actually cemented in place to the femoral stem. However, with the Mittelmeier stem, Morse tapers were employed to improve and enhance the load transmission to the ceramic ball head. In a short time it became clear that the angle of these tapers and the preciseness of the tolerances to which the tapers must be held were critical parameters. The optimum value of 6° for alumina was ascertained and efforts to standardize taper dimensions near this value were pushed in Europe (15). The load to failure values begin to drop off precipitously below the FDA minimum value of 42 kN as the angle moves further from this optimal point. In the United States, where in excess of 20 different tapers have existed, with some manufacturers having several tapers themselves, the use of ceramics must be done with caution, as the risk of getting the wrong ceramic ball head, even from the same orthopaedic device manufacturer, is possible. Most manufacturers are adopting the 12/14 taper, meaning that the trunion widens from 12 to 14 mm in diameter as one moves from proximal to distal. This creates a taper angle of approximately 6°, which optimizes the force transfer to the ceramic ball head.

Zirconia, once again, with its higher fracture toughness, could be made to fit many tapers while maintaining the load to failure at or above the FDA minimal required level. This allowed many manufacturers to offer a reduced wear ceramic solution against polyethylene as the published wear rates of this combination began to be embraced by orthopaedic surgeons. In spite of the better results, United States surgeons remained cautions about the fracture potential allowing this combination to achieve only about 9% of the market share. This is in contrast to Europe where the use of ceramic ball heads approached 50%. A survey of the members of the American association of Hip and Knee Surgeons in 1995 revealed that there had been 11 ceramic fractures out of over 5000 implanted ball heads, with three of these happening with a custom stem manufactured at the same institution. According to this survey, which demonstrates high ceramic failure rates by today's standards, these failures are more than a full order of magnitude lower than stem fractures or complete polyethylene liner failures.

With acetabular loosening becoming a major impediment to matching the long term results of the Charnley stem and other standard metal-poly bearings, new designs had to be developed. Previously cemented and uncemented monoblock designs simply did not stand the test of time, demonstrating higher rates of acetabular loosening (12). This was likely due to the biologically inert properties of alumina as well as the modulus mismatch between the ceramic component and the cement or the bone. In addition, these early designed lacked a biologically active surface for bony ingrowth. By the end of the 1980s and beginning of the 1990s, uncemented metal shells with porous surfaces were beginning to demonstrate consistent ingrowth and sustained function. It was at this time the interior of these metallic cups were modified with a taper to accept a corresponding alumina ceramic liner (Fig 7). With this new design, a major breakthrough had been reached. A metallic cup, with its exterior optimized for bone fixation with the use of porous coatings, threads, or both, could now be fitted with ceramic liners that optimized the hip system for low wear. Modularity, which had been developed to enhance intraoperative options and ease of revision when parts had worn, was now being applied in a slightly different manner, attempting to maximize the separate functions of bearing and fixation. Hip implants that used monoblock alumina components were optimized for low wear, but not fixation, and loosening subsequently occurred. In the case of cemented, all polyethylene

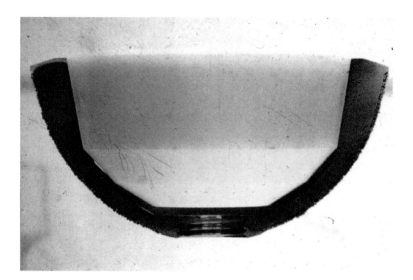

Figure 7 Modern ceramic–ceramic acetabular component. Note taper locking mechanism of the liner to the cup.

cups, although these, too, were not optimized for either fixation or wear, they represented, by far, the best material to do both jobs satisfactorily and therefore became the standard. Although a 14° taper was used initially on the cup side, difficulties with removal of the liner without cutting it with a diamond burr led to the current 6° taper which has dominated most of the current designs. This allows for a metal ring to be applied to the cup rim and impacted swiftly. The differences in the acoustic properties between the ceramic and the metal allow for the vibrations created to disrupt the Morse taper interface, and the liner "cocks" in the shell and can then be removed.

Because of their extreme inflexibility and brittleness, the manufacturing tolerances needed by the ceramic components at the taper are quite high. In an effort to achieve that goal at a reduced cost, a roughened taper is becoming the standard for many companies (Fig. 8). Much has been learned regarding tapers and the properties of ceramics. Mastering the load transfer through this interface has been the most important step forward with this technology, and a major reason why component fractures have been dramatically reduced.

The separation of bearing and fixation functions has opened up a huge opportunity for cup designs to move swiftly into the fixture with alternative bearings. There have been multiple considerations including the creation of polyethylene inserts designed as a "bail out" for a revision of a ceramic–ceramic total hip where the well in-grown cup is retained. This basic taper design with a desire of the manufacturers to offer as many choices for the surgeon as possible has been modified in so-called "second generation" cups. These cementless cups are engineered to accept not only ceramic liners, but also metal and poly liners (Fig. 9).

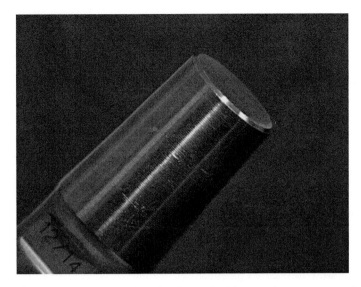

Figure 8 Typical roughened taper used with ceramic components. Impaction of the ceramic part flattens out the "peaks" and essentially "customizes" the taper for that ceramic part.

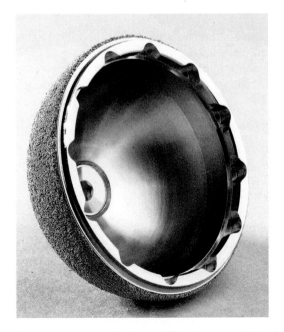

Figure 9 Modern design multibearing acetabular shell (courtesy of DePuy).

The next major technological improvement in medical grade ceramics was in the manufacturing process. Eliminating the impurities in the alumina powder though better processing and clean room implementation, and therefore inclusion bodies and stress risers sensitive to fatigue failure, improved the reliability. Hot isostatic pressing of the powder with several tons of force reduced the grain size substantially resulting in increased fracture toughness of almost 50% compared with the alumina produced in the 1970s (15). Quality control measures have also resulted in ceramic reliability. Proof testing is a process by which each ball head manufactured is subjected to a nondestructive, nondamaging overload through the taper. Components surviving this test should perform well and have a very low incident of fracture ($>1/10,000$) (15). Prior to the adoption of proof testing, only a sampling audit with destructive testing could be performed with the potential of flawed components leaving the facility for implantation.

The very low wear of ceramic bearings has also produced renewed interest in larger ball head sizes. In the past, large ball head sizes coupled with polyethylene were implicated for increased volumetric wear. This often resulted in increased osteolysis and increased loosening and failure. Smaller ball heads resulted in less volumetric wear, but were more likely to impinge or be unstable due to the reduced head/neck ratio. The poor experiences of the Autophor virtually eliminated the production of skirted ceramic ball heads for increased lengths. This requires more operative precision to be within the 8 mm range that ceramic–ceramic ball heads are offered. This is discussed further below.

Improvements in taper technology, the ceramic quality, and the quality assurance testing have significantly elevated the reliability and performance of modern ceramic components to the point that they rival or even exceed the reliability and quality of the other manufactured parts in most THR systems.

Operative Technique Considerations

The large forces needed to fracture ceramic pieces are very encouraging, but this makes the assumption that the ceramic pieces are properly installed at the time of surgery and, in the case of hip replacements, that these devices are also placed in the proper orientation.

Over the course of the last several years of implanting these devices, seven general technical considerations have been outlined to optimize the success of these implants. It is suggested that the surgeon be familiar with these guidelines as he goes to the operating room with the intention of implanting a ceramic-on-ceramic device in order to optimize the opportunity for a long-term successful outcome for him and his patient while steering clear of potential pitfalls. Ceramic–ceramic components are not yet available in the vast and variable combinations that exist for polyethylene, and, therefore, ceramic–ceramic combinations may not be the best choice for any one particular patient. This may not be apparent until the time of surgery, so corresponding standard polyethylene components should be available as well.

1. *Conservative neck cut.* At the current time ceramic ball heads are available only in a very limited range from approximately 0 to 8 mm. Since only a small range of lengths are available, it is advisable to use a conservative neck cut and remove more neck as necessary to properly restore leg length. With the use of metal ball heads surgeons would occasionally go to even longer head–neck combinations which employ skirted heads in order to reconstruct proper leg length or stability. Skirted ball heads are not available in ceramic and over resection may force the conversion to another bearing system or placing the femoral component proud. A conservative neck cut assists in avoiding problems with respect to the need for ball heads providing more than 8 mm of length.

2. *The cup in a horizontal position.* Ceramic-on-ceramic components, although very strong, should be optimally placed at 45° on the acetabular side in order to optimize the distribution of forces over the greatest amount of surface area of both the ball head and the cup. Since the greatest amounts of load take place with the hip in extension, placement of the cup in a more horizontal angle improves this load transfer. Minimizing rim overload with horizontal placement can potentially reduce any late chipping of the ceramic rim.

3. *Increased anteversion.* With increasing horizontal orientation, more of the cup is pulled from a posterior to a superior position, leaving less posterior coverage as the horizontal orientation of the cup increases. These can be compensated for by increasing the anteversion of the cup. In addition, ceramic liners are not currently available with elevated lips like they are available in the polyethylene counterparts. Therefore, further anteversion may be helpful in optimizing stability, particularly when using the posterior approach.

4. *Use of trial liners.* The tapers on the cup and stem side of the articulation are to be used only once with ceramic pieces. Therefore, it is very important that trial liners and ball heads be utilized at the time of trial reduction and that proper manipulations of these trials take place before the final implants are brought up onto the table. This may seem intuitive but many surgeons at the current time, because polyethylene is so user friendly, will impact the polyethylene liner into place and then move onto the femur. If the ceramic liner is impacted and cup orientation is suboptimal, then disimpaction of the ceramic pieces is first of all very difficult and requires special instrumentation (although this instrumentation is available and it can be done successfully), but in

addition potentially damages the taper in such a way that reimplantation or impaction of a ceramic liner or head is not advisable. Once a surgeon is satisfied with the stability and range of motion with the trials, then he or she can comfortably move on toward impaction of ceramic pieces.

5. *Removal of osteophytes and anterior acetabular wall.* (when necessary). Occasionally increased cup anteversion drops the anterior edge of the cup slightly below the top of the anterior wall or anterior osteophytes. In some instances, impingement on these anterior structures leads to a suboptimal degree of stability. In an effort to enhance the stability in this situation, careful resection of the bone responsible for impingement can be effective in optimizing stability. This maneuver may avoid the use of additional length or offset to achieve stability goals.

6. *Hand placement of the liner.* The ceramic acetabular liner can be slightly difficult to place. The relatively gentle taper can allow for "cocking" of the liner in a malposition fashion. Tools included with the set to assist in placement of the liner have in my experience been suboptimal. Placement of these liners by hand is usually relatively easy and placement can be confirmed with a simple running of the finger around the rim to be sure that the component has been evenly pressed into the taper and that no area of the taper is deeper into the cup relative to any other area. It is also important to note that as the cup size increases the possibility to malseat the liner increases. Impacting the liner in a malpositioned fashion can lead to either difficult extraction or fracture of the component. Care should be taken at this time to be sure that the liner is carefully seated.

7. *Ceramic component impaction.* At the current time the tapers on the acetabular and femoral sides have been machined with a number of grooves which on a microscopic level demonstrate a series of peaks and valleys. In order to meet the proper tolerances necessary for ceramics these grooves do it in a very efficient fashion. When the ceramic piece is inserted and subsequently impacted there is a relative flattening of the peaks and a very even distribution of the forces throughout the entire surface area circumferentially around the taper of the ceramic piece. These pieces should not be simply twisted on or placed without impaction as they can subsequently shake loose or not undergo the full seating required to optimize their force transfer.

Clinical Results and Complications

As American orthopaedic surgeons focused on improving the metal–polyethylene couple in hip replacement surgery, their European counterparts continued to refine and improve both the quality of the material and the surgical techniques employed in ceramic-on-ceramic hip arthroplasty. Their efforts have generated the majority of medium- and long-range results concerning these prostheses.

Nizard et al. (13) reported on their initial series of consecutive prostheses implanted between 1977 and 1979. Of the original 187 implants, 87 were available for review and 24 had been revised. Using revision for aseptic loosening as an endpoint, the authors found an overall survival rate of 88.57%. The majority of these revisions (15) were performed for acetabular loosening, which in retrospect is not surprising, given that all acetabula in this series were fixed to bone with cement. Other causes for revision included femoral head (3) and acetabular liner (2) fractures. The authors point out that the femoral head fractures occurred in implants manufactured prior to 1979. After this date, advances in the manufacturing process led to higher quality alumina, and no head fractures were noted in subsequent patients. The quality of bone stock at revision is not addressed, but the authors note that patients under 50 years of age tended to have a greater implant survival. In addition revisions were straightforward, and were "nearly like a primary procedure" due to the virtual absence of osteolysis in their series.

A report from Germany (30) further emphasizes the difficulties that followed the implantation of early, medical-grade alumina (31). Of the 100 hybrid devices (cemented stem with screw-in all-alumina cup) initially implanted, 77 were available for clinical and roentgenographic evaluation after 10–14 years. Over 30% (25/77) of these had been revised for mechanical failures or loosening secondary to excessive wear. Furthermore, nearly half of the retained prostheses showed migration of the cup of over 5 mm. The authors speculate that this might be due to wear, modulus mismatch, or poor host bone quality.

In the early stages of ceramic–ceramic hip replacement, the incidence of femoral head fracture has been listed as approximately 1% (32). Subsequent improvements in taper technology and in ceramic manufacturing have decreased this value to one in two thousand or less over a 10-year period (33).

Mittelmeier (34), as previously mentioned, described excellent early results for his Autophor ceramic–ceramic hip articulation. His initial design consisted of an all-alumina screw-in cup with an uncemented femoral stem. This prosthesis was also the most strongly marketed ceramic-on-ceramic device, allowing it to be used worldwide. Although a pioneering design which contributed much to the early experience with ceramic bearings, its market place domination and suboptimal results prevented universal acceptance of the ceramic–ceramic concept.

Subsequent investigators have also reported encouraging results using the same prosthesis. Huo et al. (35) reported a consecutive series of 112 THRs using the Mittelmeier Autophor prosthesis for either osteoarthritis or femoral head osteonecrosis. Ninety-three of these implants were followed for a minimum of five years. After a median follow-up of 108 months the overall mechanical failure rate (revision plus radiographic loosening) was reported as 21.5% for the cup and 22.5% for the stems; 86.5% of patients were rated as having either a good or excellent clinical result. Furthermore, even in cases requiring revision, there was no evidence of femoral or acetabular osteolysis. The authors concluded that the high failure rates were most likely due to design flaws and that the ceramic–ceramic articulation provided for decreased particle generation and periprosthetic bone loss.

Unfortunately, these results did not meet the requirement of reproducibility. Mahoney and Dimon (36) report a combined failure rate of 35% for the femoral and acetabular components after an average of over four years of follow-up. They implicate a poor prosthetic design as the primary cause of failure and state that the ceramic–ceramic articulation "performed well and did not contribute to the unsatisfactory results." Yoon et al. (37) also reporting on the Mittelmeier prosthesis, describe an incidence of pelvic osteolysis and cup migration of nearly 50% in 103 hip replacements with an average of 92 months of follow-up. Additionally, periprosthetic tissue obtained during revision surgery was analyzed histiologically and demonstrated abundant ceramic wear particles. These were felt to be the cause of the pronounced bone resorption. Once again, the Autophor with its poor track record for fixation failed to produce a long-term series with good survivorship. In fact, impingement in these chronically loose cups eventually generated enough debris to produce osteolysis.

Boehler et al. (38) reported on 67 uncemented alumina acetabular implants. After a 12 year average follow-up, 59 of the prostheses were categorized as radiographically stable while four had been revised for loosening. Two of these cups were revised within the first 18 months. The overall cup survivorship at 136 months was calculated to be 12.4%, with stem loosening given as the primary underlying problem. Sedel et al. (39) reported a 2.2% incidence of loosening in alumina sockets fixed with cement, with less than a 1% incidence of osteolysis, noted primarily in patients whose cups had tilted and led to subsequent impingement.

Advancements in taper technology allowed for ceramic cups to be implanted with a metal backing. Riska (40) compared a cemented, all-alumina acetabular prosthesis with a titanium uncemented screw cup ring and ceramic liner. The patients with an uncemented titanium screw cup were followed for an average of 3.6 years. Out of an initial 112 patients, seven required revision. Only two of these, however, were for acetabular aseptic loosening and were felt to be due to obvious technical errors. This compares with 16 revisions in 143 patients after an average of 6.7 years, with the majority (12) being performed for acetabular aseptic loosening.

More recently, press-fit acetabular components with alumina liners have been successfully implanted. Pitto et al. (41) compared a group of 50 consecutive hip implants using a modular press-fit cup. The first group of

25 hips consisted of a polyethylene liner articulating with an alumina head. The second group of hips was comprised of the same cup, but used an alumina liner. After an average of 4.5 years of follow-up, no revisions were required in either group and there was no evidence of radiographic loosening or cup migration. There was no difference in the clinical outcomes between the two groups.

Bizot et al. (42) have reported their initial results after an average of 16 months of follow-up of 96 consecutive hips using fully coated hydroxy-apatite titanium alloy stems and cups with alumina femoral heads and acetabular liners. Ninety-three hips were available for clinical and radiographic review. There was no reported incidence of alumina failure, on either the femoral or acetabular side. Radiographs revealed no osteolysis, radiolucent lines, or subsidence. Clinically, over 90% of patients reported their status as excellent. Although the follow-up time is short, these initial results are encouraging and indicative of the improvements that have been made in ceramic technology.

In the United States, data is available for the investigational device exemption granted to Wright Medical Technology (43). Of the 330 patients enrolled between 1997 and 1998, 252 have reached the two-years minimum follow-up. This group of patients demonstrated an average Harris Hip Score increase from 44 to 97. There were a total of 27 complications reported, 22 of which were hip related. Four of these complications were specifically related to the ceramic pieces and consisted of three chipped liners and one eccentric liner seating. Overall, four revisions have been performed. These early results compare favorably with other reported series.

The use of a ceramic–ceramic articulation in THR has undergone significant progress since its introduction over 30 years ago (33). The long-term clinical series have shown a very low rate of osteolysis. As the technical aspects of implant design have improved, ceramic–ceramic hip replacement offers an excellent alternative to traditional metal–polyethylene bearing surfaces, especially in younger, active patients.

FUTURE CONSIDERATIONS AND SUMMARY

As in most aspects of manufacturing and in medicine in general, improvements in current techniques and technology are constantly being sought. At the time of this writing, a new ceramic material has begun to be utilized in several of the ceramic–ceramic studies in both the United States and Europe. This material is an alumina matrix composite containing 75% alumina and 25% zirconia and other constituents (44). This material has retained the hardness and bearing properties of alumina, while the other additives have reduced the grain size and fracture toughness in the range of zirconia. As this material is fully adopted over time, fractures of alumina ceramic parts will likely occur even at a lower frequency than the current state of the art.

In addition, the improvements in the strength of this material will likely lead to its application in smaller ball and cup sizes as well as its use in joints outside the hip.

Ceramic–ceramic arthroplasty has had a long and rich history. Although always a low wear bearing, initial problems with fixation to bone and a high component fracture rate prevented this technology from offering any improvement over its metal–polyethylene counterpart. In spite of this, the technology and fixation were improved while the revisions were surprisingly routine due to the lack of significant osteolysis. With modern designs that allow for routine good initial fixation to bone with both cemented and cementless implants, improvements in long-term success and survivorship will depend primarily on a durable articulation. That durability for time frames beyond 30 years will require not just low simulator wear, but also some resilience in the face of malposition and third body wear. The ceramic–ceramic articulation with its biocompatibility and very low wear, once a technology ahead of its time, is now poised and ready to bring arthroplasty surgery at the hip and elsewhere back to the future.

REFERENCES

1. Schulte KR, Callaghan JJ, Kelley SS, Johnston RC. The outcome of Charnley total hip arthroplasty with cement after a minimum twenty-year follow-up. The results of one surgeon. J Bone Joint Surg 1993; 75-A:961–975.
2. Callaghan JJ, Albright JC, Goetz DD, Olejniczak JP, Johnston RC. Charnley total hip arthroplasty with cement. Minimum twenty-five-year follow-up. J Bone Joint Surg 2000; 82-A:487–497.
3. Smith SW, Estok DM II, Harris WH. Total hip arthroplasty with use of second-generation cementing techniques. An eighteen-year-average follow-up study. J Bone Joint Surg 1998; 80-A:1632–1640.
4. Engh Jr CA, Culpepper WJ, Engh CA. Long-term results of the anatomic medullary looking prosthesic in. Total hip Arthroplasty J Bone Joint Surg 1997; 79A:177–184.
5. Charnley J. Low Friction Arthroplasty: Theory and Practice. New York: Springer-Verlag, 1979.
6. Jones LC, Hungerford DS. Cement disease. Clin Orthop Rel Res 1987; 225: 192–206.
7. Cooper RA, McAllister CM, Borden LS, Bauer TW. Polyethylene debris-induced osteolysis and loosening in uncemented total hip arthroplasty. J Arthroplasty 1992; 7:285–290.
8. Schmalzried TP, Jasty M, Harris WH. Periprosthetic bone loss in total hip arthroplasty. Polyethylene wear debris and the concept of the effective joint space. J Bone and Joint Surg 1992; 74-A:849–863.
9. Harris WH. The problem is osteolysis. Clin Orthop Rel Res 1995; 311:46–53.
10. Charnley J. Total hip replacement by low friction arthroplasty. Clin Orthop Rel Res 1970; 72:7–21.

11. Charnley J. Tissue reactions to polytetrafluoroethylene, letters to the editors. Lancet 1992; 2:1379.
12. Boutin PM. Arthroplastie totale de la hanche par prothese en alumine frittee. Rev Chi Orthop 1992; 58:229–246.
13. Nizard RS, Sedel L, Christel P, Meuiner A, Soudry M, Witvoet J. Ten-year survivorship of cemented ceramic-ceramic total hip prosthesis. Clin Orthop Rel Res 1992; 282:53–63.
14. Malchau H, Herberts P. Prognisis of total hip replacement. Results from the Swedish National Registry, a revision-risk study of 134,056 primary operations. AAOS, Atlanta, 1996.
15. Heros RJ, Willmann W. Ceramics in total hip arthroplasty: history, mechanical properties, clinical results, and current manufacturing state of the art. Sem Arthroplasty 1998; 9:114–122.
16. Sedel L, Nizard R, Bizot P, Meunier A. Perspective on a 20-year experience with ceramic-on-ceramic articulation in total hip replacement. Sem Arthroplasty 1998; 9:123–134.
17. O'Leary JF, Mallory TH, Kraus TJ, Lombardi AV Jr, Lye CL. Mittelmier ceramic total hip arthroplasty: A retrospective study. J Arthroplasty 1988; 3:87–96.
18. Black J. Orthopaedic Biomaterials in Research and Practice. New York: Churchill Livingstone Inc., 1988:57–80.
19. Lerouge S, Yahie L, Sedel L. Alumina ceramic in total joint replacement. In: Sedel L, Cabanela ME, eds. Bioceramics 11. London: Martin Dunitz, 1998:31–40.
20. Mckellop H, Lu B. Friction, lubrication, and wear of cobalt–chromium, alumina, and zirconia hip prostheses compared on a joint simulator. Proceedings of Orthopaedic Research Society, Washington, DC 1992:402.
21. Shanbhag As, Jacobs JJ, Black J, Galante JO, Glant TT. Effects of particles on fibroblast proliferation and bone resorption in vitro. Clin Orthop Rel Res 1997; 342:205–217.
22. Böhler M, Mochida Y, Bauer T, Salzer M. Analysis of wear debris particles from alumina on alumina ceramic THA. In: Sedel L, Willman G, eds. Reliability and Long-Term Results of Ceramics in Orthopaedics: 4th International CeramTec Symposium. Stuttgart: Thieme, 1999:57–59.
23. Archibeck MJ, Jacobs JJ, Black J. Alternate bearing surfaces in total joint arthroplasty: Biologic considerations. Clin Orthop Rel Res 2000; 379:12–21.
24. Christel P. Biocompatibility of surgical-grade sense poly-crystalline alumina. Clin Orthop Rel Res 1992; 282:10–18.
25. Christel P. Ceramics for joint replacement. In: Morrey BF, ed. Biological, Material, and Mechanical Considerations of Joint Replacement. New York: Raven Press, 1993:303–317.
26. Willert HG. Reactions of the articular capsule to wear products of artificial joint prostheses. J Biomed Mater Res 1977; 11:157–164.
27. Catelas I, Huk OL, Petit A, Zukor DJ, Marchand R, Yahia L. Flow cytometric analysis of macrophage response to ceramic and polyethylene particle: effects of size, concentration, and compostion. J Biomed Mater Res 1998; 41:600–607.
28. Kubo T, Sawada K, Hirakawa K, Shimizu C, Takamatsu T, Hirasawa Y. Histiocyte reaction in rabbit femurs to UHMWPE, metal, and ceramic particles in different sizes. J Biomed Mater Res 1999; 45:363–369.

29. Ryu RK, Bovill EG Jr, Skinner HB, et al. Soft tissue sarcoma associated with aluminum oxide ceramic total hip arthroplasty. A case report. Clin Orthop Rel Res 1987; 216:207–212.

30. Winter M, Griss P, Scheller G, Moser T. Ten- to 14-year results of ceramic hip prosthesis. Clin Orthop Rel Res 1992; 282:73–79.

31. Walter IA. On the material and the tribology of alumina–alumina couplings for hip joint prostheses. Clin Orthop Rel Res 1992; 282:31–46.

32. Fritsch EW, Gleitz M. Ceramic femoral head fractures in total hip arthroplasty. Clin Orthop Rel Res 1996; 328:129–136.

33. Sedel L. Evolution of alumina/alumina implants. In: Sedel L, Willman G, eds. Reliability and Long-Term Results of Ceramics in Orthopaedics: 4th International CeramTec Symposium. Stuttgart: Thieme, 1999:2–6.

34. Mittelmeier H, Harms J. Treatment of post-traumatic hip disease by total replacement with a ceramic endoprosthesis. Unfallheilkunde 1979; 82:67–75.

35. Huo MH, Martin RP, Zatorski LE, Keggi KJ. Total hip replacements using the ceramic Mittelmeier prosthesis. Clin Orthop Rel Res 1996; 332:143–150.

36. Mahoney OM, Dimon JH. Unsatisfactory results with a ceramic total hip prosthesis. J Bone Joint Surg 1990; 72A:663–671.

37. Yoon TR, Rowe SM, Jung ST, Seon KJ, Maloney WJ. Osteolysis in association with a total hip arthroplasty with ceramic bearings surfaces. J Bone Joint Surg 1998; 80A:1459–1468.

38. Boehler M, Knahr K, Plenck H Jr, Walter A, Salzer M, Schreiber V. Long-term results of uncemented alumina acetabular implants. J Bone Joint Surg Br 1994; 76-B:53–59.

39. Sedel L, Kerboull L, Cristel P, Meunier A, Witvoet J. Alumina-on alumina hip replacement: results of survivorship in young patients. J Bone Joint Surg Br 1990; 72-B:658–663.

40. Riska EB. Ceramic endoprosthesis in total hip arthroplasty. Clin Orthop Rel Res 1993; 297:87–94.

41. Pitto RP, Schwämmlein D, Schramm M. Modular press-fit acetabular components in total hip arthroplasty. In: Willmann G, Zweymüller K, eds. Bioceramics in Hip Joint Replacement: Proceedings 5th International CeramTec Symposium. New York: Thieme, 2000:19–25.

42. Bizot P, Nizard R, Hamadouche M, Hannouche D, Sedel L. Prevention of wear and osteolysis: Alumma-on-alumina bearing. Clin Orthop Rel Res 2001; 393: 85–93.

43. Garino JP. Status and early results of modern ceramic-ceramic total hip replacement in the United States. In: Willmann G, Zweymüller K, eds. Bioceramics in Hip Joint Replacement: Proceedings 5th International CeramTec Symposium. New York: Thieme, 2000:88–91.

44. Rack R, Pfaff HG. Long term performance of the alumina matrix cocomposite biolox delta. In: Toni A, Willmann G, eds. Bioceramics in Hip Joint Arthroplasty: Proceedings 6th International CeramTec Symposium. Stuttgart, New York: Thieme, 2001:103–108.

28

Tissue Engineering Alternatives to Joint Replacement

B. Kinner

*Department of Orthopaedic Surgery, Brigham and Women's Hospital,
Harvard Medical School, Boston, Massachusetts, U.S.A. and Department of
Trauma Surgery, University of Regensburg, Regensburg, Germany*

M. Spector

*Department of Orthopaedic Surgery, Brigham and Women's Hospital,
Harvard Medical School, VA Boston Healthcare System, Boston,
Massachusetts, U.S.A.*

INTRODUCTION

Despite the success with which total joint prostheses are able to relieve pain and restore meaningful function to diseased joints, problems with joint arthroplasty remain. Concern regarding the longevity of prosthetic joints in young active patients and the profound consequences of multiple revision procedures has drawn attention to techniques for treating cartilage defects before they become symptomatic and involve the majority of the joint surface. The widespread implementation of arthroscopy and the improvements in imaging modalities have enabled the identification of defects in the articular surface that are likely to predispose to an arthritic condition. New treatment modalities hold the promise of inducing a reparative tissue in these defects that will yield pain-free function for a meaningful period, thus delaying the need for total joint arthroplasty. The early success achieved in treating these defined circumscribed lesions has also now led to a reconsideration of methodology for the treatment of the frankly arthritic joint to achieve a biological solution to the problem, as an alternative to prosthetic replacement.

Because of the public's heightened interest in tracking medical advances, patients generally have a greater awareness of new developments. It is important for the joint replacement surgeon to be prepared to respond to patients' inquiries about the meaningfulness of new treatment modalities. Patients want to know how newly developed cartilage repair procedures apply to their own joint problems. The objective of this chapter is to address the current status of, and future prospects for, cartilage repair.

The strategies being investigated in orthopaedic surgery for the regeneration of articular cartilage as an alternative to prosthetic joint replacement parallel those being implemented in other surgical disciplines for the treatment of problems in other organs. Important recent developments have been (i) the isolation of cells from tissues and expansion of their number in vitro under conditions that allow them to retain or recover their phenotypic traits, and (ii) the development of porous absorbable scaffolds into which cells can be seeded for their growth in three-dimensional culture. These developments have provided the opportunity for the formation of tissue in vitro and the formulation of cell-seeded constructs as implants to facilitate the regeneration of tissue in vivo. The former process was initially referred to as "tissue engineering" and the latter more recently has been called "regenerative medicine." However, these terms have now been used interchangeably to describe these and other methods directed toward providing a reparative tissue to restore the function of a tissue or organ.

CARTILAGE REPAIR PROCEDURES: HISTORICAL PERSPECTIVE

The limited healing potential of articular cartilage has been known for many years (1,2). However, despite intense research, the reasons are not completely understood. As with other tissues, cartilage repair depends on fibrin clot formation and the subsequent cascade of chondroprogenitor cells derived from adjacent cartilage, underlying marrow, or synovium that eventually lead to the formation of reparative tissue in the defect. Due to the rather unique anatomical and physiological characteristics of cartilage (viz., avascularity, low mitotic activity of chondrocytes, and the chondrocytic release of degrading enzymes) this process will not be initialized if the defect does not penetrate the subchondral bone.

Myriad repair procedures have been introduced in the last 30 years to overcome these limitations. Rinsing the joint, and therefore washing out debris and diluting degradative enzymes, resulted in some beneficial effect on patient symptoms. However, improvement was only found in 45% to 60% of patients and its duration was limited (3,4). Combining lavage with debridement of the defect increased the success rate to about 70% (5,6). However, overall results were generally regarded as unsatisfactory by the surgeons as by the patients. Second look arthroscopies revealed that there was some cartilage repair, but the repair tissue was limited in amount and inferior in tissue make up, since the predominant finding was fibrocartilage (6).

In the ensuing years it was learned that perforating the subchondral bone and accessing the underlying bone marrow resulted in some improvement. Chondroprogenitor cells, believed to reside within the bone marrow, were thought to infiltrate the defect and finally differentiate into chondrocytes. These cells then synthesized a durable extracellular matrix that was able to withstand mechanical loading.

Techniques implemented to provide access of bone marrow to a cartilage defect include: abrasion arthroplasty (6–9), subchondral drilling (8,10,11), spongialization (12), and fracturing the subchondral plate with special tools (13,14). The degree of damage introduced to the subchondral bone plate using these methods varies considerably. Promising results have been obtained using a technique called "microfracturing" (14). This method uses specially designed awls to make multiple perforations, or "microfractures," through the subchondral bone plate. Microfracture is minimally invasive because it is performed arthroscopicaly through standard portals in most cases. The perforations are made as close together as necessary, but not so close that one breaks into another. Consequently, the microfracture holes are approximately 3–4 mm apart (or 3–4 holes/cm^2). Importantly, the integrity of the subchondral bone plate is preserved, thus improving load-bearing characteristics following healing. No heat necrosis is introduced into the subchondral bone and marrow with microfracture. The released marrow elements form a "super clot" which provides an enriched environment for tissue regeneration. Follow-up with long-term results of more than eight years have been encouraging (14). About 67% of the patients treated by microfracture are improved with respect to their activities of daily living and ability to work. Twenty percent of patients remain unchanged and 13% are worse (15) relative to their preoperative condition.

The instruments used for microfracture, and the related depth and width of the perforation of the subchondral bone plate, are crucial (13). At the same time, however, surgical equipment and supply costs are minimal, without the need for expensive cell cultures or nonstandard apparatus. Microfracture is not overly demanding technically, but emphasis must be placed on meticulous handling of the subchondral plate and surrounding healthy cartilage and adequate debridement of unhealthy cartilage. Microfracture has been shown to be an effective tool in the treatment of chondral defects in both recreational and high-level athletes with mean follow-up of four years (16). Hence, this procedure has found widespread acceptance among orthopaedic surgeons around the world. However, no long-term outcomes or controlled studies have yet been published.

Osteochondral transplantation, another method for treating joint problems, has been used clinically for more than 25 years. Large osteochondral allografts have been applied for orthopaedic tumor surgery and to a lesser extent for repairing degenerative defects (17,18). However, for smaller defects these procedures introduced significant morbidity.

More recently osteochondral autografting has been introduced into the clinic as an alternative treatment for small or medium sized defects (19,20). Promising reports by Matsusue et al. (21) and Bobic (22) have fueled interest in this method. Matsusue was the first to harvest and implant osteochondral autografts in a patient with a cartilage defect associated with a rupture of the anterior cruciate ligament. Later Bobic (22) reported the treatment of 12 patients with multiple osteochondral transplants (5–10 mm in width and 10–15 mm in length). With this technique an osteochondral plug is harvested from a lower weight bearing area of the knee joint and transferred to the prepared defect, implanted using a press-fit technique. Using this approach, Bobic was able to treat defects up to $4 \, cm^2$.

Since 1992, Hangody et al. (23) has treated a total of 227 patients using osteochondral autografts for full-thickness lesions resulting from chondropathy, traumatic chondral defects, and osteochondritis dissecans; the procedure was evaluated in 57 patients who had more than three years of follow-up. Magnetic resonance imaging, computed tomography arthrographies, ultrasound, and arthroscopy were used to evaluate the technique. Using the modified Hospital for Special Surgery (HSS) knee scoring system, 91% of the patients achieved a good or excellent result. But there are also disadvantages: Graft matching and contouring to the recipient articular surface is difficult. The lack of available donor sites can be a limiting factor. Furthermore, the fibrocartilaginous interface between the donor and recipient site may contribute to breakdown in the long run.

Early results with osteochondral autografts are promising (22–26). However, no long-term patient outcomes or data from controlled clinical studies are available and there is limited knowledge about integration and survival of the chondral graft. Especially for larger defects, requiring the harvest of several plugs, the potential for harvest site morbidity becomes an issue. Of particular concern are cases in which there is too little donor material in the affected joint. In order to treat an osteochondritis dissecans lesion or other cartilage defect in the ankle after a traumatic injury, osteochondral plugs have usually been harvested from the knee joint (27). However, thus far no published data on this potentially valuable approach have been published. Considering the potential untoward clinical sequellae of creating donor defects in a previously healthy joint, this procedure should still be considered experimental.

For larger defects in the articular surface, osteochondral allografts can still be considered an alternative, with a 75% success rate at five years, 64% at 10 years, and 63% at 14 years. Chondrocyte viability has been shown up to 14 years (28). However, bipolar defects have a higher failure rate, as does the procedure performed in patients older than 60 years of age or with malalignment of the joint. Moreover, chondrocyte viability for cryopreserved allografts is known to be less than 10%, based on literature of tumor treatment.

CELL-BASED THERAPIES CURRENTLY EMPLOYED IN THE CLINIC

Novel techniques employing tissue engineering principles have been introduced into the clinic for the treatment of cartilage defects. These techniques are generally aimed at delivering chondrogenic cells to the cartilage defect, either in the form of tissues containing precursor cells [e.g., the periosteum (29) or the perichondrium (30)] or in the form of autologous chondrocytes isolated from a biopsy of healthy cartilage and expanded in number in vitro (31).

Autologous Periosteum Grafts

The use of autologous periosteum alone (29,32,37–40) has also been investigated for cartilage repair. Periosteal transplantation was initially described by Rubak (41). He used a periosteal flap to treat cartilage defects in rabbits. The results revealed that the defects were repaired and filled after four weeks with a hyaline-like cartilage whereas the empty control defect showed fibrocartilage-like repair tissue. The first trial in humans was published three years later by Niedermann et al. (42). They reported successful results in all of their four initially treated patients. Hoikka et al. (43) treated 13 patients, of which eight had a good results, four a fair outcome and one a poor result. O'Driscoll contributed in the following years valuable basic findings (35,37,44–46). It was found that orientation of the periosteal flap (cambium layer facing up), postoperative factors such as the use of continuous passive motion (32), and the age (44) and maturity of the experimental animal were of importance when dealing with periosteal transplants. O'Driscoll (29) himself treated approximately 40 patients, 20 of which had defects in the knee and were followed up by the author. Twelve individuals had a good outcome, four had poor results and four patients had inadequate length of follow-up. O'Driscoll also contributed valuable information on technical detail on harvesting the periosteal flap. In an animal model he could show that training the surgeon led to a significant increase of the chondrogenic potential of the harvested periosteum (47,48).

Altogether the results with periosteal grafting have been promising, but as with the other techniques, there have been no controlled studies, which would allow for comparison to other methods.

Perichondrium

Autologous perichondrium has also been employed for cartilage repair (30,49–51). Perichondrium, taken from the cartilaginous covering of the rib, is placed into the chondral defect of the affected joint. The first clinical study of this approach was performed by Homminga et al. (30). Twenty-five patients with 30 symptomatic chondral lesions received autologous perichondrial grafts taken from the costal arch and fixed to the subchondral bone with human fibrin glue. The majority of the lesions were graded Outerbridge grade III/IV and half were located on the medial femoral condyle. The opposing articulating surface had no greater than Outerbridge II changes. Preparation of the defect was performed using techniques very similar to those employed for ACI. Postoperatively, CPM was started two weeks after surgery and nonweight bearing was continued for three months. All patients were examined arthroscopically at an average of 10 months after implantation.

Of the 30 grafted defects, 27 had completely filled with tissue resembling cartilage. In two cases the defect was unchanged, and one patella graft was covered with white tissue with fibrillated surface. Three biopsies were taken at one year, two of which showed disruption of the cartilage–bone junction. Histologically, the regenerated cells appeared to be chondrocytes. Clinically, at one year the mean clinical improvement was 80%, as rated by the HSS grading scheme; 18 of the 25 patients were completely symptom free. These results remained stable even after 23.5 months, but at five years 20 of the 27 grafts were associated with pain and degeneration. A total of 88 patients were treated between 1986 and 1992 in one series (52). After a mean follow-up of four years only 38% showed a good, 8% a fair but 55% a poor result. Graft failure ranged between 33 and 62% according to the location of the defect. Only a small, carefully selected group of patients (isolated defects) showed good results in 91%.

Animal experiments subsequently demonstrated an increased calcification of the basal layer of the repair tissue (51) and this was confirmed clinically. Twenty-five out of 47 patients displayed calcification of the graft, prompting the authors to start a treatment with indomethacin (52).

One of the main shortcomings of perichondrial grafting is the limited availability of large grafts. Graft size is limited to the rib size, so that several rib perichondrial grafts have to be harvested to fill a large defect. Additionally, endochondral ossification and delamination of the cartilage from the subchondral bone plate are potentially significant limitations to the long-term efficacy of this repair.

Autologous Chondrocyte Implantation

Laboratory investigations of articular chondrocytes (viz., allogeneic cells), expanded in vitro, for cartilage repair date back more than 20 years (53), In a study in rabbits Grande et al. (54) showed that defects that had received transplants had a significant amount of cartilage reconstituted (82%), compared to ungrafted controls (18%). Brittberg et al. (55) later obtained similar results treating 51 New Zealand white rabbits. Autologous chondrocyte implantation (ACI) significantly increased the amount of newly formed repair tissue up to 52 weeks in contrast to the lack of intrinsic repair with periosteal grafts alone. However, they also noted that repair tissue tended to be incompletely bonded to the adjacent cartilage.

Subsequently, Breinan et al. (56) repeated these experiments in a canine model. They found no significant differences among the treated and control (periosteum alone and nontreated defects) groups after one year. By 18 months neither a complete filling, nor the restoration of the architecture was complete (Figs. 1 and 2) (57). Moreover, cartilage surrounding the defect showed degenerative changes, which seemed to be related to suturing of the periostel flap. These results were in contrast to the very promising result after six months where a reasonable amount of defect filling with hyaline-like articular cartilage could be seen. These contradictory results might have been due in part to differences in the animal models. Dogs have a thin subchondral bone plate that can easily be damaged. As a consequence, mesenchymal stem cells can get access to the defect and mix with the implanted chondrocytes.

Other related work showed a significant correlation between the degree to which the calcified cartilage layer and subchondral bone were disturbed and the amount of defect filling (57). Comparing microfracture treatment with ACI showed that more defect filling was achieved using microfracture technique, whereas the defect was more likely to be filled with hyaline cartilage after ACI. This work stresses the importance of an intact calcified cartilage layer for obtaining repair tissue composed mainly of articular cartilage. However, the amount of filling repair tissue is inversely related to the remaining intact calcified cartilage (Fig. 3).

Additionally, the observation that some spontaneous regeneration can occur in a canine model raised the question of the degree to which such regeneration can occur in humans (58). In a surgical created full-thickness cartilage defect (to the tide mark) in 20 adult mongrel dogs, 40% of the created defects were filled with reparative tissue, and 19% of which were found to be hyaline-like articular cartilage (58). Therefore, investigations of new modalities treating lesions in articular cartilage have to acknowledge, through careful design of controls, the potential for spontaneous regeneration (58).

On basis of promising animal studies (rabbit) ACI was introduced into the clinic. Brittberg et al. (31) were the first to publish their results on 23 patients treated in Sweden for symptomatic cartilage defects. Thirteen patients had femoral condylar defects, ranging in size from 1.6 to 6.5 cm^2, due to trauma or osteochondritis dissecans. Seven patients had patellar defects. Ten patients had previously been treated with shaving and debridement of unstable cartilage. Cartilage was harvested arthroscopically from a minimally load-bearing area of the upper aspect or the medial condyle of the affected knee. Chondrocytes were isolated and culture expanded in a cell

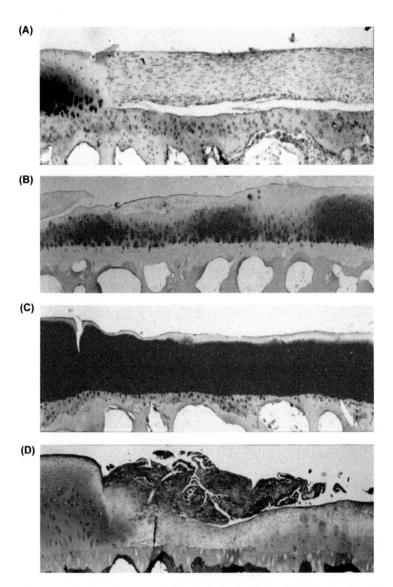

Figure 1 Light micrographs showing the healing of ACI-treated canine articular defects after, (**A**) 1.5 months, defect filled with fibrous tissue (H&E staining), (**B**) 3 months, approximately 50% of the defect is filled with repair tissue, comprising transitional tissue, hyaline cartilage and some articular cartilage (safranin O—fast green staining), (**C**) 6 months: defect filled approximately 80%, predominantly with hyaline and to some extent articular cartilage (safranin O—fast green staining), (**D**) 12 months: break down of repair tissue, note: decreased staining for gylcosaminogly-canes as present in osteoarthritis (staining shown here in gray scale). *Abbreviation*: ACI, autologous chondrocyte implantation.

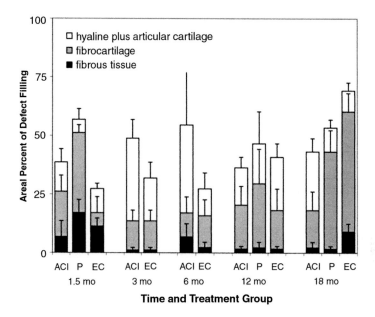

Figure 2 Results of histomorphometric evaluations of repair tissue in a canine articular cartilage defect model. *Abbreviations*: ACI, autologous chondrocytes implantation; EC, empty (untreated) control, periosteum control, mean ± SEM.

culture lab. During a second operation, the defect was debrided using a medial or lateral parapatellar incision. Then a periosteal flap was harvested and sutured to the rim of the defect. Finally, the chondrocyte suspension was injected under the periosteal flap.

The results were very promising for the condylar defects. Patients were followed for 16–66 months (mean, 39 months). Initially, the transplants eliminated knee locking and reduced pain and swelling in all patients. After three months, arthroscopy showed that the transplants were level with the surrounding tissue and spongy when probed, with visible borders. A second arthroscopic examination showed that in many instances the transplants had the same macroscopic appearance as they had earlier but were firmer when probed and similar in appearance to the surrounding cartilage. Two years after transplantation, 14 of the 16 patients with femoral condylar transplants had good-to-excellent results. Two patients required a second operation because of severe central wear in the transplants, with locking and pain. A mean of 36 months after transplantation, the results were excellent or good in two of the seven patients with patellar transplants, fair in three, and poor in two; two patients required a second operation because of severe chondromalacia. Biopsies showed that 11 of the 15 femoral transplants and one of the seven patellar transplants had the appearance

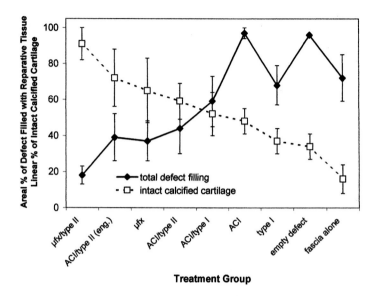

Figure 3 Graph depicting the inverse relationship between intact calcified cartilage for 15-week canine implant groups and controls. Linear regression analysis of the correlation of total filling with intact calcified cartilage $R^2 = 0.61$: µfx, microfracture, ACI, autologous chondrocyte implantation; type I and type II refer to the applied collagen matrices.

of "hyaline-like" cartilage. These results and the fact that a commercial service for culturing autologous chondrocytes was established led to a dramatic increase in the use of this cell-based therapy for cartilage repair.

While there appear to be general similarities in the procedures used by various commercial and academic laboratories for the isolation and expansion of articular chondrocytes for ACI, there may be important differences. One such difference is the use of the patient's own serum for culturing the cells, as described in the original method by Brittberg et al. (31). One commercial enterprise, Genzyme Biosurgery (Cambridge, Massachusetts, USA), uses approved and validated fetal bovine serum, instead of the patient's serum, in the culture media. Another potentially important difference is that Genzyme needs to freeze and store the isolated cells in order to allow for verification of adequate insurance coverage prior to the implantation procedure. A recent study has indicated that this freeze–thaw cycle may adversely affect the outcome of the procedure. Perka et al. (59) demonstrated that cryopreserved chondrocytes seeded into polymer scaffolds yielded a 85% repair of an osteochondral defect in rabbits, whereas 100% of the defects treated with noncryopreserved cells were filled. Additional work is necessary to more fully explore the effects of certain handling and culture procedures on the performance of monolayer-expanded chondrocytes in ACI.

ACI Procedure

Since first published in 1994, techniques of cell isolation, expansion in culture, and implantation have remained essentially the same. Cartilage (150–300 mg) is harvested arthroscopically from a minimally load-bearing area of the upper aspect or the medial condyle of the affected knee. The biopsy is then transported to a laboratory facility using transport media. Chondrocytes are isolated using standard techniques. After a certain period of cell expansion [11–21 days (60), depending upon the growth kinetics] a certain number of cells (e.g., minimally 12×10^6 for Genzyme's Carticel procedure) are provided in a serum-free and gentamycin-free transport medium.

Using a medial or lateral parapatellar incision, the defect is debrided to the level of normal-appearing surrounding cartilage. The integrity of the tidemark needs to be maintained in order to avoid infiltration of undifferentiated mesenchymal stem cells which could contribute to the formation of fibrocartilagenous repair tissue (61). A periosteal flap is harvested from the anterior aspect of the proximal tibia or distal femur, formed to the shape of the lesion, and sutured to the rim of the defect. The border of periosteal cover is then sealed using fibrin glue. The chondrocyte suspension is subsequently injected under the periosteal flap. Postoperative rehabilitation protocols generally involve continuous passive motion and limited weight bearing for an extended time. Cooperation of the patient in this respect is essential for a favorable outcome, hence, difficult to control. This contributes to the difficulty in evaluating outcome data.

Clinical Results

Follow-up investigations of the two largest patient groups have been reported: patients treated in Sweden predominately by L. Peterson, M.D., and M. Brittberg, M.D., and the Genzyme Cartilage Repair Registry. Peterson et al. (60) recently reported their 2–9 year results including clinical, arthroscopic, and histological evaluations of 101 patients. In this retrospective study, ACI yielded good results in 92% for isolated femoral lesions, 67% for multiple lesions, 89% for osteochondritis dissecans, and 65% for patella defects after an average follow-up of 4.2 years. Arthroscopically follow-up in 65 of 93 patients showed slow maturing of the tissue during the first year, however, repair tissue at the subsequent follow-ups was as firm as the adjacent tissue. Histopathologic analysis in 21 patients revealed a homogenous matrix with low cellularity considered to be "hyaline like" in 17 patients, whereas four patients showed fibrous repair tissue. Immunohistochemistry for collagen type II was positive in all of the patients with "hyaline like" repair tissue, and negative in the fibrous repair tissue. Adverse events were reported in 51% of the patients, including seven graft failures (7%) and 10 adhesions which needed arthroscopic intervention. Graft hypertrophy, attributed to the periosteal flap, was seen in 26 patients.

The last volume of the Genzyme Patient Registry Report included five-year patient outcomes for individuals treated outside of Sweden. Progressive improvement in the overall condition of the patients and in symptomatology could be demonstrated at 24, 36, 48, and 60 months. Improvement compared to baseline was 79% (78%) for all treated locations as rated by the clinician (patient). However, there was a difference between the treatment sites, with ACI being most successful at the lateral femoral condyle (100% improvement, $n = 3$) and less successful if treating a defect in the trochlea (50%, $n = 2$). Adverse events were reported in 7% of the patients ($n = 4834$). These included adhesions or fibroarthrosis in 2% and hypertrophic changes in 1.3%. The cumulative incidence of treatment failure was estimated as 3.0% at 60 months. 5.9% of the patients treated reported an operation following implantation.

Federal Regulations

Since the clinical introduction of the procedure there has been much attention paid to the standardization and validation of the cell culture procedures. In August, 1997 the United States Food and Drug Administration granted accelerated approval for Genzyme's Carticel procedure for the repair of symptomatic, cartilaginous defects of the femoral condyle, including both first and second line repairs (FDA Talk paper, T97-38). As a condition of this approval, Genzyme agreed to conduct two studies, including a multicenter, randomized controlled trial in 300 patients comparing Carticel to other primary repair techniques, to confirm the benefits of Carticel in this setting.

However, to date Genzyme has not been able to enroll an adequate number of patients in either of the planned studies. As a result Genzyme changed the product labeling, narrowing the indications for Carticel to second line therapy for the repair of cartilage defects of the femoral condyle.

Risks and Quality Control

The risks associated with ACI are unknown, but might include the following: (i) adverse effects of the harvest procedure to procure the articular cartilage tissue for cell isolation, (ii) effects of the arthrotomy currently required for the open implantation of the cells, (iii) degeneration of the adjacent articular cartilage related to the damage due to suturing, (iv) flap detachment, and (v) malignant transformation of cells in culture.

Fortunately, while there is a finite possibility (albeit small) for malignant or dysplastic transformation of cells during their in vitro expansion, no such occurrence has been reported. In addition, implantation of normal autologous chondrocytes could potentially stimulate growth of malignant cells in the area of the implant, although there have been no reported incidents in humans.

Another problem in using autologous articular chondrocytes arises on the harvest site. To obtain autologous chondrocytes, healthy cartilage must be harvested from uninvolved and principal "unloaded" areas of the femoral side of the knee. Published data on the healing of the harvest sites is scarce. For all of these techniques it is assumed that cartilage harvest does not affect overall outcome. There are no clinical studies, however, focusing on the harvest site. Harvesting cartilage for ACI makes a second operation necessary with all theoretical possibilities of complication (e.g., infection). Moreover, the harvest procedure may place the other cartilage in the joint at risk of degeneration as a recent animal study has shown (62).

Although autologous cell therapies circumvent complications like graft rejection or viral transmission, significant challenges exist in assuring a safe and reproducible product. Genzyme established a quality assurance program based on US FDA Good Manufacturing Practice regulations, which was reviewed recently (63). Process variables have to be controlled rigorously and testing stalled for sterility testing and endotoxin testing. Moreover, assessments of cell viability and growth kinetics are a crucial part of nonconformance reporting.

According to Genzyme data, 1.64% of the cartilage biopsies received were contaminated. Contamination was recorded only for 0.03% during processing and in 0.16% at release. Endotoxin content ranged between less than 0.15 and 0.5 EU/mL (allowable limit 82.5 EU/mL), and cell viability was $90.9 \pm 4.06\%$ at release. Measurement of growth kinetics revealed 0.311 doublings per day. Out of 1377 cartilage biopsies, 86 nonconformances were identified related to biopsy quality; only 12 were related to cell processing.

COMPARISON OF RESULTS FROM CARTILAGE REPAIR PROCEDURES CURRENTLY EMPLOYED IN THE CLINIC

In recent years biologic or tissue engineered therapies of cartilage defects have progressed significantly and are becoming important modalities of treatment in orthopaedic surgery. However, for all these therapies long-term outcome is unknown, and there is a lack of controlled studies comparing the different treatment options. Prospective studies are needed to better understand which of the different options will be the most suitable for specific indications.

A recent study compared the histological outcomes of different cartilage repair procedures (64). The reparative tissue was retrieved during revision surgery from full thickness chondral defects in 18 patients in whom abrasion arthroplasty ($n = 12$), grafting of perichondrial flaps ($n = 4$), and periosteal patching augmented by autologous chondrocyte implantation in cell suspension ($n = 6$) failed to provide lasting relief of symptoms. Histologic and immunohistochemical investigations showed fibrous, spongiform tissue comprising type I collagen in $22 \pm 9\%$ (mean $\pm$ standard error of the mean) of the cross-sectional area, and degenerating hyaline tissue ($30 \pm 10\%$) and fibrocartilage ($28 \pm 7\%$) with positive type II collagen staining. Three of four specimens obtained after implantation of perichondrium failed as a result of bone formation that was found in $19 \pm 6\%$ of the cross-sectional area, including areas staining positive for type X collagen, as an indicator for hypertrophic chondrocytes. Revision after autologous chondrocyte implantation was associated with partial displacement of the periosteal graft from the defect site because of insufficient ongrowth or early suture failure. When the graft edge displaced, repair tissue was fibrous ($55 \pm 11\%$), whereas graft tissue attached to subchondral bone displayed hyaline tissue (to 6%) and fibrocartilage (to 12%) comprising type II collagen at three months after surgery.

Competing and alternative techniques like osteochondral autograft transfer (21,22), mosaicplasty (23), or osteochondral paste have to be considered or included into the therapeutic algorithm (65). Not only the quality of the provided cells and the technical procedure of implanting the cells affect the outcome. Correction of predisposing factors like malalignment of the knee or maltracking of the patella has been shown to be necessary for a good clinical outcome (66).

One of the main shortcomings of comparing different cartilage repair procedures as above is that we are dealing with an array of different indications, predisposing deformities, and extent of disease or injury. However, it is crucial to exactly distinguish among the different entities of cartilage defects, and to acknowledge the size of the defect.

In recent years, important advances have been made in the arthroscopic and noninvasive diagnosis of cartilage defects. In the future diagnostics might go far beyond what is routinely done today, providing a mechanical analysis. A topographic and "biochemical" analysis of the cartilage might soon be available through improved MRT imaging techniques or optical coherence tomography (OCT). Additionally a genetic analysis might prove to be of value to improve on selecting patients for one or the other method.

In summary, not only will the development of new techniques replacing the damaged cartilage be necessary, but also an improvement of diagnostic tools and understanding of the pathological processes underlying cartilage damage and breakdown that prevent the healing of injured cartilage.

NOVEL TISSUE ENGINEERING APPROACHES FOR CARTILAGE REPAIR CURRENTLY UNDERGOING INVESTIGATION

Many basic and preclinical investigations of novel techniques are being directed toward improving cartilage repair procedures. Research concentrates on

Table 1 Summary of Cells Used for Cell-Based Cartilage Repair Procedures and Tissue Engineering Approaches

Cell type	References
Autologous chondrocytes	31,55,56,60,168,169
Allogeneic chondrocytes	119,170,171
Autologous rib/ear perichondrial cells	51,52,172,173
Mesenchymal stem cells	
Bone marrow derived	94,96,127,174,175
Adipose tissue derived	108
Trabecular bone derived	106
Muscle derived	107
Neonatal foreskin fibroblasts	76,176

the three major areas of tissue engineering: optimizing the cell source for cartilage repair, delivering the cells together with a suitable scaffold, and introducing soluble regulators into the system. There are a considerable number of parameters relating to these issues (Tables 1, 2 and 3). In the future we will have to determine which combination might be the most valuable. The following paragraphs will discuss some of these options.

Cell Sources

One decision is whether to use fully differentiated cells or precursors (e.g., isolated from a bone marrow biopsy) for tissue engineering approaches Table 1. It might also be suitable to recruit enough endogenous local cells capable of migration, proliferation, differentiation, and biosynthesis using a method similar to microfracture.

Table 2 Summary of Matrices Used for Cartilage Tissue Engineering

Matrix composition	References
Collagen, type I	82,90,119,121,177
Collagen, type II	82,90
Devitalized articular cartilage	178–180
Agarose	181
Cellulose	181,182
Coral, hydroxyapatite	130
Polylactic acid (PLA)	129,183
Polyglycolic acid (PGA)	121
PLA/PGA composite	121,125,160
Polypropylene	182
PEMA/THFMA	184

Autologous Articular Chondrocytes

The rationale for using articular chondrocytes for a cell-based therapy is that they already possess the desired phenotype (67). Chondrocytes comprise the single cellular component of adult hyaline cartilage and are considered to be terminally differentiated, thus being highly specialized. Their main function is to maintain the cartilage matrix, synthesizing—types II, IX, and XI collagen; the large aggregating proteoglycan, aggrecan; the smaller proteoglycans biglycan and decorin; and several specific and nonspecific matrix proteins that are expressed at defined stages during growth and development. Freshly isolated articular chondrocytes continue to exhibit their specific phenotype in culture for at least several days to weeks. This makes them a suitable cell type for a cell-based treatment of chondral defects.

One of the disadvantages of employing articular chondrocytes is that they do not readily proliferate in vitro. Cells from a younger population (e.g., third and fourth decades of life) have been found to undergo 0.3 doublings per day, using a standardized and validated approach for culturing cells for later implantation (63). Even lower proliferation rates are obtained in older patients and arthritic cartilage (60). Another report shows the rapid replicative senescence of articular chondrocytes (68).

Once chondrocytes are deprived of their three-dimensional environment, their phenotype switches to a more fibroblastic cell form, expressing types I and III collagen instead of cartilage specific type II collagen (69–71). The process of "de-differentiation" is known to be dependent upon culture conditions. Expression of fibroblast-like proteins and morphology can be promoted by seeding at low density and treatment with certain cytokines (70). On the other hand "re-differentiation," re-expression of cartilage-specific behavior can be accomplished: (i) using selected culture systems, including spinner flasks (72) and dishes coated with materials that prevent cell adherence—agarose or collagen gels (73); (ii) seeding in high density micromass cultures (74,75); (iii) using hypoxic culture conditions (76); and (iv) by embedding the cells in solid matrices that do not allow adherence—agarose (77), collagen, or alginate gels (78–80). The chondrocytic phenotype can also be maintained when the cells are seeded in certain sponge-like scaffolds used for tissue engineering (81,82). Additionally, different cytokines have influence on the degree of expression of cartilage specific molecules. Members of the transforming growth factor beta (TGF-β) superfamily can trigger the expression of the chondrocytic phenotype (83). Additionally, staurosporine, a protein kinase C inhibitor (75,76,84), insulin-like growth factor (IGF) with or without addition of insulin (85–87), hepatocyte growth factor (HGF), and fibroblast growth factor (FGF) (81,88) have been shown to increase the expression of cartilage specific matrix products.

Other studies propose that chondrocytes, even if dedifferentiated after a extended time in monolayer culture, re-express their chondrocytic phenotype if implanted into a cartilage defect in vivo, probably due to the release of growth and differentiation factors from the adjacent host tissue (89). However, more recent studies suggest that this process might not be occurring (90).

Other recent studies have demonstrated that as articular chondrocytes are expanded in monolayer culture a greater percentage of cells express the gene that encodes for a contractile muscle actin, a-smooth muscle actin (SMA). These studies have also demonstrated that SMA-expressing cells in articular cartilage are capable of contracting a collagen–glycosaminoglycan analog of extracellular matrix in vitro (91,92). Moreover, cells with a higher passage number express higher levels of SMA and display higher levels of contractility (92). This work raises the question of the role that SMA expression may play once the cells are injected into the cartilage defect.

Another issue in employing autologous articular chondrocytes relates to donor site morbidity. To obtain autologous chondrocytes, healthy cartilage must be harvested from uninvolved regions of the joint. Although it has been assumed that there are no major problems associated with the harvest of cartilage, evidence is scarce. There are no published clinical studies focusing on the harvest site. Harvesting cartilage for ACI makes a second operation necessary with all theoretical possibilities of complication (e.g., infection). Moreover, harvesting cartilage might initiate additional damage to the joint. A recent study in a canine animal model (62) demonstrated that the harvest of articular cartilage introduces distinct changes of the mechanical behavior of the cartilage distant from the harvest site. The articular cartilage in the harvested joint displayed a three-fold increase of dynamic stiffness and streaming potential. These changes are consistent with hypertrophic changes that may precede degeneration. Clearly, additional studies are necessary to determine the consequences of harvesting articular cartilage for the isolation of chondrocytes for cell-based therapies.

Mesenchymal Stem Cells

The difficulty in obtaining chondrocytes and maintaining differentiated cell cultures has led to research on other cell types for cell-based therapies for cartilage repair. Several studies have shown that autologous bone marrow derived progenitor cells and periosteum-derived cells are able to exhibit a chondrocytic phenotype in vivo (93) and in vitro under certain conditions (94).

Friedenstein (95,96) was the first to describe the plastic adherence of bone marrow-derived stromal cells to tissue culture plastic. Using this phenotypic characteristic he was able to easily separate mesenchymal from hematopoietic progenitor cells. Subsequently Haynesworth et al. (97), Bruder et al. (98), and Johnstone and Yoo (99) developed a culture system that facilitated the chondrogenic differentiation of bone marrow-derived mesenchymal progenitor cells. Cells obtained in bone marrow aspirates were first isolated by monolayer culture and then transferred into conical tubes and allowed to form three-dimensional aggregates in a chemically defined medium which included dexamethasone and/or TGB-β1. The chondrogenic differentiation of cells within the aggregate was evidenced by the appearance of toluidine blue metachromasia and the immunohistochemical detection of type II collagen (94). Chondrogenic differentiation in this environment seemed to recapitulate embryonic chondrogenesis.

In an undifferentiated stage bone marrow-derived cells have almost unlimited proliferative capacity without any signs of senescence as shown by unchanged telomere length (100). Because the mesenchymal stem cells (MSCs) are readily available and easy to obtain, interest in applying bone marrow-derived precursor cells for cell therapy and tissue engineering is growing. Several preclinical studies also suggest the value of hMSC for cartilage repair (101,102). Some reports even suggest a lower chondrogenic activity of articular chondrocytes compared to mesenchymal stem cells isolated from the same animal (goat model) (103).

Recent investigations carried out by Osiris therapeutics suggest that MSCs, delivered by direct injection into the osteoarthritic joint, may bind to the surface of fibrillated host tissue and potentially alter the progression of the disease (102). Murphy et al. (101) could show that injection of MSCs into destabilized, osteoarthritic joints of 24 goats resulted in marked regeneration of the medial meniscus, which had been previously excised. The neo-tissue formed had a hyaline appearance with focal areas rich in type-II collagen similar to developing meniscus. In parallel with this tissue regeneration there was a marked chondroprotective effect.

Despite promising reports of hMSC for the treatment of musculoskeletal defects, no clinical trials have yet been published. Osiris has begun a Phase 1 safety trial with autologous hMSC delivered on a hydroxyapatite matrix (OsteoCelTM) in alveolar ridge regeneration prior to dental implantation. Others have used hMSC together with bone marrow transplants to correct genetic defects like osteogenesis imperfecta (104,105).

Other approaches describe the isolation of progenitor cells, viz. cells capable of differentiation along multilineage pathways, from trabecular bone explants (106), skeletal muscle (107), and fat tissue (108). Culturing these cells at high-density or under hypoxic conditions (micromass cultures) promotes differentiation towards a chondrocytic phenotype, viz. the expression of chondrogenic genes (74,99,109). This process may also be facilitated by addition of selected cytokines including TGF-β1 or 3 and BMP-2, and perhaps by merely adding dexamethasone to the culture medium (99). The principal advantages associated with the use of these cells over autologous articular chondrocytes for cartilage repair procedures are their ready availability and minimal donor site morbidity.

Moreover, with the development of gene transfer techniques, these cells have become the targets of in vitro and in vivo gene therapy, which involves direct injection of viral and nonviral vectors carrying transgenes. Importantly, in vitro data suggest that the chondrogenic potential of these cells is maintained with virally mediated ex vivo gene transfer (110,111).

Embryonic Stem Cells

Recently also embryonic stem cells have gained interest for cell therapy and transplantation. The feasibility of isolating and culture expanding embryonic stem cells as well as their differentiation into bone and cartilage has been shown (112). However, legal and ethical issues have restricted widespread embryonic stem cell research and cell therapy approaches.

Fibroblasts

Nicoll et al. (76) described a model for the conversion of human dermal fibroblasts to chondrocyte-like cells and the potential application of this methodology to cartilage tissue engineering. Human neonatal foreskin fibroblasts were seeded in two-dimensional high-density micromass cultures in the presence of staurosporine and lactic acid to induce functional hypoxia. Cells were also seeded into three-dimensional polymer scaffolds. Northern analysis revealed aggrecan core protein expression in lactate-treated micromass cultures, and type I collagen gene expression was virtually abolished in all cultures supplemented with staurosporine. Moreover, the cells in these cultures displayed a rounded, cobblestone-shaped morphology typical of differentiated chondrocytes and were organized into nodules which stained positive with Alcian blue. When seeded on PGA/PLLA matrices a chondrocyte-like morphology was observed in cultures treated with lactate and staurosporine in contrast to the flattened sheets of fibroblast-like cells seen in untreated controls. Also this approach might hold promise for the use of readily accessible nonchondrocytic autologous cells for cartilage repair procedures.

Allogeneic Cells

From a commercial point of view the use of allogeneic cell would be desirable. Transplantation of allogeneic osteochondral grafts has been used clinically for many years (17,113,114), and several investigations have focused on studying tissue engineering using allogeneic cells (115–118). Moreover, it has been proposed (119) that allogeneic chondrocytes from amputated limbs or joint arthoplasties might play a major role in the future. However, issues related to immune response and transmission of disease make this approach currently less attractive.

On the other hand allogeneic bone marrow transplantation has been used successfully for many years. Further research is needed before allogeneic cell transplantation is applied clinically for the purpose of cartilage repair.

Matrices

As phenotypic changes of chondrocytes in monolayer culture have been shown in many studies, interest has focused on three-dimensional systems to culture and deliver the cells to the defect. These systems can act as templates for growth and hence contribute to phenotypic stability of the chondrocytes. A second important feature of a scaffolding device is the increased surface available for the cells to attach and finally participate in the repair process. Additionally the matrix, or scaffold, can have several roles in the process of tissue engineering. These roles include: (i) structural support for the defect site, (ii) barrier to the ingrowth of undesirable cell and tissue types, (iii) scaffold for cell migration and proliferation, and (iv) carrier or reservoir of cells or regulators (e.g., growth factors). A variety of scaffolds have shown promise thus far. Table 2 summarizes the matrices currently under investigation for cartilage repair.

Bell (120) described the ideal scaffold for tissue engineering as one that provides a transitional framework whereby the cells populating it create a replacement tissue as the scaffolding material disappears. Ideally this scaffold should be degraded at the same speed that the cells produce their own framework. Other studies have demonstrated that matrix composition affects cell viability, cell attachment, morphology, and synthesis of matrix components.

What is the rationale for scaffold selection? Selecting or even more designing and constructing an ideal matrix for cartilage tissue engineering requires careful consideration of numerous factors (121). Questions which need to be addressed in the near future are: Which material should be used? What should the degradation rate be? What is the optimal pore size?

The following general properties are crucial matrix requirements for tissue engineering in general (122,123):

1. Cell adhesion to the matrix.
2. Neither the polymer or degradation products must be toxic or antigenic.
3. Reproducible three-dimensional structure.
4. Porosity >90%. Maximized surface for cell–matrix interactions, allow for cell migration and the deposition of extra cellular matrix. Supporting diffusion of nutrients and gas exchange during in vitro culture.
5. Complete degradation after completing the supportive function.
6. Steady state between matrix production of the cells and degradation of the matrix.

Moreover specific requirements of a matrix for cartilage tissue engineering are necessary:

1. The matrix should support cartilage *specific* matrix production (collagen type II and aggrecan). Our previous studies showed that

there is a considerable difference between the scaffolds, even if only changing the collagen type, pore size, or method of cross-linking (82,90).

2. Matrix should provide enough mechanical support for allowing early mobilization of the treated joint (33,124).
3. Allow for cell migration of cells to achieve a good bonding to the adjacent host tissue.

The following will discuss the most commonly used matrices.

Poly alpha-hydroxy esters, specifically polylactic acid (PLA) and polyglycolic acid (PGA) and their copolymers have a long history of use as synthetic biodegradable materials, and have been used as surgical suture material, plates, and screws for fracture fixation devices. They have already been accepted by the US FDA for certain clinical applications and are therefore very attractive as biosynthetic material for cartilage tissue engineering. Degradation rate can be controlled during the fabrication process (weeks–years) and degradation products are nontoxic. However, at high concentrations the degradation products lactic and glycolic acid can cause a decrease in local pH, resulting in tissue damage (123,125).

Porous type I collagen sponge-like matrices have also been researched extensively for regeneration of skin, bone, knee meniscus articular cartilage, esophagus, and muscle. Copolymers with glycosaminoglycans have been applied for skin, bone, and cartilage regeneration. More recently type II collagen, with or without copolymers have also been investigated (82,90). Stiffness and degradation rate can be controlled by cross-linking of the collagen molecules as well as the copolymer. Cell morphology has been found to be dependent on collagen type and pore diameter. It was shown that 60% of canine chondrocytes retained their spherical shape in a collagen type II matrix, compared to 30% in the respective collagen type I matrix (82). Moreover chondrocytes in the type II matrix synthesized more glycosaminoglycans.

Pore size is especially critical to obtain a uniform cell distribution throughout the matrix. The higher the porosity the more cells are able to penetrate the matrix and finally attach to the collagen fibers.

In a comparison of several matrix materials (PGA, collagen–gel, porous collagen), Grande et al. showed a marked variability of the chondrocyte response. Bioabsorbable polymers such as PGA enhanced proteoglycan synthesis, whereas collagen matrices stimulated synthesis of collagen (121).

Not only is there a lack of clinical data on matrix applications for cartilage repair, there are also only a few preclinical studies in larger animals. Most of the in vivo work has been done in rabbits and has shown comparatively uniform good results (94,119,126–130). However, few studies have systematically compared different methods in a larger animal model. In this respect work done by Breinan et al. (57) is of importance, comparing the effects of three different treatments on the healing of articular cartilage defects in a canine model previously .developed for ACI. In the articular surface of the trochlear grooves of 12 adult mongrel dogs, two 4-mm-diameter defects were made to the depth of the tidemark. Four dogs were assigned to each treatment group: (i) microfracture treatment, (ii) microfracture with a type II collagen matrix placed in the defect, and (iii) type II matrix seeded with cultured autologous chondrocytes. After 15 weeks, the defects were studied histologically. Data quantified on histological cross sections included area or linear percentages of specific tissue types filling the defect, integration of reparative tissue with the calcified and the adjacent cartilage, and integrity of the subchondral plate. Total defect filling (i.e., the percentage of the cross-sectional area of the original defect filled with any type of reparative tissue) averaged 56–86%, with the greatest amount found in the dogs in the microfracture group implanted with a type-II collagen matrix. The profiles of tissue types for the dogs in each treatment group were similar: the tissue filling the defect was predominantly fibrocartilage, with the balance being fibrous tissue (Fig. 4). There were no significant differences in the percentages of the various tissue types among dogs in the three groups.

Taking the results of these dog experiments together and comparing the different repair methods 15 weeks postoperatively, there was a significant correlation between the degree to which the calcified cartilage layer and subchondral bone were disrupted and the amount of tissue filling. Moreover, when it formed, hyaline cartilage most frequently occurred superficial to intact calcified cartilage.

Soluble Regulators

Polypeptide growth factors play a major role in the regulation of cell behavior, including that of chondrocytes (Table 3). Among the most influential of these factors identified for articular chondrocytes are insulin-like growth factor I (IGF-β1), basic fibroblast growth factor (FGF-2), and TGF-β). Selected growth factors—individually or in combination—may be added to the growth medium (Table 3). Chondrocyte responsiveness to growth factors has been shown to change during development, and after skeletal maturity; there is a profound decline in the levels of DNA synthesis and cell replication in response to the known chondrocyte growth factors (131).

To promote matrix production, culture media can be supplemented with ascorbic acid (25 μg/mL) which has been found to increase the amount of matrix production during short-term culture. However, it was also found to inhibit the transcription of cartilage-specific matrix genes in long-term culture (132). TGF-β was found to promote differentiation of chondrocytes and thus support matrix synthesis (133–136). In addition to being a potent mitogen for articular chondrocytes, FGF-2 has been found to support their differentiated state in a three-dimensional culture system (81) and has been

(A)

(B)

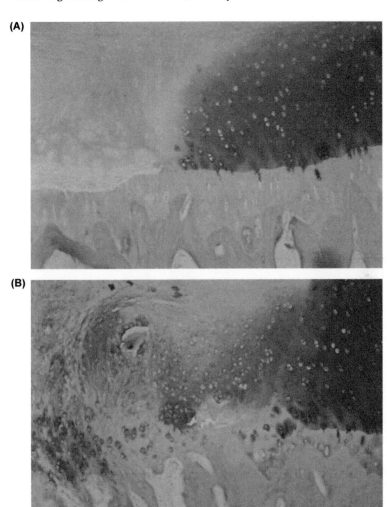

Figure 4 Light micrographs of healing full-thickness chondral articular defects in the canine trochlear groove 15 weeks after treatment (safranin O/fast green, shown here in gray scale). (**A**) Microfracture treatment resulting in fibrous tissue. No staining for glycosaminoglycanes. Portions of the repair tissue are well integrated with adjacent cartilage; however, there is no bonding to the calcified cartilage (40×), (**B**) Microfracture treatment plus type II collagen matrix. The reparative tissue, is primarily fibrocartilage, and to some extend hyaline cartilage (40×), (**C**) Results of histomorphometric evaluations of repair tissue μfx, microfracture; μfx, microfracture plus type II collagen matrix (mean ± SEM).

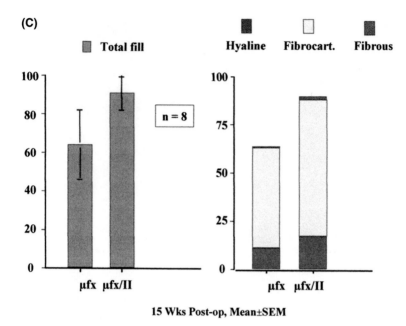

Figure 4   (*Continued*)

shown to augment articular cartilage repair in vivo. Other experiments have shown synergetic effects of TGF-β and FGF-2 (137). However, TGF-β may elicit seemingly opposite effects under different experimental conditions. These and other cytokines interact to modulate their respective actions, creating effector cascades and feedback loops of intercellular and intracellular events that control articular chondrocyte functions (138).

Because the actions of growth factors are not yet completely understood or sometimes even contradictory it is difficult to recommend a

Table 3   Summary of Soluble Regulators Used to Enhanced Matrix Production

Cytokine	References
TGF-β	94,185,186
b-FGF	81,86,88
IGF-1	86,187
PDGF-bb	85,188,189
BMP-7 (rhOP-1)	190
BMP-2	191,192

Abbreviations: TGF-β, transforming growth factor beta; b-FGF, basic fibroblast growth factor; IGF-1, insulin-like growth factor 1.

single growth factor—or a growth factor cocktail—to promote cartilage repair either during in vitro or in vivo articular cartilage tissue engineering at this point of time.

Genetically Modified Cells

In recent years interest in combining tissue engineering and gene therapy approaches has been growing. Principal applications of genetically augmented engineered tissues of the musculoskeletal system have been reviewed recently (139). A target gene, encoding a specific protein molecule, can be introduced into the cell using different vectors. There are several advantages to delivering genes, rather than the gene products, to patients, including the ability to achieve high concentrations of the gene products locally in a sustained manner for extended times. Such capabilities are likely to be especially valuable in orthopaedic tissue engineering and tissue repair, where it may be necessary to expose discrete populations of cells to various growth factors in precise anatomic locations for lengths of time that go beyond conventional means of delivery (140). Also, endogenously synthesized proteins might have greater biologic activities than exogenously administered recombinant proteins (141).

Cell therapies and tissue engineering provide the ideal partner for ex vivo gene therapy since in vivo gene transfer in humans is constrained by safety concerns and the lack of suitable vectors (140). Ex vivo gene transfer is safer because vectors are not introduced directly into the patient, and genetically modified cells can be screened extensively before they are implanted. Moreover, gene delivery to chondrocytes may require ex vivo techniques, because the dense cartilaginous matrix is likely to restrict access of vectors to the cells by in vivo delivery. Different feasibility studies delivering marker genes like the lacZ marker gene—encoding for the enzyme β-galactosidase—to different musculoskeletal tissues have been carried out (142–146). Genetically modified mesenchymal stem cells may also prove to be useful agents of tissue repair in orthopaedics (139). Moreover, recent studies have shown an increased matrix synthesis after adenoviral transfer of TGF-β1 gene to canine and human meniscal cells (146) and spinal disc cells (147).

In Vitro Tissue Engineering

So far we used our seeded scaffolds after only a limited time of culture, principally for allowing the cells to attach, viz. after 12–24 hour. Others, however were using more elaborate constructs, allowing matrix synthesis of the cells over an extended time in vitro. The goal is to finally obtain a cell-seeded implant that reaches the desired design specifications. However, these specifications have yet to be defined. In vitro attempts at engineering articular cartilage have produced tissue that is cartilage like and has some similar mechanical properties (148–152).

Kawamura et al. (119) found that culturing chondrocytes in collagen gels and allowing the accumulation of matrix molecules prior to implantation of the entire composite resulted in the implant being better protected against the in vivo mechanical loading (119).

The conditions under which cell-seeded matrices are cultured have been found to greatly affect matrix production. One advance in culture technology has been the development of rotating-wall culture vessels referred to as "bioreactors." Rotating-wall bioreactors, which randomize the gravity vector, were initially investigated as a model system in which to study microgravity (153,154). These rotating-wall vessels have the unique property of allowing for suspension of cultured substrates while reducing the shear stress applied, and they have demonstrated success for culture of matrix constructs (151,152,155). Several investigators have found that bioreactor culture of chondrocytes with and without a matrix scaffold can provide useful biologic materials for implantation into cartilage defects (156–158). Freed et al. (156) determined that the increased mass transport rates of gases and nutrients that are provided by the rotating-wall vessel enhance the proliferation and biosynthesis rates of cell–matrix constructs containing 33% as much type II collagen, 68% as much glycosaminoglycan, and cellularity comparable to normal calf articular cartilage (156).

Others have shown that the use of perfusion systems, allowing a constant supply of fresh media to the constructs, may be advantageous (159–162). Moreover, the mechanical action of shear stress on the cells, and the availability to actively transport nutrients through an increasingly dense extracellular matrix, are some of the reasons to use perfusion systems as a basic component in the in vitro engineering of cartilaginous tissue. However, optimal conditions, like flow rate [perfusion system vs. rotating vessel (151–153,155,156,158,163)], have yet to be defined.

In conclusion, in vitro attempts at engineering articular cartilage have produced tissue that is cartilage-like and has some similar mechanical properties. However, this tissue still lacks its full composition of natural cartilage and it remains to be seen how it will integrate with the host and perform in vivo. One recent report showed that when hyaline cartilage plugs formed in vitro were implanted in a defect in the articular surface of a rabbit knee, the implanted hyaline cartilage showed no signs of remodeling to articular cartilage after one year, and showed limited integration with the calcified cartilage and adjacent articular cartilage (119). Failure to integrate with the host tissue eventually results in implant instability and micromotion that will likely lead to the degradation and failure of many implants.

Regarding our design specifications, one might therefore postulate that the most efficacious implant is one that has a type II collagen and aggrecan content somewhere between 0% and 100% of mature articular cartilage, and that has mechanical features to serve as an implant but still allows remodeling to achieve the regeneration of the architecture of articular cartilage.

Loading of the Engineered Tissue

In recent years information has been made available that loading of the engineered construct in vitro as well as in vivo is of crucial importance. Articular cartilage is routinely subjected to mechanical forces and to cell-regulatory molecules. Previous studies have shown that mechanical stimuli can influence articular chondrocyte metabolic activity. Dynamic but not static compression was shown to increase the synthesis of proteoglycans (164–166).

However, when engineered tissue is transferred to the preclinical or clinical arena several issues need to be dealt with. Driesang and Hunziker (167) demonstrated that up to 100% of implanted tissue flaps utilized to cover the implant detached if the joint was not immobilized in goats. For ACI most researchers favor a prolonged immobilization.

SUMMARY

In summary, there are several issues to be resolved within the next years:

1. There is a need for controlled clinical studies concerning all of the applied methods.
2. For cell-based therapies cell biological issues like SMA enabled contraction, decreased biosynthetic activity with patient age, and increased population doubling in vitro have to be understood.
3. The pathogenesis and natural history of the specific cartilage lesion have to be taken into account.
4. The effects of additional treatments, e.g., debridement, lavage, osteotomies, etc., have to be considered and separately accounted for.

REFERENCES

1. Hunter W. Of the structure and diseases of articulating cartilages. Phil Trans R Soc Lond 1743; 42:514–522.
2. Paget J. Healing of injuries in various tissues. Lect Surg Pathol 1853; 1:262–270.
3. Jackson RW. The role of arthroscopy in the management of the arthritic knee. Clin Orthop 1974; 101(01):28–35.
4. Livesley PJ, Doherty M, Needoff M, Moulton A. Arthroscopic lavage of osteoarthritic knees. J Bone Joint Surg Br 1991; 73:922–926.
5. Jackson RW. Meniscal and articular cartilage injury in sport. J R Coll Surg Edinb 1989; 34(6):S15–S17.
6. Johnson LL. Arthroscopic abrasion arthroplasty historical and pathologic perspective: present status. Arthroscopy 1986; 2(1):54–69.
7. Singh S, Lee CC, Tay BK. Results of arthroscopic abrasion arthroplasty in osteoarthritis of the knee joint. Singapore Med J 1991; 32(1):34–37.
8. Menche DS, Frenkel SR, Blair B, Watnik NF, Toolan BC, Yaghoubian RS, Pitman MI. A comparison of abrasion burr arthroplasty and subchondral drilling in the treatment of full-thickness cartilage lesions in the rabbit. Arthroscopy 1996; 12:280–286.

9. Friedmann MJ, Berasi DO, Fox JM, Pizzo WD, Snyder SJ, Ferkel RD. Preliminary results with abrasion arthroplasty in the osteoarthritic knee. Clin Orthop 1984; 182:200–205.
10. Beiser IH, Kanat IO. Subchondral bone drilling: a treatment for cartilage defects. J Foot Surg 1990; 29(6):595–601.
11. Shamis LD, Bramlage LR, Gabel AA, Weisbrode S. Effect of subchondral drilling on repair of partial-thickness cartilage defects of third carpal bones in horses. Am J Vet Res 1989; 50:290–295.
12. Ficat RP, Ficat C, Gedeon PK, Toussaint JF. Spongialization: A new treatment for diseased patella. Clin Orthop 1984; 182:200–205.
13. Sledge SL. Microfracture techniques in the treatment of osteochondral injuries. Clin Sports Med 2001; 20(2):365–377.
14. Steadman JR, Rodkey WG, Briggs KK, Rodrigo JJ. The microfracture technic in the management of complete cartilage defects in the knee joint. Orthopade 1999; 28:26–32.
15. Steadman JR. Long-term clinical results with microcrakture (MCFR) and debridement for treatment of full-thickness chondral defects, in Annual Meeting of the American Academy of Orthopaedic Surgeons, 1998.
16. Blevins FT, Steadman JR, Rodrigo JJ, Silliman J. Treatment of articular cartilage defects in athletes: an analysis of functional outcome and lesion appearance. Orthopedics 1998; 21:761–767; discussion 767–768.
17. Gross AE, Silverstein EA, Falk J, Falk R, Langer F. The allotransplantation of partial joints in the treatment of osteoarthritis of the knee. Clin Orthop 1975; 108:7–14.
18. Gross AE, Beaver RJ, Mohammed MN. Fresh small fragment osteochondral allografts used for post traumatic defects in the knee joint. In: Fineramann GAM, Noyes FR, eds. Biology and Biomechanics of the Traumatized Synovial Joint: The Knee as a Model. Rosemount: American Academy of Orthopaedic Surgeons, 1992:123–141.
19. Meyers MH, Akeson W, Convery FR. Resurfacing of the knee with fresh osteochondral allograft. J Bone Joint Surg Am 1989; 71(5):704–713.
20. Czitrom AA, Keating S, Gross AE. The viability of articular cartilage in fresh osteochondral allografts after clinical transplantation. J Bone Joint Surg 1990; 72:574–579.
21. Matsusue Y, Yamamuro T, Hama H. Arthroscopic multiple osteochondral transplantation to chondral defect in the knee associated with anterior cruciate ligament disruption. Arthroscopy 1993; 9:318–321.
22. Bobic V. Arthroscopic osteochondral autograft transplantation in anterior cruciate ligament reconstruction: a preliminary clinical study. Knee Surg Sports Traumatol Arthroscopy 1996; 3(4):262–264.
23. Hangody L, Kish G, Karpati Z, Udvarhelyi I, Szigeti I, Bely M. Mosaicplasty for the treatment of articular cartilage defects: application in clinical practice. Orthopedics 1998; 21:1–6.
24. Hangody L, Kish G, Karpati Z, Szerb I, Udvarhelyi I. Arthroscopic autogenous osteochondral mosaicplasty for the treatment of femoral condylar defects. Knee Surg Sports Traumatol Athrosc 1997; 5:262–267.

25. Hangody L, Karpati Z, Szigeti I, Sukosd L. Clinical experience with the Mosaic Technique. Rev Osteol 1996; 4:32–36.
26. Bobic V. Autologous osteo-chondral grafts in the management of articular cartilage lesions. Orthopade 1999; 28(1):19–25.
27. Hangody L, Kish G, Karpati Z, Szerb I, Eberhardt R. Treatment of osteochondritis dissecans of the talus: use of the mosaicplasty technique—a preliminary report. Foot Ankle 1997; 18:628–634.
28. Beaver RJ, Mahomed M, Backstein D, Davis A, Zukor DJ, Gross AE. Fresh osteochondral allografts for post-traumatic defects in the knee. A survivorship analysis. J Bone Joint Surg Br 1992; 74:105–110.
29. O'Driscoll SW. Articular cartilage regeneration using periosteum. Clin Orthop 1999; 367S:S186–S203.
30. Homminga GN, Bulstra S, Bouwmeester PSM, Van Der Linden AJ. Perichondral grafting for cartilage lesions of the knee. J Bone Joint Surg 1990; 72-B:1003–1007.
31. Brittberg M, Lindahl A, Nilsson A, Ohlsson C, Isaksson O, Peterson L. Treatment of deep cartilage defects in the knee with autologous chondrocyte transplantation. N Engl J Med 1994; 331:889–995.
32. O'Driscoll SW, Keeley FW, Salter RB. The chondrogenic potential of free autogenous periosteal grafts for biological resurfacing of major full-thickness defects in joint surfaces under the influence of continuous passive motion. An experimental investigation in the rabbit. J Bone Joint Surg Am 1986; 68(7): 1017–1035.
33. O'Driscoll SW, Salter RB. The repair of major osteochondral defects in joint surfaces by neochondrogenesis with autogenous osteoperiosteal grafts stimulated by continuous passive motion. An experimental investigation in the rabbit. Clin Orthop 1986; 208:131–140.
34. O'Driscoll SW, Keeley FW. Durability of regenerated articular cartilage produced by free autogenous periostal grafts in major full thiclmess defects in joint surface under the influence of continous passive motion. J Bone Joint Surg 1988; 70-A:595–606.
35. O'Driscoll SW, Recklies AD, Poole AR. Chondrogenesis in periosteal explants. An organ culture model for in vitro study. J Bone Joint Surg Am 1994; 76(7):1042–1051.
36. O'Driscoll SW, Fitzsimmons JS, Commisso CN. Role of oxygen tension during cartilage formation by periosteum. J Orthop Res 1997; 15(5):682–687.
37. O'Driscoll SW, Saris DB, Ito Y, Fitzimmons JS. The chondrogenic potential of periosteum decreases with age. J. Orthop. Res 2001; 19:95–103.
38. O'Driscoll SW, Salter RB. The induction of neochondrogenesis in free intra-articular periostal autografts under the influence of continous passive motion. J Bone Joint Surg 1984; 66-A:1248–1257.
39. Carranza-Bencano A, Garcia-Paino L, Armas Padron JR, Cayuela Dominguez A. Neochondrogenesis in repair of full-thickness articular cartilage defects using free autogenous periosteal grafts in the rabbit. A follow-up in six months. Osteoarth Cartilage 2000; 8:351–358.
40. Zarnett R, Salter RB. Periosteal neochondrogenesis for biologically resurfacing joints: its cellular origin. Can J Surg 1989; 32(3):171–174.

41. Rubak JM. Reconstruction of articular cartilage defects with free periosteal grafts. An experimental study. Acta Orthop Scand 1982; 33(2):175–180.
42. Niedermann B, Boe S, Lauritzen J, Rubak JM. Glued periosteal grafts in the knee. Acta Orthop Scand 1985; 56:457–460.
43. Hoikka VE, Jaroma HJ, Ritsila VA. Reconstruction of the patellar articulation with periosteal grafts. 4-year follow-up of 13 cases. Acta Orthop Scand 1990; 61(1):36–39.
44. O'Driscoll SW, Saris DB, Ito Y, Fitzimmons JS. The chondrogenic potential of periosteum decreases with age. J Orthop Res 2001; 19:95–103.
45. Ito Y, Sanyal A, Fitzsimmons JS, Mello MA, O'Driscoll SW. Histomorphological and proliferative characterization of developing periosteal neochondrocytes in vitro. J Orthop Res 2001; 19:405–413.
46. Ito Y, Fitzsimmons JS, Sanyal A, Mello MA, Mukherjee N, O'Driscoll SW. Localization of chondrocyte precursors in periosteum. Osteoarth Cartilage 2001; 9:215–223.
47. O'Driscoll SW. Technical considerations in perosteal grafting for osteochondral injuries. Clin Sports Med 2001; 20(2):379–402, vii.
48. O'Driscoll SW, Fitzsimmons JS. The importance of procedure specific training in harvesting periosteum for chondrogenesis. Clin Orthop 2000; 380: 269–278.
49. Homminga GN, van der Linden TJ, Terwindt-Rouwenhorst WAW, Drukker J. Repair of articular cartilage defects by perichondrial grafts. Experiments in the rabbit. Acta Orthop Scand 1989; 60:326–329.
50. Homminga GN, Linden van der TJ, Terwindt-Rouwenhorst EA, Drukker J. Repair of articular defects by perichondrial grafts. Experiments in the rabbit. Acta Orthop Scand 1989; 60:326–329.
51. Homminga GN, Bulstra SK, Kuijer R, van der Linden AJ. Repair of sheep articular cartilage defects with a rabbit costal perichondrial graft. Acta Orthop Scand 1991; 62:415–418.
52. Bouwmeester SJM, Beckers JMH, Kuijer R, van der Linden AJ, Bulstra SK. Long-term results of rib perichondrial grafts for repair of cartilage defects in the human knee. Int'l Orthop 1997:313–317.
53. Green WT Jr. Articular cartilage repair. Behavior of rabbit chondrocytes during tissue culture and subsequent allografting. Clin Orthop 1977; 124: 237–250.
54. Grande DA, Singh IJ, Pugh J. Healing of experimentally produced lesions in articular cartilage following chondrocyte transplantation. Anat Rec 1987; 218:142–148.
55. Brittberg M, Nilsson A, Lindahl A, Ohlsson C, Peterson L. Rabbit articular cartilage defects treated with autologous cultured chondrocytes. Clin Orthop 1996; 326:270–283.
56. Breinan HA, Minas T, Hsu H-P, Nehrer S, Sledge CB, Spector M. Effect of cultured autologous chondrocytes on repair of chondral defects in a canine model. J. Bone Joint Surg 1997; 79-A:1439–1451.
57. Breinan HA, Martin SD, Hsu H-P, Spector M. Healing of canine articular cartilage defects treated with microfracture, a type II collagen matrix, or cultured autologous chondrocytes. J Orthop Res 2000; 18:781–789.

58. Wang Q, Breinan HA, Hsu HP, Spector M. Healing of defects in canine articular cartilage: Distribution of nonvascular alpha-smooth muscle actin-containing cells. Wound Repair Regen 2000; 8:145–158.
59. Perka C, Sittinger M, Schultz O, Spitzer R-S, Schlenzka D, Burmester GR. Tissue engineered cartilage repair using cryopreserved and noncryopreserved chondrocytes. Clin Orthop 2000; 378:245–254.
60. Peterson L, Minas T, Brittberg M, Nilsson A, Sjogren-Jansson E, Lindahl A. Two- to 9-year outcome after autologous chondrocyte transplantation of the knee. Clin Orthop 2000; 374:212–234.
61. Brittberg M. Autologous chondrocyte transplantation. Clin Orthop Res, 1999; 367S:147–155.
62. Lee CR, Grodzinsky AJ, Hsu H-P, Martin SD, Spector M. Effects of harvest and selected cartilage repair procedures on the physical and biochemical properties of articular cartilage in the canine knee. J Orthop Res 2000; 18:790–799.
63. Mayhew TA, Williams GR, Senica MA, Kuniholm G, Du Moulin GC. Validation of a quality assurance program for autologous cultured chondrocyte implantation. Tissue Eng 1998; 4:325–334.
64. Nehrer S, Spector M, Minas T. Histologic analysis of tissue after failed cartilage repair procedures. Clin Orthop 1999; 365:149–162.
65. Minas T. The role of cartilage repair techniques, including chondrocyte transplantation, in focal chondral knee damage. Instr Course Lect 1999; 48: 629–643.
66. Minas, T, Neher S. Current concepts in the treatment of articular cartilage defects. Orthopaedics 1997; 20:525–538.
67. Lee CR, SM. Status of articular cartilage tissue engineering. Cur Opin Orthop 1998; 9(IV):88–93.
68. Martin JA, Buckwalter JA. Telomere erosion and senescence in human articular cartilage chondrocytes. J Gerontol A Biol Sci Med Sci 2001; 56(4):B172–B179.
69. Goldring MB, Sandell LJ, Stephenson ML, Krane SM. Immune interferon suppresses levels of procollagen mRNA and type II collagen synthesis in cultured human articular and costal chondrocytes. J Biol Chem 1986; 261:9049–9055.
70. Goldring MB, Birkhead J, Sandell LJ, Kimura T, Krane SM. Interleukin 1 suppresses expression of cartilage-specific types II and IX collagens and increases types I and III collagens in human chondrocytes. J Clin Invest 1988; 82:2026–2037.
71. Saadeh PB, Brent B, Mehrara BJ, Steinbrech DS, Ting V, Gittes GK, Longaker MT. Human cartilage engineering: chondrocyte extraction, proliferation, and characterization for construct development. Ann Plast Surg 1999; 42:509–513.
72. Norby DP, Malemud CJ, Sokoloff L. Differences in the collagen types synthesized by lapine articular chondrocytes in spinner and monolayer culture. Arthritis Rheum 1977; 20(2):709–716.
73. Watt FM, Dudhia J. Prolonged expression of differentiated phenotype by chondrocytes cultured at low density on a composite substrate of collagen and agarose that restricts cell spreading. Differentiation 1988; 38(2):140–147.
74. Denker AE, Nicoll SB, Tuan RS. Formation of cartilage-like spheroids by micromass cultures of murine C3H10T1/2 cells upon treatment with transforming growth factor-beta 1. Differentiation 1995; 59(1):25–34.

75. Kulyk WM, Reichert C. Staurosporine, a protein kinase inhibitor, stimulates cartilage differentiation by embryonic facial mesenchyme. J Craniofac Genet Dev Biol 1992; 12(2):90–97.

76. Nicoll SB. Induction of a chondrocyte-like phenotype in human dermal fibroblasts: Application to cartilage tissue engineering, 24th Annual Meeting of the Society for Bio-Materials, San Diego, California, U.S.A., 1998. In: Trans Soc for Biomat, 1998;p 236.

77. Benya PD, Shaffer JD. Dedifferentiated chondrocytes reexpress the differentiated collagen phenotype when cultured in agarose gels. Cell 1982; 30:215–224.

78. Guo JF, Jourdian GW, MacCallum DK. Culture and growth characteristics of chondrocytes encapsulated in alginate beads. Connect Tissue Res 1989; 19:277–297.

79. Häuselmann HJ, Femandes RJ, Mok SS. Phenotypic stability of bovine articular chondrozytes after long-term culture in alginate beads. J Cell Sci 1994; 107:17–27.

80. Häuselmann HJ, Masuda K, Hunziker EB, Neidhardt M, Mok SS, Beat A, Thonar EJ. Adult human chondrocytes cultured in alginate form a matrix similar to native human articular cartilage. Am J Physiol 1996; 271:C742–C752.

81. Martin I, Vunjak-Novakovic G, Yang J, Langer R, Freed LE. Mammalian chondrocytes expanded in the presence of fibroblast growth factor 2 maintain the ability to differentiate and regenerate three-dimensional cartilaginous tissue. Exp Cell Res 1999; 253:681–688.

82. Nehrer S, Breinan HA, Ramappa A, Shortkroff S, Young G, Minas T, Sledge CB, Yannas IV, Spector M. Canine chondrocytes seeded in type I and type II collagen implants investigated in vitro. J Biomed Mater Res (Appl. Biomat.) 1997; 38:95–104.

83. Frenkel SR, Saadeh PB, Mehrara BJ, Chin GS, Steinbrech DS, Brent B, Gittes GK, Longaker MT. Transforming growth factor beta superfamily members: role in cartilage modeling. Plast Reconstr Surg 2000; 105:980–990.

84. Kulyk WM, Franklin JL, Hoffman LM. Sox9 expression during chondrogenesis in micromass cultures of embryonic limb mesenchyme. Exp Cell Res 2000; 255(2):327–332.

85. Chopra R, Anastassiades T. Specificity and synergism of polypeptide growth factors in stimulating the synthesis of proteoglycans and a novel high molecular weight anionic glycoprotein by articular chondrocyte cultures. J Rheumatol 1998; 25(8):1578–1584.

86. Dunham BP, Koch RJ. Basic fibroblast growth factor and insulinlike growth factor I support the growth of human septal chondrocytes in a serum-free environment. Arch Otolaryngol Head Neck Surg 1998; 124(12):1325–1330.

87. Goto K, Yamazaki M, Tagawa M, Goto S, Kon T, Moriya H, Fujimura S. Involvement of insulin-like growth factor I in development of ossification of the posterior longitudinal ligament of the spine. Calcif Tissue Int 1998; 62: 158–165.

88. Fujisato T, Sajiki T, Liu Q, Ikada Y. Effect of basic fibroblast growth factor on cartilage regeneration in chondrocyte-seeded collagen sponge scaffold. Biomat 1996; 17:155–162.

89. Shortkroff S, Barone L, Hsu H-P, Wrenn C, Gagne T, Chi T, Breinan H, Minas T, Sledge CB, Tubo R, Spector M. Healing of chondral and osteochondral defects in a canine model: the role of cultured autologous chondrocytes in regeneration of articular cartilage. Biomat 1996; 17:147–154.

90. Nehrer S, Breinan HA, Ramappa A, Young G, Shortkroff S, Louie L, Sledge CB, Yannas IV, Spector M. Matrix collagen type and pore size influence behaviour of seeded canine chondrocytes. Biomat 1997; 18:769–776.

91. Lee CR, Breinan HA, Nehrer S, Spector M. Articular cartilage chondrocytes in type I and type II collagen-GAG matrices exhibit contractile behavior in vitro. Tiss Engr 2000; 6:555–565.

92. Kinner B, Spector M. Smooth muscle actin expression by human articular chondrocytes and their contraction of a collagen–glycosaminoglycan matrix in vitro. J Orthop Res 2001; 19:233–241.

93. Wakitani S, Goto T, Pineda SJ, Young RG, Mansour JM, Caplan AI, Goldberg VM. Mesenchymal cell-based repair of large, full-thickness defects of articular cartilage. J Bone Joint Surg 1994; 76-A:579–592.

94. Johnstone B, Hering TM, Caplan AI, Goldberg VM, Yoo JU. In vitro chondrogenesis of bone marrow-derived mesenchymal progenitor cells. Exp Cell Res 1998; 238:265–272.

95. Friedenstein AJ, Gorskaja JF, Kulagina NN. Fibroblast precursors in normal and irradiated mouse hematopoietic organs. Exp Hematol 1976; 4(5):267–274.

96. Friedenstein AJ, Chailakhyan RK, Gerasimov UV. Bone marrow osteogenic stem cells: in vitro cultivation and transplantation in diffusion chambers. Cell Tissue Kinet 1987; 20(3):263–272.

97. Haynesworth SE, Goshima J, Goldberg VM, Caplan AI. Characterization of cells with osteogenic potential from human marrow. Bone 1992; 13:81–88.

98. Bruder SP, Fink DJ, Caplan AI. Mesenchymal stem cells in bone development, bone repair, and skeletal regeneration therapy. J Cell Biochem 1994; 56(3):283–294.

99. Johnstone B, Yoo JU. Autologous mesenchymal progenitor cells in articular cartilage repair. Clin Orthop 1999; 367S:S156–S162.

100. Reyes M, Verfaillie CM. Characterization of multipotent adult progenitor cells, a subpopulation of mesenchymal stem cells. Ann NY Acad Sci 2001; 938:231–233; discussion 233–235.

101. Murphy M, Kavalkovich K, Fink D, Hunziker E, Barry F. Injected mesenchymal stem cells stimulate meniscal repair and protection of articular cartilage. In: 47th Annual Meeting, Orthopaedic Research Society, San Francisco, 2001; p.193.

102. Murphy M, Kavalkovich K, Barry F. Distribution of injected mesenchymal stem cells in the osteoarthritic knee. 47th Annul Meeting, Orthopaedic Research Society. San Francisco, 2001.

103. Kavalokovich, K Murphy M, Barry F. Chondrogenic activity of mesenchymal stem cells compared to articular chondrocytes. 47th Annual Meeting, Orthopedic Research Society. San Francisco, 2001.

104. Horwitz EM, et al. Transplantability and therapeutic effects of bone marrow-derived mesenchymal cells in children with osteogenesis imperfecta. Nat Med 1999; 5(3):309–313.

105. Horwitz EM, Prockop DJ, Gordon PL, Koo WW, Fitzpatrick LA, Neel MD, McCarville ME, Orchard PJ, Pyeritz RE, Brenner MK. Clinical responses to bone marrow transplantation in children with severe osteogenesis imperfecta. Blood 2001; 97:1227–1231.

106. Noth U, Osyczka A, Tuli R, Danielson KG, Tuan RS. Multipotential mesenchymal cell cultures derived from human trabecul bone. In: 47th Annual Meeting, Orthopaedic Research Society, San Francisco, California, 2001; February 25–28, p. 310.

107. Bosch P, Musgrave DS, Lee JY, Cummins J, Shuler T, Ghivizzani TC, Evans T, Robbins TD, Huard J. Osteoprogenitor cells within skeletal muscle. J Orthop Res 2000; 18:933–944.

108. Zuk PA, Zhu M, Mizuno H, Huang J, Futrell JW, Katz AJ, Benhaim P, Lorenz HP, Hedrick MH. Multilineage cells from human adipose tissue: implications for cell- based therapies. Tiss. Eng 2001; 7:211–228.

109. Denker AE, Haas AR, Nicoll SB, Tuan RS. Chondrogenic differentiation of murine C3H10T1/2 multipotential mesenchymal cells: I. Stimulation by bone morphogenetic protein-2 in high-density micromass cultures. Differentiation 1999; 64:67–76.

110. Yoo JU, Mandell I, Angele P, Johnstone B. Chondrogenitor cells and gene therapy. Clin Orthop 2000; 379(Suppl):S164–S170.

111. Evans CH, Ghivizzani SC, Smith P, Shuler FD, Mi Z, Robbins PD. Using gene therapy to protect and restore cartilage. Clin Orthop 2000; 379(suppl): S214–S219.

112. Thomson JA, Itskovitz-Eldor J, Shapiro SS, Waknitz MA, Swiergiel JJ, Marshall VS, Jones JM. Embryonic stem cell lines derived from human blastocysts. Science 1998; 282:1145–1147.

113. Ghazavi MT, Pritzker KP, Davis AM, Gross AE. Fresh osteochondral allografts for post-traumatic osteochondral defects of the knee. J Bone Jt Surg 1997; 79-B:1008–1013.

114. McDermott AG, Langer F, Pritzker KP, Gross AE. Fresh small-fragment osteochondral allografts. Long-term follow-up study on first 100 cases. Clin Orthop 1985; 197:96–102.

115. Schreiber RE, Ilten-Kirby BM, Dunkelman NS, Symons KT, Rekettye LM, Willoughby J, Ratcliffe A. Repair of osteochondral defects with allogeneic tissue engineered cartilage implants. Clin Orthop 1999; 367S:S382–S395.

116. Peretti GM, Randolph MA, Villa MT, Buragas MS, Yaremchuk MJ. Cell-based tissue-engineered allogeneic implant for cartilage repair. Tissue Eng 2000; 6:567–576.

117. Rahfoth B, Weisser J, Sternkopf F, Aigner T, von der Mark K, Brauer R. Transplantation of allograft chondrocytes embedded in agarose gel into cartilage defects of rabbits. Osteoarthr Cart 1998; 6:50–65.

118. Wakitani S, Goto T, Young RG, Mansour JM, Goldberg VM, Caplan AI. Repair of large full-thickness articular cartilage defects with allograft articular chondrocytes embedded in a collagen gel. Tiss Eng 1998; 4:429–444.

119. Kawamura S, Wakitani S, Kimura T, Maeda A, Caplan AI, Shino K, Ochi T. Articular cartilage repair. rabbit experiment with a collagen gel-biomatrix and chondrocytes cultured in it. Acta Orthop Scand 1998; 69:56–62.

120. Bell E. Strategy for the selection of scaffolds for tissue engineering. Tissue Eng 1995; 1:163–179.
121. Grande DA, Halberstadt C, Naughton G, Schwartz R, Manji R. Evaluation of matrix scaffolds for tissue engineering of articular cartilage grafts. J Biomed Mater Res 1997; 34:211–220.
122. Freed LE, Grande DA, Lingbin Z, Emmanual J, Marquis JC, Langer R. Joint resurfacing using allograft chondrocytes and synthetic biodegradable polymer scaffolds. J Biomed Mater Res 1994; 28:891–899.
123. Freed LE, Vunjak-Novakovic G, Biron RJ, Eagles DB, Lesnoy DC, Barlow SK, Langer R. Biodegradable polymer scaffolds for tissue engineering. 1994; 12: 689–693.
124. Delaney IP, O'Driscoll SW, Salter RB. Neochondrogenesis in free intraarticular periosteal autografts in an immobilized and paralyzed limb. An experimental investigation in the rabbit. Clin Orthop 1989; 248:278–282.
125. Athanasiou KA, Agrawal CM, Barber FA, Burkhart SS. Orthopaedic applications for PLA-PGA biodegradable polymers. Arthroscopy 1998; 14:726–737.
126. Grande DA, Pitman MI, Peterson L, Menche D, Klein M. The repair of experimentally produced defects in rabbit articular cartilage by autologous chondrocyte transplantation. J Orthop Res 1989; 7:208–218.
127. Ponticiello MS, Schinagl RM, Kadiyala S, Barry FP. Gelatin-based resorbable sponge as a carrier matrix for human mesenchymal stem cells in cartilage regeneration therapy. J Biomed Mater Res 2000; 52:246–255.
128. Dounchis JS, Bae WC, Chen AC, Sah RL, Coutts RD, Amiel D. Cartilage repair with autogenic perichondrium cell and polylactic acid grafts. Clin Orthop 2000; 377:248–264.
129. von Schroeder HP, Kwan M, Amiel D, Coutts RD. The use of polylactic acid matrix and periosteal grafts for the reconstruction of rabbit knee articular defects. J Biomed Mater Res 1991; 25:329–339.
130. van Susante JL, Buma P, Homminga GN, van den Berg WB, Veth RP. Chondrocyte-seeded hydroxyapatite for repair of large articular cartilage defects. A pilot study in the goat. Biomat 1998; 19:2367–2374.
131. Guerne PA, Blanco F, Kaelin A, Desgeorges A, Lotz M. Growth factor responsiveness of human articular chondrocytes in aging and development. Arthritis Rheum 1995; 38:960–968.
132. Sandell LJ, Daniel JC. Effects of ascorbic acide on collagen mnRNA levels in short term chondrocyte cultures. Connect Tissue Res 1988; 17:11–22.
133. van Osch GJ, et al. Effect of transforming growth factor-beta on proteoglycan synthesis by chondrocytes in relation to differentiation stage and the presence of pericellular matrix. Matrix Biol 1998; 17(6):413–424.
134. Redini F, Galera P, Mauviel A, Loyau G, Pujol JP. Transforming growth factor beta stimulates collagen and glycosaminoglycan biosynthesis in cultured rabbit articular chondrocytes. FEBS Lett 1988; 234:172–176.
135. Livne E. In vitro response of articular cartilage from mature mice to human transforming growth factor beta. Acta Anat 1994; 149(3):185–194.
136. Bujia J, Pitzke P, Kastenbauer E, Wilmes E, Hammer C. Effect of growth factors on matrix synthesis by human nasal chondrocytes cultured in monolayer and in agar. Eur Arch Otorhinolaryngol 1996; 253:336–340.

137. Mattey DL, Dawes PT, Nixon NB, Slater H. Transforming growth factor beta 1 and interleukin 4 induced alpha smooth muscle actin expression and myofibroblast-like differentiation in human synovial fibroblasts in vitro: modulation by basic fibroblast growth factor. Ann. Rheum. Dis 1997; 56:426–431.

138. Trippel SB. Growth factor actions on articular cartilage. J Rheumatol Suppl 1995; 43:129–132.

139. Evans CH, Robbins PD. Genetically augmented tissue engineering of the musculoskeletal system. Clin Orthop 1999; 367S:S410–S418.

140. Kang R, Ghivizzani SC, Muzzonigro TS, Herndon JH, Robbins PD, Evans CH. Orthopaedic applications of gene therapy: from concept to clinic. Clin Orthop 2000; 375:324–337.

141. Sandhu JS, Gorczynski RM, Waddell J, Nguyen H, Squires J, Boynton EL, Hozumi N. Effect of interleukin-6 secreted by engineered human stromal cells on osteoclasts in human bone. Bone 1999; 24:217–227.

142. Kang R, Marui T, Ghivizzani SC, Nita IM, Georgescu HK, Shu JK, Robbins PD, Evans CH. Ex vivo gene transfer to chondroycytes in full-thickness articular cartilage defects: a feasibility study. Osteoarth Cart 1997; 5:139–143.

143. Gerich TG, Fu FH, Robbins PD, Evans CH. Prospects for gene therapy in sports medicine. Knee Surg Sports Traumatol Arthrosc 1996; 4:180–187.

144. Lou J, Tu Y, Ludwig FJ, Zhang J, Manske PR. Effect of bone morphogenetic protein-12 gene transfer on mesenchymal progenitor cells. Clin Orthop 1999; 369:333–339.

145. Nakamura N, Timmermann SA, Hart DA, Kaneda Y, Shrive NG, Shino K, Ochi T, Frank CB. A comparison of in vivo gene delivery methods for antisense therapy in ligament healing. Gene Ther 1998; 5:1455–1461.

146. Goto H, Shuler FD, Lamsam C, Moller HD, Niyibizi C, Fu FH, Robbins PD, Evans CH. Transfer of lacZ marker gene to the meniscus. J Bone Joint Surg Am 1999; 81:918–925.

147. Nishida K, Kang JD, Gilbertson LG, Moon SH, Suh JK, Vogt MT, Robbins PD, Evans CH. Modulation of the biologic activity of the rabbit intervertebral disc by gene therapy: an in vivo study of adenovirus-mediated transfer of the human transforming growth factor beta 1 encoding gene. Spine 1999; 24: 2419–2425.

148. Freed LE, Marquis JC, Nohria A, Emmanual J, Mikos AG, Langer R. Neocartilage formation in vitro and in vivo using cells cultured on synthetic biodegradable polymers. J Biomed Mater Res 1993; 27:11–23.

149. Freed LE, Martin I, Vunjak-Novakovic G. Frontiers in tissue engineering. In vitro modulation of chondragenesis. Clin Orthop 1999; 367S:S46–S58.

150. Martin I, Obradovic B, Treppo S, Grodzinsky AJ, Langer R, Freed LE, Vunjak-Novakovic G. Modulation of the mechanical properties of tissue engineered cartilage. Biorheology 2000; 37:141–147.

151. Obradovic B, Carrier RL, Vunjak-Novakovic G, Freed LE. Gas exchange is essential for bioreactor cultivation of tissue engineered cartilage. Biotechnol Bioeng 1999; 63:197–205.

152. Vunjak-Novakovic G, et al. Bioreactor cultivation conditions modulate the composition and mechanical properties of tissue-engineered cartilage. J Orthop Res 1999; 17(1):130–138.

153. Freed LE, Langer R, Martin I, Pellis NR, Vunjak-Novakovic G. Tissue engineering of cartilage in space. Proc. Natl. Acad. Sci. USA 1997; 94:13885–13890.
154. Freed LE, Vunjak-NovakovicG. Microgravity tissue engineering. In Vitro Cell Dev Biol Anim 1997; 33(5):381–385.
155. Wu F, Dunkelman N, Peterson A, Davisson T, De La Torre R, Jain D. Bioreactor development for tissue-engineered cartilage. Ann N Y Acad Sci 1999; 875:405–411.
156. Freed LE, A.P. H, Martin I, Barry JR, Langer R, G. V-N. Chondrogenesis in a cell-polymer-bioreactor system. Exp. Cell Res 1998; 240:58–65.
157. Freed LE, Marquis JC, Nohria A, Emmanual J, Mikos AG, Langer R. Neocartilage formation in vitro and in vivo using cells cultured on synthetic biodegradable polymers. J Biomed Mater Res 1993; 27:11–23.
158. Freed LE, Vunjak-Novakovic G, Langer R. Cultivation of cell polymer cartilage implants in bioreactors. J Cell Biochem 1993; 51:257–264.
159. Minuth WW, Sittinger M, Kloth S. Tissue engineering: generation of differentiated artificial tissues for biomedical applications. Cell Tissue Res 1998; 291(1):1–11.
160. Rotter N, Aigner J, Naumann A, Planck H, Hammer C, Burmester G, Sittinger M. Cartilage reconstruction in head and neck surgery: comparison of resorbable polymer scaffolds for tissue engineering of human septal cartilage. J Biomed Mater Res 1998; 42:347–356.
161. Sittinger M, Perka C, Schultz O, Haupl T, Burmester GR. Joint cartilage regeneration by tissue engineering. Z Rheumatol 1999; 58:130–135.
162. Sittinger M, Schultz O, Keyszer G, Minuth WW, Burmester GR. Artificial tissues in perfusion culture. Int J Artif Organs 1997; 20:57–62.
163. Potter K, Butler JJ, Horton WE, Spencer RG. Response of engineered cartilage tissue to biochemical agents as studied by proton magnetic resonance microscopy. Arthritis Rheum 2000; 43:1580–1590.
164. Mauck RL, Soltz MA, Wang CCB, Wong DD, Chao P-HG, Valhmu WB, Hung CT, Ateshian GA. Functional tissue engineering of articular cartilage through dynamic loading of chondrocyte-seeded agarose gels. J Biomech Eng 2000; 122:252–260.
165. Chen AC, Sah RL. Effect of static compression on proteoglycan biosynthesis by chondrocytes transplanted to articular cartilage in vitro. J Orthop Res 1998; 16(5):542–550.
166. Sah R, Doong J, Grodzinsky A, Plaas A, Sandy J. Effects of compression on the loss of newly synthesized proteoglycans and proteins from cartilage explants. Arch Biochem Biophys 1991; 286:20–29.
167. Driesang IM, Hunziker EB. Delamination rates of tissue flaps used in articular cartilage repair. J Orthop Res 2000; 18(6):909–911.
168. Wright JG. Autologous chondrocyte transplantation. N Eng J Med 1995; 332:540.
169. Minas T. Chondrocyte implantation in the repair of chondral lesions of the knee: Economics and quality of life. Am J Orthop 1998; 27:739–744.
170. Rahfoth B, Weisser J, Sternkopf F, Aigner T, von der Mark K, Brauer R. Transplantation of allograft chondrocytes embedded in agarose gel into cartilage defects of rabbits. Osteoarthr Cart 1998; 6:50–65.

171. Baragi VM, Renkiewicz RR, Qiu L, Brammer D, Riley JM, Sigler RE, Frenkel SR, Amin A, Abramson SB, Roessler BJ. Transplantation of adenovirally transduced allogeneic chondrocytes into articular cartilage defects in vivo. Osteoarthritis Cart 1997; 5:275–282.

172. Bulstra SK, Himinga GN, Buurman WA, Terwindt-Rouwenhorst E, van der Linden AJ. The potential of adult human perichondrium to form hyalin cartilage in vitro. J Orthop Res 1990; 8:328–335.

173. Chu CR, Dounchis JS, Yoshioka M, Sah RL, Coutts RD, Amiel D. Osteochondral repair using perichondrial cells: a 1-year study in rabbits. Clin Orthop 1997; 340:220–229.

174. Prockop DJ. Marrow stromal cells as stem cells for nonhematopoietic tissues. Science 1997; 276(5309):71–74.

175. Martin I, Padera RF, Vunjak-Novakovic G, Freed LE. In vitro differentiation of chick embryo bone marrow stromal cells into cartilaginous and bone-like tissues. J Orthop Res 1998; 16:181–189.

176. Mizuno S, Glowacki J. Chondroinduction of human dermal fibroblasts by demineralized bone in three-dimensional culture. Exp Cell Res 1996; 227(1): 89–97.

177. Frenkel SR, Toolan B, Menche D, Pitman MI, Pachence JM. Chondrocyte transplantation using a collagen bilayer matrix for cartilage repair. J Bone Joint Surg 1998; 79-B:831–836.

178. Peretti GM, Bonassar LJ, Caruso EM, Randolph MA, Trahan CA, Zaleske DJ. Biomechanical analysis of a chondrocyte-based repair model of articular cartilage. Tissue Eng 1999; 5:317–326.

179. Peretti GM, Randolph MA, Caruso EM, Rossetti F, Zaleske DJ. Bonding of cartilage matrices with cultured chondrocytes: an experimental model. J Orthop Res 1998; 16:89–95.

180. Toolan B, Frenkel S, Pereira DS, Alexander H. Development of a novel osteochondral graft for cartilage repair. J Biomed Mater Res 1998; 41:244–250.

181. Matthew IR, Browne RM, Frame JW, Millar BG. Subperiosteal behaviour of alginate and cellulose wound dressing materials. 1995; 16:275–278.

182. Cook JL, Kreeger JM, Payne JT, Tomlinson JL. Three-dimensional culture of canine articular chondrocytes on multiple transplantable substrates. Am J Vet Res 1997; 58:419–424.

183. Chu CR, Monosov AZ, Amiel D. In situ assessment of cell viability within biodegradable polylactic acid polymer matrices. Biomaterials 1995; 16(18): 1381–1384.

184. Wyre RM, Dowries S. An in vitro investigation of the PEMA/THFMA polymer system as a biomaterial for cartilage repair. Biomaterials 2000; 21(4):335–343.

185. Dounchis JS, Goomer RS, Harwood FL, Khatod M, Coutts RD, Amiel D. Chondrogenic phenotype of perichondrium-derived chondroprogenitor cells is influenced by transforming growth factor-beta 1. J Orthop Res 1997; 15: 803–807.

186. Tajima K, Yamakawa M, Katagiri T, Sasaki H. Immunohistochemical detection of bone morphogenetic protein-2 and transforming growth factor beta-1 in tracheopathia osteochondroplastica. Virchows Arch 1997; 431:359–363.

187. Loeser RF, Shanker G. Autocrine stimulation by insulin-like growth factor 1 and insulin-like growth factor 2 mediates chondrocyte survival in vitro. Arthritis Rheum 2000; 43(7):1552–1559.
188. Kieswetter K, Schwartz Z, Alderete M, Dean DD, Boyan BD. Platelet derived growth factor stimulates chondrocyte proliferation but prevents endochondral maturation. Endocrine 1997; 6:257–264.
189. Lohmann CH, Schwartz Z, Niederauer GG, Carnes DL, Jr. Dean DD, Boyan BD. Pretreatment with platelet derived growth factor-BB modulates the ability of costochondral resting zone chondrocytes incorporated into PLA/PGA scaffolds to form new cartilage in vivo. Biomaterials 2000; 21:49–61.
190. Klein-Nulend J, Louwerse RT, Heyligers IC, Wuisman PI, Semeins CM, Goei SW, Burger EH. Osteogenic protein (OP-1, BMP-7) stimuates cartilage differentiation of human and goat perichondrium tissue in vitro. J Biomed Mater Res 1998; 40:614–620.
191. Sellers RS, Peluso D, Morris EA. The effect of recombinant human bone morphogenetic protein-2 (rhBMP-2) on the healing of full-thickness defects of articular cartilage. J Bone Joint Surg Am 1997; 79(10):1452–1463.
192. Sellers RS, Zhang R, Glasson SS, Kim HD, Peluso D, D'Augusta DA, Beckwith K, Morris EA. Repair of articular cartilage defects one year after treatment with recombinant human bone morphogenetic protein-2 (rhBMP-2). J Bone Joint Surg Am 2000; 82:151–160.

29

Enhancing Cementless Fixation

Dale R. Sumner, Amarjit S. Virdi, and Robert M. Leven
Department of Anatomy and Cell Biology,
Rush University Medical Center, Chicago, Illinois, U.S.A.

Kevin E. Healy
Departments of Bioengineering and Materials Science and Engineering,
University of California at Berkeley, Berkeley, California, U.S.A.

INTRODUCTION

Enhancing cementless fixation is defined here as accelerating or augmenting bone formation in the porous coating or on the surface of an orthopaedic implant (see chap. 2 for a review of the basic concepts underlying cementless fixation.). As a matter of definition, we will restrict use of the term "bone ingrowth" in the rest of this chapter to porous coatings, where bone grows into the interstices of the implant surface (e.g., into the void spaces of a porous surface made from beads or fiber metal). We will use the term "bone ongrowth" to describe situations in which there is no surface macroporosity and at the level of the light microscope the bone often appears to be directly attached to the implant material

   The early studies of retrieved implants suggested that bone ingrowth was only obtained sporadically. These observations motivated many of the initial efforts to augment cementless fixation, including bone ingrowth and ongrowth enhancements. As implant designs improved and the retrieval analyses focused on post-mortem cases where the implants had apparently functioned well (see chap. 2), it became apparent that in most cases some degree of bone ingrowth occurred. Nevertheless, the need remains to reduce the time required to obtain secure mechanical fixation of the implant to the host bone or to ensure that fixation occurs in situations where it otherwise would be problematic (e.g., revision joint replacement).

It is important to emphasize that, with a few apparent exceptions noted below, no enhancing agent can be expected to overcome poor initial mechanical fixation of the implant to the host bone (i.e., excessive relative motion between the implant and bone) or an implant with an inappropriately designed surface (e.g., excessively small pore sizes in a porous-coated implant). As we will review, at least some of these agents are very effective in promoting bone ingrowth in the presence of impaired fixation induced by the presence of interface gaps. Although not studied in the context of implant fixation, certain growth factors can block or abrogate the negative effects of other impairing factors such as irradiation, steroid treatment, or induced diabetes (1–4), and potentially could play a similar role in improving implant fixation.

There is a long history of attempting to enhance cementless fixation (5). Some of this work involves the appropriate design of the porous coating (in cases of porous-coated implants), use of implant surface treatments such as hydroxyapatite or other calcium phosphate coatings, use of various grafting agents, use of physical modalities such as electrical stimulation and ultrasound, and so forth. In this chapter, we focus on two topics, which appear to be particularly promising in enhancing bone ingrowth and ongrowth. The first approach relies on the use of biological agents, especially growth factors and other signaling peptides that are known bone anabolic factors. The second approach relies on treating the surface to create a topography or chemical composition that enhances bone ongrowth. The second approach, if proven successful, may allow implant manufacturers to eliminate the use of porous coatings altogether. The use of biological agents has already been shown in pre-clinical studies to enhance fixation with porous-coated implants and could have similar effects on implants relying on bone ongrowth.

CELLULAR ENVIRONMENT OF FIXATION

The fact that bone tissue has the inherent capacity to respond to local demands for repair or regeneration is beyond question. The use of prosthetic devices in orthopaedics and dentistry fully exploits this property to restore function. The role of the cellular component surrounding the prosthesis is pivotal in determining the fate of the implant. This role is in turn completely under the influence of the milieu composed of signals provided by local and circulating hormones and growth factors. In this section, the discussion is focused on the osteogenic cells within the bone marrow which are known to bring about changes leading to implant fixation.

The marrow system of bone consists of two well-defined compartments, such as the hematopoietic and the stromal (6). By definition, the stromal component provides an environment conducive to hematopoiesis, the main function attributed to the marrow tissue. The bone marrow is perhaps the only tissue that contains two such independent and yet interdependent systems. This relationship between them is the underlining factor that governs the normal function of bone and marrow. This observation is not new. In fact, Aristotle described the relationship in an eloquent fashion (7):

> ... as it is necessary that animals shall have bones ... it is also a matter of necessity that some of these bones shall contain marrow; for the substance contained within the bones is the nutriment out of which these are formed

Cell lineages within the two systems are determined by the hierarchical order from the stem cell to the fully differentiated cells performing their function. It is now common knowledge that in the postnatal animal cells associated with bone formation, the osteoblasts arise from the stromal component and that the bone resorbing cells, the osteoclasts, have their origin in the hematopoietic component (8). Although the current flurry of research interest in stem cell biology, in particular the stromal stem cells, has provided tremendous amounts of information, our knowledge and understanding of the biological control of stem cells under specific conditions is still limited. It is crucial that we elucidate these control mechanisms if we plan to modulate their response by applying exogenous stimuli in order to gain heightened fixation of implants. In the musculoskeletal system, this stimulus can be applied in a variety of different forms including mechanical, electrical, chemical, and biological. In each and every case, the conversion of a stimulus into tissue function is brought about by the cells responsible for the maintenance of skeletal structure and function.

Osteogenic Stem Cell

Since the early time, the stromal system of bone has been under investigation because of its critical involvement in the formation of the hematopoietic microenvironment. It was, however, the pioneering works of Alexander Friedenstein (Moscow, U.S.S.R.) and Maureen Owen (Oxford, England) and their coworkers (9–11) that led to the current concept of the bone marrow stromal stem cell in postnatal animals with multilineage characteristics. Their investigations were based on methods of isolation and in vitro culturing of fibroblastic cells from the whole marrow and their transplantation in in vivo models. These studies, spanning a period of three decades, yielded the characteristics that compose the marrow stroma that contains within it a population of cells referred to as the stem cell of the stromal system. This now universally accepted model of the bone marrow stromal stem cell, also commonly known as the mesenchymal stem cell (MSC), dictates that different cell lineages, including osteogenic, chondrogenic, and adipocytic, can be derived from a common stem cell when subjected to appropriate conditions (12). Recent enthusiasm in adult stem cell biology has prompted the emergence of new methodologies describing the isolation, purification, and expansion of adult MSCs for future clinical use for bone repair and enhanced implant fixation (13). Not only has the expansion potential of these cells in vitro been demonstrated to be enormous, up to 30 doublings (a billion-fold increase), but also their capacity to retain the multipotentiality for differentiation (14,15). Studies have also shown that the fully differentiated progeny of MSCs can switch between lineages. For example, adipocytes can be directed to osteogenic differentiation, which forms bone tissue when placed in vivo (16,17). Fully differentiated chondrocytes in vitro can de-differentiate to exhibit more fibroblastic characteristics and then shift to the osteogenic phenotype (18,19). This inter-conversion of phenotypes across distinct differentiation lineages of a common stem cell is referred to as plasticity. Furthermore, recent reports have shown that stem cells residing in the bone marrow can give rise to cell lineages of developmentally unrelated tissue. Bone marrow has been shown to contain progenitor cells giving rise to skeletal, smooth and cardiac muscle, astrocytes and neurons (20–23). These results reinforce the concept that adult stem cells from certain tissues, including MSCs, have a broad developmental potential or are able to acquire this potential under appropriate conditions. It is this vigor for proliferation and the plasticity of phenotype that makes MSCs an attractive candidate for cell-based therapies in the medical field.

Control of Osteogenic Cells

Development of a fully differentiated osteogenic cell from its stem cell is a complex process involving a number of stages which are critically controlled to maintain the desired outcome. This process begins with asymmetric division of the stem cell to give a daughter cell and self-renewal to restore itself. The daughter cell then becomes the main source of cell progeny to follow a lineage-specific pathway. Phases which the cells of the osteogenic lineage, the osteoprogenitors, pass through include chemotaxis, adhesion, proliferation and differentiation. Various factors have been identified which act during each phase to guide the cell through (Table 1). Some of these factors are brought to the site via systemic circulation and others are produced locally either by osteogenic cells themselves or by other cells in the vicinity. In any case, the cells express receptors for these factors on their surfaces to respond to the signaling molecule. This provides the cell an additional point of control in regulating the signal by modulating the level of receptor expression.

Table 1 Influence of Local Stimuli During Different Phases of Osteogenic Lineage in Regenerating Bone Tissue

Phase	Stimulus
Chemotaxis	IGF-I
	IGF–II
	TGF-α
	TGF-β
	IL-4
	IL-13
	PDGF
	VEGF
	FGF
	BMP-2
	BMP-4
Adhesion	PDGF
	TGF-β
	FGF
	BMP-2
Proliferation	IGF-I
	IGF–II
	TGF-β
	IL-1
	PDGF
	FGF
	BMP-7
	GH
	PGE$_1$
	PGE$_2$
Inhibitors	*BMP-3*
	Hypoxia
	GM-CSF
Differentiation	BMP–2
	BMP-7
	BMP-3
	FGF
	GH
	PGE$_2$
	GM-CSF
Inhibitors	*TGF-β*
	FGF

Abbreviations: BMP, bone morphogenetic protein; GH, growth hormone; FGF, fibroblast growth factor; GM-CSF, granulocyte-macrophage colony-stimulating factor; IGF, insulin-like growth factor; IL, interleukin; PDGF, platelet derived growth factor; PGE, prostaglandin E; TGF, transforming growth factor; VEGF, vascular endothelial growth factor.
Source: From Refs. 38, 39, 145–177.

The growth factors that have been shown to exert some action on the osteogenic cells, either in vitro or in vivo, are too numerous to discuss here. The list includes, but is not limited to, fibroblast growth factor (acidic and basic), platelet derived growth factor, insulin like growth factor, epidermal growth factor, and members of the transforming growth factor-beta (TGF-β) superfamily, including TGF-β and the bone morphogenetic proteins (BMPs). It suffices to say that their action can be placed in two main categories— promote or prevent proliferation, and enhance or inhibit differentiation.

In the context of bone ingrowth and implant fixation, it is appropriate to elaborate on the role of TGF-β and related growth factors, considered to be principal local regulators, on osteogenic cells. At least during skeletal development, these molecules have unique functions and act sequentially to modulate chondrocyte and osteoblast differentiations. TGF-β has been reported to exhibit bifunctional effects in various osteoprogenitor systems. The action may be inhibitory or stimulatory on cell proliferation and differentiation depending on concentration, species, and model system used (24). For example, TGF-β has been shown to enhance osteoblast differentiation by increasing the expression of associated markers such as alkaline phosphatase, type I collagen, and osteonectin (25), and also to inhibit the expression of type I collagen, alkaline phosphatase, osteopontin, osteocalcin, and BMP-2 (26). In addition, these molecules have also been shown to have negative effects on adipocyte differentiation, thus promoting osteogenesis at the expense of adipogenesis (27,28). The decline in the amount of TGF-β resident in human bone matrix with age may contribute to the accumulation of adipose tissue at the expense of osteogenesis in the bone marrow of older individuals. Studies of TGF-β action in vivo have demonstrated increased bone formation in a variety of models. Locally applied TGF-β promoted bone healing in fractures and skull defects and similar results were observed when TGF-β was administered by continuous infusion (24,29–32). Delivery of TGF-β to the site of bone regeneration around implants, by loading the growth factor on the implant, results in an enhanced ingrowth of bone and fixation of the implant (33–36), as discussed in more detail elsewhere in this chapter.

Bone morphogenetic proteins are members of the TGF-β superfamily due to their structural relationship. Originally discovered for their ability to induce endochondral bone formation in non-skeletal tissues (37), BMPs are now known to have roles in the development of a wide variety of tissues in the body. Their actions regulate morphogenesis and growth in hair follicles, heart, kidney, tooth buds, prostate, and central nervous system. Although this subfamily is composed of at least 15 different molecules, BMP-2, BMP-4 and BMP-7 (osteogenic protein-1; OP-1) are the most extensively studied members. BMP-2 has been shown to enhance osteoblast differentiation in vitro as evidenced by an increase in the expression of alkaline phosphatase activity, osteocalcin and osteonectin, all markers of mature osteoblasts (38,39). Similar results were also reported with BMP-7 (40). Use of BMPs in clinically relevant models has been demonstrated in a number of reports including fracture repair, bone non-unions, and spine fusion (2,41–52).

As stated above, the fate of osteogenic cells is under the influence of exogenous signals. The profile of these signals is altered in disease and repair processes. Further, this delicate control is also affected over time during aging, especially after menopause, when imbalance between bone formation and resorption leads to net bone loss. This decrement is thought to be the consequence of increased resorption at trabecular and cortical bone and decreased bone formation. In addition, the population of osteoblasts is thought to be decreased. Investigators have attempted to elucidate the role of osteoblasts in this process by assessing the number of osteoprogenitors in the bone marrow. Studies performed in animals have shown a reduction in the number of osteoprogenitors and also decreased expression of alkaline phosphatase (53–56) when comparing marrow from young and old animals. In humans, however, such studies have been contradictory. Some authors have reported a decrease in the number of osteoprogenitors (57,58) and the expression of alkaline phosphatase. Yet others have shown that there is no change in the number of osteoprogenitors in the aged, but that there is a decline in the rate of cell proliferation (59,60). While there is a lack of consensus on the in vitro potential of the stromal cells, there is a common understanding that osteoprogenitors from older individuals respond differently to growth factors and culture conditions than those from younger individuals. This observation leads itself to future studies on the responsiveness of aged MSC and information thus obtained will prove invaluable in treating the elderly population for skeletal disorders.

Despite these in vitro age-related differences and the general clinical impression that fracture healing or bone repair is delayed in the elderly (61,62), only one animal model has shown a negative effect (63), while several have reported no effect (64–67) of aging on bone repair. We have recently shown that the responsiveness of aged as opposed to young adult canines to exogenous TGF-β in the repair of a skeletal defect is minimal when assessed in terms of the amount of newly regenerated bone (68). At the most effective dose studied (which was the same in the young adult and aged animals), there was a three-fold enhancement of bone regeneration irrespective of age. The older animals did have about 10% less regenerated bone whether or not the growth factor was given compared to the younger animals, although this difference was not statistically significant. In addition, the older animals had regenerated trabeculae that were thinner and more closely spaced and had a greater increase in osteoid (unmineralized bone matrix) than the younger animals.

This review of the context in which bone ingrowth and ongrowth occurs reinforces the idea that cementless implant fixation depends upon osteoblast function and in particular, having an adequate number of cells and appropriate bone matrix formation, maturation, and mineralization (69). As we will see in the following sections, some of the gene products that are up-regulated during bone formation are now under investigation as enhancing agents, especially the transforming growth factor-β superfamily (including TGF-β and BMP). A critical step in cell proliferation is cell attachment, and there is growing interest in using cell signaling molecules such as oligopeptides containing arginine–glycine–aspartate. This amino acid sequence is commonly referred to by its abbreviation RGD and oligopeptides containing such sequences are being considered to promote osteoprogenitor cell attachment in the hopes of stimulating bone ingrowth and ongrowth (70). As a general concept, likely candidates for enhancement appear to be factors that up-regulate osteoprogenitor proliferation without depressing matrix formation, maturation or mineralization.

USE OF GROWTH FACTORS

Recombinant growth factors are now being tested as enhancing agents for bone ingrowth and ongrowth. In particular, most studies of direct relevance to joint replacement involve members of the TGF-β superfamily, such as TGF-β1, TGF-β2, and BMP-2. It is already apparent that these factors have a dose response in vivo. Although little is known about the mechanisms of action of these growth factors at the cellular and molecular levels in the context of implant fixation, they apparently function by stimulating the intramembranous bone formation pathway rather than bringing endochondral bone formation into play. Thus, as studied so far, they do not alter the fundamental mechanisms of implant fixation by bone ingrowth or ongrowth.

Animal models to test for enhancement with growth factors typically involve use of a non-weight-bearing model in which a gap of less than 1 to as large as 3 mm is present between the implant surface and host bone (71) (Fig. 1). When the implant is treated with TGF-β1 (33–35,72,73), TGF-β2 (36,68) or BMP-2 (74) bone formation in the surrounding gap is enhanced. In most of these studies, bone ingrowth into a porous coating or bone ongrowth has also been studied and found to be stimulated. In addition, in a few of the studies implant fixation has been examined and found to be enhanced.

The degree of enhancement can be substantial (Fig. 2). For instance, in our original study of TGF-β1 at four weeks in a model that had a 3 mm gap between the implant surface and host bone, we found that the volume fraction of bone ingrowth was over 25% at the most effective dose studied (i.e., more than 25% of the void space within the porous coating was filled with mineralized bone) (35). This figure is quite impressive compared to bone ingrowth of approximately 10% when the gap was treated with autogenous cancellous bone graft and less than 5% when the gap was untreated

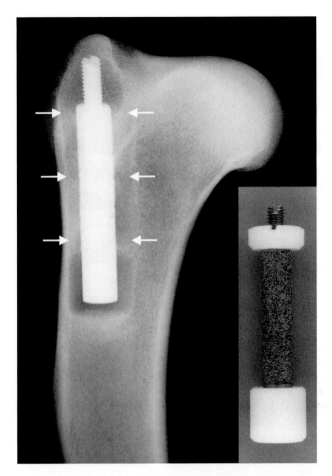

Figure 1 Contact radiograph depicting placement of a porous-coated non-weight-bearing implant (see inset) in the canine proximal humerus. The arrows indicate the margins of the gap between the host bone and surface of the implant. This gap is maintained by proximal and distal spacers that hold the surface of the porous coating 3 mm from the prepared bone surface. Implant models of this type are useful for testing the effects of various graft materials, bone graft substitutes and implant treatments on bone regeneration in the gap and bone ingrowth into the porous coating. *Source*: Modified from Ref. 36.

(75). Interestingly, in this model system in which implants are placed bilaterally, but only one implant is treated with growth factor, the contralateral "control" site can also show enhanced bone formation compared to animals in which no growth factor was used (36,74). While this observation may have interesting implications for identification of circulating factors that

(A) No Autograft or Growth Factor Treatment

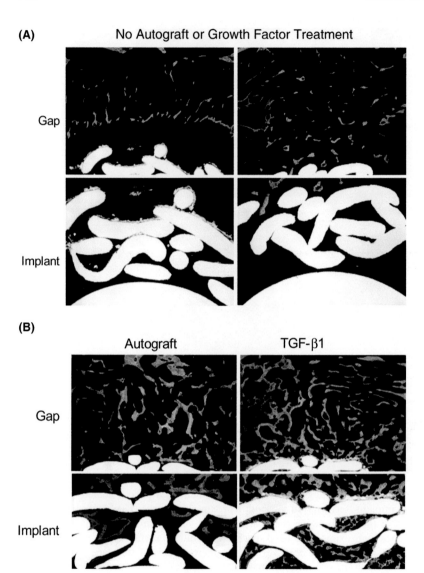

(B)

Autograft   TGF-β1

Figure 2 Backscatter scanning electron micrographs depicting bone formation in the gap and implant. (**A**) When neither autograft or growth factors are used, a variable amount of bone forms in the gap with only occasional areas of bone ingrowth. (**B**) When the gap is grafted with autogenous cancellous bone, there is enhanced bone formation in the gap and implant and when the implant is pre-treated with TGF-β1 there is considerable enhancement of bone formation in the gap and implant. All photomicrographs are backscatter SEMs in the canine 3 mm gap model at 4 weeks (original magnification 25× for the gap and 40× for the implant). *Abbreviation*: TGF, transforming gowth factor.

enhance bone formation, it also means that researchers need to use true controls in addition to contralateral controls.

To illustrate the dose response, we have compiled data from several of our canine studies using TGF-β (Fig. 3). These studies used models in which the volume of the defect varied. Ignoring this difference between models, it appears that doses of 10–300 μg are effective (Fig. 3, top panel). When the volume of the defect is considered or the nominal outer surface area of the implant is considered (Fig. 3, middle and bottom panels, respectively), it appears that there may be more of a threshold effect. Taken together, these studies indicate that treating the implant with doses ranging from roughly 0.005 to 0.12 μg/mm^3 of surrounding gap (or, alternatively, 0.025–0.5 μg/mm^2 of nominal implant surface area) are stimulatory. Of course, this precise dose response may only be valid for the delivery vehicle used in our studies (a hydroxyapatite/tricalcium phosphate coating applied to the implants). We would expect other delivery vehicles to have different release kinetics (36,76–79) and the exact dose response would need to be studied.

Although the molecular mechanisms of action of these growth factors in the context of joint replacement have not been investigated in vivo, there is now some insight on cell kinetics. Specifically, the fraction of the regenerating bone surfaces occupied by osteoblasts is greatly enhanced in the presence of exogenous TGF-β (68). Given that there are also more of these surfaces when the growth factor is administered, it is now apparent that TGF-β either enhances proliferation or suppresses death of cells in the osteogenic lineage. BMP-2 may have similar actions, but this remains to be investigated.

The presence of a dose response in which the highest doses tested were not the most stimulatory indicates that high doses may actually be inhibitory to some extent. The mechanism of high dose-induced inhibition of bone ingrowth compared to the optimum dose appears to be different for TGF-β and BMP. In the former case, our observations suggest that mineralization is inhibited (35,36,68), but in the case of BMP-2 an initial phase of bone resorption appears to be the cause (74). Although studies were not done specifically in the context of joint replacement, a similar phenomenon has been noted by others in studying BMP-2 (80–82) and BMP-7 (osteogenic protein-1) (83,84).

IMPLANT SURFACE MODIFICATION

Implant surface characteristics are critical in determining the nature of the tissue response adjacent to the implant and, presumably, the clinical success of an implant. There has been extensive work done with various calcium phosphate coatings, in particular plasma flame sprayed hydroxyapatite [reviewed in detail recently (85)], showing that various calcium phosphate coatings are stimulatory. In addition, bioglass is also stimulatory (86). Many

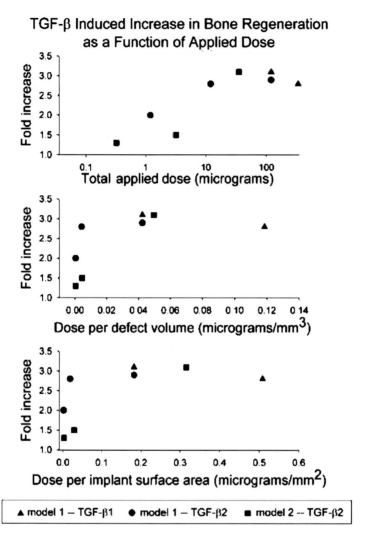

Figure 3 Graphs summarizing the increase in bone formation in the gap between the implant surface and host bone in canine models, expressed as a function of applied dose (*top panel*), per defect volume (*middle panel*) and implant surface area (*lower panel*). The fold increase for model 1 implants was based on comparison with a group that received no growth factor and the fold increase for model 2 implants was based on the contralateral control. This difference in controls was necessitated by the presence of a systemic effect in studies using model 1 implants that was not apparent in the model 2 implants. An example of a model 1 implant is shown in Figure 1. Model 2 implants were smaller to accommodate use of smaller animals. *Source*: From Refs. 35, 36, 68.

other studies suggest that an important surface characteristic is surface topography (87–89). Although it is clear that surface roughness does affect implant integration, why this is the case is not clearly understood.

Results from in vivo studies testing pull out strength, push out failure load and bone-implant contact have demonstrated that greater surface roughness correlates with a stronger interaction between bone and implant (90–94). Although rough surfaces allow for a greater surface area of contact between bone and implant, the stronger interaction seen with rougher surfaces may also be attributed to variation in local tissue strains that result from differences in surface topography (95,96). The effect of roughness may be site-dependent, as increased implant roughness was found to increase osseointegration of tibial diaphyseal but not femoral condyle implants (97).

Several in vitro studies have analyzed the response to surface roughness at the cellular level. Cell attachment is increased on titanium surfaces, hydroxyapatite-reinforced polyethylene composite surfaces, and bioactive glass surfaces when surface roughness is increased (98–102), although there are also studies that have found no effect of roughness on cell attachment (103–108). Cell attachment to rougher surfaces could be a result of an increase of focal contact density in cells at the region of contact with the edge of grooves (109,110), and also the ability of cells to form a three-dimensional cell matrix on roughened surfaces.

The effect of surface roughness on cell differentiation has also been investigated. Alkaline phosphatase or osteocalcin expression and cell proliferation have been found to increase in cells cultured on titanium or HA coated titanium implants as surface roughness increases (100,105,111), though in some studies alkaline phosphatase activity was found to be unaffected by surface roughness (105). Other studies have also found evidence of greater differentiation of marrow stromal cells on smoother titanium surfaces (112). Epiphyseal plate chondrocyte maturation and proliferation in vitro has also been shown to be altered by surface roughness, though the effects were also dependent on the precise anatomical region of origin of the epiphyseal plate chondrocytes (113). It is also interesting to note that osteoclast activity may be increased by greater surface roughness (114). In addition to the biologic effect of surface roughness, the fatigue life of titanium implant may also be decreased with increased surface roughness (115). Considering the variable response of different cells to surfaces of different roughness as well as the physical changes that different roughness may cause, the resultant effect of surface roughness on implant fixation is likely to be dependent on multiple factors whose mechanisms still remain obscure.

In addition to surface roughness, it has been demonstrated that cell attachment, growth, and differentiation on common implant materials such as commercially pure titanium, the titanium alloy Ti–6Al–4V, the cobalt alloy CoCrMo, stainless steel, hydroxyapatite, and bioactive glass differ

(116–120). As with surface roughness, results vary depending on the material, cell type, and culture conditions. Cell adhesion on these different metal surfaces has been found to be similar and also greater than on HA (121) while others have found greater cell adhesion to Ti–6Al–4V than to CoCrMo (118). In contrast to this finding, it has also been reported that HA coating of titanium implants causes an increase in cell adhesion (122). Differentiation has been found to be greater on commercially pure titanium than on stainless steel or CoCrMo and to vary on different grades of commercially pure titanium, although this may be related to the roughness of these different grades (123). Chemical modification of HA, tantalum, and alumina have also been shown to alter cell attachment or osteoblastic differentiation of cells (120,124,125).

The design and synthesis of biomimetic polymers that actively regulate the response of mammalian cells is a novel approach to integrate biomaterials with biological systems through either a molecular or cellular pathway (126–128). Introduction of bioactive signals into an implant first requires that the base material prevents non-specific interactions with constituents of the biologic environment (e.g., proteins, lipids, and cells). Ultra thin ($\sim 7\,nm$) polymer coatings that minimize protein adsorption and subsequently eliminate cell interaction have now been developed. These interpenetrating polymer networks (IPNs) have been grafted to both metal oxides (e.g., TiO_2) and polymers (129–132).

Coatings such as the IPN can be applied to standard implant materials to render them minimally interactive with proteins and amenable for subsequent modification with biological signals. Approaching the presentation of the biological ligand in this manner leads to presentation of the signal from a substrate (IPN) that prevents non-specific protein adsorption that would ordinarily foul the signal. For example, grafting peptides, containing the cell-binding (Cys–Gly–Gly–Asn–Gly–Glu–Pro–Arg–Gly–Asp–Thr–Tyr–Arg–Ala–Tyr, -RGD-) and heparin-binding (Cys–Gly–Gly–Phe–His–Arg–Arg–Ile–Lys–Ala, -FHRRIKA-) domains present in bone sialoprotein, to the IPN has affected cell adhesion, proliferation, and matrix mineralization in vitro in a ligand and surface density dependent manner (133–135). Peptide-modified IPNs exploiting the -RGD- and -FHRRIKA- signals have also enhanced bone formation surrounding metallic implants in vivo in a preliminary study (70). Preferential bone formation surrounding peptide-modified IPN coated titanium implants compared to uncoated control implants in a rat model was evident and is under further investigation (Fig. 4). Thus, the combination of a bioactive signal grafted to a non-fouling base, such as an IPN, may serve as an effective way to transform a material to possess growth factor-like qualities in controlling the behavior of mammalian cells and tissue formation surrounding an implant in vivo.

Despite the wealth of information on the interaction of osteogenic cells with implant surfaces, the use of a variety of cell lines and culture conditions

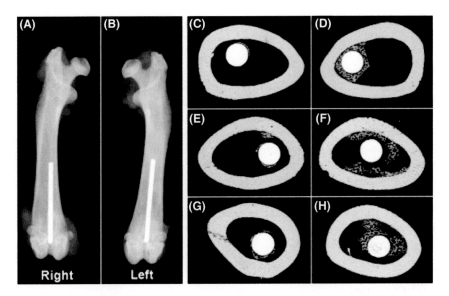

Figure 4 Use of a rat model to test peptide-grafted titanium rods. Panels (**A**) and (**B**) are contact radiographs made 1 week after implantation of control (*right*) and treated (*left*) implants. Panel (**C**) through (**H**) are backscatter scanning electron micrographs depicting control implants from 3 animals (**C, E** and **G**) and 50:50-RGD-FHRRIKA-modified implants from 3 animals (**D, F** and **H**). Note the increased bone formation in the vicinity of the treated implants. *Abbreviations*: RGD, amino acid containing arginine-glycine-aspartate oligopeptides; FHRRIKA, phenylalanine, histidine, arginine, isoleucine lysine, alanine. *Source*: From Ref. 70.

and the sometimes contradictory results observed make it difficult to predict the in vivo response of cells to different surfaces or materials. It should also be noted that although most in vitro studies focus on the effect of different surfaces on cell maturation, growth or adhesion, there is little information to indicate how the in vitro changes in cell activity relate to differences in implant performance in vivo.

OTHER ENHANCING AGENTS

Other modalities can also have enhancing effects on bone ingrowth or ongrowth. Mechanical signals to the bone may be stimulatory as evidenced by a recent study of extremely low amplitude mechanical strains in an avian model in which the implant was functionally isolated from other mechanical signals (136) and in two studies of low intensity ultrasound in canine models (137,138). One of the bisphosphonates that is being used in the treatment of osteoporosis has also been investigated in the context of implants. In canines with a total hip replacement and treated with oral alendronate, bone ingrowth into the periphery of the porous coated acetabular components was nearly doubled at six months (139). While the drug was administered based on the human clinical dose for post-menopausal osteoporosis, increased gastrointestinal absorption in canines resulted in effective over-dosing. When this effect is compensated for by administering the drug subcutaneously, another canine model found no effect on integration of host bone onto textured surfaces in ovariectomised canines on low calcium diets (140). In a third canine model, the bone surrounding alendronate-coated dental implants had higher formation rates than controls and alendronate-coated titanium implants had enhanced bone contact at four weeks (141). These are some of the more recent novel treatment possibilities. For a fuller review of the history of cementless implant fixation, the reader is referred to other reviews (5,71,142,143).

CONCLUSION

For cementless fixation, it is uncertain how rapidly an agent needs to act to be effective. Under ideal conditions in canine models, the static strength of fixation of implants reaches a plateau by approximately two weeks, in contrast to achievement of a fixation strength plateau within hours in the case of cemented implants. Undoubtedly, on a longer time scale (months to years), as the tissue matures and adapts to its new mechanical environment the strength of fixation increases over time, but this has received little attention. Clinically, there is often a period of restricted weight-bearing, frequently on the order of 6 to 12 weeks, based on the presumption that the interface needs to be protected, although even this precaution may not always be necessary (144).

It is clear that there are several biological approaches to enhancing cementless fixation, including altering the implant surface and stimulating the local environment with growth factors. Some of these treatment strategies are now coming into play clinically for other indications (e.g., spine fusion). Presumably, some of these approaches will eventually be used clinically for joint replacement. While enhancement of cementless fixation seems advantageous even in the context of primary joint replacement, perhaps, the first widespread use of these agents will be in revision joint replacement, a situation where bone stock is poor and the regeneration potential of the host skeleton may be compromised.

ACKNOWLEDGMENTS

NIH Grants AR42862 and AR43187, Grainger Foundation.

REFERENCES

1. Wurzler KK, DeWeese TL, Sebald W, Reddi AH. Radiation-induced impairment of bone healing can be overcome by recombinant human bone morphogenetic protein-2. J Craniofac Surg 1998; 9:131–137.
2. Luppen CA, Blake CA, Ammirati KM, Stevens ML, Seeherman HJ, Wozney JM, Bouxsein ML. Recombinant human bone morphogenetic protein-2 enhances osteotomy healing in glucocorticoid-treated rabbits. J Bone Miner Res 2002; 17:301–310.
3. Thaller SR, Lee TJ, Armstrong M, Tesluk H, Stern JS. Effect of insulin-like growth factor type 1 on critical-size defects in diabetic rats. J Craniofac Surg 1995; 6:218–223.
4. Thaller SR, Salzhauer MA, Rubinstein AJ, Thion A, Tesluk H. Effect of insulin-like growth factor type I on critical size calvarial bone defects in irradiated rats. J Craniofac Surg 1998; 9:138–141.
5. Sumner DR, Galante JO. Bone ingrowth. In: Evarts CM, ed. Surgery of the Musculoskeletal System. New York: Churchill Livingstone, 1990:151–176.
6. Owen M. Lineage of osteogenic cells and their relationship to the stromal system. In: Peck WA, ed. Bone and Mineral Research. Amsterdam: Elsevier, 1985:1–25.
7. Barnes J. The Complete Works of Aristotle: the Revised Oxford Translation: Princeton University Press, 1984.
8. Waller EK, Olweus J, Lund-Johansen F, Huang S, Nguyen M, Guo GR, Terstappen L. The "common stem cell" hypothesis reevaluated: human fetal bone marrow contains separate populations of hematopoietic and stromal progenitors. Blood 1995; 85:2422–2435.
9. Friedenstein AJ, Deriglasova UF, Kulagina NN, Panasuk AF, Rudakowa SF, Luria EA, Ruadkow IA. Precursors for fibroblasts in different populations of hematopoietic cells as detected by the in vitro colony assay method. Exp Hematol 1974; 2:83–92.
10. Owen M. Marrow stromal stem cells. J Cell Sci (suppl) 1988; 10:63–76.
11. Owen M, Friedenstein AJ. Stromal stem cells: marrow-derived osteogenic precursors. Ciba Found Symp 1988; 136:42–60.
12. Triffitt JT. The stem cell of the osteoblast. In: Bilizekian J, Raisz L, Rodan G, eds. Principles of Bone Biology. San Diego: Academic Press, 1996:39–50.
13. Pittenger MF, Mackay AM, Beck SC, Jaiswal RK, Douglas R, Mosca JD, Moorman MA, Simonetti DW, Craig S, Marshak DR. Multilineage potential of adult human mesenchymal stem cells. Science 1999; 284:143–147.
14. Bruder SP, Fox BS. Tissue engineering of bone. Cell based strategies. Clin Orthop 1999; 367(suppl):S68–S83.
15. Goshima J, Goldberg VM, Caplan AI. The osteogenic potential of culture-expanded rat marrow mesenchymal cells assayed in vivo in calcium phosphate ceramic blocks. Clin Orthop 1991:298–311.
16. Bennett JH, Joyner CJ, Triffitt JT, Owen ME. Adipocytic cells cultured from marrow have osteogenic potential. J Cell Sci 1991; 99(Pt 1):131–139.
17. Zuk PA, Zhu M, Mizuno H, Huang J, Futrell JW, Katz AJ, Benhaim P, Lorenz HP, Hedrick MH. Multilineage cells from human adipose tissue: implications for cell-based therapies. Tissue Eng 2001; 7:211–228.

18. Galotto M, Campanile G, Robino G, Cancedda FD, Bianco P, Cancedda R. Hypertrophic chondrocytes undergo further differentiation to osteoblast-like cells and participate in the initial bone formation in developing chick embryo. J Bone Miner Res 1994; 9:1239–1249.

19. Gentili C, Bianco P, Neri M, Malpeli M, Campanile G, Castagnola P, Cancedda R, Cancedda FD. Cell proliferation, extracellular matrix mineralization, and ovotransferrin transient expression during in vitro differentiation of chick hypertrophic chondrocytes into osteoblast-like cells. J Cell Biol 1993; 122:703–712.

20. Reyes M, Lund T, Lenvik T, Aguiar D, Koodie L, Verfaillie CM. Purification and ex vivo expansion of postnatal human marrow mesodermal progenitor cells. Blood 2001; 98:2615–2625.

21. Ferrari G, Cusella-De Angelis G, Coletta M, Paolucci E, Stornaiuolo A, Cossu G, Mavilio F. Muscle regeneration by bone marrow-derived myogenic progenitors. Science 1998; 279:1528–1530.

22. Kopen GC, Prockop DJ, Phinney DG. Marrow stromal cells migrate throughout forebrain and cerebellum, and they differentiate into astrocytes after injection into neonatal mouse brains. Proc Natl Acad Sci USA 1999; 96:10,711–10,716.

23. Mezey E, Chandross KJ, Harta G, Maki RA, McKercher SR. Turning blood into brain: cells bearing neuronal antigens generated in vivo from bone marrow. Science 2000; 290:1779–1782.

24. Centrella M, Horowitz MC, Wozney JM, McCarthy TL. Transforming growth factor-beta gene family members and bone. Endocr Rev 1994; 15:27–39.

25. Ingram RT, Bonde SK, Riggs BL, Fitzpatrick LA. Effects of transforming growth factor beta (TGF beta) and 1,25 dihydroxyvitamin D3 on the function, cytochemistry and morphology of normal human osteoblast-like cells. Differentiation 1994; 55:153–163.

26. Harris SE, Bonewald LF, Harris MA, Sabatini M, Dallas S, Feng JQ, Ghosh-Choudhury N, Wozney J, Mundy GR. Effects of transforming growth factor β on bone nodule formation and expression of bone morphogenetic protein 2, osteocalcin, osteopontin, alkaline phosphatase, and Type I collagen mRNA in long-term cultures of fetal rat calvarial osteoblasts. J Bone Miner Res 1994; 9:855–863.

27. Ahdjoudj S, Lasmoles F, Holy X, Zerath E, Marie PJ. Transforming growth factor beta 2 inhibits adipocyte differentiation induced by skeletal unloading in rat bone marrow stroma. J Bone Miner Res 2002; 17:668–677.

28. Locklin RM, Oreffo RO, Triffitt JT. Effects of TGF beta and βFGF on the differentiation of human bone marrow stromal fibroblasts. Cell Biol Int 1999; 23:185–194.

29. Joyce ME, Jingushi S, Bolander ME. Transforming growth factor-beta in the regulation of fracture repair. Orthop Clin North Am 1990; 21:199–209.

30. Beck LS, Amento EP, Xu Y, Deguzman L, Lee WP, Nguyen T, Gillett NA. TGF-β_1 induces bone closure of skull defects: temporal dynamics of bone formation in defects exposed to rhTGF-β_1. J Bone Miner Res 1993; 8:753–761.

31. Rosen D, Miller SC, DeLeon E, Thompson AY, Bentz H, Mathews M, Adams S. Systemic administration of recombinant transforming growth factor

beta 2 (rTGF-β2) stimulates parameters of cancellous bone formation in juvenile and adult rats. Bone 1994; 15:355–359.

32. Lind M, Schumacker B, Søballe K, Keller J, Melsen F, Bünger C. Transforming growth factor-beta enhances fracture healing in rabbit tibiae. Acta Orthop Scand 1993; 64:553–556.

33. Lind M, Overgaard S, Nguyen T, Ongpipattanakul B, Bünger C, Søballe K. Transforming growth factor-β stimulates bone ongrowth: hydroxyapatite-coated implants studied in dogs. Acta Orthop Scand 1996; 67:611–616.

34. Lind M, Overgaard S, Ongpipattanakul B, Nguyen T, Bünger C, Søballe K. Transforming growth factor-β1 stimulates bone ongrowth to weight-loaded tricalcium phosphate coated implants. J Bone Joint Surg Br 1996; 78-B: 377–382.

35. Sumner DR, Turner TM, Purchio AF, Gombotz WR, Urban RM, Galante JO. Enhancement of bone ingrowth by transforming growth factor beta. J Bone Joint Surg Am 1995; 77-A:1135–1147.

36. Sumner DR, Turner TM, Urban RM, Leven RM, Hawkins M, Nichols EH, McPherson JM, Galante JO. Locally delivered rhTGF-β2 enhances bone ingrowth and bone regeneration at local and remote sites of skeletal injury. J Orthop Res 2001; 19:85–94.

37. Urist MR. Bone: formation by autoinduction. Science 1965; 150:893–899.

38. Rickard DJ, Sullivan TA, Shenker BJ, Leboy PS, Kazhdan I. Induction of rapid osteoblast differentiation in rat bone marrow stromal cell cultures by dexamethasone and BMP-2. Dev Biol 1994; 161:218–228.

39. Fromigue O, Marie PJ, Lomri A. Bone morphogenetic protein-2 and transforming growth factor-beta2 interact to modulate human bone marrow stromal cell proliferation and differentiation. J Cell Biochem 1998; 68:411–426.

40. Yeh LC, Mallein-Gerin F, Lee JC. Differential effects of osteogenic protein-1 (BMP-7) on gene expression of BMP and GDF family members during differentiation of the mouse MC615 chondrocyte cells. J Cell Physiol 2002; 191: 298–309.

41. Nilsson OS, Urist MR, Dawson EG, Schmalzried TP, Finerman GAM. Bone repair induced by bone morphogenetic protein in ulnar defects in dogs. J Bone Joint Surg Br 1986; 68-B:635–642.

42. Lovell TP, Dawson EG, Nilsson OS, Urist MR. Augmentation of spinal fusion with bone morphogenetic protein in dogs. Clin Orthop 1987; 243:266–274.

43. Heckman JD, Boyan BD, Aufdemorte TB, Abbott JT. The use of bone morphogenetic protein in the treatment of non-union in a canine model. J Bone Joint Surg Am 1991; 73-A:750–764.

44. Yasko AW, Lane JM, Fellinger EJ, Rosen V, Wozney JM, Wang EA. The healing of segmental bone defects, induced by recombinant human bone morphogenetic protein (rhBMP-2). J Bone Joint Surg Am 1992; 74-A:659–670.

45. Gerhart TN, Kirker-Head CA, Kriz MJ, Holtrop ME, Hennig GE, Hipp J, Schelling SH, Wang E. Healing segmental femoral defects in sheep using recombinant human bone morphogenetic protein. Clin Orthop 1993; 293: 317–326.

46. Toriumi DM, Kotler HS, Luxenberg DP, Holtrop ME, Wang EA. Mandibular reconstruction with a recombinant bone-inducing factor: functional,

histologic, and biomechanical evaluation. Arch Otolaryngol Head Neck Surg 1993; 117:1101–1112.

47. Cook SD, Wolfe MW, Salkeld SL, Rueger DC. Effect of recombinant human osteogenic protein-1 on healing of segmental defects in non-human primates. J Bone Joint Surg Am 1995; 77-A:734–750.

48. Bostrom M, Lane JM, Tomin E, Browne M, Berberian W, Turek T, Smith J, Wozney J, Schildhauer T. Use of bone morphogenetic protein-2 in the rabbit ulnar nonunion model. Clin Orthop 1996; 327:272–282.

49. Ripamonti U, van den Heever B, Sampath TK, Tucker MM, Rueger DC, Reddi AH. Complete regeneration of bone in the baboon by recombinant human osteogenic protein-1 (h)OP-1, bone morphogenetic protein-7). Growth Factors 1996; 13:273–289.

50. Sandhu HS, Kanim LD, Toth JM, Kabo JM, Liu D, Delamarter RB, Dawson EG. Experimental spinal fusion with recombinant human bone morphogenetic protein-2 without decortication of ossesous elements. Spine 1997; 22:1171–1180.

51. Welch RD, Jones AL, Bucholz RW, Reinert CM, Tjia JS, Pierce WA, Wozney JM, Li XJ. Effect of recombinant human bone morphogenetic protein-2 on fracture healing in a goat tibial fracture model. J Bone Miner Res 1998; 13:1483–1490.

52. Den Boer FC, Bramer JA, Blokhuis TJ, Van Soest EJ, Jenner JM, Patka P, Bakker FC, Burger EH, Haarman HJ. Effect of recombinant human osteogenic protein-1 on the healing of a freshly closed diaphyseal fracture. Bone 2002; 31:158–164.

53. Bergman RJ, Gazit D, Kahn AJ, Gruber H, McDougall S, Hahn TJ. Age-related changes in osteogenic stem cells in mice. J Bone Miner Res 1996; 11:568–577.

54. Tsuji T, Hughes FJ, McCulloch CAG, Melcher AH. Effects of donor age on osteogenic cells of rat bone marrow in vitro. Mech Aging Dev 1990; 51: 121–132.

55. Quarto R, Thomas D, Liang CT. Bone progenitor cell deficits and the age-associated decline in bone repair capacity. Calcif Tissue Int 1995; 56:123–129.

56. Egrise D, Martin D, Vienne A, Neve P, Schoutens A. The number of fibroblastic colonies formed from bone marrow is decreased and the in vitro proliferation rate of trabecular bone cells increased in aged rats. Bone 1992; 13:355–361.

57. Nishida S, Endo N, Yamagiwa H, Tanizawa T, Takahashi HE. Number of osteoprogenitor cells in human bone marrow markedly decreases after skeletal maturation. J Bone Miner Metab 1999; 17:171–177.

58. Muschler GF, Nitto H, Boehm CA, Easley KA. Age- and gender-related changes in the cellularity of human bone marrow and the prevalence of osteoblastic progenitors. J Orthop Res 2001; 19:117–125.

59. Oreffo RO, Bord S, Triffitt JT. Skeletal progenitor cells and ageing human populations. Clin Sci 1998; 94:549–555.

60. Shigeno Y, Ashton BA. Human bone-cell proliferation in vitro decreases with human donor age. J Bone Joint Surg Br 1995; 77-B:139–142.

61. Cornell CN. Management of fractures in patients with osteoporosis. Orthop Clin N Am 1990; 21:125–139.

62. Lane JM, Cornell CN, Healey JH. Osteoporosis: the structural and reparative consequences for the skeleton. Instr Course Lect 1987; 36:71–83.

63. Aronson J, Gao GG, Shen XC, McLaren SG, Skinner RA, Badger TM, Lumpkin CK Jr. The effect of aging on distraction osteogenesis in the rat. J Orthop Res 2001; 19:421–427.

64. Bak B, Andreassen TT. The effect of aging on fracture healing in the rat. Calcif Tissue Int 1989; 45:292–297.

65. Meyer RA Jr, Tsahakis PJ, Martin DF, Banks DM, Harrow ME, Kiebzak GM. Age and ovariectomy impair both the normalization of mechanical properties and the accretion of mineral by the fracture callus in rats. J Orthop Res 2001; 19:428–435.

66. Tonna EA, Cronkite EP. Changes in the skeletal cell proliferative response to trauma concomitant with aging. J Bone Joint Surg Am 1962; 44-A:1557–1568.

67. Street JT, Wang JH, Wu QD, Wakai A, McGuinness A, Redmond HP. The angiogenic response to skeletal injury is preserved in the elderly. J Orthop Res 2001; 19:1057–1066.

68. Sumner DR, Turner TM, Cohen M, Losavio P, Urban RM, Nichols EH, McPherson JM. Aging does not lessen the effectiveness of TGF-β_2 enhanced bone regeneration. J Bone Miner Res 2003; 18:730–736.

69. Stein GS, Lian JB. Molecular mechanisms mediating proliferation-differentiation interrelationships during progressive development of the osteoblast phenotype: update 1995. Endocr Rev 1995; 4:271–289.

70. Harbers GM, Barber TA, Stile RA, Sumner DR, Healy KE. Mimetic peptide modified materials for control of cell differentiation. In: Dillow AK, Lowman A, eds. Biomimetic Materials and Design: Interactive Biointerfacial Strategies, Tissue Engineering and Drug Delivery. New York: Marcel Dekker, 2001:55–89.

71. Sumner DR, Turner TM, Urban RM. Animal models of bone ingrowth and joint replacement. In: An YH, Friedman RJ, eds. Animals Models in Orthopedic Research. Boca Raton, Fla: CRC Press, 1999:407–425.

72. Lind M, Overgaard S, Søballe K, Nguyen T, Ongpipattanakul B, Bünger C. Transforming growth factor-$\beta 1$ enhances bone healing to unloaded tricalcium phosphate coated implants: an experimental study in dogs. J Orthop Res 1996; 14:343–350.

73. Zhou H, Choong PC, Chou ST, Kartsogiannis V, Martin TJ, Ng KW. Transforming growth factor $\beta 1$ stimulates bone formation and resorption in an in vivo model in rabbits. Bone 1995; 17:443S–448S.

74. Sumner DR, Turner TM, Urban RM, Turek T, Seeherman H, Wozney JM. Locally delivered rhBMP-2 enhances bone ingrowth and gap healing in a canine model. J Orthop Res 2004; 22:58–65.

75. Kienapfel H, Sumner DR, Turner TM, Urban RM, Galante JO. Efficacy of autograft and freeze-dried allograft to enhance fixation of porous coated implants in the presence of interface gaps. J Orthop Res 1992; 10:423–433.

76. Ongpipattanakul B, Nguyen T, Zioncheck TF, Wong R, Osaka G, Deguzman L, Lee WP, Beck LS. Development of tricalcium phosphate/amylopectin paste combined with recombinant human transforming growth factor beta 1 as a bone defect filler. J Biomed Mater Res 1997; 36:295–305.

77. Nicoll SB, Radin S, Santos EM, Tuan RS, Ducheyne P. In vitro release kinetics of biologically active transforming growth factor-β1 from a novel porous glass carrier. Biomaterials 1997; 18:853–859.

78. Gombotz WR, Pankey SC, Bouchard LS, Phan DH, Puolakkainen P. Stimulation of bone healing by transforming growth factor-beta$_1$ released from polymeric or ceramic implants. J Appl Biomater 1994; 5:141–150.

79. Gombotz WR, Pankey SC, Bouchard LS, Ranchalis J, Puolakkainen P. Controlled release of TGF-β_1 from a biodegradable matrix for bone regeneration. J Biomater Sci, Polymer Edition 1993; 5:49–63.

80. Wikesjo UM, Guglielmoni P, Promsudthi A, Cho KS, Trombelli L, Selvig KA, Jin L, Wozney JM. Periodontal repair in dogs: effect of rhBMP-2 concentration on regeneration of alveolar bone and periodontal attachment. J Clin Periodontol 1999; 26:392–400.

81. Toriumi DM, O'Grady K, Horlbeck DM, Desai D, Turek TJ, Wozney J. Mandibular reconstruction using bone morphogenetic protein 2: long-term follow-up in a canine model. Laryngoscope 1999; 109:1481–1489.

82. Rodeo SA, Suzuki K, Deng XH, Wozney J, Warren RF. Use of recombinant human bone morphogenetic protein-2 to enhance tendon healing in a bone tunnel. Am J Sports Med 1999; 27:476–488.

83. Laursen M, Hoy K, Hansen ES, Gelineck J, Christensen FB, Bunger CE. Recombinant bone morphogenetic protein-7 as an intracorporal bone growth stimulator in unstable thoracolumbar burst fractures in humans: preliminary results. Eur Spine J 1999; 8:485–490.

84. Cook SD, Barrack RL, Santman M, Patron LP, Salkeld SL, Whitecloud TS. Strut allograft healing to the femur with recombinant human osteogenic protein-1. Clin Orthop 2000; 47–57.

85. Sun L, Berndt CC, Gross KA, Kucuk A. Material fundamentals and clinical performance of plasma-sprayed hydroxyapatite coatings: a review. J Biomed Mater Res 2001; 58:570–592.

86. Wheeler DL, Montfort MJ, McLoughlin SW. Differential healing response of bone adjacent to porous implants coated with hydroxyapatite and 45S5 bioactive glass. J Biomed Mater Res 2001; 55:603–612.

87. Li J, Liao H, Fartash B, Hermansson L, Johnsson T. Surface-dimpled commercially pure titanium implant and bone ingrowth. Biomaterials 1997; 18:691–696.

88. Wong M, Eulenberger J, Schenk R, Hunziker E. Effect of surface topology on the osseointegration of implant materials in trabecular bone. J Biomed Mater Res 1995; 29:1567–1575.

89. Ogawa T, Ozawa S, Shih JH, Ryu KH, Sukotjo C, Yang JM, Nishimura I. Biomechanical evaluation of osseous implants having different surface topographies in rats. J Dent Res 2000; 79:1857–1863.

90. Baker D, London RM, O'Neal R. Rate of pull-out strength gain of dual-etched titanium implants: a comparative study in rabbits. Int J Oral Maxillofac Implants 1999; 14:722–728.

91. Trisi P, Rao W, Rebaudi A. A histometric comparison of smooth and rough titanium implants in human low-density jawbone. Int J Oral Maxillofac Implants 1999; 14:689–698.

92. Nishiguchi S, Kato H, Neo M, Oka M, Kim HM, Kokubo T, Nakamura T. Alkali- and heat-treated porous titanium for orthopedic implants. J Biomed Mater Res 2001; 54:198–208.

93. Buser D, Schenk RK, Steinemann S, Fiorellini JP, Fox CH, Stich H. Influence of surface characteristics on bone integration of titanium implants. A histomorphometric study in miniature pigs. J Biomed Mater Res 1991; 25:889–902.

94. Klokkevold PR, Nishimura RD, Adachi M, Caputo A. Osseointegration enhanced by chemical etching of the titanium surface. A torque removal study in the rabbit. Clin Oral Implants Res 1997; 8:442–447.

95. Simmons CA, Meguid SA, Pilliar RM. Differences in osseointegration rate due to implant surface geometry can be explained by local tissue strains. J Orthop Res 2001; 19:187–194.

96. Wiskott HW, Belser UC. Lack of integration of smooth titanium surfaces: a working hypothesis based on strains generated in the surrounding bone. Clin Oral Implants Res 1999; 10:429–444.

97. Hayakawa T, Yoshinari M, Nemoto K, Wolke JG, Jansen JA. Effect of surface roughness and calcium phosphate coating on the implant/bone response. Clin Oral Implants Res 2000; 11:296–304.

98. Bowers KT, Keller JC, Randolph BA, Wick DG, Michaels CM. Optimization of surface micromorphology for enhanced osteoblast responses in vitro. Int J Oral Maxillofac Implants 1992; 7:302–310.

99. Qu J, Chehroudi B, Brunette DM. The use of micromachined surfaces to investigate the cell behavioural factors essential to osseointegration. Oral Dis 1996; 2:102–115.

100. Korovessis PG, Deligianni DD. Role of surface roughness of titanium versus hydroxyapatite on human bone marrow cells response. J Spinal Disord Tech 2002; 15:175–183.

101. Itala A, Ylanen HO, Yrjans J, Heino T, Hentunen T, Hupa M, Aro HT. Characterization of microrough bioactive glass surface: surface reactions and osteoblast responses in vitro. J Biomed Mater Res 2002; 62:404–411.

102. Dalby MJ, Kayser MV, Bonfield W, Di Silvio L. Initial attachment of osteoblasts to an optimised HAPEX topography. Biomaterials 2002; 23:681–690.

103. Mustafa K, Wroblewski J, Hultenby K, Lopez BS, Arvidson K. Effects of titanium surfaces blasted with TiO2 particles on the initial attachment of cells derived from human mandibular bone. A scanning electron microscopic and histomorphometric analysis. Clin Oral Implants Res 2000; 11:116–128.

104. Lumbikanonda N, Sammons R. Bone cell attachment to dental implants of different surface characteristics. Int J Oral Maxillofac Implants 2001; 16: 627–636.

105. Mustafa K, Wennerberg A, Wroblewski J, Hultenby K, Lopez BS, Arvidson K. Determining optimal surface roughness of TiO(2) blasted titanium implant material for attachment, proliferation and differentiation of cells derived from human mandibular alveolar bone. Clin Oral Implants Res 2001; 12: 515–525.

106. Kononen M, Hormia M, Kivilahti J, Hautaniemi J, Thesleff I. Effect of surface processing on the attachment, orientation, and proliferation of human gingival fibroblasts on titanium. J Biomed Mater Res 1992; 26:1325–1341.

107. Richards RG. The effect of surface roughness on fibroblast adhesion in vitro. Injury 1996; 27(suppl 3):SC38–SC43.
108. Lauer G, Wiedmann-Al-Ahmad M, Otten JE, Hubner U, Schmelzeisen R, Schilli W. The titanium surface texture effects adherence and growth of human gingival keratinocytes and human maxillar osteoblast-like cells in vitro. Biomaterials 2001; 22:2799–2809.
109. Schmidt C, Kaspar D, Sarkar MR, Claes LE, Ignatius AA. A scanning electron microscopy study of human osteoblast morphology on five orthopedic metals. J Biomed Mater Res 2002; 63:252–261.
110. Eisenbarth E, Linez P, Biehl V, Velten D, Breme J, Hildebrand H. Cell orientation and cytoskeleton organisation on ground titanium surfaces. Biomol Eng 2002; 19:233–237.
111. Lohmann CH, Sagun R Jr, Sylvia VL, Cochran DL, Dean DD, Boyan BD, Schwartz Z. Surface roughness modulates the response of MG63 osteoblast-like cells to 1,25-$(OH)_2D_3$ through regulation of phospholipase A_2 activity and activation of protein kinase A. J Biomed Mater Res 1999; 47:139–151.
112. Ter Brugge PJ, Wolke JG, Jansen JA. Effect of calcium phosphate coating crystallinity and implant surface roughness on differentiation of rat bone marrow cells. J Biomed Mater Res 2002; 60:70–78.
113. Boyan BD, Lincks J, Lohmann CH, Sylvia VL, Cochran DL, Blanchard CR, Dean DD, Schwartz Z. Effect of surface roughness and composition on costochondral chondrocytes is dependent on cell maturation state. J Orthop Res 1999; 17:446–457.
114. Matsunaga T, Inoue H, Kojo T, Hatano K, Tsujisawa T, Uchiyama C, Uchida Y. Disaggregated osteoclasts increase in resorption activity in response to roughness of bone surface. J Biomed Mater Res 1999; 48:417–423.
115. Bapna MS, Lautenschlager EP, Moser JB. The influences of electrical potential and surface finish on the fatigue life of surgical implant materials. J Biomed Mater Res 1975; 9:611–621.
116. Merklein F, Hendrich C, Noth U, Kochinki G, Rader CP, Schutze N, Thull R, Eulert J. Standardized tests of bone implant surfaces with an osteoblast cell culture system. I. Orthopedic standard materials. Biomed Tech (Berl) 1998; 43:354–359.
117. Shah AK, Sinha RK, Hickok NJ, Tuan RS. High-resolution morphometric analysis of human osteoblastic cell adhesion on clinically relevant orthopedic alloys. Bone 1999; 24:499–506.
118. Sinha RK, Morris F, Shah SA, Tuan RS. Surface composition of orthopaedic implant metals regulates cell attachment, spreading, and cytoskeletal organization of primary human osteoblasts in vitro. Clin Orthop 1994; 305:258–272.
119. Mayr-Wohlfart U, Fiedler J, Gunther KP, Puhl W, Kessler S. Proliferation and differentiation rates of a human osteoblast-like cell line (SaOS-2) in contact with different bone substitute materials. J Biomed Mater Res 2001; 57:132–139.
120. Zreiqat H, Howlett CR. Titanium substrata composition influences osteoblastic phenotype: in vitro study. J Biomed Mater Res 1999; 47:360–366.
121. Puleo DA, Holleran LA, Doremus RH, Bizios R. Osteoblast responses to orthopedic implant materials in vitro. J Biomed Mater Res 1991; 25:711–723.

122. Takebe J, Itoh S, Okada, Ishibashi K. Anodic oxidation and hydrothermal treatment of titanium results in a surface that causes increased attachment and altered cytoskeletal morphology of rat bone marrow stromal cells in vitro. J Biomed Mater Res 2000; 51:398–407.

123. Ahmad M, Gawronski D, Blum J, Goldberg J, Gronowicz G. Differential response of human osteoblast-like cells to commercially pure (cp) titanium grades 1 and 4. J Biomed Mater Res 1999; 46:121–131.

124. Ohgaki M, Kizuki T, Katsura M, Yamashita K. Manipulation of selective cell adhesion and growth by surface charges of electrically polarized hydroxyapatite. J Biomed Mater Res 2001; 57:366–373.

125. Kato H, Nakamura T, Nishiguchi S, Matsusue Y, Kobayashi M, Miyazaki T, Kim HM, Kokubo T. Bonding of alkali- and heat-treated tantalum implants to bone. J Biomed Mater Res 2000; 53:28–35.

126. Healy KE, Rezania A, Stile RA. Designing biomaterials to direct biological responses. Ann N Y Acad Sci 1999; 875:24–35.

127. Healy KE, Harbers GM, Barber TA, Sumner DR. Osteoblast interactions with engineered surfaces. In: Davies JE, ed. Bone Engineering. Toronto: Em squared, 2000; 268–281.

128. Healy KE. Molecular engineering of materials for bioreactivity. Current Opinions in Solid State Materials Science 1999; 875:24–35.

129. Bearinger JP, Castner DG, Chen J, Hubchak S, Golledge SL, Healy KE. P(AAm-*col*-EG) interpenetrating polymer networks grated to oxide surfaces: surface characterization, protein adsorption, and cell detachment studies. Langmuir 1997; 13:5175–5183.

130. Thomas CH, Lhoest JB, Castner DG, McFarland CD, Healy KE. Surfaces designed to control the projected area and shape of individual cells. J Biomech Eng 1999; 121:40–48.

131. Barber TA, Golledge SL, Castner DG, Healy KE. Peptide-modified p(AAm-co-EG/AAc) IPNs grafted to bulk titanium modulate osteoblast behavior in vitro. Biomed J Mater Res 2000 (In press).

132. Bearinger JP, Castner DG, Healy KE. Biomolecular modification of p(AAm-co-EG/AA) IPNs supports osteoblast adhesion and phenotypic expression. J Biomater Sci Polym Ed 1998; 9:629–652.

133. Rezania A, Healy KE. Biomimetic peptide surfaces that regulate adhesion, spreading, cytoskeletal organization, and mineralization of the matrix deposited by osteoblast-like cells. Biotechnol Prog 1999; 15:19–32.

134. Rezania A, Healy KE. The effect of peptide surface density on mineralization of a matrix deposited by osteogenic cells. J Biomed Mater Res 2000; 52:595–600.

135. Rezania A, Healy KE. Integrin subunits responsible for adhesion of human osteoblast-like cells to biomimetic peptide surfaces. J Orthop Res 1999; 17:615–623.

136. Rubin CT, McLeod KJ. Promotion of bony ingrowth by frequency-specific, low-amplitude mechanical strain. Clin Orthop 1994; 298:165–174.

137. Tanzer M, Harvey E, Kay A, Morton P, Bobyn JD. Effect of noninvasive low intensity ultrasound on bone growth into porous-coated implants. J Orthop Res 1996; 14:901–906.

138. Tanzer M, Kantor S, Bobyn JD. Enhancement of bone growth into porous intramedullary implants using non-invasive low intensity ultrasound. J Orthop Res 2001; 19:195–199.

139. Shanbhag AS, May D, Cha C, Kovach C, Hasselman CT, Rubash HE. Enhancing net bone formation in canine total hip components with bisphosphonates. Trans Orthop Res Soc 1999; 255.

140. Frenkel SR, Jaffe WL, Valle CD, Jazrawi, Wright A. The effect of alendronate (Fosamaxtrade mark) and implant surface on bone integration and remodeling in a canine model. J Biomed Mater Res 2001; 58:645–650.

141. Meraw SJ, Reeve CM, Wollan PC. Use of alendronate in peri-implant defect regeneration. J Periodontol 1999; 70:151–158.

142. Bauer TW, Schils J. The pathology of total joint arthroplasty. I. Mechanisms of implant fixation. Skeletal Radiol 1999; 28:423–432.

143. Kienapfel H, Sprey C, Wilke A, Griss P. Implant fixation by bone ingrowth. J Arthrop 1999; 14:355–368.

144. Woolson ST, Adler NS. The effect of partial or full weight bearing ambulation after cementless total hip arthroplasty. J Arthroplasty 2002; 17:820–825.

145. Panagakos FS. Insulin-like growth factors-I and -II stimulate chemotaxis of osteoblasts isolated from fetal rat calvaria. Biochim 1993; 75:991–994.

146. Lind M, Deleuran B, Thestrup-Pedersen K, Søballe K, Eriksen EF, Bünger C. Chemotaxis of human osteoblasts. Effects of osteotropic growth factors. APMIS 1995; 103:140–146.

147. Panagakos FS. Transforming growth factor–alpha stimulates chemotaxis of osteoblasts and osteoblast-like cells in vitro. Biochem Mol Biol Int 1994; 33:643–650.

148. Pfeilschifter J, Wolf O, Naumann A, Minne HW, Mundy GR, Ziegler R. Chemotactic response of osteoblastlike cells to transforming growth factor beta. J Bone Miner Res 1990; 5:825–830.

149. Hughes FJ, Aubin JE, Heersche JN. Differential chemotactic responses of different populations of fetal rat calvaria cells to platelet-derived growth factor and transforming growth factor beta. Bone Miner 1992; 19:63–74.

150. Lind M, Deleuran B, Yssel H, Fink-Eriksen E, Thestrup-Pedersen K. IL-4 and IL-13, but not IL-10, are chemotactic factors for human osteoblasts. Cytokine 1995; 7:78–82.

151. Tsukamoto T, Matsui T, Fukase M, Fujita T. Platelet-derived growth factor B chain homodimer enhances chemotaxis and DNA synthesis in normal osteoblast-like cells (MC3T3-E1). Biochem Biophys Res Commun 1991; 175:745–751.

152. Fiedler J, Roderer G, GuntherK-P, Brenner RE. BMP-2, BMP-4 and PDGF-bb stimulate chemotactic migration of primary mesenchymal progenitor cells. J Cell Biochem 2002; 87:305–312.

153. Mayr-Wohlfart U, Waltenberger J, Hausser H, Kessler S, Gunther KP, Dehio C, Puhl W, Brenner RE. Vascular endothelial growth factor stimulates chemotactic migration of primary human osteoblasts. Bone 2002; 30:472–477.

154. Lind M, Eriksen EF, Bünger C. Bone morphogenetic protein-2 but not bone morphogenetic protein-4 and -6 stimulates chemotactic migration of human osteoblasts, human marrow osteoblasts, and U2-OS cells. Bone 1996; 18:53–57.

155. Park YJ, Lee YM, Lee JY, Seol YJ, Chung CP, Lee SJ. Controlled release of platelet-derived growth factor-BB from chondroitin sulfate-chitosan sponge for guided bone regeneration. J Control Release 2000; 67:385–394.

156. Park YJ, Lee YM, Park SN, Sheen SY, Chung CP, Lee SJ. Platelet derived growth factor releasing chitosan sponge for periodontal bone regeneration. Biomaterials 2000; 21:153–159.

157. Nesti LJ, Caterson EJ, Wang M, Chang R, Chapovsky F, Hoek JB, Tuan RS. TGF-beta 1 calcium signaling increases alpha 5 integrin expression in osteoblasts. J Orthop Res 2002; 20:1042–1049.

158. Lai CF, Feng X, Nishimura R, Teitelbaum SL, Avioli LV, Ross FP, Cheng SL. Transforming growth factor-beta up-regulates the beta 5 integrin subunit expression via Sp1 and Smad signaling. J Biol Chem 2000; 275:36,400–36,406.

159. Debiais F, Lemonnier J, Hay E, Delannoy P, Caverzasio J, Marie PJ. Fibroblast growth factor-2 (FGF-2) increases N-cadherin expression through protein kinase C and Src-kinase pathways in human calvaria osteoblasts. J Cell Biochem 2001; 81:68–81.

160. Shah AK, Lazatin J, Sinha RK, Lennox T, Hickok NJ, Tuan RS. Mechanism of BMP-2 stimulated adhesion of osteoblastic cells to titanium alloy. Biol Cell 1999; 91:131–142.

161. Jia D, Heersche JN. Insulin-like growth factor-1 and -2 stimulate osteoprogenitor proliferation and differentiation and adipocyte formation in cell populations derived from adult rat bone. Bone 2000; 27:785–794.

162. Kawakami A, Nakashima T, Tsuboi M, Urayama S, Matsuoka N, Ida H, Kawabe, Sakai H, Migita K, Aoyagi T, Nakashima M, Maeda K, Eguchi K. Insulin-like growth factor I stimulates proliferation and Fas-mediated apoptosis of human osteoblasts. Biochem Biophys Res Commun 1998; 247:46–51.

163. Langdahl BL, Kassem M, Moller MK, Eriksen EF. The effects of IGF-I and IGF-II on proliferation and differentiation of human osteoblasts and interactions with growth hormone. Eur J Clin Invest 1998; 28:176–183.

164. Lundy MW, Hendrix T, Wergedal JE, Baylink DJ. Growth factor-induced proliferation of osteoblasts measured by bromodeoxyuridine immunocytochemistry. Growth Factors 1991; 4:257–264.

165. Kim CH, Kang BS, Lee TK, Park WH, Kim JK, Park YG, Kim HM, Lee YC. IL-1beta regulates cellular proliferation, prostaglandin E2 synthesis, plasminogen activator activity, osteocalcin production, and bone resorptive activity of the mouse calvarial bone cells. Immunopharmacol Immunotoxicol 2002; 24:395–407.

166. Yang D, Chen J, Jing Z, Jin D. Platelet-derived growth factor (PDGF)-AA: a self-imposed cytokine in the proliferation of human fetal osteoblasts. Cytokine 2000; 12:1271–1274.

167. Tang KT, Capparelli C, Stein JL, Stein GS, Lian JB, Huber AC, Braverman LE, DeVito WJ. Acidic fibroblast growth factor inhibits osteoblast differentiation in vitro: altered expression of collagenase, cell growth-related, and mineralization-associated genes. J Cell Biochem 1996; 61:152–166.

168. Knutsen R, Wergedal JE, Sampath TK, Baylink DJ. Osteogenic protein-1 stimulates proliferation and differentiation of human bone cells in vitro. Biochem Biophys Res Commun 1993; 194:1352–1358.

169. Kassem M, Blum W, Ristelli J, Mosekilde L, Eriksen EF. Growth hormone stimulates proliferation and differentiation of normal human osteoblast-like cells in vitro. Calcif Tissue Int 1993; 52:222–226.
170. Conconi MT, Tommasini M, Baiguera S, De Coppi P, Parnigotto PP, Nussdorfer GG. Effects of prostaglandins E1 and E2 on the growth and differentiation of osteoblast-like cells cultured in vitro. Int J Mol Med 2002; 10:451–456.
171. Amedee J, Bareille R, Rouais F, Cunningham N, Reddi H, Harmand MF. Osteogenin (bone morphogenic protein 3) inhibits proliferation and stimulates differentiation of osteoprogenitors in human bone marrow. Differentiation 1994; 58:157–164.
172. Steinbrech DS, Mehrara BJ, Saadeh PB, Chin G, Dudziak ME, Gerrets RP, Gittes GK, Longaker MT. Hypoxia regulates VEGF expression and cellular proliferation by osteoblasts in vitro. Plast Reconstr Surg 1999; 104:738–747.
173. Postiglione L, Domenico GD, Montagnani S, Spigna GD, Salzano S, Castaldo C, Ramaglia L, Sbordone L, Rossi G. Granulocyte-macrophage colony-stimulating factor (GM-CSF) induces the osteoblastic differentiation of the human osteosarcoma cell line SaOS-2. Calcif Tissue Int 2002.
174. Spinella-Jaegle S, Roman-Roman S, Faucheu C, Dunn FW, Kawai S, Gallea S, Stiot V, Blanchet AM, Courtois B, Baron R, Rawadi G. Opposite effects of bone morphogenetic protein-2 and transforming growth factor-beta 1 on osteoblast differentiation. Bone 2001; 29:323–330.
175. Sampath TK, Maliakal JC, Hauschkas PV, Jones WK, Sasak H, Tucker RF, White KH, Coughlin JE, Tucker MM, Pang RHL et al. Recombinant human osteogenic protein-1 (hOP-1) induces new bone formation in vivo with a specific activity comparable with natural bovine osteogenic protein and stimulates osteoblast proliferation and differentiation in vitro. J Biol Chem 1992; 267:20,352–20,362.
176. Scutt A, Bertram P. Basic fibroblast growth factor in the presence of dexamethasone stimulates colony formation, expansion, and osteoblastic differentiation by rat bone marrow stromal cells. Calcif Tissue Int 1999; 64:69–77.
177. Laitinen M, Halttunen T, Jortikka L, Teronen O, Sorsa T, Lindholm TS. The role of transforming growth factor-beta on retarded osteoblastic differentiation in vitro. Life Sci 1999; 64:847–858.

30

Genome Sciences in Clinical Orthopaedics

**Arun Shanbhag, Grant E. Garrigues, Adam M. Kaufman,
and Harry E. Rubash**
*Department of Orthopaedic Surgery, Massachusetts General Hospital,
Harvard Medical School, Boston, Massachusetts, U.S.A.*

INTRODUCTION

In 1868, the Swiss Biologist Friedrich Miescher isolated an acidic substance from the nuclei of pus cells in discarded surgical bandages. The material he referred to as "nuclein" is now known to be deoxyribonucleic acid (DNA), the genetic blueprint for life. Thus the discovery of nucleic acids and its revolutionary effects on molecular biology can be traced to a humble surgical by-product. Fifty years ago another biological revelation came as Watson and Crick exposed the double helix structure of nucleic acids (1). Today, with the entire human genome sequenced, DNA is moving out of the basic science laboratory and returning to the operating room with a great deal more fanfare, impacting surgery and patient care in ways that were inconceivable just a few decades ago.

DNA has been recognized as the starting point for all cellular and therefore, all living processes. Its efficient replication ensures each somatic and reproductive cell in an organism has nearly the same genetic library. DNA dictates cellular action by what has become known as the "central dogma" of molecular biology, detailing the conversion of DNA's genetic message into function (Fig. 1). Though there are exceptions, the general flow of information in the cell is that DNA is first transcribed into ribonucleic

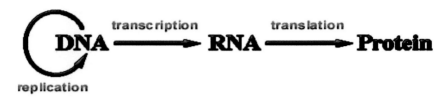

Figure 1 The central dogma of molecular Biology. Though some exceptions have been found, the general flow of information in living cells is diagrammed above. DNA replication allows for cells to copy the genome before division. When genes are activated, transcription creates messenger RNA from DNA. From this RNA template, the genetic code is translated into a string of amino acids and eventually, a functioning protein. *Abbreviations*: DNA, deoxyribonucleic acid; RNA, ribonucleic acid.

acid (RNA), a messenger intermediate that exits the nucleus and is in turn translated into proteins, the functional unit of the cell (2). Protein transcription factors ultimately close the loop by altering DNA transcription and replication according to the needs of the living organism.

Thus, the basic structure of proteins is determined by the DNA sequence, which codes for the string of amino acids comprising the polypeptide backbone. Post-translational modifications such as cleavage, phosphorylation, glycosylation, and chaperone-guided folding can lead to variations in protein structure independent of the DNA sequence. For these cases, studying all proteins directly, known as proteomics, becomes an important adjunct to studies of the genetic code. However, the fundamental inherited differences between each individual's proteins and his or her disease susceptibility arise from disparities in their coding DNA sequences. While the DNA makeup of each cell in an organism remains unchanged, the RNA and protein levels fluctuate according to cell type and environment, yielding a diversity of tissues and functions.

Advances in molecular biology, genetics, bioinformatics, and related fields have made it possible to monitor each step in the process of DNA replication, gene expression, and protein translation. DNA can now be easily sequenced and specific genes can be mapped on their chromosomes. Further downstream, RNA levels can be determined using Northern blotting, microarrays, and RT-PCR and individual strands of RNA can be localized within tissues and cells using in situ hybridization. Proteins can be identified and quantified using the Enzyme Linked Immunosorbent Assay (ELISA), Western blotting, mass spectroscopy, immunohistochemistry and most recently with protein chips. Scientists can even observe protein location and movement within a cell using fluorescence labeling and modern microscopic methods.

The most recent revolution in biology has come with the sequencing of all genes in the human genome. In March of 2001, McPherson et al. and Venter et al. (3,4) identified the order of the three billion chemical bases making up the complete sequence of the estimated 35,000 genes in the human DNA. The sequence of the genome represents a valuable resource of detailed information about the structure, organization, and function of human DNA and essentially constitutes the complete set of inherited "instructions" for the development and functioning of a human being. An important hope of this sequencing effort is that by knowing all the genes involved in normal human function, we will then be able to understand the mechanisms of many of our human diseases, which in turn will permit us to target appropriate molecules and develop cures for these maladies.

The current technology employs the latest optics, robotics, chemistry, and engineering techniques to create high throughput systems that generate phenomenally large amounts of data (5). The field of bioinformatics, a melding of computer science, statistics, and mathematics is growing to manage this rush of data (6). While high throughput technologies make it feasible to extract information on a genomic scale, bioinformatics has made it possible to analyze, organize, and interpret this information. Public access to such powerful resources as the human genome[a] and a complete database of genes with their biological functions and role in human disease[b] is already a reality. If medical advances over the last few decades are any indication, larger, faster and more precise experiments have the potential to improve patient care in a myriad of ways.

MODERN GENOMIC TECHNIQUES

Gene Therapy

With this increased knowledge of the genome, clinicians and researchers are now searching for the genetic causes for specific aliments. New technologies in genetics and genomics have helped identify specific variations that are responsible for specific characteristics or outcomes. A classic example is sickle-cell anemia, where a single nucleotide mutation in codon 6 of the β-globin gene causes the disease. With this knowledge, researchers are now using viral vectors to insert functional genes lacking this mutation, into stem cells. These cells are placed back into the patient with the ability to generate healthy red blood cells (7). This process of inserting genes for a therapeutic effect is known as "gene therapy." While it may seem futuristic, gene therapy is reality in the armamentarium of today's physicians.

Gene therapy intially began as a way to introduce a functional gene in place of a non functional one, but the applications have extended as many

---

[a] http://public.celera.com/cds/login.cfm, http://genome.ucsc.edu, http://www.ensembl.org/genome/central, http://www.ncbi.nlm.nih.gov/genome/guide/central.html.

[b] http://www.ncbi.nih.gov/entrez/query.fcgi?CMD=search&DB=omin, http://www.ncbi.nlm.nih.gov/omin.

diseases can benefit from gene therapy, even in the absence of underlying gene mutations. Osteoprotegerin (OPG) is a natural decoy receptor for RANKL that inhibits osteoclast activation and bone resorption. Investigators used gene therapy to introduce the *OPG* gene into myocytes in a wear debris-induced osteolysis model. The resulting OPG sythesis and release effectively absorbed the RANKL and successfully inhibited osteolysis (8).

Recombinant Factors

Gene therapy uses insertion of genes to provide a sophisticated drug delivery system. For diseases where a gene product is known to have therapeutic benefits, a more common practice is the production of protein product by recombinant genetic techniques and then using more traditional drug delivery methods. Recombinant DNA technology allows clinicians to harness the generative powers of micro-organisms by the insertion of excised human genes into a bacterial or yeast cell. The transcription and translation capabilities of these organisms can yield high levels of human proteins without the risk of infectious contamination found in animal or cadaveric sources.

Recombinant insulin-like growth factors and growth hormone are already in use to increase longitudinal bone growth in children falling below their growth curves. Other skeletal growth factors, such as the bone morphogenetic proteins involved in skeletogenesis, are produced and used in a similar manner. Human recombinant bone morphogenetic protein-2 (hrBMP-2, American Home Products, Madison, New Jersry U.S.A.) and erythropoietin alpha (Procrit, Johnson & Johnson, New Brunswick, New Jersey U.S.A.) are already FDA approved for clinical use.

Other recombinant proteins appear poised to impact orthopaedics specifically. For example, osteoprotegerin and other inhibitors of osteoclast activity might be used to alleviate bone-loss in a variety of pathologic conditions, including osteolysis and osteoporosis (9). The drawback of recombinant DNA technology is that the product drugs are peptides, which are generally poor therapeutic agents with short half-lives, difficult injections, and possible immune response.

Polymerase Chain Reaction

As advances of molecular biology have an increasing impact on clinical orthopaedics, clinicians must be facile with the science behind the technology. The Polymerase Chain Reaction (PCR) has an increadible impact on the laboratory and the clinic. Perfected in the mid-1980s, PCR allows the rapid amplification of DNA through a simple automated system. A small amount of isolated DNA is placed in a tube with a thermostable DNA polymerase, deoxynucleoside triphosphates, and an excess of short oligonucleotide primers that match the ends of the target DNA sample (Fig. 2). The solution is heated, causing the double stranded target DNA to dissociate.

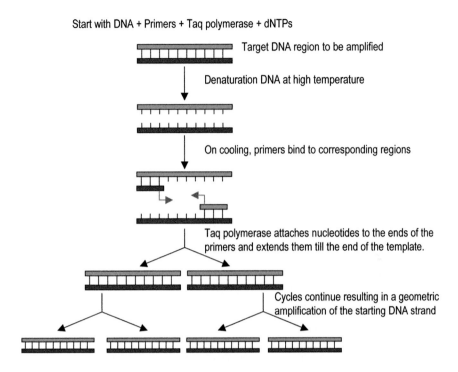

Start with DNA + Primers + Taq polymerase + dNTPs

Target DNA region to be amplified

Denaturation DNA at high temperature

On cooling, primers bind to corresponding regions

Taq polymerase attaches nucleotides to the ends of the primers and extends them till the end of the template.

Cycles continue resulting in a geometric amplification of the starting DNA strand

After 30 cycles, there is a 10^9 fold amplification of the DNA segment of interest.

Figure 2 PCR. As DNA is heated, its strands fall apart like ice melting. When cooling in the presence of numerous copies of complementary primers, the target DNA strands hybridize to the primers, providing a starting point for DNA replication by Taq DNA polymerase. The number of copies of the DNA region flanked by the primers is doubled with each cycle, resulting in a rapid ($2\times$) amplification. *Abbreviations*: PCR, Polymerase Chain Reaction; DNA, deoxyribonucleic acid.

As the solution is cooled, most DNA strands hybridize to the single-stranded oligonucleotides, which now act as primers for DNA polymerase. This enzyme then adds nucleotides until a new double-stranded molecule is formed, identical to the original strand. This cycle can be repeated for n cycles and a geometric amplification of 2^n.

A similar procedure, known as reverse transcriptase polymerase chain reaction (rtPCR) can amplify DNA from an mRNA source. First, the enzyme reverse transcriptase binds to an oligo (dT) primer and forms a strand complementary to the isolated mRNA. Then simple modifications to the normal PCR technique can amplify the resulting cDNA.

PCR and rtPCR have facilitated work in the research environment and have gained widespread use in molecular medicine. For instance,

PCR followed by Southern or Northern blotting, allows the amplification of even picograms of DNA to the visible and quantifiable level. The analysis of restriction fragment length polymorphisms (RFLP) and sequencing of DNA are also reliant on this technique. In a clinical environment, PCR can be used to detect minute amounts of nucleic acid, facilitating the diagnosis of viral RNA in an HIV infection and preimplantation diagnosis for in vitro fertilization clinics. In addition, the reaction is used to detect a variety of mutations including those responsible for Duchene type muscular dystrophy, cystic fibrosis, and mutations associated with myocardial infarction and cancer. As the genes causing orthopaedic maladies are discovered, our ability to detect and study diseases such as osteogenesis imperfecta, familial osteoarthrosis, osteopetrosis, hereditary osteoporosis, and a variety of connective tissue diseases becomes possible. In addition to unraveling diseases with clear genetic causes, researchers are also studying the more subtle roles genes play in diseases with more complex etiologies such as rheumotoid arthritis and osteoarthritis (10).

Genetic Basis of Diseases

The simplest way to determine the correlation between genetics and disease is to follow the inheritance of simple traits through generations as Gregor Mendel did in the 1860s (11). An inherited trait can be located by observing nearby polymorphic markers to confirm that the gene in question is inherited with the disease. These genetic variations between individuals are hypothesized to represent the process of phenotypically silent mutations being passed down and reshuffled at every generation. Polymorphic markers near each other are more likely to remain together in the reshuffling process than those that are distant. Thus, markers that are always found in family members with the disease are near to the gene causing the dysfunction. This process allows researchers to focus in on the location of an inherited disease gene (12).

Research begins by determining the particular markers and alleles that differentiate a patient, a process known as genotyping. A variety of techniques involved in genotyping include karyotyping, hybridization, RFLP analysis, and single nucleotide polymorphism (SNP) analysis. Karyotyping refers to the study of the chromosome structure, where cells are osmotically swollen so the nuclei break open. The chromosomes are stained with various dyes and the resulting banding patterns can be read by trained specialists to reveal gross chromosomal abnormalities. Although the strands of genomic DNA are arranged in ever increasing levels of superstructure, slight differences in the DNA sequence often have visible effects on the chromosome structure. In addition, many deletions and translocations can be seen under the microscope, along with any aneuploidy, or abnormal number of chromosomes (13).

The use of hybridization probes allows the observation of specific DNA sequences. A short stretch of nucleotides can be synthesized and labeled with a fluorescent or radioactive marker. The target DNA helix is peeled apart and exposed to these labeled probes that bind only to complementary nucleotide sequences. The ability to label DNA sequences has resulted in the techniques of fluorescence in situ hybridization (FISH) and genotyping microarrays (14,15).

Many bacteria synthesize enzymes called restriction fragment endonucleases, which can cleave human DNA at specific recognition sequences. Cleavage of a sample with a restriction enzyme will give a unique panoply of fragments called RFLP, depending where the sites are present (16). Though these cleavage sites may not be in protein coding regions of the genome, they are inherited just like any other genetic sequence. This type of genotyping has been widely used in the past 15 years, with applications as far reaching as the "DNA fingerprinting" in forensic science.

The most common type of markers are SNPs or "snips." SNPs occur in nearly all genes and represent variations of a single base pair at a given site (17). These genetic differences, like RFLPs, most often do not lead to differences in protein structure, as they often occur in noncoding regions of the genome, code for the same amino acid as the original nucleotide, or code for an amino acid that does not change the protein appreciably (18). Of the approximately 1,190,295 SNPs located by the human genome project, only about 0.04% are predicted to have any functional effects. Like all genetic material, SNPs are inherited and can therefore be used as markers to hone in on disease causing genes. This is the brute-force technique being used by scientists working on the Human Genome Project to identify genetic differences and correlate them with disease states (19). In the realm of orthopaedics, SNP analysis has helped highlight seven chromosomal regions that may contain osteoarthritis susceptibility genes (20).

cDNA Microarrays

DNA technologies described above are used to investigate the genetic code. Further downstream, changes in RNA and protein concentrations contribute to phenotypic differences not explained by the DNA template. Traditional research techniques rely on a combination of intuition and luck in order to isolate the key pathways involved in a pathological process. Only a handful of molecules could be studied at one time, meaning one would have to screen approximately 35,000 genes to understand each trait. Microarray technology now makes it possible to look at the RNA expression of every gene in the genome in a single experiment. The expression of every gene, whether hypothesized to be involved or not, can be studied simultaneously. In DNA microarray technology, all of the RNA species in a given population of cells are reverse transcribed to create cDNA and then tagged with radioisotopes or fluorescent labels. This labeled hybridization cocktail encompasses the RNA from all of the genes being transcribed at that time. The tagged cDNA copies of the cells' messenger RNA are then hybridized to a microarray or gene chip. Microarrays are a grid of short nucleic acid segments, or oligonucleotide probes, specifically complementary to each gene in the genome and located in predefined portions of the array. Each microarray chip contains probes for thousands of genes, even the entire genome. By visualizing the intensity of each spot with bound sample, a quantitative and comprehensive snapshot of gene expression is obtained.

In most variations of nucleotide microarray technology, RNA is extracted, labeled and allowed to hybridize to its complementary nucleotide probes bound to the array chip. Photolithography, the same technology used to manufacture computer chips, is one of the advances that has made high-density synthesis and localization of oligonucleotides possible (21–23). A very similar array technology uses cDNA products placed on a glass slide by a robot "spotter" instead of in situ synthesis of the probes as in the oligonucleotide arrays (24).

Protein Microarrays

cDNA microarrays only monitor RNA species; they cannot take into account downstream changes that do not affect gene transcription, such as alternative RNA splicing, post-translational modifications, or protein–protein interactions like phosphorylation/dephosphorylation. In cells, RNA from different genes can be differentially translated and degraded, meaning RNA levels do not always approximate protein levels. Because of these variables, precise methods to monitor protein levels themselves are being developed. While mass spectrometry and 2D gel electrophoresis are among the most commonly used methods to date, emerging protein array technology has the power to truly revolutionize proteomics, the study of all the proteins to unravel biological processes. Protein microarrays are fabricated and function in a manner similar to DNA arrays; the probes in this case may be monoclonal antibodies instead of complementary nucleic acid sequences. Along with the quantification of proteins, this technique allows the detection of protein-antibody, protein–protein, protein–drug, protein–ligand, and enzyme–substrate interactions. Using minimal sample amounts, protein arrays could facilitate pharmaceutical discovery with high-throughput screening of bioactive molecules and help define changes in a cell's protein make-up under different conditions. In the field of orthopaedics, such technology may provide a much better picture of cellular interaction and expression in bones and joints and a better understanding of disease pathogenesis (25). In our laboratory, we are evaluating a newly developed protein biochip (Zyomyx, Hayward, California, U.S.A) which quantifies 29 inflammatory cytokines in a tiny 40 µL sample. We have used this technology to explore the protein profile of clinical cases of osteolysis and the preliminary results are very exciting and offer opportunities to re-assess this clinical pathology (26).

These genomic and proteomic techniques are vital to the future of orthopaedics and must be appreciated by the modern clinician. Such advances have already impacted the treatment of rheumatoid arthritis, for example. Using genomic technology, researchers discovered the central role tumor necrosis factor-α (TNF-α) plays in the pathogenesis of rheumatoid arthritis as a potent autocrine and paracrine inducer of inflammatory cytokines and cartilage degradation. In culture and in humans, antibodies against TNF-α reduced the ability of synovial cells to produce these inflammatory interleukins. A variety of therapies have since been developed to alleviate the symptoms of rheumatoid arthritis: etanercept (Enbrel, Wyeth) is a dimeric TNF-α receptor, infliximab (Remicade, Centocor) is a chimeric monoclonal antibody against TNF-α, D2E7 is a human antibody against TNF-α, and various other interleukin receptor antagonists have been developed. Gene therapies for rheumatoid arthritis have now entered clinical trials, one of the most promising being retrovirus-expressing IL-1 receptor antagonists (27). With clinical follow-up of less than five years, the long-term clinical effectiveness of these treatments remains to be determined. These studies however represent the diversity and potential of modern genomic therapies.

UNDERSTANDING THE PATHOGENESIS OF OSTEOARTHRITIS

While ailments like cystic fibrosis and hemophilia can be traced to a single, genetic origin, most orthopaedic disorders represent a complicated interplay of genetic, lifestyle, and environmental contributions. In conditions like osteoarthritis, gene–gene and gene–environment interactions, as well as purely environmental factors complicate genetic research. In addition to confounding environmental factors such as a history of joint trauma, there are many genes associated with an increased risk for this condition, but not necessarily causally. For example, it is well known that obesity is a risk factor linked to osteoarthritis. As such, genes causing conditions associated with obesity, such as hypertension, Type II diabetes mellitus, fat storage and hormonal mediators of satiety, are expected to correlate with the development of osteoarthritis. These genes are not directly involved in the disease pathogenesis; they only increase the development of comorbidity and obesity, which often lead to osteoarthritis through the local effect of increased stresses upon the articular cartilage and a putative systemic factor present in the obese (28).

In a different example, cigarette smoking has been shown to have a negative association with hip (29) and knee (30) osteoarthritis. This lifestyle anticorrelation, however, does not imply "anticausation," or protection, because cigarette smoking is known to cause a lower body mass index (BMI) and, when adjusted for BMI, cigarettes appear to have no effect on osteoarthritis (30). A mechanistic understanding along with careful statistical and epidemiological analyses is required to transform the results of studies to show genetic correlation into knowledge of actual risk factors (31). Other osteoarthritic patients may have developed their disease due to trauma destabilizing or initiating a degenerative process in the joint (30). These patients clearly do not have "genetic osteoarthritis," but if osteoarthritis genes are located, they may provide insight into pathogenesis and treatment, as they have with rheumatoid arthritis. Such knowledge would enhance the wide scope of medicine, affecting diagnosis, treatment, and eventually screening and prevention of orthopaedic disorders.

Due to the interaction of multiple genes and environmental factors making diagnosis and treatment difficult, very large-scale studies are required to determine the genetic correlations of osteoarthritis. These large-scale trials are often done with short-lived organisms (e.g., yeast, worms, and flies) to allow monitoring and breeding over many generations, but decreasing the results' applicability to humans. deCODE Genetics has collected genetic material from the Icelandic population to overcome these problems in large-scale studies of osteoarthritis genes. With the country's genetic homogeneity and small population, the Icelandic people represent ideal participants for investigation. In addition, the Icelandic people maintain detailed genealogical records tracing back over 1100 years (19) (www.deCODE.com). With this ideal population, deCODE has mapped three genes linked to osteoarthritis and has isolated a mutation in the MATN3 gene that cosegregates with hand osteoarthritis (32). Despite these positive results, the homogeneity of the Icelandic population may also limit the applicability of deCODE's findings to the heterogeneous world population.

There is good evidence to indicate that osteoarthritis has a genetic component. Studies performed on twins indicate as much as 65% of osteoarthritis may be due to genetic influences (33). Genes for some familial forms of osteoarthritis have already been localized, but the most common form of familial osteoarthritis, primary generalized osteoarthritis, remains elusive. Some studies have shown that HLA-A1B8, HLA-B8, and certain alpha 1 antitrypsin isoforms are associated with primary generalized osteoarthritis (34,35). Some families also show primary generalized osteoarthritis linked to alleles of the gene for type II procollagen (COL2A1) (36,37). Another inherited osteoarthritic condition is Sickler syndrome, or hereditary arthro-ophthalmopathy. This autosomal dominant disease occurs in approximately 1 in 10,000 and has also been linked to COL2A1 in up to one half of all families (34,38). The role of type II collagen in hyaline cartilage is somewhat clear, making this association relatively easy to find. This intuitive approach has led to associations of articular diseases with other cartilage and extracellular matrix components (39). More esoteric gene suspects will require large studies, strengthening statistical predictions in the absence of intuitive answers.

Once genes associated with osteoarthritis are identified, genetic treatments can be developed. Small molecules might be used to block adverse effects of an overactive osteoarthritic gene as is the strategy with rheumatoid arthritis. Here, IL-1 has been identified as the main catabolic cytokine of the arthritic joint, stimulating the synthesis of proteinases which break down the cartilage extracellular matrix. Simply blocking the IL-1 receptor with IL-1 receptor antagonist acts to inhibit such cartilage loss (20). Alternately, gene therapy can restore a functional copy of a missing or dysfunctional gene. For instance, certain patients with osteogenesis imperfecta have a null allele in the type I procollagen gene which causes a 50% drop in collagen production. A patient with this disorder could have a functional copy of procollagen I inserted into his or her cultured cells, usually accomplished using attenuated viruses (40). Since a viable copy of the affected gene can be nearly identical to the endogenous copy, there would be no inherent immunological side effects when implanting the cultured cells back into the patient. Tissue engineers seek to insert such genes in vitro, into pluripotent stem cells or tissue explants, to restore normal function (41). Such a procedure exemplifies the essence of gene therapy, the transfer of genes to patients for the therapeutic benefit of their product proteins (42).

The field of pharmacogenetics seeks to identify certain genes or mutations associated with disease and determine how genetics alters drug response. While the full therapeutic power of pharmacogenetics might not be realized for many years, the elucidation of genes involved in osteoarthritis may have an immediate impact on the orthopaedic community. For example, patients with a family history of osteoarthritis can be screened for genes known to increase the risk of osteoarthritis. For individuals genetically prone to osteoarthritis, prophylactic pharmaceutical interventions, dietary modifications, and lifestyle changes such as weight loss, could be taken for the early prevention of articular cartilage loss.

Diversity in disease and treatment response stem from differences in both an individual's genetic makeup and environment. Orthopaedic researchers and clinicians have gained a strong understanding of the environmental pathogenesis of osteoarthritis; the diagnosis and treatment of stress and trauma-related osteoarthritis is routine. What is lacking is a clear understanding of the genetic origins of osteoarthritis. If the allelic variations leading to osteoarthritis are identified, knowledge of these genes will be a powerful tool for future therapies aimed at prevention and treatment of osteoarthritis.

DIAGNOSIS BY GENE EXPRESSION PROFILING

A gene expression profile is the specific pattern of RNA transcription from DNA, that defines a certain cell type. The particular pattern of gene expression is analogous to the way a trained pathologist recognizes a cell type from a constellation of features. In this case, those features are the approximately 35,000 genes that make up the human genome, or a smaller set, from a few genes to a few hundred genes, made up of genes with expressions that correlated most strikingly with the cell type. Microarrays, as measures of

RNA expression for each gene in the genome, are ideally suited to assay a cell's gene expression profile.

Investigators at Harvard Medical School and the Whitehead Institute have pioneered the concept of "diagnosis by microarray" using a variety of cancer types including brain, lung, breast and prostate cancer, Ewing's sarcoma, and a variety of leukemias and lymphomas (43–51). One of the most intriguing gene expression profiling studies is the seminal work by Golub et al. (52) on acute lymphoblastic leukemia (ALL) and acute myeloid leukemia (AML). These two leukemias are very similar with respect to histochemistry, immunophenotyping, cytogenetic analysis, and histomorphology, and require a highly trained hematopathologist to ensure an accurate diagnosis (49,52). Classifying the patient's disease correctly is crucial because AML and ALL have drastically different chemotherapy regimens and prognoses. Using a process known as "clustering" to apply powerful, but simple, pattern finding algorithms to the microarray gene expression data from patient blood samples, they were able not only to distinguish the AML from the ALL samples, but also to categorize new patient samples based on the closest gene expression profile, and diagnose the leukemias with 100% accuracy (52). Thus the gene expression profiles of these two subtly different leukemias provided a molecular signature that allowed correct differentiation and classification of each patient sample. It is only a matter of time before such "diagnosis by microarray" is applied to orthopaedic oncology as well as to other diseases where similar clinical manifestations arise from different disease processes.

In a similar manner, a future physician might run a microarray analysis on a small sample of a patient's blood or biopsy cells and the results used to categorize the patient as high or low risk for developing osteoarthritis, osteoporosis, fracture nonunions, or other maladies. Microarray analysis can also indicate appropriate treatments for the diseased and prophylaxis for the at-risk patients. In addition, we may find that diseases listed separately under our current nosology may have multiple subtypes when viewed in the context of gene expression. This marvelous future is made possible by the comprehensive nature of microarray studies and the sophisticated analytical tools, such as clustering, that make understanding the significant patterns in the data possible.

The power of genomics can not only be used to understand why joint replacements are needed and to motivate new therapies for osteoarthritis, it can also improve existing treatments of osteolysis and avoid peri-implant bone loss. The global look at how cells or tissues respond to a specific stimulus or condition that microarrays reveal can increase our understanding of how macrophages respond to particulate biomaterials, how chondrocytes and osteocytes respond to mechanical load and many other orthopaedically relevant concerns. For instance, in our recent publication, we monitored the reaction of macrophages to wear particles from conventional implants

(Figs. 3 and 4) (53). Using microarrays to monitor RNA level, we were able to identify "discriminators," genes (Table 1) that had very altered expression upon exposure to wear particles (53). In studying thousands of genes we were able to get a more comprehensive picture of the mechanisms of osteolysis that included both genes known to be involved, and new genes with plausible roles in the pathogenesis. Experiments are also currently underway to compare linear, aseptic loosening to focal osteolysis through gene expression profiling of interfacial membrane tissue. If radiographically distinct types have identical genetic profiles, then differences must be due to variations in particle dispersion, not cellular mechanisms. Genetically identical ailments might not necessitate different treatments or pharmaceutical intervention. On the other hand, the different patterns of bone resorption might represent different cellular pathogeneses with different genetic profiles, as in AML and ALL. In this case, the two pathologies would represent two different diseases with possibly different treatments. Either way, knowing the important genes involved in osteolysis will open the door for new gene targets and pathways for therapeutic benefit.

IMPROVING ORTHOPAEDIC IMPLANTS

One of the benefits of genomic research for the orthopaedic surgeon will likely be in the form of improved joint replacement prostheses. Current orthopaedic implants are plagued by problems of interfacial instability from osteolysis and aseptic loosening. These diseases are widely thought to be caused by the generation of wear particles; consequently, the latest implant technologies are aimed at decreasing this debris. Other interface problems include stress shielding caused by mismatches in elastic moduli and changes in osteogenesis caused by the protheses' electric fields (54,55). With a greater understanding of cell–materials interaction, biomaterials can be optimized with respect to biocompatibility and mechanical strength.

One route to this improvement is to minimize the interaction of the patient with the biomaterial. This reasoning gave rise to polyethylene cross-linking technology, shown to decrease the release of wear particles and minimize the associated inflammatory response. In a complete paradigm shift, tissue engineers seek to *maximize* the patient–biomaterial interaction by harnessing the body's regeneration and remodeling response. The manipulation of an implant's surface chemistry, architecture, and strength profile can vastly alter the body's reaction to a material. In hopes of accommodating the wide array of biomaterials applications, developers of polymeric biomaterials are now creating combinatorial libraries of compounds, each with slightly different properties. Some implants are even being coated with biomolecules, like proteins or growth factors, to fine tune cellular adhesion and differentiation. For orthopaedic surgeons, this promises an increased viability of engineered tissues. Regenerative bioactive materials seek to combine the positive structural

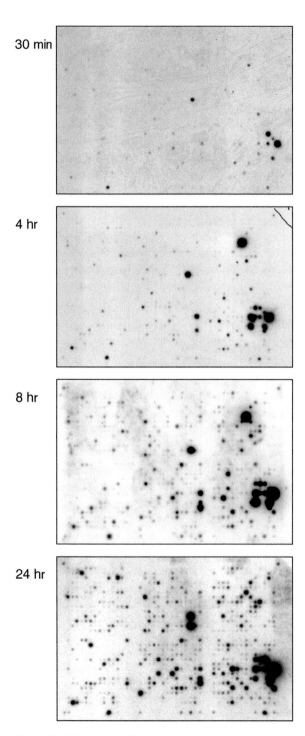

30 min

4 hr

8 hr

24 hr

Figure 3 (*Caption on facing page*)

elements of inert biomaterials with the versatility and biocompatibility of tissue engineered implants. With biologically active glasses and ceramics, for example, presurgical seeding with stem cells allows direct bonding between the implant and the surrounding bone or connective tissue (54). This type of interaction is the goal of tissue engineers; because osteogenic stem cells are present over the entire bone surface, simply providing the correct osteoconductive scaffold and growth factors, could allow the patients to act as the bioreactor (40). For any of these strategies to work however, we must determine which implant characteristics elicit a specific cellular response, desirable or undesirable. Genome-wide studies of the genetic and molecular causes of osteogenesis can help provide such an understanding.

Modern molecular biology may impact orthopaedic implants in ways other than engineered prostheses. Xenografts, tissue transfers from another species, represent a potential abundance of replacement organs, including bone, cartilage, and soft tissues. Bovine bone substitutes are in routine use, and genetic alteration of transplantable tissues from other species could further alleviate organ shortage problems entirely (54). These tissues can also be nonliving, chemically treated grafts, but exhibit the same drawbacks inherent in all allografts such as dystrophic calcification, infection, pathogen transfer, and religious implications (54). Attempts to create animal organs that will allow xenografting with less immunosuppression are currently under way. This advance requires the introduction of genes into the foreign tissue, making it appear "more human," limiting the body's immune response, and protecting the graft from apoptosis and necrosis (56–58).

PHARMOGENOMICS

Medical treatments of orthopaedic problems will also be impacted by pharmacogenomics: the study of how genetic variations affect patients' responses to drugs (59). One of the first great physicians, Galen, once said, "All who drink of this remedy recover in a short time, except those whom it does not help, who all die. Therefore, it is obvious that it fails only in incurable cases." (http://www.acponline.org/cgi-bin/medquotes.pl?subject=Drugs) Patients react differently to the same medical interventions. This differential response to treatments is not just due to variations in the extent of the

---

Figure 3 (*Facing page*) cDNA microarray of human monocytes. Monocytes were stimulated with various types of submicron particles and the interactions terminated after 30 minute, 4, 8, and 24 hour. The mRNA was extracted, reverse transcribed, radioactively labeled and hybridized to the Clontech cDNA microarray. In the example shown for monocyte interaction after stimulation with UHMWPE particles, within 30 minute more than 50 genes are upregulated. The intensity of the genes and the number of genes increase to more than 500 genes by 24 hour after culture. *Source*: From Ref. 53.

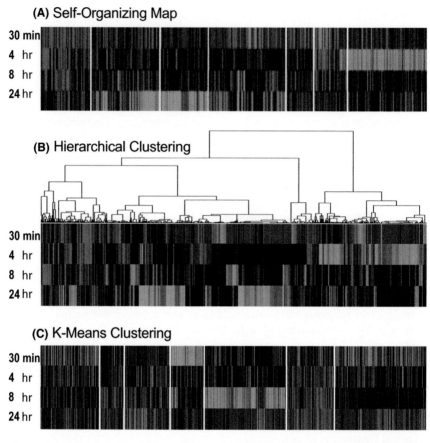

Figure 4 Clustering algorithms. These graphical representations show the clustering results for four nucleotide microarrays, each one representing gene expression of about 1100 genes at each of four time points. Genes are arrayed horizontally, while the microarrays for each time point are stacked vertically. A red bar represents gene up-regulation compared to control, while a green bar represents down-regulation. Black bars represent genes which did not deviate from control. Vertical white bars separate distinct clusters. Notice the fine structure provided by hierarchical clustering while the dendrogram cluster tree completely clusters all elements and does not provide a rough cluster grouping. The K-means clustering has the opposite effect of providing only a rough cluster grouping, without any ordering of the genes or the clusters. The self-organizing map is helpful in that it provides both a smooth ordering of genes and clusters and parcels the genes into distinct clusters. (*See color insert.*)

disease, but also to the way the drugs operate in different patients. The thrust of pharmacogenomics is to understand the genetic variations giving rise to these disparities. Pharmacogenomics could allow the categorization of patients by genetics, creating treatments tailor made for a patient's genome.

Table 1 Discriminator Analysis of Gene Regulation After Interaction with Biomaterials

	LPS	UHMWPE	TiAlV
Up-regulated	GTP binding protein ß3	Acidic fibroblast growth factor (4 hr)	Acyl-CoA-binding protein
	TATA-box factor	Acidic fibroblast growth factor (8 hr)	Cadherin 2 (24 hr)
		ADP-ribosylation factor 1	
		Apoptosis regulator bcl-x	
		Aquaporin 9 (24 hr)	
		CACCC-box DNA binding protein	
		c-cbl proto-oncogene	
		CD19	
		c-rel (24 hr)	
		GAP-associated protein	
		Glucagon precursor	
		Glycogen synthase kinase 3 ß	
		IL-1α	
		IL-3	
		IL-5 (24 hr)	
		IL-9	
		IL-15	
		Integrin alpha 7B	
		MAP kinase 2	
		MAP kinase kinase kinase 5 (24 hr)	
		NF-kappa B	
		Protein phosphatase 2Cα	
		Ski oncogene	
		Uromodulin	
Unchanged	Alpha-1 antitrypsin	Cdc25	Calpain (0.5 hr)
	Delta-like protein precursor (24 hr)	Cyclin dependent kinase 2	Cdc2-related protein
	IEX-1L anti-death protein	Serotonin receptor channel	c-src
			Cyclin K
			DNA excision repair protein

(Continued)

Table 1 Discriminator Analysis of Gene Regulation After Interaction with Biomaterials (*Continued*)

	LPS	UHMWPE	TiAlV
			GTP binding protein α-S
			HMG-1
			IGF II receptor
			IL-6
			Ink adapter protein
			Integrin alpha X
			Integrin alpha 5
			Leukocyte janus kinase
			Placenta growth factors 1, 2
Down-regulated	c-myc		Aurora-related kinase 1
	GABA$_A$ receptor β1 subunit		C enhancer binding prot α (24 hr)
	IGF binding protein 2		Calpain (24 hr)
	Ini 1		Cyclin D3
	Orphanin FQ receptor		Cyclin-dependent kinase4inhib
	ProstaglandinE2 receptorEP3		MAP kinase assoc. protein
			MAP kinase kinase 5 (24 hr)

Gene responses were divided into three rough categories of upregulated by >2-fold, unchanged or downregulated by >2 fold. Genes where the response was in the same category for two conditions, but differed for the third condition were termed "discriminators." While the macrophage response was generally similar under all conditions, these genes could potentially be used to investigate key differences and help explain variations in biologic activity of different biomaterials. Genes represented in "*italic*" discriminate at 24 hour, thus representing more chronic differences. *Source*: From Ref. 53.

Advances could revolutionize the pharmaceutical industry, where countless drugs are denied FDA approval because they are ineffective for a small, genetically identifiable group (60). Pharmacogenomics could also reduce the morbidity and mortality of drug side effects by avoiding administration in patients likely to have serious adverse events.

Two current examples of the medical value of this information come from pharmacogenetics. Malignant hyperthermia during general anesthesia is a life-threatening genetic trait that only becomes evident during surgery.

Inherited mutations in the ryanodine receptor calcium release channel cause skeletal muscle contraction and hypermetabolic crisis after anesthesia with halogenated drugs and depolarizing muscle relaxants (61). Presurgical screening for this mutation can all but eliminate this risk. Another genetic disease, aminoglycoside antibiotic induced deafness, is often dose dependant, but patients with a mutation in the mitochondrial translation machinery are highly susceptible. Because almost all mitochondria derive from the oocyte, this disease is transmitted to all offspring of an affected mother (62). Knowing the genotype of patients makes it possible to avoid these types of calamities when a different anesthesia or drug treatment can be easily substituted.

A subfield of pharmacogenomics is pharmacokinetics, the study of how medications are absorbed, distributed, and cleared from the body. Not surprisingly, some of the most relevant genes in pharmacokinetics are the oxygenases of the cytochrome p450 system, enzymes which act as membrane transported proteins in the conjugation system (59). Polymorphisms in the p450 system, for example, cause "poor metabolizers," patients who metabolize drugs very slowly. Even with identical dosages, the level of drug in these patients remains high, imparting an increased risk of side effects (60). All of these kinetic factors will affect how long a drug remains in an active state at its sight of action, a key parameter in drug response variation.

In the realm of orthopaedics, pharmacogenomics is approaching rapidly. For example, the discovery of a variety of hypercoagulable states may one day make screening for these disorders part of a routine pre-operative work up. As treatments for each disease are worked out, anticoagulant therapy could be tailored toward an individual's specific genetic makeup. Pharmacogenomics offers the ability to tailor our pharmaceutical therapies to each patient—a strategy that will maximize the benefit and minimize side effects.

SUMMARY

Over the last fifty years, scientific knowledge has progressed from the discovery of DNA to our present familiarity with cellular functions and molecular mechanisms. Utilizing current technology, researchers can precisely monitor the inner workings of cells in ways unfathomable only a few decades ago. Genomics has allowed the sequencing of the entire human genome and tools like microarrays yield precise quantifications of RNA and protein. These advances will permit a truer understanding of the disease process and allow revolutionary treatments in all fields of medicine.

Genomics is already beginning to impact both the surgical and medical treatment of orthopaedic ailments. Creating bioinert implants by understanding the cell–biomaterial interaction, harnessing the inherent ability of cells to repair and remodel, and raising animals to grow humanized organs for xenotransplantation are the next steps in surgical orthopaedics. Medically, genomics research is providing new targets for use with powerful recombinant DNA to use unicellular systems for high-volume synthesis of specific and potent human proteins. Medical treatments will also be aided by pharmacogenomics, which promises rational drug design and prescription through an improved understanding of individual drug metabolism.

Physicians use the most up to date epidemiological data and diagnostic techniques to make the proper diagnoses, and then prescribe the most efficacious pharmaceutical and surgical treatment to heal the patient. Now that the genomics revolution is upon us, this paradigm will continue on in a more streamlined manner. Epidemiology and conventional diagnostic techniques can be replaced by knowledge of a patient's genomic sequence. It holds the keys to understanding disease susceptibility and diagnosis. To new healing treatments unimagined just a few decades ago, the genome is giving up its secrets, and the scientist and physicians communities are steadily stepping into the future.

REFERENCES

1. Watson JD, Crick FH. Molecular structure of nucleic acids; a structure for deoxyribose nucleic acid. Nature 1953; 171(4356):737–738.
2. Crick FHC. The Biological Replication of Macromolecules. Symposium of the Society of Experimental Biology 1958; 7:138.
3. McPherson JD, Marra M, Hillier L, et al. A physical map of the human genome. Nature 2001; 409(6822):934–941.
4. Venter JC, Adams MD, Myers EW, et al. The sequence of the human genome. Science 2001; 291(5507):1304–1351.
5. Houston JG, Banks M. The chemical-biological interface: developments in automated and miniaturised screening technology. Curr Opin Biotechnol 1997; 8(6):734–740.
6. Luscombe NM, Greenbaum D, Gerstein M. What is bioinformatics? A proposed definition and overview of the field. Methods Inf Med 2001; 40(4): 346–358.
7. Pawliuk R, Westerman KA, Fabry ME, Payen E, Tighe R, Bouhassira EE, Acharya SA, Ellis J, London IM, Eaves CJ, Humphries RK, Beuzard Y, Nagel RL, Leboulch P. Correction of sickle cell disease in transgenic mouse models by gene therapy. Science 2001; 294(5550):2368–2371.
8. Ulrich-Vinther M, Carmody EE, Goater JJ, balle S, O'Keefe RJ, Schwarz EM. Recombinant adeno-associated virus-mediated osteoprotegerin gene therapy inhibits wear debris-induced osteolysis. J Bone Joint Surg Am 2002; 84-A(8): 1405–1412.
9. Puzas JE, O'Keefe RJ, Lieberman JR. The orthopaedic genome: what does the future hold and are we ready? J Bone Joint Surg Am 2002; 84-A(1):133–141.
10. Evans CH, Robbins PD. Possible orthopaedic applications of gene therapy. J Bone Joint Surg Am 1995; 77(7):1103–1114.

11. Weiling F. Historical study: Johann Gregor Mendel 1822–1884. Am J Med Genet 1991; 40(1):1–25.

12. Mustafa Z, Chapman K, Irven C, Carr AJ, Clipsham K, Chitnavis J, Sinsheimer JS, Bloomfield VA, McCartney M, Cox O, Sykes B, Loughlin J. Linkage analysis of candidate genes as susceptibility loci for osteoarthritis-suggestive linkage of COL9A1 to female hip osteoarthritis. Rheumatology (Oxford) 2000; 39(3):299–306.

13. Bridge JA. Cytogenetic and molecular cytogenetic techniques in orthopaedic surgery. J Bone Joint Surg Am 1993; 75(4):606–614.

14. McKenzie SE, Mansfield E, Rappaport E, Surrey S, Fortina P. Parallel molecular genetic analysis. Eur J Hum Genet 1998; 6(5):417–429.

15. Lepretre F, Montpellier C, Delannoy V, Froguel P, Vasseur F. Molecular and cytogenetic characterisation of a small interstitial de novo 20p13– > p12.3 deletion in a patient with severe growth deficit. Cytogenet Cell Genet 2001; 94(3-4):142–146.

16. Kant JA. DNA restriction enzymes and RFLPs in medicine. Methods Biochem Anal 1992; 36:129–149.

17. Shastry BS. SNP alleles in human disease and evolution. J Hum Genet 2002; 47(11):561–566.

18. Chang H, Fujita T. PicSNP: a browsable catalog of nonsynonymous single nucleotide polymorphisms in the human genome. Biochem Biophys Res Commun 2001; 287(1):288–291.

19. Wade N. A Genomic Treasure Hunt May Be Striking Gold. The New York Times 2002 Jun 18.

20. Loughlin J, Dowling B, Mustafa Z, Chapman K. Association of the interleukin-1 gene cluster on chromosome 2q13 with knee osteoarthritis. Arthritis Rheum 2002; 46(6):1519–1527.

21. Wodicka L, Dong H, Mittmann M, Ho MH, Lockhart DJ. Genome-wide expression monitoring in Saccharomyces cerevisiae. Nat Biotechnol 1997; 15(13):1359–1367.

22. DeRisi JL, Vishwanath RI, Brown PO. Exploring the Metabolic and Genetic Control of Gene Expression on a Genomic Scale. Science 1997; 278:680–686.

23. Lander ES. Array of hope. Nat Genet 1999; 21(1 Suppl):3–4.

24. DeRisi J, Penland L, Brown PO, Bittner ML, Meltzer PS, Ray M, Chen Y, Su YA, Trent JM. Use of a cDNA microarray to analyse gene expression patterns in human cancer. Nat Genet 1996; 14(4):457–460.

25. Service RF. Biochemistry. Protein arrays step out of DNA's shadow. Science 2000; 289(5485):1673.

26. Shanbhag AS, Kaufman AM, Agarwal S, Hayata K, Decker J, Kawashima M, Freiberg A, Grills G, Rubash HE. Critical Insights into osteolysis using protein microarrays: The importance of IL-6 and T-cell Activation. Trans Orthop Res Soc 2005; 30:148.

27. Bessis N, Doucet C, Cottard V, Douar AM, Firat H, Jorgensen C, Mezzina M, Boissier MC. Gene therapy for rheumatoid arthritis. J Gene Med 2002; 4(6):581–591.

28. Felson DT. The Epidemiology of Osteoarthritis in the Peripheral Joints: Does excess weight cause osteoarthritis and, if so, why?. Annals of the Rheumatic Diseases 1996; 55(9):668–670.

29. Cooper C, Inskip H, Croft P, Campbell L, Smith G, McLaren M, Coggon D. Individual risk factors for hip osteoarthritis: obesity, hip injury, and physical activity. Am J Epidemiol 1998; 147(6):516–522.

30. Hart DJ, Spector TD. Cigarette smoking and risk of osteoarthritis in women in the general population: the Chingford study. Ann Rheum Dis 1993; 52(2): 93–96.

31. Edelman ER. On causes: Hippocrates, Aristotle, Robert Koch, and the Dread Pirate Roberts. Circulation 2001; 104(21):2509–2512.

32. Stefansson SE, Jonsson H, Ingvarsson T, Manolescu I, Jonsson HH, Olafsdottir G, Palsdottir E, Stefansdottir G, Sveinbjornsdottir G, Frigge ML, Kong A, Gulcher JR, Stefansson K. Genomewide scan for hand osteoarthritis: a novel mutation in matrilin-3. Am J Hum Genet 2003; 72(6):1448–1459.

33. Spector TD, Cicuttini F, Baker J, Loughlin J, Hart D. Genetic influences on osteoarthritis in women: a twin study. BMJ 1996; 312(7036):940–943.

34. Cicuttini FM, Spector TD. Genetics of osteoarthritis. Ann Rheum Dis 1996; 55(9):665–667.

35. Pattrick M, Manhire A, Ward AM, Doherty M. HLA-A, B antigens and alpha 1-antitrypsin phenotypes in nodal generalised osteoarthritis and erosive osteoarthritis. Ann Rheum Dis 1989; 48(6):470–475.

36. Palotie A, Vaisanen P, Ott J, Ryhanen L, Elima K, Vikkula M, Cheah K, Vuorio E, Peltonen L. Predisposition to familial osteoarthrosis linked to type II collagen gene. Lancet 1989; 1(8644):924–927.

37. Knowlton RG, Katzenstein PL, Moskowitz RW, Weaver EJ, Malemud CJ, Pathria MN, Jimenez SA, Prockop DJ. Genetic linkage of a polymorphism in the type II procollagen gene (COL2A1) to primary osteoarthritis associated with mild chondrodysplasia. N Engl J Med 1990; 322(8):526–530.

38. Francomano CA, Liberfarb RM, Hirose T, Maumenee IH, Streeten EA, Meyers DA, Pyeritz RE. The Stickler syndrome: evidence for close linkage to the structural gene for type II collagen. Genomics 1987; 1(4):293–296.

39. Williams CJ, Jimenez SA. Heritable diseases of cartilage caused by mutations in collagen genes. J Rheumatol Suppl 1995; 43:28–33.

40. Oreffo RO, Triffitt JT. Future potentials for using osteogenic stem cells and biomaterials in orthopedics. Bone 1999; 25(2 Suppl):5S–9S.

41. Musgrave DS, Fu FH, Huard J. Gene therapy and tissue engineering in orthopaedic surgery. J Am Acad Orthop Surg 2002; 10(1):6–15.

42. Evans CH, Robbins PD. Gene therapy in orthopaedics. Orthop Nurs 2000; 19(1):16–22.

43. Ramaswamy S, Golub TR. DNA microarrays in clinical oncology. J Clin Oncol 2002; 20(7):1932–1941.

44. Ramaswamy S, Tamayo P, Rifkin R, Mukherjee S, Yeang CH, Angelo M, Ladd C, Reich M, Latulippe E, Mesirov JP, Poggio T, Gerald W, Loda M, Lander ES, Golub TR. Multiclass cancer diagnosis using tumor gene expression signatures. Proc Natl Acad Sci U S A 2001; 98(26):15149–15154.

45. Bhattacharjee A, Richards WG, Staunton J, Li C, Monti S, Vasa P, Ladd C, Beheshti J, Bueno R, Gillette M, Loda M, Weber G, Mark EJ, Lander ES, Wong W, Johnson BE, Golub TR, Sugarbaker DJ, Meyerson M. Classification of human lung carcinomas by mRNA expression profiling reveals distinct

adenocarcinoma subclasses. Proc Natl Acad Sci U S A 2001; 98(24): 13790–13795.

46. Pomeroy SL, Tamayo P, Gaasenbeek M, Sturla LM, Angelo M, McLaughlin ME, Kim JY, Goumnerova LC, Black PM, Lau C, Allen JC, Zagzag D, Olson JM, Curran T, Wetmore C, Biegel JA, Poggio T, Mukherjee S, Rifkin R, Califano A, Stolovitzky G, Louis DN, Mesirov JP, Lander ES, Golub TR. Prediction of central nervous system embryonal tumour outcome based on gene expression. Nature 2002; 415(6870):436–442.

47. Singh D, Febbo PG, Ross K, Jackson DG, Manola J, Ladd C, Tamayo P, Renshaw AA, D'Amico AV, Richie JP, Lander ES, Loda M, Kantoff PW, Golub TR, Sellers WR. Gene expression correlates of clinical prostate cancer behavior. Cancer Cell 2002; 1(2):203–209.

48. Lessnick SL, Dacwag CS, Golub TR. The Ewing's sarcoma oncoprotein EWS/FLI induces a p53-dependent growth arrest in primary human fibroblasts. Cancer Cell 2002; 1(4):393–401.

49. Armstrong SA, Staunton JE, Silverman LB, Pieters R, Den Boer ML, Minden MD, Sallan SE, Lander ES, Golub TR, Korsmeyer SJ. MLL translocations specify a distinct gene expression profile that distinguishes a unique leukemia. Nat Genet 2002; 30(1):41–47.

50. Tamayo P, Slonim D, Mesirov J, Zhu Q, Kitareewan S, Dmitrovsky E, Lander ES, Golub TR. Interpreting patterns of gene expression with self-organizing maps: methods and application to hematopoietic differentiation. Proc Natl Acad Sci U S A 1999; 96(6):2907–2912.

51. Tibshirani R, Hastie T, Narasimhan B, Chu G. Diagnosis of multiple cancer types by shrunken centroids of gene expression. Proc Natl Acad Sci U S A 2002; 99(10):6567–6572.

52. Golub TR, Slonim DK, Tamayo P, Huard C, Gaasenbeek M, Mesirov JP, Coller H, Loh ML, Downing JR, Caligiuri MA, Bloomfield CD, Lander ES. Molecular classification of cancer: class discovery and class prediction by gene expression monitoring. Science 1999; 286(5439):531–537.

53. Garrigues GE, Cho DR, Rubash HE, Goldring SR, Herndon JH, Shanbhag AS. Gene expression clustering using self-organizing maps: analysis of the macrophage response to particulate biomaterials. Biomaterials 2005; 26(16):2933–2945.

54. Hench LL. Biomaterials: a forecast for the future. Biomaterials 1998; 19(16):1419–1423.

55. McLeod KJ, Rubin CT. The effect of low-frequency electrical fields on osteogenesis. J Bone Joint Surg Am 1992; 74(6):920–929.

56. Li TS, Hamano K, Kajiwara K, Nishida M, Zempo N, Esato K. Prolonged survival of xenograft fetal cardiomyocytes by adenovirus- mediated CTLA4-Ig expression. Transplantation 2001; 72(12):1983–1985.

57. Gojo S, Cooper DK, Iacomini J, LeGuern C. Gene therapy and transplantation. Transplantation 2000; 69(10):1995–1999.

58. Contreras JL, Bilbao G, Smyth C, Eckhoff DE, Xiang XL, Jenkins S, Cartner S, Curiel DT, Thomas FT, Thomas JM. Gene transfer of the Bcl-2 gene confers cytoprotection to isolated adult porcine pancreatic islets exposed to xenoreactive antibodies and complement. Surgery 2001; 130(2):166–174.

59. Altman RB, Klein TE. Challenges for biomedical informatics and pharmacoge-
    nomics. Annu Rev Pharmacol Toxicol 2002; 42:113–133.
60. Branca M. FDA Fosters Pharmacogenomics. BioIT World. 6–12–2002.
61. Louis CF, Balog EM, Fruen BR. Malignant hyperthermia: an inherited disor-
    der of skeletal muscle Ca+ regulation. Biosci Rep 2001; 21(2):155–168.
62. Fischel-Ghodsian N. Genetic factors in aminoglycoside toxicity. Ann N Y Acad
    Sci 1999; 884:99–109.

Index